THE
CANCER
DICTIONARY

Third Edition

Michael J. Sarg, M.D.

Associate Chief of Medical Oncology,
St. Vincent's Hospital, New York City
Member of the teaching faculty
of the St. Vincent's Hospital
Comprehensive Cancer Center

Associate Professor of Clinical Medicine,
New York Medical College

Ann D. Gross, M.A., Gerontology

Medical Writer
A. D. Gross & Company, New York

Checkmark Books®
An imprint of Infobase Publishing

The Cancer Dictionary, Third Edition

Checkmark Books
An imprint of Infobase Publishing
132 West 31st Street
New York NY 10001

ISBN-10: 0-8160-6412-1
ISBN-13: 978-0-8160-6412-0

Gross, Ann D.
The cancer dictionary / Ann D. Gross, Michael J. Sarg.—Third. ed.
p. cm.
Includes bibliographical references and index.
ISBN 0-8160-6411-3 (hc: alk. paper).—ISBN 0-8160-6412-1 (pbk: alk. paper)
1. Cancer—Dictionaries. I. Sarg, Michael. II. Title. RC262.A39 1999
616.99/4003 22—DC21 99-21201

Text design by Cathy Rincon
Cover design by Salvatore Luongo
Illustrations on pages 43–46, 66, 111, and 183 by Jeremy Eagle
Illustrations on pages 38 and 164 by Sholto Ainslie

Printed in the United States of America

VB Hermitage 10 9 8 7 6 5 4 3 2 1

This book is printed on acid-free paper.

This third edition of *The Cancer Dictionary* is dedicated to the
fond memory of Roberta Altman, who left us in 2001,
overtaken by a major recurrence of her breast cancer.
To the final days she was passionate about living and
about her cause to educate people on resisting and doing battle with a
disease she fought with courage and with a determination to
strengthen others by providing them with in-depth information.

CONTENTS

ACKNOWLEDGMENTS

Ongoing thanks to Laurie Likoff at Facts On File for her understanding of the pressing need to update this *Cancer Dictionary;* she continues to show a commitment that carries the project. Thanks also to agent Joe Vallely and to Janis Vallely for their encouragement and help. Our gratitude also goes out to the hundreds of organizations dedicated to the palliation and cure of cancer and related diseases and the remarkable resources they have put into creating Web sites that are comprehensive, interactive, invaluable tools for researchers, patients, and practitioners alike. And thanks, too, to our spouses, and to Natalie Berger, who understood that work on this third edition would be a long project requiring many hours of excused absences at events and encouraged us to persevere and complete this book in the most thorough way that would be a true service to our readers.

INTRODUCTION TO THE THIRD EDITION

There is no question that the pursuit of a cure for cancer—or at least the means of turning it into a chronic disease we can live with for decades—continues to be a national priority. The National Cancer Institute estimated that it would spend some $4.9 billion in fiscal year 2005, in addition to all the money that private industry and other state and federal agencies spent in search of the means to vanquish an enemy that still manages to exact its toll on too many of all ages. In fact, since the publication of the last edition, Roberta Altman, who was the primary force in creating the prior editions of this book, succumbed to her long battle with breast cancer.

However, the world of cancer care and therapy continues to progress at lightning speed. No sooner did we publish the revised edition of *The Cancer Dictionary* than advances in the management of cancers of many organs—including breast, prostate, and lung cancer, as well as some of the leukemias—burst onto the scene. In this, the third edition, my coauthor, Ann Gross, and I found ourselves writing and making entries almost up to the moment when the book had to go to print. Each time we reviewed the material, theoretically for a "last glance," we found we were e-mailing and faxing each other the latest articles in the treatment of so many different cancers, including cancers of the breast, lung, and, most recently, in January 2006, ovarian cancer. And with each new FDA approval, we both felt strongly that we could not let the book be issued without adding "just this one new drug."

As such, I am happy to report that you will find in this third edition entries for more theapeutic modalities than ever before.

— Michael J. Sarg, M.D.

INTRODUCTION TO THE PREVIOUS EDITION

The last five years have seen an explosion of new concepts in basic molecular biology and technology that have been widely discussed and disseminated by the media. Many of these new developments in understanding have led to practical applications—new drugs, new treatments and treatment strategies, etc. All of this has been amplified and dispersed by the growth of the World Wide Web.

Many patients, as well as their friends and relatives, use the Internet to search for the very latest information and treatment options. However, for many the plethora of previously inaccessible information has created even greater confusion, frequently making it difficult to resolve the issues of choice. Information, while often invaluable, is not of itself a treatment for a serious illness.

Over the past years, there has been a rebirth of interest in medical ethics, stimulated by major trends in health care, including awareness of economic concerns, issues of access to competent care for all Americans, and multiple issues concerning end-of-life care. At medical schools, more attention is being given to integrating courses in humanism and medical ethics into the already crowded curriculum to help future physicians and other health-care workers properly frame these difficult questions.

Among workers in the field of cancer care, there is evident a real sense of optimism related to the application of state-of-the-art care as well as to new prevention strategies. The tide in the "war on cancer" may finally be turning.

— Michael J. Sarg, M.D.

INTRODUCTION TO THE
FIRST EDITION

CANCER!

Few other words in our common experience are so feared, dreaded, and charged with emotion. Growing up in the late forties, I can recall my family whispering about the disease, to avoid using the word. They referred to "it" in hushed tones with looks of dismay. To me, those afflicted with it seemed doomed, the ultimate unfortunate ones. Their illness was itself unspeakable, treatment was "mysterious" and thought to be ineffective, and their future was to confront unspeakable horror until they finally died. If they didn't die, they would be disfigured—unable to live any kind of normal life. They were "better off dead."

For many, the cause of such monumental misfortunes, such as cancer, was based on religious beliefs. "Bad" people got cancer. And of course if you "got" cancer, your morality was questioned. Although there are still some people who believe this, the number (fortunately) is dwindling.

Many of the old cancer myths—cancer is a death sentence; cancer is contagious; cancer only happens to "bad" people—have been dispelled in the face of tremendous advances in communication and technology. Those advances have affected medical care in ways hardly even imagined, and nowhere more so than in the field of cancer. Fifty years ago, there was no hope for a child diagnosed with leukemia. Virtually no children diagnosed with leukemia survived. Today, more than half the children survive and are free of disease five years after their initial diagnosis. That is a dramatic, but not unique, example. Today, as a society, we are

more interested than ever before in good health in general and in cancer in particular. There is still fear; there is still dread; and there is still a great amount of emotion surrounding cancer. But there is also encouragement, hope, and optimism.

Cancer has come out of the closet. Hardly a day goes by that there isn't some report on television, on the radio, and in all the newspapers on the progress that is being made—the newest drug for cancer treatment; the newest way to detect it; what one can do to prevent it; and the newest way to "cure" cancer. The media are full of articles; talk show hosts openly discuss with their guests the battle they fought with cancer. While much of this may be attributed to our obsession with "news," there is no doubt that there is an ever-increasing abundance of information on cancer that is truly newsworthy.

The mass media exposure of cancer has resulted in a more informed public and has played a role in dispelling some of the cancer myths. In the past, many people would wait before consulting a doctor. Their thinking was, "If I've got 'it,' there's nothing that can be done anyway; I'm just going to die." And they would die, because the more advanced any cancer is when it's diagnosed, the less likely it is that it can be cured. The importance of early detection and treatment is now more widely known and understood—and that is resulting in more cures. It has also resulted in a greater quest for information. There is less hesitation to ask questions, and there is less fear of the answers.

The media have also focused a tremendous amount of attention on prevention—the role that environmental factors (radon and radiation exposure, hazardous-waste sites, asbestos, the diminishing ozone layer, etc.) and life-style factors (smoking, diet, sun "tanning," etc.) play in the development of cancer. Cities and states have passed laws prohibiting smoking, a known carcinogen, in public places; a major fast-food chain has decreased the amount of fat in its burgers; and sunscreen lotion is a big seller. People have become more health conscious. They want to protect themselves and their loved ones and will change long-ingrained habits to accomplish that. There is an unprecedented demand for accurate, helpful, and understandable information.

Practicing medicine at a major hospital in a large urban area, I find that many of my patients are fairly sophisticated and well educated. But when cancer strikes, they are suddenly "illiterate." Many are frightened and feel out of control. They come into my office with lists of questions. They want to know what their options are; just how successful a particular treatment has been for their cancer; what the "state-of-the-art" treatment is. They do not hesitate to ask questions.

The most difficult question I am asked by patients is, "What would you do if it were you?" The answer is not simple. But I believe any decision I would make would be based on having accurate, understandable information.

The question that follows is obvious. "Where can I find information? I want to, have to, become as well informed as possible." Today, hundreds of books on cancer are available—ranging from personal life stories, to self-help techniques, to books with textbook-like explanations. There are several books I would suggest to patients, but I was never really satisfied with any of them. One would be good in one area, another in another area. But there was not one "comprehensive" book on cancer that I could recommend, a basic book that covered the topic from A to Z.

Some years ago, I was talking with one of my patients, a journalist who suddenly became very "cancer educated" when she was diagnosed with recurrent breast cancer. She was telling me about the hard time she had tracking down the information she needed for her battle against the disease. "You know," she said, "*you* ought to write a book that is easy to use and that anyone can understand."

Much of medical science is admittedly "mysterious" and difficult to understand. In *The Cancer Dictionary,* my co-author (journalist and patient) Roberta Altman and I have attempted to demystify it as much as possible. On the other hand, as mystifying as modern medicine and cancer may be, at no time has society been as ready and eager to seek accurate information for personal and family health (as well as for the health of the nation).

Our premise is that knowledge *does* make a difference in the course of one's life, that ignorance is not bliss. For a newly diagnosed cancer patient, the terror can be enormous. Emotions run the gamut from fear to denial to guilt to depression to anger. After the initial shock of discovering that one has cancer, most people come to the resolution that they have to "do something." For most people, understanding what's going on, what is going to happen or is likely to happen, can alleviate a lot of the fear. Learning about the disease can help the patient make informed choices. It can also enable the patient to feel a little more in control in a situation that very often seems totally out of his or her control.

The Cancer Dictionary is meant to provide the cancer patient and general public with easy access to areas of information that are often hard to locate, or when found are hard to understand. In writing it our goal was twofold: to include *every* word that the average person might come across in the course of his or her illness; and to define each word in layperson's language, so that it would be understandable to the person without a medical background while at the same time providing enough information to be truly helpful. I believe we have accomplished that. (My patients will let me know!)

The Cancer Dictionary contains the latest information available at the time of publication. However, from the moment this book appears in bookstores and libraries, new discoveries will continue to be made. But how exciting and encouraging that concept really is! The ever-quickening pace of progress in cancer research is apparent to all of us. But, despite that, the basic information in this dictionary will stand up to the storms of change. (On the other hand, I shall be delighted when that ultimate obsolescence occurs, the discovery of a cure that banishes *The Cancer Dictionary* to the archives.) In the meantime, *The Cancer Dictionary* will, I hope, be of help and possibly some comfort to cancer patients, family members, their friends, and the general public.

— Michael J. Sarg, M.D.

HOW TO USE THIS BOOK

The Cancer Dictionary is designed to be "user friendly." It is for the layperson. Words in small capital letters in an entry are defined elsewhere in the book. Pronunciation is included for any word that we thought might be unfamiliar. Alphabetization follows the letter-by-letter system; word spaces and punctuation other than a comma are ignored. Entry words preceded by numbers are alphabetized according to how the numbers appear spelled out. Where numbers follow identical entry words, terms are listed in numerical sequence. Acronyms are alphabetized letter for letter.

Everything is cross-referenced. Because so many drugs, treatments, tests, sites, and so forth in cancer go by multiple names, we tried to define the word that we believed to be the most common and most well-known. For example, drugs usually have more than one name. If you were to look up the drug Adriamycin (a very widely used chemotherapy drug), you would find the definition as well as the information that it is also known as "DOX" and "doxorubicin." (Multiple names are given in brackets.) Doxorubicin is not capitalized because it is the chemical and not the brand name. If you looked up "doxorubicin," you would be directed to "see Adriamycin." In breast cancer treatment, removal of just the malignant tumor is called a "lumpectomy" as well as "breast conservation," "excisional biopsy," "wedge excision," "local wide excision," "partial mastectomy," "quadrantectomy," "quadrant excision," "hemimastectomy," and "tylectomy." We defined lumpectomy. If you look up any of the other names, you will be referred to lumpectomy. A little confusing? Yes . . . but we have organized the book, we hope, to eliminate as much confusion as possible!

When we questioned whether we should include a word, we usually included it. We felt it was better to have too much information than not enough.

At the time we revised the book, our intention was to include in the third edition of *The Cancer Dictionary* virtually any word you might hear in connection with cancer, including

- the individual cancers—causes, incidence, symptoms, diagnosis, stages, and treatment
- diagnostic tests
- surgical procedures
- therapeutic drugs
- types of radiation therapy
- biological therapy
- side effects
- risk factors
- carcinogens
- prevention
- supportive services and medical support staff
- organizations

We have listed symptoms that may be present for a particular cancer and many side effects that may accompany treatments. It is important to note that many signs or symptoms can occur with *many other disorders* besides cancer and usually people *do not have all* the side effects of a particular therapeutic drug or radiation therapy.

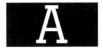

ABCD an acronym for the warning signs of MELANOMA. The following changes in a mole may signal a transformation to cancer:

- Asymmetry—the shape of one half does not match the other
- Border—edges that are ragged, notched, or blurred
- Color—uneven with shades of black, brown, or tan; areas of red, white, or blue may be seen
- Diameter—a change in size

abdomen the part of the body below the diaphragm between the thorax (chest) and the pelvis. The organs of the digestive and urinary systems—bladder, kidneys, liver, colon (which is part of the large intestine), stomach, and small intestine—are located in the abdomen. The abdomen is lined by the peritoneum, a smooth, transparent membrane. See entries for each organ for incidence of cancer.

abdominal cancer (ab-dom′ĭ-nal) a general term for a number of different cancers that occur in the area of the body between the diaphragm and pelvic bones, including cancer of the COLON/RECTUM (colorectal cancer), BLADDER, KIDNEY, STOMACH, LIVER, PANCREAS and the SMALL INTESTINE.

abdominoperineal resection (APR) (ab-dom′ĭ-no-per′ĭ-ne′al) the surgical removal of the anus (out-let of the bowel) and the lower part of the rectum. This operation is performed as a cure for RECTAL CANCER. It is done by cutting into the abdomen and the perineum (the space between the anus and the scrotum (in men) or vulva (in women). Then a STOMA (opening on the outside of the body) is made through which waste can leave the body (usually on the left side). This is known as a COLOSTOMY and requires a special bag to be worn to collect body wastes. For many years this was the only surgical treatment for rectal cancer. However, in recent years the development of other surgical procedures has resulted in a substantial reduction in the number of patients requiring a permanent colostomy, and every effort is made to avoid it whenever possible. In most patients with rectal cancer an APR is not required.

ABMT See AUTOLOGOUS BONE MARROW TRANSPLANT.

Abraxane [paclitaxel] protein-bound particle for injection. A new formulation (as of 2005) of PACLITAXEL, eliminating the hypersensitivity reaction caused by the solvent vehicle (chremophor) in standard paclitaxel preparation. The INDICATION is for treatment of BREAST CANCER after failure of COMBINATION THERAPY. The major side effect remains sensory NEUROPATHY.

ABVD a combination of the anticancer drugs ADRIAMYCIN, BLEOMYCIN, VINBLASTINE, and DTIC used primarily in the curative treatment of HODGKIN'S DISEASE as well as some other cancers. This combination of drugs was developed in the 1970s as a "salvage" therapy for patients with Hodgkin's disease who relapsed and were not responding to MOPP therapy. It is now the first treatment chosen by many doctors. ABVD is also being used in combination with MOPP, thus exposing the Hodgkin's tumor to eight active agents. See individual drug listings for side effects.

See also COMBINATION CHEMOTHERAPY.

AC   a combination of anticancer drugs ADRIAMYCIN and CYTOXAN most commonly used in the treatment of breast cancer. See individual drug listing for side effects.

See also COMBINATION CHEMOTHERAPY.

Accutane [isotretinoin]   an artificial form of vitamin A widely used for the treatment of acne. Accutane is under investigation for its role as possible ADJUVANT THERAPY to suppress second primary tumors in people with SQUAMOUS CELL CARCINOMA of the head and neck. Accutane is also being investigated as a CHEMOPREVENTIVE agent. In one study, people who were at risk of developing cancer of the lung, throat, or mouth as a result of having had larynx, pharynx, or mouth cancer were given high doses of Accutane or a placebo. The patients treated with Accutane had a lower incidence of secondary tumors.

Side effects associated with high doses of Accutane may include dry skin, chapped lips, and eye inflammation.

acetaminophen (as-ēt″ĕ-min′o-fen)   The generic name for an analgesic (pain killer), and antipyretic (fever reducer), nonprescription drug for pain that may be used instead of aspirin. Brand names include Tylenol or Datril. It is the weakest of the analgesics but may be effective when the pain is mild or moderate. Because acetaminophen does not contain aspirin, which can exacerbate bleeding problems, it can be used more safely by people experiencing a decrease in their PLATELETS (cells needed by the blood for clotting). A decrease in the blood platelet level is a not uncommon side effect of treatment with anticancer drugs. Acetaminophen is also less likely to irritate the stomach. It has few side effects, although prolonged daily use may cause liver or kidney damage.

Acetaminophen can be taken in pill, capsule, or liquid form. For patients receiving CHEMOTHERAPY (anticancer drugs) whose platelet level may be compromised, most physicians would recommend acetaminophen over aspirin as a safety measure.

See also ANALGESIC and NONOPIOIDS.

acetazolamide (as″et-ah-zol′ah-mīd)   a DIURETIC that may be used to reduce pressure within the eye. Possible side effects may include loss of appetite, weight loss, nausea, vomiting, diarrhea, weakness, depression, and dizziness.

achlorhydria (ah″klor-hi′dre-ah)   the absence of hydrochloric acid in the stomach. This can cause a nutritional deficiency and puts a person at a higher risk of stomach cancer than the general population.

acid phosphatase test (fos′fah-tās) [prostatic acid phosphatase]   a test once used in the diagnosis of prostate cancer. Its use virtually ended when the prostate specific antigen (PSA) test became available.

See also PROSTATE-SPECIFIC ANTIGEN TEST.

acinar cell carcinoma (as′i-nar kar″sin-o″mah)   a rare form of exocrine pancreatic cancer. See PANCREATIC CANCER.

ACOPP   a combination of the anticancer drugs ADRIAMYCIN, CYTOXAN, Oncovin (VINCRISTINE), PROCARBAZINE, and PREDNISONE sometimes used in the treatment of childhood HODGKIN'S DISEASE. See individual drug listings for side effects.

See also COMBINATION CHEMOTHERAPY.

acoustic neuroma (ah-kūs′tik ner-o′mah) [schwannoma, neurinoma]   a benign (noncancerous) brain tumor of the hearing nerve. It is the most common neuroma to occur in the brain, most frequently affecting middle-aged adults. Symptoms may include a loss of hearing in the ear, buzzing or ringing in the ear, and occasionally some dizziness. If the tumor has spread, there may be some facial paralysis, difficulty in swallowing, loss of sensation in the face, impaired eye movement, and unsteadiness. This tumor can usually be completely removed by surgery.

See also NEUROMA and BRAIN CANCER.

acquired immune deficiency (immunodeficiency) syndrome See AIDS.

acral-lentiginous melanoma (ak'ral len-tij'i-nus) one of four types of MELANOMA. It appears as a dark mark on the palms of the hand, soles of the feet, or around the nails.

ACTA (automatic computerized transverse axial) scan See CT SCAN.

Actimmune See INTERFERON GAMMA 1-B.

actinic keratosis (ak-tin'ik ker"ah-to'sis) [solar keratosis] a premalignant (precancerous) stage of SQUAMOUS CELL CARCINOMA OF THE SKIN. It looks like rough, red raised spots on the skin. It usually occurs on skin that has been exposed to the sun, but it can appear elsewhere. It occurs most often in older Caucasians but may also develop in younger people exposed to ULTRAVIOLET RADIATION over a long period of time (e.g., people who work outdoors). Most affected are people with fair complexions. It is very rare for people of African descent to develop actinic keratosis. If actinic keratosis is not treated, up to 10% of these may evolve into squamous cell carcinoma of the skin, a very common condition.

actinomycin D See COSMEGEN.

Actiq a raspberry-flavored "lollipop" that contains the powerful narcotic fentanyl citrate. It is a pain medication prescribed for cancer patients whose extreme pain cannot be controlled by oral narcotics. It takes about 15 minutes for a patient to consume the lozenge, which is on the end of a stick. Pain relief can occur while the lozenge is being consumed and can last for several hours. To prevent possible misuse, prescriptions are accompanied by a lock for the medicine chest and the childproof packages can only be opened with scissors.

acupressure a noninvasive treatment based on the same principles as ACUPUNCTURE, but using fin-gertips rather than needles. The tip of the thumb or forefinger is used to apply pressure to trigger points in the body to reduce or eliminate pain. The pressure is exerted until a sharp twinge is felt. Then the spot is massaged for as long as four minutes. The procedure is repeated at the same location on the opposite side of the body.

acupuncture an ancient Chinese form of therapy used to treat pain and other conditions with needles inserted into the body. It is based on the philosophy that a cycle of energy flowing through the body in meridians, or channels, controls health, and that a disturbance in the flow results in pain and disease.

Acupuncturists insert long, thin needles into the body at specific points along those meridians (there are as many as 1,000). Each point controls a different part of the body. Once the needles are in place, they are rotated gently back and forth; they may also be charged with a small electric current for a short period of time. Acupuncture is usually administered as a series of treatments. Acupuncture is also used as a method of anesthesia. In late 1997 a National Institutes of Health (NIH) Consensus Development Conference on acupuncture cosponsored by the Office of Alternative Medicine and the Office of Medical Applications of Research concluded that in cancer treatment, the procedure was an effective treatment for nausea caused by CHEMOTHERAPY for some patients. (The Office of Alternative Medicine is now known as the National Center for Complementary and Alternative Medicine.)

Considered an alternative treatment, acupuncture is gaining acceptance for treating pain.

acute a term used to describe an illness that appears suddenly, has a short course, and may have severe symptoms. There are a number of cancers that are described as acute. Some cancers can be either acute or CHRONIC. For example, LEUKEMIA is classified as both acute (ACUTE LYMPHOCYTIC LEUKEMIA, or ALL, and ACUTE NONLYMPHOCYTIC LEUKEMIA, or ANLL) and CHRONIC (CHRONIC LYMPHOCYTIC LEUKEMIA and CHRONIC MYELOGENOUS LEUKEMIA). Conditions that are chronic may also be associated with abrupt DECOMPENSATION. The term *acute* can also be used to describe pain that is sharp and relatively short-lived.

acute erythroleukemia (e-rith″ro-lu-ke′me-ah) a rare form of ACUTE MYELOGENOUS LEUKEMIA (AML). The predominant MALIGNANT (cancerous) cell in this illness is an early RED BLOOD CELL precursor (erythroblast).

See also ANLL and LEUKEMIA.

acute granulocytic leukemia (gran″u-lo-sit′ik) See ANLL and LEUKEMIA.

acute lymphatic leukemia (lim-fat′ik) See ALL and LEUKEMIA.

acute lymphoblastic leukemia (lim″fo-blas′tik) See ALL and LEUKEMIA.

acute lymphocytic leukemia (lim″fo-sit′ik) See ALL and LEUKEMIA.

acute monocytic leukemia (mon″o-sit′ik) See ANLL and LEUKEMIA.

acute myelocytic leukemia (mi″ĕ-lo-sit′ik) See ANLL and LEUKEMIA.

acute myelogenous leukemia (AML) (mi″ĕ-loj′e-nus) See ANLL and LEUKEMIA.

acute myelomonocytic leukemia (mi″ĕ-lo-mon″o-sit′ik) See ANLL and LEUKEMIA.

acute nonlymphocytic leukemia See ANLL and LEUKEMIA.

acute promyelocytic leukemia (pro-mi″ĕ-lo-sit″ik) See ANLL and LEUKEMIA.

adamantinoma (ad″ah-man″tĭ-no′mah) cancer of the long bones in the body, usually the shinbones. It is a rare cancer.

See BONE CANCER.

ADCC See ANTIBODY-DEPENDENT CELL-MEDIATED CYTOTOXICITY.

additives See FOOD ADDITIVES.

adenocarcinoma (ad″en-o-kar″sĭ-no′mah) a cancer made up of abnormal gland (adeno means "gland") cells on the lining or inner surface of an organ. It can develop in virtually any part of the body. Adenocarcinomas may develop in the lung, pancreas, breast, prostate, esophagus, stomach, vagina, urethra, and small intestine, among others.

adenocarcinoma of the lung (ad″en-o-kar″sĭ-no′mah) one type of NON-SMALL CELL LUNG CANCER that often develops along the outer edges of the lung and under the membranes lining the bronchi. A subtype is BRONCHIOLOALVEOLAR CARCINOMA OR ALVEOLAR LUNG CANCER.

See also LUNG CANCER.

adenoid cystic carcinoma (ad′ĕ-noid sis′tik kar″sĭ-no′mah) an uncommon cancer arising in one of the minor salivary glands. Generally the treatment is surgical removal. This cancer may recur in the local area or in a distant site. It is not unusual for the recurrence to appear after many years. It is because of the long latency that medical cancer specialists, who are controlling the spread of the disease with chemotherapy, are particularly interested in it.

adenoma (ad″ĕ-no′mah) a benign (noncancerous) tumor or growth arising in the lining or inner surface of an organ. It can grow to be several inches in size. Because cancer cells may eventually grow in adenomas, they should be removed when they are found. They are most commonly formed in the large bowel or large intestine (the colon and rectum). It is believed that COLON CANCER and RECTAL CANCER develop from adenomas. Occasionally tumors in the lung are found to be adenomas, but that is very rare. Adenomas may also occur in many other parts of the body such as the breast, ADRENAL gland, etc.

adenomatous hyperplasia (ad″ĕ-nom′ah-tus hi″per-pla′ze-ah) a type of endometrial hyperplasia, abnormal or heavy bleeding during menopause caused by an overgrowth of the uterine lining. Adenomatous hyperplasia may precede ENDOMETRIAL CANCER.

adenomatous polyps (ad″ĕ-nom′ah-tus pol′ips) small, spontaneous (not inherited), noncancerous growths in the intestines. They occur in up to 15%

of the adult population in the United States. They usually do not cause symptoms, but if they are large and obstruct the passage of waste material, they can cause intermittent bleeding. Invasive cancer develops in roughly 5% of adenomatous polyps.

adjuvant therapy (ad′ju-vant) treatment (CHEMO-THERAPY, RADIATION, HORMONAL THERAPY, or BIO-LOGICAL THERAPY) used in addition to and following the primary treatment (generally surgery) to cure, reduce, control, or palliate (see PALLIATIVE TREATMENT) the cancer. This is usually prescribed when there is any indication that there are still cancer cells in the body. However, it is not uncommon for there to be microscopic cancer cells remaining in the body at the time of DIAGNOSIS and follow-up tests that are simply too small to be seen.

Although it may seem obvious that additional treatment would be beneficial, it is only in recent years that strong evidence of the benefits of adjuvant therapy has emerged. CLINICAL TRIALS using adjuvant therapy in the treatment of many common cancers have shown that in some patients adjuvant therapy will prevent the RECURRENCE (the return of the cancer locally or to a district site) of cancer; or, to put it another way, adjuvant therapy will cure some patients.

In the late 1980s and early 1990s the most widely known example of adjuvant therapy was its use in the treatment of early BREAST CANCER. In the past, it was common for a woman who had a MAS-TECTOMY (surgical removal of the breast) to be treated with chemotherapy (anticancer drugs) only if breast cancer cells were found in nearby LYMPH NODES. Since finding cancer cells in the lymph nodes is a good indication that other cancer cells may be circulating in the body, chemotherapy was administered to fight the remaining cancer. However, the women whose nodes were negative (no cancer cells found) were not advised to have adjuvant chemotherapy, a potentially toxic treatment. Today, many of those same women *would be advised* to have adjuvant chemotherapy because of the studies that show a reduced risk of a recurrence when adjuvant chemotherapy is administered.

Although many studies have established the benefits of adjuvant therapy, in some instances it remains a controversial issue. For example, in breast cancer, many women with negative nodes do not have a recurrence after primary treatment; therefore, of the relatively large number of women who undergo adjuvant chemotherapy, a relatively small number will actually benefit from it. There are some doctors who think the reduced risk of a recurrence after adjuvant therapy is so small that the adjuvant therapy is not really warranted. Other doctors feel just as strong that the adjuvant therapy may be curative and should be administered. The consensus, overall, is that the benefit does outweigh the risk in properly chosen women who receive adjuvant chemotherapy. Ultimately, the decision whether to undergo adjuvant chemotherapy rests with the patient, who must decide whether the often unpleasant, and at times debilitating, side effects—immediate as well as short- and long-term—are outweighed by the possible benefits. In an effort to make that clearer, investigations are focusing on finding tests that would identify those women at a greater risk of breast cancer recurrence after PRIMARY TREATMENT.

Another example of adjuvant therapy in breast cancer is the use of radiation therapy to the breast following a LUMPECTOMY (surgical removal of only the cancer tumor in the breast). This adjuvant therapy is not controversial and is accepted as standard treatment.

See also NEOADJUVANT THERAPY and PROPHYLACTIC THERAPY.

adoptive immunotherapy (ĭ-mu″no-ther′-ah-pe) a procedure under investigation for use in boosting a cancer patient's IMMUNE SYSTEM so it can more effectively fight CANCER CELLS. The essential concept is to transfer to the host (patient) cells that have "antitumor" activity. Large doses of IL-2 (INTERLEUKIN-2), which stimulate the production of LYMPHOCYTES (white blood cells that fight foreign substances), are injected into the patient's bloodstream. Then lymphocytes are removed from the body, bathed in more IL-2, and returned to the body as LAK CELLS (LYMPHOKINE-ACTIVATED KILLER CELLS), which have the potential to destroy cancer cells. In the early 1990s, adoptive immunotherapy appeared to be most useful in the treatment of kidney cancer and melanoma. The use of this technique in humans is relatively new and is being actively investigated as cancer therapy. This treatment has been pioneered by physicians at the

National Cancer Institute (NCI). TUMOR-INFILTRAT-ING LYMPHOCYTE (TIL) therapy is another type of adoptive immunotherapy still being investigated by the NCI.

adrenal cancer (ah-dre'nal)   cancer of the small ADRENAL GLANDS located above the kidneys. Most abnormal growths in the adrenal glands are benign (noncancerous). There are two types of malignant (cancerous) growths, both of which are very rare: ADRENOCORTICAL CANCER, which arises in the cortex (the outer shell of the gland), and PHEOCHRO-MOCYTOMA, which arises on the medulla (the inner core of the gland).

adrenal glands (ah-dre'nal) [suprarenal glands] a pair of small organs located above the kidneys. The adrenal glands produce HORMONES known as CORTICOSTEROIDS, which help control the metabolism of protein, fat, and carbohydrates; they also regulate the amount of sodium and potassium in body fluids. The glands produce small amounts of the sex hormones ESTROGEN and ANDROGEN. The adrenal glands also secrete the hormones epinephrine and norepinephrine, which help regulate the part of the nervous system that controls the heart muscles, and the digestive and respiratory systems.

adrenal medullary tumors (ah-dre'nal med'u-lar"e)   tumors that may arise with, before, or after development of FAMILIAL MEDULLARY CANCER, one type of THYROID CANCER. They may produce an excess of adrenalin-like substances in the blood, causing a rise in blood pressure.

adrenalectomy (ah-dre"nal"ek'to-me)   surgical removal of the ADRENAL GLANDS (located above the kidneys), which produce a wide variety of corticosteroid hormones, including androstenedione, a male hormone. Many years ago it was observed that removal of the adrenal glands slowed the spread of recurrent breast cancer in older women. This occurred because the hormone-producing gland that stimulated cancer growth was removed.

Surgical removal of the adrenal glands is rarely performed today. In the contemporary treatment of breast cancer a medication known as AMINOG-LUTETHIMIDE, which blocks hormone production

by the adrenal glands, may be administered to postmenopausal women who have breast cancer that is estrogen dependent. This is a form of "medical" adrenalectomy, which has served to eliminate the need for an adrenalectomy in most instances.

adrenocortical cancer (ad-re"no-kor'te-kal)   cancer of the adrenal cortex, the outer layer of the ADRENAL GLANDS, located above each kidney. It is a rare tumor and usually appears in adults, generally between the ages of 40 and 50. Between 75 and 115 new cases a year are diagnosed in the United States.

Symptoms of adrenocortical cancer may include abdominal pain, weakness, weight loss, high blood pressure because of retention of salt, and a variety of hormone-related symptoms. In men there may be loss of sex drive, impotence, or enlargement of the breasts resulting from an overproduction of hormones caused by the cancer. It may be more common in men who developed sexually at an early age. In women, the overproduction of hormones can cause a deepening of the voice, unusually oily skin, excessive hairiness, or enlargement of the clitoris. Other possible symptoms include Cushing's syndrome (fat deposits forming along the center of the upper back and the face), mild diabetes, and softening of the bones. Many adrenocortical tumors do not produce extra hormones and are called nonfunctioning tumors.

Procedures used in the diagnosis and evaluation of adrenocortical cancer may include blood and urine tests to check hormone levels, endocrine studies, CT SCANS, MRI, ANGIOGRAPHY, and adrenal venography (contrast X-ray of the veins).

Following is the NATIONAL CANCER INSTITUTE'S (NCI) STAGING of adrenocortical carcinoma:

- Stage I—tumor is less than five CENTIMETERS (cm), with NEGATIVE LYMPH NODES, no LOCAL invasion, no METASTASES
- Stage II—tumor is more than 5 cm, with negative lymph nodes, no local invasion, no metastases
- Stage III—there is local invasion and/or positive lymph nodes, no metastases
- Stage IV—there are distant metastases
- Recurrent—the cancer has returned to the same area or to a different part of the body after treatment.

Treatment depends on the STAGE of the disease, the general state of health of the patient, and other factors. It usually includes surgical removal of the adrenal glands along with any tissue around the glands (such as kidney, liver) that contains cancer. LYMPH NODES may also be removed. CHEMOTHERAPY—and/or RADIATION THERAPY—may also be used. Treatment may also be given to prevent or modify symptoms caused by the extra hormones produced by the cancer. For information on the current state-of-the-art treatment, by stage of the disease, call NCI's Cancer Information Service at 1-800-4-CANCER (1-800-422-6237), or for a TTY: 1-800-332-8615.

adrenocorticoids (ad-re″no-kor′tĕ-coids) [adrenocortical hormone]   a class of hormonal agents produced naturally by the adrenal cortex, the outer layer of the ADRENAL GLANDS. It also refers to a synthetic substance modeled after the secretion of the adrenal cortex, hydrocortisone, first synthesized in 1950.

Adrenocorticoids may be used in the treatment of some cancers, including lymphomas, leukemias, Hodgkin's disease, and multiple myeloma (in addition to noncancerous conditions such as arthritis and autoimmune disorders). Some agents may be used to prevent and treat GRAFT VERSUS HOST DISEASE. Several are used as ANTIEMETICS in cancer treatment, and adrenocorticoids are used to reduce swelling in the brain or around the nerves.

Among the adrenocorticoids used in the treatment of cancer are cortisone, hydrocortisone, PREDNISONE, prednisolone, methylprednisolone, MEDROL, triamcinolone, paramethasone, fluprednisole, dexamethasone, betamethasone, fludrocortisone, and DECADRON. They are usually taken by mouth and occasionally by IV (injected into a vein).

Common side effects may include an increased appetite, weight gain, fluid retention, mood changes, acne, increased blood pressure, elevated blood sugar, intestinal ulcers, lowered resistance to infection, and gastrointestinal upset.

Adrenocorticoids have become very important agents in the treatment of cancer.

Adriamycin (a″dre-ah-mi′sin) [DOX, doxorubicin]   a major ANTIBIOTIC anticancer drug used frequently in the treatment of many cancers, including cancer of the breast, bladder, thyroid, lung, and ovary and WILMS' TUMOR, NEUROBLASTOMA, RHABDOMYOSARCOMA, EWING'S SARCOMA, RETINOBLASTOMA, and KAPOSI'S SARCOMA. It is given by IV (injected into a vein). Its administration must be done with great care since the drug can cause severe skin damage if it leaks out of the vein. Patients receiving Adriamycin should drink a lot of fluids. Producing more urine can prevent bladder and kidney problems.

The most common side effects of Adriamycin may include nausea, vomiting, fever (short term), red urine (which can stain clothing), hair loss (usually reversible), and temporary bone marrow depression. Side effects that are rare but which require immediate medical attention include unusually fast or irregular heartbeat, shortness of breath, wheezing, pain at the injection site, and swelling of the feet and lower legs. Other rare side effects in which medical attention should be sought include fever, chills, sore throat, sores in the mouth and on the lips, side or stomach pain, joint pain, unusual bleeding or bruising, and skin rash or itching.

The most significant side effect of Adriamycin is cardiomyopathy, direct damage to individual muscle cells of the heart. This is related to the total cumulative lifetime dose. In 1995 the drug ZINECARD was approved as a cardioprotective agent to be given immediately before administration of Adriamycin to prevent or reduce the incidence and severity of doxorubicin cardiomyopathy. It may be given to women whose doctors feel they would benefit from continuing therapy with Adriamycin.

Adrucil   See 5-FU.

adult Hodgkin's disease   See HODGKIN'S DISEASE.

adult non-Hodgkin's lymphoma   See NON-HODGKIN'S LYMPHOMA/ADULT.

adult soft tissue sarcoma   See SOFT TISSUE SARCOMA/ADULT.

adult T-cell leukemia   See CLL and LEUKEMIA.

adult T-cell leukemia-lymphoma (ATLL)   See ATLL.

advance directive   specific written instructions provided by a patient to be used in decision making and setting limits on future care in the event he or she is no longer capable of making decisions.

advanced cancer   an expression used when the disease is considered widespread and usually incurable. The cancer can neither be cured nor controlled and life expectancy may be very short. However, many people with advanced cancer have lived far longer than expected.

See also HOSPICE.

Advil   See NONSTEROIDAL ANTI-INFLAMMATORY DRUG.

AFP test   See ALPHA-FETOPROTEIN TEST.

after loading   a technique used in RADIATION THERAPY to direct radiation to a local site in the body. A catheter, tube, or needle is placed in the proximity of the target and then loaded with radioactive material. After an appropriate time of exposure, the tube is removed from the patient's body.

See BRACHYTHERAPY.

AG 013736   an investigational agent (in 2005) targeting multiple receptor tyrosine kinases, undergoing trials in the treatment of kidney cancer and other cancers.

age-adjusted rate   an incidence or mortality rate that has been adjusted to reduce the effects of age on statistics and make them more meaningful. It is compounded by weighting the age-specific rates by the proportions of people in the same age groups within a standard population. For example, the overall rate for breast cancer deaths in women between 1983 and 1987 was 27.2 per 100,000 women. However, if you adjust for age, there is a rate of 16.8 for women under the age of 65 and 122.1 for women 65 and over.

Agent Orange   a toxic herbicide containing DIOXIN used by American soldiers during the Vietnam War. Some 36,000 Vietnam veterans have claimed they have suffered various health effects, including cancer, from its use.

aggressive non-Hodgkin's lymphoma   (lim-fo′mah) a group of NON-HODGKIN'S LYMPHOMAS (NHLs) characterized by the rapid growth of tumor cells.

(Another type of non-Hodgkin's lymphoma is called INDOLENT NON-HODGKIN'S LYMPHOMA.) About half the people who get non-Hodgkin's lymphoma get the aggressive form. Aggressive non-Hodgkin's lymphoma is the most common form of lymphoma in children. If left untreated, aggressive non-Hodgkin's lymphoma can spread rapidly and become fatal. In patients with the aggressive form a complete remission achieved with therapy may be associated with a cure.

Among the aggressive non-Hodgkin's lymphomas are nodular HISTIOCYTIC lymphoma, diffuse histiocytic lymphoma, diffuse mixed LYMPHOCYTIC histiocytic lymphoma, diffuse undifferentiated lymphoma, and diffuse LYMPHOBLASTIC LYMPHOMA. (See the entry on non-Hodgkin's lymphoma for descriptions of these types.) In the diagnosis of non-Hodgkin's lymphoma, determining the type plays a significant role in the choice of treatment.

agranulocytosis   See NEUTROPENIA.

AGT   See CYTADREN.

AIDS (acquired immune deficiency [immunodeficiency] syndrome)   a disease in which the destruction of white blood cells (LYMPHOCYTES) results in the breakdown and eventual failure of the body's immune system. People who are HIV positive and have a T-cell count under 200 are generally thought to have AIDS. With an impaired immune system, which is the body's main line of defense against disease, the body cannot fight infections that would ordinarily be warded off. People with AIDS are therefore much more susceptible to infections; and although AIDS is not cancer, it has been associated with the development of several different cancers, including KAPOSI'S SARCOMA (a form of skin cancer), SQUAMOUS CELL CARCINOMA OF THE SKIN, NON-HODGKIN'S LYMPHOMA, BURKITT'S LYMPHOMA, primary brain cancer and lymphoma, and CERVICAL CANCER. AIDS-related cancers seem to be increasing in the general population.

AIDS was first recognized in the United States in 1981, although researchers later found that there were cases of AIDS in the United States years earlier. It has been present in other areas, parts of Africa and possibly the Caribbean, for a much greater period of time. It is at epidemic proportions around the world.

AIDS is caused by the human T cell lymphotropic virus III (HTLV-III) or HIV. It destroys one type of lymphocyte known as the T4, or "helper cell." Helper cells protect the body against infections and some cancers. It is possible, although highly unlikely, that a person who tests positive for the HTLV-III virus may never develop symptoms and may carry the virus for the rest of his or her life. Someone with the AIDS virus may develop an AIDS-related condition (ARC), such as swollen glands and a high fever.

In an early stage of AIDS, the body may be able to fight back. But as the condition worsens, more and more of the helper cells are destroyed, making the person far more susceptible to other, much more serious disorders.

AIDS can be transmitted in several ways, including through genital or anal sex. It is also possible for a woman to acquire the AIDS virus if the semen she receives during artificial insemination is infected. The unborn child may also become infected. AIDS can also be transmitted through body fluids such as blood. For example, a razor, syringe, or needle that has been used by someone with the AIDS virus can infect another person if it comes in contact with his or her blood; a person can also be infected by receiving a transfusion of blood or transplanted organ from someone with the AIDS virus. In 1985 the United States started screening prospective blood donors for the AIDS virus using the HIV test.

Treatment of HIV infection is best accomplished by use of combinations of antiretroviral agents, the most potent being a category known as protease inhibitors. HAART (highly active antiretroviral therapy) can dramatically lower measurable virus particles in the blood. The U.S. death rate from AIDS has begun to decline slightly for the first time. People with HIV are living longer, which has led to some optimism. To date, however, AIDS is not considered curable.

AIDS is not spread by ordinary social contact—such as shaking hands, hugging, kissing, working together, nursing a patient, using someone else's towel in a gym, etc.

Anyone can get HIV—young and old, men and women, straight, gay, and bisexual, rich and poor,

and all racial and ethnic groups—but not everyone faces the same risk. At highest risk are people who have sex and/or share needles with someone who is infected; someone who is "infected" could be carrying the virus and not show any signs/symptoms of it. The number of heterosexual, nondrug users in the United States diagnosed with AIDS has been increasing.

There are several measures that can be taken to prevent AIDS:

- avoid sex with any person who has AIDS, including those carrying the AIDS virus, even if they show now signs of AIDS-related illness
- request that a potential sexual partner be tested for presence of the AIDS virus prior to engaging in sexual intercourse of any kind with him/her, and use condoms with spermicide if there are any doubts about whether the sexual partner has AIDS
- never share a needle or syringe
- when giving first aid to someone, wear rubber gloves; if blood gets on the skin, wash it off immediately; blood from a person with AIDS can only be harmful if it enters the body through a break in the skin, or mucous membranes (such as the mouth or eyes).

Symptoms of AIDS include weight loss, fever, swollen glands, weakness, headaches, drowsiness, confusion, and chest, skin, or mouth infections. However, these symptoms can be signs of *many other disorders.*

A definitive diagnosis of AIDS is by a blood test for the AIDS virus.

Research to develop a vaccine to prevent AIDS as well as antiviral drugs to fight it is continuing. The National AIDS Hotline number is 1-800-342-AIDS. See Appendix I for other support organizations for AIDS.

AIPC (androgen-independent prostate cancer)   a metastatic disease not subject to hormonal manipulation and control.

air-contrast X-rays   an X-RAY that uses inflation with air to obtain a better outline of some parts of the body. The air can be inhaled, swallowed, injected, or ingested by drinking a carbonated beverage, after which the X-ray is taken. For example, when a chest X-ray is done, the patient is told to "take a deep breath and hold it." This allows for maximum inflation of the air sacs that make up the lung tissue. Any abnormality in the lung tissue would then be highlighted.

albinism (al′bĭ-nizm)   a condition in which people have very small amounts of melanin (pigment) in their skin, making them more sensitive to ULTRAVIOLET RADIATION from the Sun and therefore placing them at a higher risk of getting skin cancer.

ALCL (anaplastic large cell lymphoma)   a distinct NON-HODGKIN'S LYMPHOMA (NHL), defined in 1985. ALCL represents approximately 3% of adult and 10–30% of childhood NHLs. Among this group, ALK(+) gene presence has the best prognosis. Overall ALCL behaves as an aggressive, high-grade LYMPHOMA, for which the treatment is CHEMOTHERAPY.

alcohol   a drug that may play a role in the development of a number of different cancers, including cancer of the breast, liver, esophagus, pharynx, larynx, and mouth and colon/rectal cancer. Epidemiological studies have indicated an increased risk of cancer with high alcohol consumption. Based on numerous epidemiological studies, the International Agency for Research on Cancer has categorized alcoholic beverages as carcinogenic. Alcohol's cancer-causing risk appears to increase if a person smokes as well.

aldesleukin   See INTERLEUKIN-2.

alemtuzumab [Campath]   a recombinant humanized monoclonal antibody directed against the CD52 surface protein expressed on most normal and malignant B and T lymphocytes. It is given intravenously and is characterized as a biological response modifier. It is indicated in patients with relapsed and/or refractory B-CELL chronic lymphocytic LEUKEMIA. These patients usually have failed alkylating agents and fludarabine therapy. It is also indicatred in patients with T-CELL prolymphocytic leukemia. Usefulness in other settings is being explored. Because of its broad spectrum of anti-lymphocyte activity, significant immunosuppression and infection are its major adverse consequences, especially with opportunistic infections.

aleukemia (ah″lu-ke′me-ah)   a condition in which the BONE MARROW has an abnormally high number of cancerous WHITE BLOOD CELLS, but where the white blood cells are not entering the bloodstream. Aleukemia occurs in about 30% of all patients with LEUKEMIA, regardless of the specific type. When a patient is aleukemic, the leukemia is not behaving in the usual way, i.e., with an overwhelming number of early white blood cells in the blood. A person with aleukemic leukemia will have a normal or low white blood count. This condition does not alter the prognosis.

Alferon   See ALPHA INTERFERON and INTERFERON.

Alimta [pemetrexed]   an injectable chemotherapeutic agent approved for the treatment of malignant pleural mesothelioma.

alkaline phosphatase (al′kah-l-īn fos′fah-tās″)   an ENZYME produced primarily by bone and liver tissue. Elevations of alkaline phosphatase may appear in the blood in a wide variety of conditions affecting these organs, including cancer.

alkaline phosphatase test (al′kah-l-īn fos′fah-tās″)   one of a number of tests using a TUMOR MARKER in the diagnosis of cancers that commonly spread to the bone such as prostate, kidney, breast, thyroid, and lung cancer; it is also used to investigate abnormalities or cancers of the liver or bile duct system. Elevated levels of the enzyme may result from a bone's effort to repair itself from damage caused by either progressive cancer or a BENIGN (noncancerous) injury such as a fracture. The alkaline phosphatase test is an important marker of tumor activity in patients with OSTEOSARCOMA (bone cancer). The alkaline phosphatase test is not "cancer specific" but may be used by doctors to evaluate patients.

alkaloids (al′kah-loids″) [plant alkaloids]   one type of anticancer drug developed from plant alkaloids, organic compounds containing nitrogen. Alkaloids act on cells in different phases of the cell cycle. Examples of some alkaloids are VINCRISTINE and VINBLASTINE (products of the periwinkle family of plants) and VP-16 (from the mandrake plant). They are used in the treatment of many cancers including BREAST and LUNG CANCERS, HODGKIN'S DISEASE, LYMPHOMAS, and LEUKEMIAS.

Alkeran (al-ker'an) [L-PAM, melphalan, L-phenyl-alanine mustard, L-sarcolysin] an ALKYLATING anti-cancer drug sometimes used in the treatment of BREAST and OVARIAN CANCER and MYELOMA. It is taken by mouth. Common side effects may include mild nausea and vomiting. Side effects that are not common but that you should tell your doctor about include black, tarry stools, fever, chills or sore throat, unusual bleeding or bruising, side or stomach pain, joint pain, and sores in the mouth and on the lips. Uncommon side effects that require immediate medical attention include sudden skin rash. The more serious and rare side effects may include temporary BONE MARROW depression (especially PLATELETS), second malignancies (cancers), lung problems (scarring of the lungs, which may be fatal), menstrual irregularities, hair loss (usually reversible), and temporary mouth sores. Alkeran is one of the more commonly used chemotherapy drugs and is very important in the treatment of cancer.

See also CARCINOGENS.

alkylating (al'kīla"ting) a characteristic of a major group of drugs used to treat cancer. They interfere with the division process of cancer cells, slowing or stopping their growth and reproduction. They cause the greatest damage to cells that are in any active phase of the CELL CYCLE; in high enough doses they can also kill cells in their "resting" phase. Alkylating agents are effective against many different cancers, including breast and lung cancer, LEUKEMIAS, and LYMPHOMAS. Alkylating agents can occasionally cause sterility, and when used over a long period of time, they slightly increase the risk of leukemia. Some examples of alkylating agents are MUSTARGEN, LEUKERAN, CYTOXAN, THIOTEPA, STREPTOZOCIN, and BUSULFAN.

ALL (acute lymphocytic leukemia) (lim"fo-sit'ik) [ACUTE LYMPHATIC LEUKEMIA, ACUTE LYMPHOBLASTIC LEUKEMIA, ACUTE LEUKEMIA, ACUTE] one of the four basic types of LEUKEMIA. It is characterized by the abnormal production of immature LYMPHOCYTES, one type of white blood cell. As a result, there is an accumulation of those abnormal cells in the bone marrow, bloodstream, and LYMPH system.

Of all the leukemias, ALL occurs most frequently. It is the most common childhood leukemia, peaking between the ages of two and nine years, and may be referred to as "childhood leukemia." A much smaller percentage of people (mostly male) get ALL in old age. In 1999 there were 3,100 new cases and 1,400 deaths according to the American Cancer Society. Twenty years ago most patients with ALL lived for just a few months. In the late 1980s the potential cure rate was 50%.

The term ALL refers to a number of different leukemias listed below:

• common acute lymphocytic leukemia—the most predominant form of ALL, occurring in about 75% of the children and more than 50% of adults
• B-CELL (also called BURKITT CELL ALL)—the rarest form of ALL, occurring in both older children and older adults
• T-CELL—predominantly occurs in older teens and young adults, with a slightly higher incidence among men, and accounting for about 12% of all ALL
• NULL-CELL (also called undifferentiated ALL)—affecting primarily older children and adults and making up about 8% of the cases of ALL.

The general symptoms for ALL may occur suddenly and progress rapidly. Symptoms may include fever and flu-like symptoms including chills and respiratory discomfort, enlarged lymph nodes (especially in children), spleen and liver enlargement causing a protrusion and pain, bone and joint pain, paleness, weakness, tendency to bleed or bruise easily, loss of appetite, heavy menstrual periods, blood in the stool, and frequent infections. These can also be symptoms for many other disorders, however.

The only definitive diagnosis is by BONE MARROW BIOPSY, which is usually done after a suspicious blood test. After a positive diagnosis, a sample of cerebrospinal fluid is examined for leukemia in the central nervous system.

There is no clear-cut staging for either adult or childhood acute lymphocytic leukemia. The NATIONAL CANCER INSTITUTE (NCI) breaks it down in the following way:

• untreated—there has been no treatment except to treat symptoms (blood products, antibiotics, etc.); there are too many white blood cells in the blood and bone marrow; there may be no other signs or symptoms of leukemia

- in remission—the number of white blood cells and other blood cells in the blood and marrow is normal following treatment; there are no signs or symptoms of leukemia
- relapsed/refractory—the leukemia has recurred (come back) after going into remission; refractory means it has failed to go into remission after treatment.

Currently, the most effective treatment for adult acute lymphocytic leukemia is CHEMOTHERAPY. The treatment of childhood acute lymphocytic leukemia is usually chemotherapy. RADIATION THERAPY is also sometimes used.

Treatment consists of three phases:

- induction—intensive treatment over four to six weeks to kill as many of the leukemic cells as possible
- consolidation—additional chemotherapy to wipe out remaining leukemic cells that had become resistant to the drugs used in induction therapy
- maintenance therapy—lower doses of chemotherapy for a longer period of time, two to three years, to wipe out any remaining leukemic cells and keep the cancer from recurring (coming back).

Another treatment that may be used is central nervous system (CNS) preventive therapy to prevent a recurrence in the CNS. This generally consists of whole brain irradiation along with chemotherapy. BONE MARROW TRANSPLANTATION (BMT) is another possible treatment for both adult and childhood ALL.

allogeneic bone marrow transplant (al″o-jĕ-ne′ik)   replacing a patient's bone marrow with the healthy marrow of someone who is not genetically identical, such as a parent, sibling, or unrelated donor. Special blood tests are done to determine how closely the potential donor marrow matches the bone marrow of the recipient. The success of the transplant depends, in large part, on how close the match is. Allogeneic transplants are at greater risk of rejection than the two other types of transplants SYNGENEIC transplants (identical twins) and

AUTOLOGOUS transplants (the patient's own marrow is used).

See also BONE MARROW TRANSPLANTATION.

allogeneic stem cell transplant   transplantation of stem cells from a donor who is not genetically identical to the recipient.

allopurinol sodium (al-o-pure′ĭ-nōl) [Zyloprim] a drug given to some cancer patients as premedication before administration of CHEMOTHERAPY (anticancer drugs) to reduce some toxic side effects of the chemotherapy. It is taken by mouth. Possible side effects may include rashes, fever, nausea, diarrhea, abdominal pain, and drowsiness.

allovectin-7   a gene product injected directly into a tumor to enhance immunologic destruction. It is undergoing investigation in the treatment of METASTATIC MELANOMA.

all-trans retinoic acid [Vesanoid, tretinoin] Usually referred to as "ATRA." A derivative of vitamin A, it works by prodding MALIGNANT LEUKEMIC cells to differentiate or "mature" into normal cells, which subsequently die. It is being used as the standard treatment of patients with ACUTE PROMYELOCYTIC LEUKEMIA (APL). Common side effects may include headaches and bone pain. Less common side effects may include retinoic acid syndrome, a shock-like state characterized by fever, DYSPNEA, weight gain, PULMONARY INFILTRATES, and pleural or pericardial EFFUSIONS. RETINOIC ACID SYNDROME can be fatal. All-trans retinoic acid is taken orally in pill form.

alopecia (al″o-pe′she-ah)   the loss of hair. For cancer patients, this can be a side effect of CHEMOTHERAPY (anticancer drugs) or RADIATION THERAPY to the head. The hair generally grows back either during or following treatment, although there are rare instances when the hair does not return.

Alopecia occurs because of damage to the very delicate hair follicles that are susceptible to the toxic chemicals in the chemotherapy drugs or to the direct effect of radiation treatment. The hair loss does not occur instantly. It can take two to three weeks from the time of exposure.

Though physically painless, alopecia can cause enormous distress to patients. Great strides have been made in the development of effective and attractive hair prostheses (wigs) for patients. Most insurance companies will reimburse patients for a prosthesis. It is frequently recommended to patients that they get a wig before they lose their hair. There are some patients who will simply wear a hat or scarf until their hair grows back.

alpha-fetoprotein (al′fah fē″to-pro′tēn) [(AFP) test] an examination of blood for levels of alpha-fetoprotein, a specific protein found in embryonic tissue and the blood. Alpha-fetoprotein is one of the oncofetal antigens, a substance present in childhood development and rarely in healthy adult tissue. Elevated levels in the blood may be an indication of some cancers, including testicular, liver, stomach, pancreatic, lung, and ovarian cancer as well as other conditions. This is a TUMOR MARKER that may be used in the diagnosis of cancer as well as in follow-up to evaluate the effectiveness of treatment and the presence of recurrent disease. However, a raised AFP level is just a possible indicator and cannot be used for a definitive diagnosis. An elevated level can be caused by many other conditions.

alpha interferon (in″ter-fēr′on) [human leukocyte interferon] a "type 1" INTERFERON derived from the white blood cells called leukocytes and other sources. In 1986 the Food and Drug Administration licensed alpha interferon for the treatment of HAIRY CELL LEUKEMIA. Since then it has been approved for treating KAPOSI'S SARCOMA, CHRONIC MYELOGENOUS LEUKEMIA, and MULTIPLE MYELOMA. It was the first BIOLOGICAL RESPONSE MODIFIER to be licensed for cancer treatment in the United States. Alpha interferon appears to work best in people with early-stage disease and whose immune systems are not severely impaired.

alternative treatment generally refers to treatments that are used instead of conventional treatments. Alternative treatments have generally not been studied for safety and effectiveness through a rigorous scientific process, including clinical trials with large numbers of patients, as have conventional treatments. When alternative treatments are used with conventional ones they are considered to be "complementary." See National Center for Complementary and Alternative Medicine (http://nccam.nih.gov).

altretamine See HEXAMETHYLMELAMINE.

alveolar cell lung cancer See BRONCHIOLOALVEOLAR LUNG CANCER.

alveolar ridge cancer a head/neck cancer involving tissue lining the mandible (jawbone). These are squamous cell cancers, primarily treated by surgery.

alveolar soft part sarcoma (al-ve′o-lar) an uncommon malignant (cancerous) tumor having a unique microscopic appearance. It occurs primarily in the thighs of adults and in the neck area of children. Its primary treatment is surgery.

See also SOFT TISSUE SARCOMA/ADULT and SOFT TISSUE SARCOMA/CHILDHOOD.

alveoli (al-ve′o-li) tiny air sacs at the end of the bronchioles.

American Board of Surgeons an organization that grants BOARD CERTIFICATION to surgeons. Physicians who have had full training in approved surgical residencies must then pass rigorous written and oral tests to become board certified. The American Board of Surgery was founded in 1937 by a group of prominent American surgeons.

amethopterin (am-eth-op′ter-in) See METHOTREXATE.

aminoglutethimide (ah-me″no-gloo-teth′-ĭ-mīd) See CYTADREN.

amifostine See ETHYOL.

AML (acute myelogenous leukemia) See also ANLL.

AMSA See M-AMSA.

amsacrine See M-AMSA.

amyloidosis (am″ĭ-loi-do′sis) a condition in which deposits of insoluble protein fragments can occur in a number of different parts of the body, including the tongue, heart, gastrointestinal tract, muscles, and ligaments, especially the carpal tunnel area of the hand. That can result in carpal tunnel syndrome—pain, numbness, and/or tingling in the fingers and hands. Other symptoms include weakness, weight loss, shortness of breath, or light-headedness. Amyloidosis affects about 15% of people with MULTIPLE MYELOMA. The treatment for amyloidosis with myeloma is essentially the treatment for multiple myeloma.

anagrelide See ARGYLIN.

anal cancer a gastrointestinal cancer of the anus (the outlet of the bowel) that is fairly rare and often curable. It is usually a SQUAMOUS CELL CARCINOMA. Cancer in the outer part of the anus is more likely to occur in men; cancer in the inner part of the anus is more likely to occur in women. Anal cancer has been shown to be associated with HPV (human papilloma virus), leading many to consider it a form of STD (sexually transmitted disease).

Symptoms may include bleeding from the rectum (even a small amount), pain or pressure in the area around the anus, itching or discharge from the anus, or a lump near the anus.

Diagnostic procedures may include a rectal exam by the doctor and a biopsy (microscopic examination of tissue for cancer cells). The doctor will remove a small amount of tissue from the area for the biopsy if he or she sees or feels anything that is not normal.

Following is the NATIONAL CANCER INSTITUTE's (NCI) STAGING for anal cancers:

- Stage 0—carcinoma in situ; a very early cancer that has not spread below the limiting membrane of the first layer of anal tissue
- Stage I—cancer is less than two CENTIMETERS (cm) in size and has not spread anywhere else; there is no sphincter involvement
- Stage II—cancer is more than two cm in size but does not involve lymph nodes or other organs
- Stage III—cancer has spread to the lymph nodes and/or to adjacent organs
   IIIA—cancer has spread to nearby lymph nodes or has spread to nearby organs such as the vagina, urethra, or bladder or
   IIIB—cancer has spread to nearby lymph nodes and to adjacent organs

- Stage IV—cancer has spread to the sacrum (part of the spine), to distant lymph nodes within the abdomen far away from the original cancer, or other organs in the body
- Recurrent—cancer has returned to the same site or spread to another part of the body after treatment

Treatment depends on the type and stage of the disease as well as other factors and may include surgery, radiation, and chemotherapy. The goal of the treatment is to preserve function while improving the cure rate. In the past, many patients were cured by a large operation to remove the rectum and anus, an ABDOMINOPERINEAL RESECTION (APR). Current programs combining combination chemotherapy (anticancer drugs) and radiation therapy may eliminate the need for the surgical removal of the organ. For specific information on the latest state-of-the-art treatment for anal cancer, by stage, call NCI's Cancer Information Service at 1-800-4-CANCER (1-800-422-6237), or for a TTY: 1-800-332-8615.

analgesic (an"al-je'zik) a drug that gives relief from pain. Analgesics are the major type of drug used for the control of pain in cancer. There are three basic categories of analgesics: nonprescription (over-the-counter) drugs; NONSTEROIDAL ANTI-INFLAMMATORY DRUGS (NSAIDs); and NARCOTIC DRUGS, which must be obtained with a doctor's prescription.

The most well-known nonprescription analgesic is ASPIRIN. Aspirin can be quite effective in treating mild or moderate cancer pain (as well as other pains, of course, including arthritis) if taken correctly, as it has anti-inflammatory properties. Side effects, more common with high doses of aspirin, include mild headaches, ringing in the ears, excessive sweating, nausea, vomiting, or diarrhea. Much less common but more serious side effects are bleeding problems and ulcers.

Cancer patients taking anticancer drugs are usually advised to use another main type of analgesic, ACETAMINOPHEN, instead of aspirin. Tylenol and Datril are two brand names of acetaminophen. Acetaminophen differs from aspirin in two major ways: It as it does not have anti-inflammatory properties, it does not reduce swelling caused by inflammation, nor does it cause bleeding problems. Side effects are very rare, although large doses or extended use can cause kidney or liver damage.

The long-term use of nonprescription analgesics is limited by the side effects described above. Patients do not become addicted to analgesics nor do they develop a drug tolerance to them.

When NSAIDs like Motrin and Nuprin were introduced in the early 1970s, they were only available with a doctor's prescription. Today, however, the NSAID ibuprofen (common brand names are Advil and Nuprin) is available without a prescription. It acts in a way similar to aspirin, reducing inflammation and pain. Possible side effects include stomach irritation and water retention.

A doctor's prescription is always needed for the narcotic drugs, which are the strongest painkillers. The most common narcotics include CODEINE, MORPHINE, fentanyl citrate, PERCODAN (oxycodone or oxycontin), DILAUDID (hydromorphone), METHADONE (Dolophine), DEMEROL (meperidine), LEVO-DROMORAN (levorphanol), NUMORPHAN (oxymorphone), Roxicet (acetaminophen and oxycodone), and Vicodin (hydrocodone). HEROIN, a well-known narcotic, is not legally available in the United States.

Some common side effects of narcotics include sedation, nausea, vomiting, constipation, and depressed respiration.

Analgesics work most quickly when injected into a vein and take the longest time to be effective when taken by mouth. New and more effective ways of delivering drugs are being developed. One new method is the ANALGESIC PUMP, or the PCA pump (patient-controlled analgesia pump) which allows the patient to regulate administration of pain medication.

analgesic pump (an″al-je′zik) [patient-controlled analgesia, PCA pump] a device that contains a narcotic solution to control pain and may be operated by the patient. It was first marketed in 1974. The analgesic pump is hooked up to an intravenous line in the patient's arm. It is then set, by computer, so that by pressing a button, the patient can deliver a premeasured dose of the drug into his or her bloodstream. The patient may press the button as often as needed, but a control in the pump sets a safety limit.

The analgesic pump has a number of advantages, not the least of which is the psychological boost to many patients, who may, for the first time, feel they have some control over their pain—and over their cancer. Another major advantage is that the patient does not have to wait for a nurse to come with another dose of medication (it also saves time for the nursing staff). The analgesic pump can be set to meet the needs of the individual patient. Because the analgesic is delivered directly into the bloodstream, it works very quickly.

See also PAIN MANAGEMENT, PCA PUMP, and INFUSION PUMP.

anaplasia (an″ah-pla′ze-ah) [anaplastic] cells in a cancer tumor that lack an organized structure and that have reversed to a "primitive" state.

anaplastic (an″ah-plas′tik) See ANAPLASIA.

anaplastic astrocytoma (an″ah-plas′tik as″tro-si-to′mah) a grade III ASTROCYTOMA, a type of brain tumor that is relatively fast growing. Its cells look very different from normal cells. See BRAIN CANCER.

anaplastic oligodendroglioma (an″ah-plas′tik ol″ĭ-go-den″dro-gli-o′mah) See BRAIN CANCER.

anaplastic thyroid carcinoma (an″ah-plas′tik) [undifferentiated thyroid carcinoma] one type of THYROID CANCER representing 18% of the total number of thyroid cancers. It is quite aggressive and largely untreatable.

anastomosis (ah-nas″to-mo′sis) reattaching the ends of two parts of a body structure—two nerves, two blood vessels, or other tissues. For example, when a tumor is removed from the large intestine, an anastomosis is performed so that the intestine (though shorter) will continue to function.

anastrozole See ARIMIDEX.

androgen (an′dro-jen) a male hormone, such as testosterone and androsterone, produced in the testes, and to a lesser extent in the ADRENAL GLANDS. The androgens are responsible for male characteristics. Females also produce androgens, but in very small amounts.

Androgens used in the treatment of cancer include:

- testosterone propionate (Neohombreol, Oraton)
- floxymesterone (Halotestin, Ora-Testryl)

- nandrolone decanoate (Deca-Durabolin)
- calusterone (Methosarb)
- dromostanolone propionate (Drolban, Masteril, Macleron, Permastril)

anecdotal evidence   word-of-mouth descriptions or testimonials based on individual cancer cases. For example, a person may know someone who was told that his or her cancer could be cured and, after sitting out in the sun for seven days straight, or eating a diet of cherries and brown rice, or walking three and a half miles a day, or any one of a number of other things, was suddenly cured. Anecdotal evidence is not considered to be scientific support for a type of treatment. However, a group of cases with similar components may eventually be investigated in a controlled study to determine whether there is any merit to the claims. See CLINICAL TRIALS.

anemia (ah-ne′me-ah)   a condition in which there is a deficit of RED BLOOD CELLS that are produced by the BONE MARROW. There are many reasons for this, both hereditary (e.g., sickle cell anemia) and acquired. Slow bleeding of a small amount of blood daily over months can lead to significant anemia that may be a sign of COLON CANCER. Anemia can also be the result of cancer treatment (CHEMOTHERAPY and RADIATION THERAPY).

Symptoms of anemia can include fatigue, dizziness, pale skin color, weakness, heart palpitations, lack of energy, and a tendency to feel cold. Without enough red blood cells to carry oxygen to the tissues in the body that require it, it is difficult for the body to get all the oxygen it needs.

The treatment of anemia depends on its cause. For cancer patients whose treatment is the primary cause of anemia, blood transfusions are often administered. The risk of AIDS, however, has caused major concern on the part of many patients, who may accept blood transfusions only when absolutely necessary. ERYTHROPOIETIN, a COLONY-STIMULATING FACTOR (CSF) that stimulates the production of blood cells, may play a role in the correction of this form of anemia.

anesthesia (an″es-the′ze-ah)   a state of total or partial loss of consciousness and sensation, especially pain, induced in a patient for any painful pro-

cedure, usually a surgical procedure. Anesthesia may be achieved with one drug or a combination of drugs. Anesthesia can be administered in the following ways:

- topical—injected, sprayed, or painted directly onto the area involved
- local—confined to a specific part of the body; used for many minor surgical procedures
- regional—affecting a large part of the body; more extensive than a "local"
- total—affecting the entire body; done for major surgical procedures; a total loss of consciousness and sensation

anesthetic (an″es-thet′ik)   an agent that induces a state of ANESTHESIA.

aneuploid (an′u-ploid)   of cancer cells that have abnormal amounts of DNA. Most cancer cells are aneuploid, and the more aneuploid they are, the more aggressive the cancer is. TUMOR CELLS that have a normal amount of DNA are called DIPLOID.

See also PLOIDY.

angiogenesis   the complex process involving the formation of new blood vessels. Research scientists have found some evidence that agents that block tumor angiogenesis will be useful as treatment. See ANTIANGIOGENESIS AGENTS.

angiogenesis inhibitors   See ANTIANGIOGENESIS agents.

angiogram (an′je-o-gram″)   See ANGIOGRAPHY.

angiography (an″je-og′rah-fe) [arteriography]   a diagnostic procedure that examines the blood vessels leading to an organ or area of concern as well as the blood distribution within the organ. A contrast agent that will show up on an X-RAY is injected into the blood vessels, usually through a catheter or tube. These X-rays, called an angiogram, can then show structural abnormalities or disorders. Angiography is used most frequently in the evaluation of liver, pancreatic, kidney, or brain cancer.

angiosarcoma (an″je-o-sar-ko′mah)   a MALIGNANT (cancerous) tumor originating in a BLOOD VESSEL. This is a very rare SOFT TISSUE SARCOMA.

angiostatin and endostatin   two antiangiogenic (see ANGIOGENESIS and ANTIANGIOGENESIS) agents identified by Dr. Judah Folkman; they are proteins that stop the development of new blood vessels, thereby interfering with the blood supply needed by tumors to survive and grow. When used together experimentally in mice, the drugs have eliminated tumors. Once eradicated, the tumors have not returned. Angiostatin is a part of a very common protein called PLASMINOGEN that the body used in blood clotting. Endostatin is a part of the protein collagen 18 that is in all blood vessels but by itself has no effect on cancer. The mice had no adverse side effects from angiostatin and endostatin whereas they suffer many side effects when given chemotherapy. And they did not become resistant to the drugs. These drugs are the only ones ever tested that seem able to eliminate all tumors in mice, regardless of the size of the tumor. There is much promise for their use in humans. They have generated tremendous excitement and optimism in the cancer community. However, because of difficulty with preparation and purification of these agents, clinical trials in humans are in the very early stages with conflicting results (2005).

ANLL (acute nonlymphocytic leukemia)   a MALIGNANT—(cancerous) disorder in which abnormal, immature WHITE BLOOD CELLS are produced in the BONE MARROW. The result is an excessive accumulation of those cells in the bloodstream and bone marrow.

ACUTE MYELOGENOUS LEUKEMIA (AML) is the most common kind of ANLL. AML is a major form of LEUKEMIA, accounting for about 35% of all diagnosed cases in the United States, most frequently affecting people aged 40 and over. In children, it is the second most common leukemia. AML is also referred to as ACUTE MYELOCYTIC LEUKEMIA, ACUTE MYELOBLASTIC LEUKEMIA, and ACUTE GRANULOCYTIC LEUKEMIA. Because it is the major type of ANLL, AML is frequently used instead of ANLL, which can be confusing. In 1999, there were approximately 10,100 new cases of AML diagnosed and 6,900 deaths attributed to the disease.

ANLL has other subtypes that are very rare and account for less than 10% of the diagnosed cases. The other types are:

- ACUTE MONOCYTIC LEUKEMIA—characterized by the overproduction of the white blood cells monocytes and monoblasts
- acute promyelocytic leukemia—characterized by the overproduction of promyelocytes (primitive granulocytes)
- acute erythroleukemia leukemia—characterized by the overproduction of immature red cells mixed with a variety of immature white cells
- acute myelomonocytic leukemia—characterized by the overproduction of monocytes and myelocytes (an intermediate stage monocyte)
- acute megakaryoblastic leukemia—characterized by the overproduction of a rare white blood cell in its earliest, most immature state

Symptoms of ANLL may include fatigue, infections, flu-like symptoms including high fever and chills, respiratory discomfort, weakness, irritability, loss of appetite, and unexplained weight loss. Excessive bleeding may occur after a minor injury, and the skin may bruise easily or develop purplish red blotches. The gums or nose may bleed with no apparent cause, and women may experience unusually heavy menstrual periods. Occasionally there is bone or joint pain. These symptoms may also be signs of many other disorders.

The only definitive diagnosis is by BONE MARROW BIOPSY, which is usually done after a suspicious blood test. After a positive diagnosis, a sample of CEREBROSPINAL FLUID (CSF) may be examined for leukemia in the central nervous system.

There is no clear-cut staging system for adult or childhood ANLL. The National Cancer Institute (NCI) breaks it down in the following way for adult ANLL:

- untreated—there has been no treatment except to treat symptoms (blood products, antibiotics, etc.); there are too many white blood cells in the blood and bone marrow; there may be no other signs or symptoms of leukemia
- in remission—the number of white blood cells and other blood cells in the blood and marrow is normal following treatment; there are no signs or symptoms of leukemia
- relapsed/refractory—the leukemia has recurred (come back) after going into remission; refractory means it has failed to go into remission after treatment.

NCI breaks down childhood ANLL in the following way:

- untreated—there has been no treatment other than supportive care (blood products, antibiotics, allopurinol)
- in remission—blood counts are normal, bone marrow is normal, and there are no signs or symptoms of the disease following radiation remission induction treatment
- relapsed—leukemia has come back following remission

Treatment depends on the type and stage of the disease and other factors. ANLL may be treated with combination chemotherapy. Bone marrow transplantation is a treatment under evaluation, as are biological therapies. For specific information on the latest state-of-the-art treatment for ANLL, call the NCI's Cancer Information Service at 1-800-4-Cancer (1-800-422-6237), or for a TTY: 1-800-332-8615.

anorexia (an″o-rek′se-ah) loss of appetite frequently experienced by cancer patients, which can be caused by the cancer itself or its treatment. A patient may experience a lack of appetite or a change in the way things taste; a condition in the mouth, such as sores, may develop and make eating painful; or experiencing pain generally can cause a patient to lose his or her appetite. Anorexia can result in CACHEXIA (severe protein loss). Good nutrition is an essential ingredient in recovery, enabling the body to repair normal cells that have been damaged by cancer treatment and giving the patient a sense of well-being. Good nutrition is also important to keep the immune system operating at the most optimal level possible. It is important, therefore, that the cancer patient gets the required nutrients.

Anorexia can cause intense family distress. It is natural to equate eating and appetite with health. Attempts to alleviate this condition are directed at its cause if at all possible. The agent MEGACE (MEG) is being widely used to increase the appetite and promote weight gain in anorexic patients. Marinol (MARIJUANA) has been of some help to some patients.

Following are some tips for patients experiencing a lack of appetite:

- eat small frequent meals
- keep nutritious snacks available for eating throughout the day
- eat foods high in calories and protein
- avoid empty calories like water, diet soda, etc.
- schedule meals to coincide with the times during the day when you're feeling best
- stimulate appetite with light exercise or a glass of wine
- boost caloric and protein intake by adding skim milk, butter, etc. to foods
- take medications with drinks high in calories
- make changes in the foods—try new recipes, spices, consistencies, etc.
- change the place where you eat—eat at a friend's home, at a favorite restaurant
- serve food in as attractive and appetizing way as possible

It is not uncommon to develop an aversion to meats. Following are some tips for patients experiencing a change in taste:

- substitute chicken, fish, eggs, and cheese for red meat
- marinate meats with sweet marinades or sauces
- serve meats cold instead of at hot temperatures
- use extra seasonings, spices, garlic, and onions to flavor foods
- substitute milk shakes, puddings, ice cream, cheeses, and other high-protein foods for meats
- rinse mouth before eating
- use lemon flavored drinks to stimulate the taste buds

Anorexia should not be confused with anorexia nervosa, which is caused by psychological problems.

anoscopy (ah-nos′ko-pe) an examination of the rectum. Anoscopy is a diagnostic procedure for RECTAL CANCER. Using an anoscope, the doctor sees inside the rectum. An anoscope is a smaller version of a SIGMOIDOSCOPE, which is used for the same purpose in a SIGMOIDOSCOPY.

anterior exenteration (eks-en″ter-ā′shun) surgical removal of the urethra, bladder, and vagina. This may be done in the treatment of URETHRAL CANCER.

anthracycline one of hundreds of antibiotics that are synthesized or made from *Streptomyces,* a mold-like bacteria. Anthracyclines are an important source of antibiotics used to fight cancer tumors. Adriamycin is probably the best-known CHEMOTHERAPY that falls into this category.

antiandrogen (an″tĭ-an′dro-jen) an agent used to block the function of the male hormones (androgens) in the body. Antiandrogens may be used in the treatment of PROSTATE CANCER. They inhibit the action of TESTOSTERONE on prostate cancer cells that are stimulated to grow by ANDROGENS. Antiandrogen drugs may also increase the effectiveness of other hormone therapies by blocking the small amount of testosterone made by the adrenal gland. Antiandrogens currently in use include flutamide (Eulexin) and Casodex (bicalutamide). Some steroids—megestrol (MEGACE), cyproterone, and MEDROXYPROGESTERONE (Depo-Provera)—function as antiandrogens.

antiangiogenesis agents [angiogenesis inhibitors] molecules that interfere with production of new blood vessels (ANGIOGENESIS) thus cutting off the nutrition and other signals needed by TUMORS or METASTASES to survive and grow. Years of research investigating angiogenesis has identified the major pathway involved in the process to be the VEGF family of proteins and receptors. Most of these agents remain investigational and offer much promise (2005). Antiangiogenesis agents constitute an intense area of pharmaceutical drug development interest. The seminal work in this area came from Dr. Judah Folkman, who identified two substances (endostatin and angiostatin) as key components of curative therapy, at least in animal models.

Some agents currently in clinical trials (2005) include:

SU 5416
SU 11248
PTK 787
marimastat
primomastat
neovastat
endostatin
angiostatin

See ANGIOSTATIN and ENDOSTATIN.

antibiotic (an″tĭ-bi-ot′ik) a substance used to treat infectious diseases. Antibiotics are a substance derived from a living organism such as mold, bacteria, or other types of microorganisms. When used in the treatment of cancer, antibiotics interfere with or inhibit cell division. Antibiotic drugs used in cancer treatment are far more TOXIC than the average antibiotic, such as penicillin, and are generally not used to treat infections because of their toxicity. Among the more common antibiotics used in the treatment of cancer are ADRIAMYCIN, BLEOMYCIN, PAUNOMYCIN, and MUTAMYCIN.

antibody (an′tĭ-bod″e) [immunoglobulin] a PROTEIN produced by the body's IMMUNE SYSTEM to fight infection or harmful foreign substances (ANTIGENS). Antibodies are secreted by B CELLS that are found in the BONE MARROW and the LYMPHATIC SYSTEM. Some are produced naturally and some are

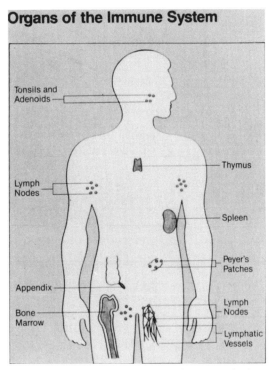

The body's immune system produces antibodies.
Courtesy National Cancer Institute (NCI).

produced in response to ANTIGENS, which stimulate the production of specific antibodies that attack them. Researchers estimate that the body produces more than 10 million antibodies. Each antibody can target a specific antigen.

Antibodies float freely in the body fluids. They destroy or disable their prey in a number of different ways. Antibodies can block viruses from entering healthy cells or they can set in motion a chain reaction, killing the foreign substance after which scavenger cells destroy them and cart them away. Antibodies cannot penetrate living cells, which makes them ineffective against microorganisms inside living cells.

See also MONOCLONAL ANTIBODIES.

antibody-dependent cell-mediated cytoxicity (ADCC) (an″tǐ-bod″e si″tok-sis′ǐ-te) a response by the IMMUNE SYSTEM to specific foreign cells. This requires both parts of the immune system working together. The antibody coats the "target" cell, which makes it vulnerable to attack by immune cells.

anticipatory nausea and vomiting (ANV) a conditioned response in which any cues associated with the CHEMOTHERAPY treatment (smell, the door of the doctor's office, etc.) set off the same physical response as the actual treatment. As many as 44% of patients receiving chemotherapy at some point experience ANV. Since this is not really caused by the chemotherapy itself, the use of an antiemetic to reduce the feeling of nausea is generally not effective.

The main treatment for ANV has been behavioral techniques employing either distraction and/or counter-conditioning. Guided imagery or relaxation may be used in distraction. Guided imagery, relaxation exercises, hypnosis, and desensitization may be used in counterconditioning (behavior modification). Another approach that has proved useful with some patients is informing them in advance about what to expect from chemotherapy—what it will feel like, how they may be affected. These techniques appear to be most effective when used early in treatment before ANV has become firmly established.

antidepressant drug medication to relieve feelings of depression, despair, and hopelessness. Antidepressants can also help a cancer patient whose fear and anxiety is keeping him or her from getting needed sleep.

antiemetic (an″tǐ-e-met′ik) a medication to prevent or reduce nausea and vomiting, a fairly common side effect of CHEMOTHERAPY (anticancer drugs) and RADIATION THERAPY. Whenever possible, doctors use antiemetics to *prevent* nausea from occurring rather than treating it once it has occurred.

A wide variety of antiemetics are available. Many act by suppressing the CHEMORECEPTOR TRIGGER ZONE (CTZ) in the brain. They are usually given six to 12 hours before the chemotherapy. They may be given repeatedly as long as the nausea and/or vomiting persists.

Some widely used antiemetics are Aprepitant, Compazine, DECADRON, Toracen, Tigan, Thorazine, Reglan (metoclopramide), ATIVAN, Valium, Marinol, dronabinol, Kytrel, Anzemet, and ZOFRAN. If one is not helpful to the patient, another might work very well. A combination of antiemetics may be given in the form of an "antiemetic cocktail."

Antiemetics can be given by IV (injected into a vein), taken by mouth, and in some cases as a rectal suppository.

Investigations in this area progressed rapidly in the 1980s because of the need to develop useful antiemetics to deal with the newer anticancer drugs, especially the platinum compounds like CISPLATIN.

antiestrogen   See TAMOXIFEN.

antigen (an′tǐ-jen) a foreign substance in the body such as protein, bacteria, virus, pollen, and other material. Antigens stimulate the body to produce ANTIBODIES, which then fight them. Tissues or cells from another person's body, such as in a transplant, can act as antigens in the recipient's body. This can play a role in the rejection of the transplanted organ or marrow.

antimetabolite (an″tǐ-mě-tab′o-lǐt) one kind of CHEMOTHERAPY (anticancer drug) that works by interrupting cellular reproduction. Because the antimetabolite drug resembles a nutrient, the cancer cell is deceived into ingesting it. Antimetabolites interrupt the reproduction of the cancer cell at one short, specific time in its reproduction cycle.

Therefore, the longer the period of time over which an antimetabolite is given, the greater the number of cells the drug will be able to destroy. In some cases, antimetabolites may be administered over hours, days, or even weeks. Over time, cancer cells can become resistant to a particular antimetabolite. Examples of some antimetabolites are ARA-C, 5 FU, and METHOTREXATE.

antineoplastic   An agent used to inhibit or prevent the growth of tumors, that is, to prevent the maturation and proliferation of cancer cells.

antineoplastons   See BURZYNCKI, STANISLAW.

antioxidant (an″tĭ-ok′sĭ-dent)   a substance added to products to prevent or delay their deterioration by exposure to air. There are more than two dozen antioxidants approved for use in foods, including vitamin C (ascorbate) and vitamin E (tocopherol). One group of antioxidants that has generated a lot of controversy and some regulation is the sulfites, which can cause adverse reactions in people. The Food and Drug Administration requires airlines and other interstate carriers to inform their customers if they are using sulfites.

Two other antioxidants in wide use are BHA and BHT. Animals fed large amounts of BHT developed *less cancer* when exposed to carcinogens and lived longer than animals not given BHT.

antipyretic (an″tĭ-pi-ret′ik)   an agent that relieves or reduces fever.

antiretroviral therapy   treatment with drugs that inhibit the ability of the human immunodeficiency virus (HIV) or other types of retroviruses to multiply in the body.

antisense therapy   a form of treatment for genetic disorders or infections. Antisense therapy is being researched as a potential treatment for lung and other cancers.

See AUGMEROSEN.

antiserotonin   See SEROTONIN ANTAGONISTS.

antithymocyte globulin (an″tĭ-thi′mo-sīt glob′u-lin)   a protein preparation used to prevent and treat GRAFT VERSUS HOST DISEASE.

antiviral (an″tĭ-vi′ral)   an agent that destroys viruses or suppresses their replication. There are many antivirals being used in the treatment of AIDS.

anus   the opening at the end of the large intestine through which body waste passes.

ANV   See ANTICIPATORY NAUSEA AND VOMITING.

Anzemet [dolasetron]   an antiemetic drug used to prevent or reduce nausea and vomiting. It can be given orally or by IV (injected into a vein).

AP   a combination of the anticancer drugs ADRIAMYCIN and CISPLATIN sometimes used in the treatment of OVARIAN CANCER. See individual drug listings for side effects. See also COMBINATION CHEMOTHERAPY.

APC 8015 [a vaccine]   a fusion protein of PAP/GMCSF being investigated in 2005 as a form of immunotherapy for treating prostate cancer.

apheresis   the procedure whereby STEM CELLS are extracted from the blood that has been removed by use of a cell separator in stem cell harvesting for a peripheral blood stem cell transplantation.

APL (acute promyelocytic leukemia)   See ANLL. This is a distinct form of ANLL (acute nonlymphocytic leukemia) with a specific cytogenetic (pertaining to chromosomes) feature and clinical course. The clinical use of ATRA (all trans-retinoic acid) plus chemotherapy can lead to a high complete remission rate (85%), mostly maintained. Arsenic trioxide is used for relapse. One characteristic clinical feature of APL is DIC (disseminated intravascular coagulopathy), which can cause serious, often fatal, bleeding.

aplasia (ah-pla′zhe-ah)   the lack of development of an organ or tissue or of the products of an organ or tissue. This can occur in virtually any part of the body.

aplastic (ah-plas′tik)   a condition in which a body organ or tissue, or its cells, is not fully developed.

aplastic anemia (ah-plas′tik ah-ne′me-ah)   a rare condition in which the BONE MARROW does not produce enough blood cells. When not enough RED BLOOD CELLS are being produced, the person may experience the common symptoms of ANEMIA; when not enough WHITE BLOOD CELLS are being produced, the person is more susceptible to infections; and when there are not enough PLATELETS, there is a greater chance of spontaneous bruising and bleeding.

Aplastic anemia is a serious condition often occurring spontaneously without known cause, or following exposure to a drug. The most successful therapies developed to treat it are BONE MARROW TRANSPLANTATION of another person's marrow, or IMMUNE THERAPY.

apoptosis   a term used in cell biology related to programmed cell death. See BCL-2 and P53 GENE.

appendix   a narrow projection from the large intestine, considered a remnant from an earlier developmental stage. It has no known function in the body.

appetite loss   See ANOREXIA.

APR   See ABDOMINOPERINEAL RESECTION.

aprepitant   the generic name for Emend, an ANTIEMETIC, that is always used in combination with other ANTIEMETIC agents.

arabinosyl cytosine   See ARA-C.

ara-C (air'ah-se) [cytarabine, cytosine arabinoside, Cytosar-U, arabinosyl cytosine] an ANTIMETABOLITE anticancer drug sometimes used in the treatment of acute LEUKEMIA and LYMPHOMAS. It is given by IV (injection into a vein).

Common side effects may include nausea, vomiting, diarrhea, and anemia. Occasional or rare side effects may include bone marrow depression, liver damage, ulcers, dizziness, headache, and lung problems.

Side effects requiring medical attention, as soon as possible, include fever, chills, sore throat, unusual bleeding or bruising, side or stomach pain, joint pain, numbness or tingling in the fingers, toes, or face, sores in the mouth and on the lips, swelling of the feet and lower legs, tiredness, black tarry stools, bone or muscle pain, chest pain,

cough, difficulty in swallowing, fainting spells, general feeling of body discomfort or weakness, heartburn, irregular heartbeat, pain at place of injection, reddened eyes, shortness of breath, skin rash, unusual decrease in urination, weakness, and yellowing of eyes and skin. Patients receiving ara-C should drink a lot of fluids. Producing more urine can prevent bladder and kidney problems.

Ara-C is one of the more important CHEMOTHERAPY drugs used in the treatment of cancer.

Aredia [pamidronate disodium]   a drug used in the treatment of HYPERCALCEMIA. Its use was approved by the Food and Drug Administration (FDA) in 1991. It is administered INTRAVENOUSLY (into a vein), one dose over 24 hours. In 1995 it was approved by the FDA for the treatment of bone METASTASES in patients with MULTIPLE MYELOMA and in 1996 for BREAST CANCER patients with METASTASIS to the bone who are receiving CHEMOTHERAPY and/or HORMONE THERAPY.

areola (ah-re'o-lah)   the circular area of dark-colored skin surrounding the nipple on the breast.

Argylin [anagrelide]   a PLATELET lowering agent used to treat patients with chronic MYELOPROLIFERATIVE disorders associated with elevated PLATELET counts. It is taken orally. See CHRONIC MYELOPROLIFERATIVE DISORDER.

Arimidex [anastrozole]   a drug used in postmenopausal women with BREAST CANCER whose disease has progressed despite treatment with TAMOXIFEN. It is taken orally.

aromatase inhibitor (AI)   a class of drugs used in the hormonal management of postmenopausal women with estrogen receptor positive (ER+) BREAST CANCER. They reduce the level of circulating estrogen in these patients. In METASTATIC disease, the results are equal to or superior to TAMOXIFEN. A special panel of ASCO (in 2005) recommended that optimum ADJUVANT THERAPY for postmenopausal women with ER+ breast cancer includes an AI as initial therapy, or after a period of treatment with tamoxifen to lower the recurrence rate. In 2005, Femara was (approved for post-tamoxifen therapy) The side effect profile includes osteoporosis and fracture, but lower incidence of UTERINE CANCER and thromboembolic disease (clots) than tamoxifen. (See also ARIMDEX, EXEMUSTANE, AND FEMARA, members of this class of drugs).

arsenic a chemical used in pesticides, herbicides, the manufacture of glass and ceramics, smelting of metal ores, and in food and drinking water. Arsenic is no longer being manufactured in the United States but it is still being imported. The National Institute for Occupational Safety and Health (NIOSH), estimates that some 1.5 million industrial workers are potentially exposed to arsenic. People may be exposed to small amounts through food, drinking water, air emissions from pesticide manufacturing sites, cotton gins, glass manufacturing operations, cigarette tobacco, burning of fossil fuels, and other sources. Exposure to arsenic may put people at a greater risk of developing LUNG CANCER, SKIN CANCER, LIVER CANCER, and other CANCERS.

See also CARCINOGENS.

arsenic trioxide [Trisenox] an IV chemotherapy and inducing agent that is FDA-approved for treatment of APL (acute promyelocytic leukemia). As a side effect, it can cause heart rhythm disturbances and an APL (acute promyelocytic leukemia) differentiation syndrome similar to the RETINOIC ACID syndrome.

arterial embolization (ar-te'rĭ-al) a procedure in which vessels that supply blood (nourishment) to a TUMOR are blocked by injecting a special substance into the renal area (kidneys) through a CATHETER. Arterial embolization may be used in patients with KIDNEY CANCER to shrink the tumor and make it more amenable to surgery before a RADICAL NEPHRECTOMY is done. Other uses for arterial embolization may be developed in the future for cancer and other disorders.

See also CHEMOEMBOLIZATION.

arteriography (ar″te-re-og′rah-fe) See ANGIOGRAPHY.

artificial sweeteners low- or no-calorie agents used as a sweetener in place of sugar and other nat-ural sweeteners high in calories. The three major artificial sweeteners are aspartame (Nutrasweet), which is a nutritive sweetener (has some food value), saccharin, a nonnutritive sweetener (has no food value), and Splenda, a no-calorie sweetener that is made from sugar and is designated as suitable for people with diabetes. Saccharin is the oldest alternative sweetener in the United States and is used in a large number of different products besides food, including cosmetic and toiletry products, tobacco, and drugs. Aspartame was approved for use in 1974. The approval was put on hold in order to conduct further research on its safety. In 1981 the marketing stay was lifted. Another artificial sweetener, cyclamate, has been banned in the United States because of an association with bladder tumors in animals. Artificial sweeteners are not considered to be CARCINOGENIC (cancer causing).

asbestos a group of naturally occurring mineral fibers found in rocks and used in a variety of products and building materials. Asbestos fibers are fire resistant and not easily destroyed or degraded by natural processes. Minuscule asbestos fibers cannot be seen or smelled, but they can be inhaled and absorbed by the skin. Exposure to asbestos has been linked to a number of diseases, including lung cancer, MESOTHELIOMA (cancer of the membrane lining the chest or lung), and other cancers and ASBESTOSIS (a noncancerous respiratory disease).

Asbestos first came into use in the early 1900s. By the early 1970s, the United States was using about 800,000 tons a year. However, in the 1970s, as people became more and more aware of its hazards, the government started restricting its use. In 1990, a six-year program began that would ban about 84% of the asbestos products made in the United States.

Asbestos has been used in many different products. It is estimated that more than 5,000 patents have been issued for products containing asbestos, including brake linings, clutch pads, floor tiles, paints, table pads, roofing materials, and insulation. Asbestos becomes a hazard when it is damaged and releases fibers into the air.

See also CARCINOGENS.

asbestosis (as″bĕ-sto′sis) a lung disease caused by inhaling fibers of ASBESTOS. Although exposure to asbestos can cause lung cancer, asbestosis is not cancer.

ascites (ah-si'tēz)   an accumulation of fluid in the abdomen that can cause swelling. It may occur in BENIGN (noncancerous) conditions such as liver cirrhosis and in people with different types of cancer. It is not unusual for fluid containing cancer cells to be found in the lining of the wall of the abdomen in a late stage of the cancer. When that occurs, it can be difficult to treat. Ascites can cause a number of symptoms, including a feeling of pressure, loss of appetite, and difficulty in breathing and walking.

Ascites can occur in a number of different ways. Cancer cells, or a TUMOR, can block the normal channels for draining fluids. In OVARIAN CANCER, the illness often spreads widely along tissue planes in the abdominal cavity, resulting in the secretion of fluid. In liver cancer, there can be a fluid buildup as a result and tissue blockage and a decrease in the production of the protein albumin. Ascites may also be caused by therapeutic radiation implants on the lining of the abdominal cavity, which can result in fluid buildup by mechanical irritation.

Methods used to manage ascites include the use of DIURETICS, a diet low in salt, surgical removal of fluid (PARACENTESIS), systemic chemotherapy, instillation of the chemotherapy into the cavity (INTRA-PERITONEAL CHEMOTHERAPY), and peritoneovenous shunting, which attempts to channel the fluid from the cavity back into the venous blood circulation by way of a surgically implanted catheter. It is unusual for any method to be 100% successful. Frequently a combination of methods will be used to achieve maximum control as well as patient comfort.

See also INTERNAL RADIATION and INTERSTITIAL RADIATION.

ASCO (American Society of Clinical Oncology) the professional organization founded in 1964 with the goal of improving cancer care and prevention. ASCO has seen tremendous growth, and now has a significant international role in the cancer community and is a multidisciplinary organization. It was instrumental in assisting the American Board of Internal Medicine in certifying medical oncology as a board specialty in 1979. Its large annual meeting in May regularly generates multiple news releases as it is widely followed by the media and may influence the standard of care. (See the ASCO Web site www.asco.org).

ASH (American Society of Hematology) the dominant professional organization of hematologists founded to focus on diseases of the blood, such as leukemia, and the various kinds of anemias and bleeding/clotting diseases. Its membership is international and multidisciplinary.

ASHAP a combination of the anticancer drugs ADRIAMYCIN, SOLUMEDROL, high-dose ARA-C, and platinum (CISPLATIN) sometimes used in the treatment of NON-HODGKIN'S LYMPHOMA. See individual drug listings for side effects.

See also COMBINATION CHEMOTHERAPY.

ASP   See L-ASPARAGINASE.

asparaginase   See L-ASPARAGINASE.

aspartame (ah-spar'tām)   See ARTIFICIAL SWEETENERS.

aspiration (as"pĭ-rā'shun)   removal of fluid or a small sample of tissue cells from a body cavity or tumor by suction, generally using a syringe. The cells may then be microscopically examined for cancer. Whenever possible, an aspiration is done to obtain cells for a biopsy. It is simpler, less expensive, less time consuming, and less dangerous than a larger surgical procedure using a scalpel.

See also NEEDLE ASPIRATION BIOPSY, BONE MARROW ASPIRATION, and ENDOMETRIAL ASPIRATION.

aspiration biopsy   See NEEDLE ASPIRATION BIOPSY.

aspiration bone marrow   See BONE MARROW ASPIRATION.

aspiration curettage   See ENDOMETRIAL ASPIRATION.

aspiration cytology   the microscopic examination of fluid or tissue obtained by ASPIRATION using a needle or syringe.

aspirin (as'pĭ-rin)   an over-the counter ANALGESIC drug widely used for pain relief or control. It appears to work by reducing inflammation and inhibiting the action of prostaglandins (a group of natural substances in the body that cause inflammation and pain).

Aspirin has been used for more than 100 years and is the "first line of defense" against pain. Although it is available without a doctor's prescription and can be purchased widely, it is a very effective pain medication for many people. It can be taken alone or in combination with other pain medication for extended periods of time.

Aspirin has minimal side effects. After a single dose, from one to three hours later there may be some temporary stomach discomfort. Occasional or rare side effects from regular long-term use may include ringing in the ears or hearing loss; unusual sweating; headache, dizziness, dimness of vision, confusion, fever, or drowsiness; rapid breathing; rapid heartbeat; thirst; diarrhea; and nausea and vomiting.

Aspirin is also known to cause bleeding. Anticancer drugs can cause BONE MARROW DEPRESSION, which can result in a lowered platelet count (platelets are the blood-clotting factor in the blood). For that reason, patients being treated with anticancer drugs are frequently told not to take aspirin and are advised to take ACETAMINOPHEN (e.g., Tylenol) instead.

assay a procedure where the concentration of a component part of a mixture is determined. There are numerous applications of an assay, such as an antigen capture assay, an immunoassay, a stem cell assay, and many others.

Astler Coller staging one way of STAGING the extent of COLON-RECTAL CANCER. Developed in 1974, it is not in wide use today.

astrocytoma (as″tro-si-to′mah) a brain tumor that can be benign (noncancerous) or malignant (cancerous). It arises in the supportive (glial) tissue of the brain. Astrocytomas account for 10% of all brain tumors. In adults, astrocytomas are relatively slow growing; in children, they can be slow or fast growing. Astrocytomas generally have a relatively low degree of malignancy. In children, astrocytomas can cause movement disorders. Adults can have vague symptoms that can go undiagnosed for years. Treatment for malignant astrocytomas is commonly surgical removal followed by radiation therapy.

See also BRAIN CANCER.

asynchronous disease (a-sin′kro-nus) a primary cancer that appears in two or more places at the same time in the same organ. This is *not* metastatic disease, in which cancer spreads from an original site to other parts of the body.

ataxia telangiectasia (ah-tak′se-ah tel-an″je-ek-ta′ze-ah) an inherited disease that damages the nerves. People who have it are at a higher risk for getting leukemia, Hodgkin's disease, medulloblastoma, and kidney and stomach cancer as well as other forms of cancer.

ATBC (alpha-tocopherol beta-carotene) study the final (1996) report addressed the rates of lung cancer in Finland. Lung cancer incidence was not affected by alpha tocopherol. BETA-CAROTENE supplements appeared to significantly increase the rates of lung cancer especially in those people who were the heaviest smokers and who drank the most alcohol.

Ativan [lorazepam] an antianxiety agent.

ATLL (adult T-cell leukemia-lymphoma) a rare form of LYMPHOMA that has been linked with a virus called HTLV-1. ATLL occurs infrequently in the United States. It is much more prevalent in Caribbean countries, parts of South America, and southern Japan, where in some areas more than 50% of adult lymphomas are linked to HTLV-1. It is believed that the HTLV-1 virus is transmitted sexually or by blood transfusions.

ATRA See ALL-TRANS RETINOIC ACID.

atrophy (at′ro-fe) shrinking or wasting away of a body part or tissue due to disease or lack of use. Although atrophy is not solely associated with cancer, muscle atrophy can occur in a cancer patient who is bedridden. Another possible cause of atrophy in the cancer patient is neurological damage caused by the tumor or surgery.

AUC a pharmacological expression of the area under the drug concentration-time curve, providing a measure of total drug exposure. It is used primarily in calculating the dose of CARBOPLATIN.

augmerosen [Genasense, Bcl-2 Antisense] an investigational agent being studied to treat MULTIPLE MYELOMA and MELANOMA, as well as for leukemia, lymphoma, and cancers of the lung, prostate, and colon.

autoantibody (aw"to-an'tĭ-bod"e) See AUTO-IMMUNE.

autoimmune (aw"to-im-ūn') [autoantibody] a condition in which a person's normal IMMUNE SYSTEM manufactures ANTIBODIES against components of his or her own body. Systemic lupus erythematosus (SLE) and rheumatoid arthritis, identified as autoimmune diseases, are thought to be conditions associated with this process. Researchers are trying to develop cancer treatments based on this principle, to induce the patient's own immune system to manufacture antibodies against his or her own cancer.

autologous blood transfusion (aw-tol'o-gus) the use of one's own blood for a transfusion. The blood is removed from a person, stored, and then transfused back to the person when needed.

autologous bone marrow transplant (ABMT) (aw-tol'o-gus) transplantation of a patient's own bone marrow that has been removed and stored. See BONE MARROW TRANSPLANTATION.

autologous transplant (aw-tol'o-gus) using the patient's own body tissue or blood in a transplant treatment. For example, skin from one part of the body may be grafted to another part of the body from which cancer has been removed. *Autologous transplant* can also refer to the use of a patient's bone marrow or stem cells as a support during high-dose chemotherapy or radiation for various cancers, such as breast or ovarian.

automatic computerized transverse axial (ACTA) See CT SCAN.

automatic computerized transverse axial scanner See CT SCAN.

Avastin [bavacizumab] An antiangiogenesis agent administered IV (via intravenous injection) approved for first-line therapy of metastatic colorectal cancer when used with 5-FU-based regiments. It was the first antiangiogenesis agent in its class to be approved by the FDA (which took place in 2004). It is also active in BREAST and LUNG CANCER. It is thought to bind and neutralize VEGF and thus acts as an ANTIANGLOGENESIS AGENT.

AVDP a combination of the anticancer drugs L-ASPARAGINASE, VINCRISTINE, doxorubicin (ADRIAMYCIN), and PREDNISONE sometimes used in the treatment of ALL. See individual drug listings for side effects.

See also COMBINATION CHEMOTHERAPY.

axillary dissection (ak'sĭ-lar"e) removal of the LYMPH NODES under the arm. The AXILLARY NODES are generally removed during a MODIFIED RADICAL MASTECTOMY or during breast conservation procedures such as a LUMPECTOMY. Axillary dissection may also be performed in the therapy and staging of MELANOMA arising in the skin of the arm or shoulder.

See also SENTINEL LYMPH NODE BIOPSY.

axillary lymph nodes (ak'sĭ-lar"e) the LYMPH NODES located in the armpit. These are normal structures that respond to areas of local infection or injury in the arm, hand, and in the surrounding chest wall and breast. In melanoma of the skin of the arm, they may be the first place to which cancer cells metastasize (spread). Therefore, a complete axillary surgical dissection (removal of the lymph nodes) may be performed as part of the treatment.

In breast cancer, the staging is critically dependent on whether the axillary lymph nodes are involved. The standard curative operations in breast cancer include removal of these glands since further therapy and prognosis are very dependent on whether the glands are positive (cancerous) or negative (noncancerous). Axillary dissection is generally performed during a MASTECTOMY and also during breast conservation (LUMPECTOMY) procedures.

The normal number of axillary lymph nodes is between 30 and 40. The pathological report from a lymph node dissection will indicate the number and location of these nodes for future treatment planning.

See also SENTINEL LYMPH NODE BIOPSY.

Azacitidine (AZC) [Vidaza] the first chemo-therapy drug FDA-approved (2004) for treatment of MDS. It is given intravenously.

azathioprine   See CARCINOGENS.

azidothymidine   See AZT.

AZT (azidothymidine) [zidovudine, ZDV, Retrovir] an antiviral drug sometimes used in the treatment of acquired immune deficiency syndrome (AIDS). At present, it has been shown to prolong the life of patients with early stages of AIDS. It is made from thymidine, one of the normal components of DNA, the molecule needed by normal cells to reproduce. Common side effects may include nausea, mild headaches, and a lowered red blood count. The prescribed dose required for AZT's most beneficial effect has been reduced since it was first used. AZT remains an important drug in the treatment of AIDS.

B cell [B lymphocytes]   one of the two major types of lymphocytes, which are white blood cells. (The other major type is the T CELL.) B cells are part of the immune system and secrete ANTIBODIES into the body fluid to fight foreign substances that could cause infections, disease, or poisoning. Each B cell is programmed to make one specific antibody. For example, one B cell may produce antibodies to fight a particular bacterium and another may produce antibodies to fight a different bacterium.

B lymphocytes   See B CELL.

Bacillus Calmette-Guérin   See BCG.

BACON   a combination of the anticancer drugs BLEOMYCIN, ADRIAMYCIN, CCNU, Oncovin (VIN-CRISTINE), and NITROGEN MUSTARD (MUSTARGEN). See individual drug listings for side effects.
See also COMBINATION CHEMOTHERAPY.

BACOP   a combination of the anticancer drugs BLEOMYCIN, ADRIAMYCIN, Cytoxan, Oncovin (VIN-CRISTINE), and PREDNISONE sometimes used in the treatment of NON-HODGKIN'S DISEASE. See individual drug listings for side effects.
See also COMBINATION CHEMOTHERAPY.

bacteria   one-celled microscopic organisms that may cause disease. Many bacteria are harmless, and many are even beneficial. Cancer patients may be more susceptible to the effects of bacteria as a result of their treatment (which may compromise the immune system) or the cancer itself.

barium   a contrast medium used in a GI series.

barium enema (BE)   See LOWER GI SERIES.

barium milkshake   See UPPER GI SERIES.

barium swallow   See UPPER GI SERIES.

Barrett's esophagus (ĕ-sof'ah-gus)   Barrett's esophagus is the most severe complication of chronic gastroesophageal reflux disease (GERD) and is important because of its well-recognized association with ADENOCARCINOMA of the esophagus. The incidence of adenocarcinoma of the esophagus due to Barrett's esophagus and GERD is on the rise. Current strategies for improved survival in patients with esophageal adenocarcinoma focus on cancer detection at an early and potentially curable stage. For unknown reasons, Barrett's esophagus is found three times more often in males than in females. People with Barrett's usually have symptoms similar to those produced by chronic GERD, such as heartburn and reflux of stomach acid into the mouth. Some people may also suffer from other complications of GERD, such as esophageal peptic ulcers and stricture—narrowing of the esophagus—that comes from scarring. Diagnosis of Barrett's esophagus requires an examination called upper endoscopy or EGD (ESOPHAGOGASTRODUODENOSCOPY).

basal cell (bā'sal)   a small, round cell found in the lower part, or base, of the epidermis (surface layer of the skin).

basal cell carcinoma of the eye   See EYE CANCER.

basal cell carcinoma of the skin (bā'sal kar″sĭ-no'mah) [basal cell skin cancer]   the most common and least lethal form of skin or other cancers. In the United States, basal cell cancer accounts for 90% of all skin cancers in the southern states, and 479% in the northern states. It occurs most frequently in people over 45 years of age, and almost twice as often in men as in women. The incidence of basal cell skin cancer is far more prevalent among whites in the United States. It occurs less often in Asians and rarely among blacks. The risk of getting skin cancer is related to the amount of exposure to the sun and the amount of pigmentation in the skin. The longer the exposure to the sun and the lighter the skin, the greater the risk of developing skin cancer.

The main cause of basal cell carcinoma of the skin is ULTRAVIOLET RADIATION from the Sun. The earth's ozone layer offers protection from UV radiation by blocking it. However, depletion of the ozone layer since the late 1970s has increased the risk of damage to the skin that can result in cancer. Ongoing clinical trials are trying to determine if this skin cancer can be prevented.

Basal cell carcinoma (basal cells form the lowest level of skin) usually develops on areas of the skin exposed to sunlight, including the face, head, neck, arms, hands, and back. It can look many different ways. It commonly appears as a small, nodular bump that is raised from the surrounding skin and has a pearly quality. It can also appear as a scar-like, firm patch on the skin. Basal cell skin cancer is very slow growing and seldom fatal.

Diagnosis requires the removal of some tissue for a biopsy, a microscopic examination for cancer cells. Frequently, if it is a small cancer, the biopsy also removes the cancer. However, if the area is sizable, more tissue may have to be removed until there are "clean margins." Treatment depends on the size of the tumor, the type of tumor, and the general health of the patient. Treatment is generally surgery to remove the cancer. There are several ways the surgery may be performed:

- electrodesiccation and curettage—the cancer is burned and removed with a sharp instrument
- cryosurgery—the cancer is killed by freezing it
- excision—the cancer is cut from the skin along with some healthy tissue around it
- micrographic surgery—the cancer is cut from the skin along with some healthy tissue around it, after which the doctor uses a microscope to examine the area for any remaining cancer cells
- laser surgery—a narrow beam of light is used to remove the cancer.

Other treatments for basal cell skin cancer include radiation therapy, the application of topical chemotherapy to the cancer site, and MOHS' MICROGRAPHIC SURGERY. BIOLOGICAL THERAPY is being investigated. The aim of the treatment is the removal of the cancer with the least disfigurement. Depending on where on the body the cancer is and its size, the doctor may recommend that the cancer be removed by a plastic surgeon. For the latest state-of-the-art treatment for basal cell skin cancer, call the National Cancer Institute's (NCI) Cancer Information Service 1-800-4-CANCER (1-800-422-6237), or for a TTY: 1-800-332-8615.

See also SKIN CANCER and EYE CANCER.

basal cell skin cancer   See BASAL CELL CARCINOMA OF THE SKIN.

basaloid carinoma   See CLOACOGENIC CANCER.

baseline mammogram   See MAMMOGRAPHY.

basophil (ba'so-fil)   a white blood cell that makes up less than 1% of the WHITE BLOOD CELLS in the body. It plays a special role in allergic reactions.

BAY43-9006 [Sorafenib]   a new agent with antiangiogenesis properties in clinical trials against a variety of cancers.

B-cell acute lymphocytic leukemia (lim″fo-sit'ik) [B-cell ALL] [Burkitt cell acute lymphocytic leukemia]   the rarest form of acute lymphocytic leukemia (ALL), accounting for 5% of the cases of the disease. It affects immature stem cells that have started to mature along the B-cell line of development. It occurs in older children and older adults, and more frequently in males.

See also LEUKEMIA.

B-cell stimulatory factor-1   See INTERLEUKIN-4.

B-cell stimulatory factor-2   See INTERLEUKIN-6.

Bcl-2 (B-cell lymphoma/leukemia-associated gene 2)   This gene produces a protein that regulators APOPTOSIS (programmed cell death). The gene is overexpressed in many tumors and this is thought to maintain the viability of cancer cells (Bcl-2 is anti-apoptotic), and is related to drug resistance.

BCG (bacillus Calmette-Guérin) (bah-sil'lus kal'met ga-ran') [TheraCys]   a vaccine originally developed in 1906 in France to immunize people against tuberculosis. BCG was originally investigated for its use in the treatment of cancer in the late 1950s and early 1960s. Those investigations led to the discovery of the TUMOR NECROSIS FACTOR (TNF). When mice were injected with large doses of BCG, they produced TNFs, which act against the tumor. In 1990 BCG was approved by the Food and Drug Administration as a treatment for bladder cancer. It appears to be highly effective against early stage bladder cancer, especially carcinoma-in-situ. BCG is administered directly into the bladder through a catheter, where it remains for two hours, causing an inflammation that destroys many of the cancer cells. This procedure is repeated over a period of time. Common side effects may be flu-like symptoms and bladder discomfort as a result of the inflammation.

BCNU   [Carmustine, BiCNU, Gliadel Wafer] an alkylating anticancer drug sometimes used in the treatment of cancers of the brain and lung, HODGKIN'S DISEASE and other lymphomas, and multiple myeloma. It is given by IV (injection into a vein). Common side effects may include nausea, vomiting, and swelling and burning of the vein. Occasional and rare side effects may include lowered blood count, lung problems, facial flushing, liver problems, dizziness, and eye problems.

This drug can also be administered in the form of a quarter-sized wafer called a Gliadel Wafer, which contains BCNU. The wafer is implanted in the surgical cavity of patients with recurrent glioblastoma multiforme (brain). The wafer is a delivery vehicle for the anticancer drug.

BCP   combination of the anticancer drugs BCNU, CYTOXAN, and PREDNISONE sometimes used in the treatment of MYELOMA. See individual drug listings for side effects.

See also COMBINATION CHEMOTHERAPY.

BCPT   See BREAST CANCER PREVENTION TRIAL.

B-DOPA   a combination of the anticancer drugs BLEOMYCIN, DTIC, Oncovin (VINCRISTINE), PREDNISONE, and ADRIAMYCIN sometimes used in the treatment of Hodgkin's disease. See individual drug listings for side effects.

See also COMBINATION CHEMOTHERAPY.

BE (barium enema)   See LOWER GI SERIES.

Bence-Jones protein   a protein found in the urine of most patients with MYELOMA. It is occasionally found in the urine of patients with other cancers. This represents part of the immunoglobulin protein (antibodies) being abnormally manufactured due to the underlying illness.

bendamustine   an investigational treatment, given intravenously, that is related to nitrogen mustard, an alkylating agent, being studied in hematological malignancies.

benign prostatic hyperplasia (BPH) (be-nīn' prostat'ik hi"per-pla'ze-ah) [prostatic hypertrophy]   a noncancerous enlargement of the prostate that is common in older men. It is estimated that more than half of the men in the United States over the age of 40 have an enlarged prostate gland. It has been suggested that this may be a precursor of prostate cancer. Studies to date have produced conflicting results.

benign tumor (be-nīn′) an abnormal, non-cancerous growth of tissue that does not spread to other parts of the body, as a cancerous tumor can do. Though generally not life threatening (except for a brain tumor), benign tumors can cause a whole range of problems and side effects, some quite serious. As benign tumors grow larger, they can affect body functions and cause pain by exerting pressure on various organs and nerves and blocking access routes in the body. Some benign tumors may become cancerous.

benign uterine tumor   See FIBROID TUMOR.

benzene   See CARCINOGENS.

benzidine   See CARCINOGENS.

beta-carotene (ba′tah kar′o-tēn)   a dietary source of vitamin A. Beta-carotene is derived from leafy green or yellow vegetables and converted to, or absorbed as, vitamin A in the digestive tract.
   Results published in the July 23, 2003 *Journal of the American Medical Association* reported that ATBC (Alpha-Tocopherol, Beta Carotene Cancer Prevention Trial) researchers found that men who took beta-carotene had an 18 percent increase in the incidence of lung cancers and an 8 percent increased overal mortality.
   See also VITAMINS.

betamethasone   See ADRENOCORTICOIDS.

bevacizumab   See AVASTIN.

Bexxar [tositumomab]   the therapeutic regimen combining Tositumomab (a monoclonal antibody), and the same agent tagged with a radioactive material. This was FDA-approved (2003) for the treatment of advanced, refractory follicular B-cell NHL (NON-HODGKINS LYMPHOMA). This antineoplastic RADIOPHARMACEUTICAL is administered IV in two discrete steps. The dosimetry (see RADIATION THERAPY) phase is followed by the therapeutic step. It is administered by one trained in nuclear medicine and may involve a brief hospital stay to ensure safety. Since I^{31} also targets normal thyroid tissue, medication is given days before to block this unwanted effect. Successful use of Bexxar as initial

therapy of advanced follicular NHL has also been reported. The goal of Bexxar is to have the radioactive MONOCLONAL ANTIBODY deliver high does of radiation to the target (the CD20 receptor on malignant B CELLS that make up the lymphoma). The methodology described (above) requires several days to deliver the optimum amount of radiation to the desired place. Side effects are generally mild and related to BONE MARROW suppression.

BHD   a combination of the anticancer drugs BCNU, HYDREA, and DTIC sometimes used in the treatment of MELANOMA. See individual drug listings for side effects.
   See also COMBINATION CHEMOTHERAPY.

bicalutamide   See CASODEX.

BiCNU   See BCNU.

bilateral mastectomy (mas-tek′to-me)   surgical removal of both breasts. This may be performed in the unusual occurrence of cancer arising simultaneously in both breasts. It may also be done as a "preventive" measure. A woman at a greater-than-average risk of developing breast cancer may opt to have both breasts removed when cancer is discovered in one breast. Some symptom-free women, at a high risk of developing breast cancer, decide to have their breasts removed purely as a preventive measure.
   See also PREVENTIVE MASTECTOMY.

bilateral nephrectomy   surgical removal of both kidneys. This is only done if a PARTIAL NEPHRECTOMY cannot be performed. A bilateral nephrectomy requires a kidney transplant or dialysis (removal of body wastes previously removed by the kidneys).

bilateral orchiectomy (or″ke-ek′to-me)   removal of both testicles (the male reproductive glands).
   See also ORCHIECTOMY.

bilateral pedal lymphangiography (lim-fan″je-og′rah-fe)   a procedure that detects enlarged LYMPH NODES in the area of the body known as the retroperitoneum in the abdominal cavity. It may be used in the diagnosis of HODGKIN'S DISEASE. An

iodized substance is injected into the lymphatic passages of the legs. It is then followed by X-RAY as it
moves through the passages and into the abdomen.
Its use in STAGING Hodgkin's disease has been
replaced by CT SCAN.

bilateral   salpingo-oophorectomy   (BSO)   (sal-
ping′go o″of-o-rek′to-me)   surgical removal of the
uterus, both ovaries, and fallopian tubes, sometimes performed in the treatment of ENDOMETRIAL
CANCER.

bile duct cancer [extrahepatic bile duct cancer]
a relatively rare form of cancer in the tube system
that drains bile from the liver to the intestine.
There are two kinds: distal and proximal.

The most common symptom of bile duct cancer
(as well as other, noncancerous conditions) may be
jaundice, a yellowing of the skin sometimes noticed
first in the white parts of the eyes. Other symptoms
may include itchy skin, urine that is a dark red or
wine color, pain in the abdomen, fever, and stool
that is light and clay colored.

Procedures that may be used in the diagnosis
and evaluation of bile duct cancer include X-rays,
ultrasound, MRI, an ERCP (endoscopic retrograde
cholangiopancreatography), percutaneous transhepatic cholangiography, and CT scans. Definitive
diagnosis may require abdominal surgery.

The NATIONAL CANCER INSTITUTE (NCI) stages
bile duct cancer as "localized" or "unresectable"
People with the localized stage have cancer that can
be completely resected (removed by surgery). They
represent a minority of cases of bile duct cancer
overall, with most resectable lesions arising in the
distal duct. People with the unresectable stage have
cancer that cannot be completely removed by
surgery. They represent the majority of cases of bile
duct cancer. Often the cancer invades directly into
the adjacent liver or along the common bile duct
and to adjacent lymph nodes. Spread to distant
parts of the body is not common; intra-abdominal
spread does occur.

Treatment depends on the stage of the disease
and other factors. Treatments used for bile duct
cancer include surgery and radiation. For specific
information on the latest state-of-the-art treatment,
by stage, for bile duct cancer, call NCI's Cancer
Information Service at 1-800-4-CANCER (1-800-
422-6237), or for a TTY: 1-800-332-8615.

bilobectomy (bi″lo-bek′to-me)   removal of more
than one lobe of a lung. The lung has five major
lobes.

biofeedback   a method of learning to control the
body's automatic functions such as heartbeat, blood
pressure, muscle tension, etc. Electrical machinery,
wired to the body, gives visual or auditory signals
that serve as "feedback." (A person can learn to
control a bodily function by controlling the signal.)
For some people this can be an effective way of
controlling pain.

biological response modifiers (BRM)   any agent
that boosts the body's IMMUNE SYSTEM by stimulating it, modifying it, or restoring it. There are many
types of BRMs, some produced naturally in the
body, others made in labs.

The 1980s saw an increasing interest in BRMs
and an increasing optimism that they may soon
become a main treatment of cancer. There are many
ongoing clinical trials exploring the use and effectiveness of BRMs in BIOLOGICAL THERAPY to treat
many different cancers.

The major biological response modifiers are ANTI-
BODIES, MONOCLONAL ANTIBODIES, VACCINES, COLONY-
STIMULATING FACTORS (CSF), and CYTOKINES, which
include the INTERFERONS and INTERLEUKINS.

biological response modifiers program (BRMP)
[biomodulation]   a program established in 1981
by the NATIONAL CANCER INSTITUTE (NCI) to identify and promote the study of new BIOLOGICAL
RESPONSE MODIFIERS to fight cancer. It also coordi-
nates laboratory and clinical studies of these substances. NCI has developed the following three-
step program to evaluate the potential usefulness of
BRMs in the treatment of cancer:

• the agent is tested in a lab on various immune
  cells and cancer cells
• agents that had an effect during one or more of
  the tests are then used on animals with cancer
  that occurred spontaneously or was implanted
  by the researchers

- the researchers may induce cancers in animals by exposure to ultraviolet light or a known carcinogen and then test the substance on that animal.

If the agent proves effective through the three steps, it may undergo the NCI's standard evaluation procedure. It is first tested on mice for toxicity. If the side effects are tolerable, the NCI may use it in CLINICAL TRIALS with patients.

biological therapy [immunotherapy]   the newest anticancer treatment, still primarily investigational, which uses BIOLOGICAL RESPONSE MODIFIERS (BRMs), the body's own immune system, to fight cancer. Substances, some occurring naturally in the body and others made in a lab, are used to boost, direct, or restore normal defenses of the body in the following ways:

- enhancing the immune system so that it can fight cancer more effectively; eliminating, regulating, or suppressing body responses that permit cancer growth
- making a cancer cell more sensitive to destruction by the immune system
- stimulating a cancer cell to become a less harmful or a normal cell
- blocking the process that makes a normal or precancerous cell become a cancer cell
- enhancing the body's ability to repair normal cells damaged by other forms of cancer treatment.

For more than 100 years researchers have been trying to find ways to stimulate the body's own immune system to fight cancer successfully. Although there is still a long way to go, tremendous progress has been made since the early 1970s. In 1976, the T-cell growth factor, INTERLEUKIN-2 was discovered. The first trials of a biological response modifier in humans were in 1978. The agent tested was ALPHA INTERFERON, which was first isolated in 1956. In 1979 the National Cancer Institute committed $9 million for human interferon studies. The American Cancer Society invested another $2 million. Another major step was made in 1981, when RECOMBINANT DNA TECHNOLOGY made it possible to "mass-produce" alpha interferon at a reasonable cost. In the 1980s, many other biological anticancer agents became available for testing in humans because of recombinant DNA technology. There was

also rapid growth of another biological therapy agent in the 1980s, MONOCLONAL ANTIBODIES.

Researchers continue to study the best way to use BRMs. It is believed that many may be most effective when used along with other treatment—surgery, chemotherapy (anticancer drugs), and radiation. BRMs appear to have the potential of treating cancer with fewer side effects and less damage to the normal cells.

biologically guided chemotherapy   an UNCONVENTIONAL TREATMENT METHOD developed by Emanuel Revici, M.D., a Romanian immigrant who practiced medicine in New York. He claimed this treatment could be used for cancer as well as a wide range of other disorders including AIDS, arthritis, chronic pain, and schizophrenia. Revici wrote that his treatment "when correctly applied . . . can, in many cases, bring under control even-far-advanced malignancies." In 1965, nine physicians evaluated Revici's method of treating cancer. Their finding that the method is without value in the treatment of cancer was published in the *Journal of the American Medical Association*. In 1988, the New York State Board for Professional Medical Conduct recommended that Revici be placed on probation for a period of five years. There has not been a controlled CLINICAL TRIAL to evaluate the safety and efficacy of biologically guided chemotherapy. Revici died in 1998.

biomodulation   See BIOLOGICAL RESPONSE MODIFIERS.

biopsy (bi′ŏp-se)   the microscopic examination of tissue or cells removed from the body to determine if cancer cells are present. The pathologist (a doctor who specializes in the study of body tissues) examines the tissue or fluid under a microscope to see if there are any cancer cells, and if there are, the type. The material used for the biopsy may also be processed for special studies, or stained to get more information on the prognosis and guide treatment. In most cases a biopsy is the only way to reach a *definitive* diagnosis of cancer. In some instances, the biopsy removes the cancer itself—for example, an excisional biopsy in breast cancer. For other patients, total removal of the lump, which is also (and more commonly) called a LUMPECTOMY, may end up being the primary treatment.

There are many different ways of performing biopsies. The choice of which procedure is used depends on a number of different factors, including the area of the body where it is to be performed, the actual location of the tumor, and the health of the patient.

Among the more common biopsies are the NEEDLE ASPIRATION BIOPSY (also called an aspiration biopsy, fine needle biopsy, suction biopsy, and fine needle aspiration); CORE NEEDLE BIOPSY (needle biopsy, widecore biopsy); SHAVE BIOPSY; EXCISIONAL BIOPSY (punch biopsy, surgical biopsy); INCISIONAL BIOPSY; BONE MARROW BIOPSY; and SPINAL TAP. Other procedures done in the diagnosis of cancer, such as an ENDOSCOPY, can, at the same time, obtain tissue or fluid for a biopsy.

Many biopsies can be done in a doctor's office or on an outpatient basis at a hospital. Most require some kind of anesthesia. Preliminary results can be obtained, practically on the spot, by doing a FROZEN SECTION BIOPSY. A PERMANENT SECTION BIOPSY, which can take several days for results, is usually done after the frozen section to verify the results. A permanent section is more accurate than a frozen section and can be given to other pathologists for a second opinion and review.

biotechnology the use of living organisms or their products to make or modify a substance. It includes genetic engineering and HYBRIDOMA TECHNOLOGY. This area of research, investigation, and production expanded greatly during the 1980s and continues to do so.

Birt Hogg Dubé (BHD) an inherited familial syndrome in which affected individuals develop unusual, small BENIGN SKIN TUMORS and are at an increased risk for renal tumors both benign and malignant. The gene has been located on chromosome 17 and is thorught to act as a tumor suppressor gene. Thus mutations are associated with the tumor.

bis [chloromethyl ether] See CARCINOGENS.

bisphosphonate a class of drugs used to strengthen bone.

bladder cancer the presence of malignant (cancerous) cells in the bladder. Bladder cancer is the cancer most frequently found cancer of the urinary tract. In 1999 about 54,200 people were diagnosed

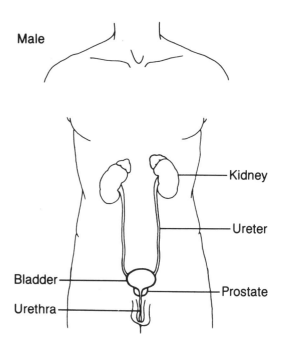

The female and male urinary systems. Courtesy NCI.

with bladder cancer in the United States, and about 12,100 died from the disease. Bladder cancer occurs most frequently in white adults between the ages of 50 and 70, with men developing it about three times more often than women.

The most common type of bladder cancer is TRANSITIONAL CELL CARCINOMA (90%), which arises from the transitional epithelial cells that line the bladder. The other types of bladder cancer include papillary, SQUAMOUS CELL CARCINOMA, and ADENOCARCINOMA.

Scientists believe that bladder cancer develops over many years as a gradual change in bladder cells. The precise cause of bladder cancer is still not known. However, several risk factors have been identified. It is estimated that smoking is a contributing factor in as many as half the bladder cancers in men and a third of the bladder cancers in women. Smokers have a two to three times greater risk of developing bladder cancer. Exposure of workers in the dye industries is thought to be a contributing factor in bladder cancer. Other occupations that have been linked to an increased risk of bladder cancers include those in the rubber, leather, textile, and chemical industries, as well as hairdressers, machinists, metalworkers, painters, printers, and truck drivers. A bladder infection caused by the parasitic flatworm *Schistosoma haematobium* increases the risk of squamous cell bladder cancer. Other urinary infections may also increase the risk.

Some medical treatments may present a risk as well. The Food and Drug Administration has banned the use of PHENACETIN, which has been associated with bladder cancer, in painkillers. Studies have shown an increased risk of bladder cancer as a result of treatment with the anticancer drug CYCLOPHOSPHAMIDE (Cytoxan). Some studies have shown an association between radiation therapy to the pelvis and bladder cancer.

The most common symptom of bladder cancer is blood in the urine, usually associated with increased frequency of urination. Other symptoms may include painful urination or a feeling of urgency to urinate. On rare occasion there may be retention of urine or incontinence. (However, all of these may be symptomatic of other conditions.)

Among the procedures that may be used in the diagnosis and evaluation of bladder cancer are a rectal or vaginal physical examination, urinalysis, a CT SCAN, FLOW CYTOMETRY, CYSTOSCOPY, an intravenous pyelogram (IVP), and a cystoscopic surgical BIOPSY.

Following is the National Cancer Institute's (NCI) staging for bladder cancer:

- Stage 0 or CARCINOMA IN SITU—cancer found only on the inner lining of the bladder; after the cancer is removed, no swelling or lumps are felt during an internal examination
- Stage I—cancer cells have spread a little deeper into the inner lining of the bladder but have not spread to the muscular wall of the bladder
- Stage II—cancer cells have spread to the inside lining of the muscles lining the bladder
- Stage III—cancer cells have spread throughout the muscular wall of the bladder and/or to the layer of tissue surrounding the bladder and/or to the nearby reproductive organs; there may be a swelling or lumps after surgery for removal of the cancer
- Stage IV—cancer cells have spread to the nearby reproductive organs or to the lymph nodes in the area and/or other places far from the bladder
- Recurrent—the cancer has returned to the same site or to another part of the body after being treated.

Another way of staging bladder cancer is the JEWETT & STRONG method, which characterizes the cancer as superficial, deep, or METASTATIC CANCER.

Treatment of bladder cancer depends on the stage of the disease, the general state of health of the patient, and other factors. Surgery is a common treatment—including the following procedures: TRANSURETHRAL RESECTION, SEGMENTAL CYSTECTOMY, CYSTECTOMY, RADICAL CYSTECTOMY, and URINARY DIVERSION. RADIATION THERAPY, CHEMOTHERAPY (anticancer drugs), and BIOLOGICAL THERAPY may also be used. Reconstructive techniques may eliminate the need for external drainage devices. For specific information on the latest state-of-the-art treatment, by stage, call NCI's Cancer Information Service at 1-800-4-CANCER (1-800-422-6237), or for a TTY: 1-800-332-8615.

bladder-sparing in bladder cancer, a strategy using combined CHEMORADIOTHERAPY (chemotherapy plus radiotherapy given at the same time, also called "chemorads") in treating disease that has invaded the muscle wall; the intent of bladder sparing is to make surgical removal of the bladder unnecessary.

blast cells [leukemia cells]   abnormal cells found in the blood that are undifferentiated (immature). They normally reside in the bone marrow as a precursor cell. See LEUKEMIA.

blast crisis   the transformation of chronic myelogenous leukemia to acute myelogenous leukemia. Blast crisis is the development of a more accelerated phase of chronic myelogenous leukemia, signaling a change to the acute, fatal form of the disease. BONE MARROW TRANSPLANTATION is widely used during the chronic phase of the illness in order to prevent the natural progression to an acute phase.

See also LEUKEMIA.

Blenoxane (blen-oks′ān)   See BLEOMYCIN.

BLEO   See BLEOMYCIN.

bleomycin (ble-o-mi′sin) [Blenoxane, BLEO]   an ANTINEOPLASTIC, anticancer drug sometimes used in the treatment of cancers of the head, neck, penis, vulva, cervix, skin, testes, kidney, lung, and esophagus and lymphomas, SOFT TISSUE SARCOMAS, KAPOSI'S SARCOMA, and MELANOMA. It is given by IV (injection into a vein), IM (injection into a muscle), subcutaneously (under the skin), or by regional arterial infusion (injection into an artery). Bleomycin was approved in 1996 as a sclerosing agent to control malignant (cancerous) pleural effusions (fluid in the lining of the lungs) by direct instillation into the pleural cavity to decrease production of the fluid.

Common side effects may include nausea, vomiting, fever, and chills. Side effects that should be brought to the attention of the doctor may include a cough, shortness of breath, and sores in the mouth and on the lips. Side effects needing *immediate medical attention* may include fever and chills (occurring within three to six hours after administration of the drug), faintness, confusion, sweating, and wheezing. Occasional and rare side effects may include skin rash, darkening, discoloration, peeling, or tenderness of skin, chronic lung problems, hair loss, headache, swelling and pain in joints, unusual taste sensation, and loss of appetite. Another rare but possible dangerous side effect may be pulmonary toxicity.

Bleomycin plays an important role in the treatment of cancer. It is one of the more commonly used anticancer drugs.

blood-brain barrier   a thin membrane that can prevent harmful substances from getting into the central nervous system (the spinal fluid and brain). This "barrier" can also keep some chemotherapy (anticancer drugs) from getting through to a tumor in the brain. Research is being done to find ways to temporarily disrupt the barrier so that chemotherapy can penetrate it. Among the procedures being used and or investigated are the use of the drug mannitol (and others) to temporarily allow the medication to enter the tumor site, HYPERTHERMIA (raising the body's temperature), and administration of the chemotherapy into an artery or spinal fluid rather than into a vein. (The testicles in men have a similar barrier that blocks chemotherapy.)

blood cancer   See LEUKEMIA.

blood count   See COMPLETE BLOOD COUNT.

blood stool test   See OCCULT BLOOD STOOL TEST.

blood test   a diagnostic test; examination of a sample of blood taken from a vein, usually in the arm. The blood is generally sent to a laboratory for analysis, and these results can help in the diagnosis and management of a host of conditions. Blood tests of various types are commonly used in the diagnosis of many different types of cancer. Levels of various TUMOR MARKERS found in the blood can be an indication of the presence of cancer or the recurrence of cancer. Blood tests are also used to monitor a patient's progress once in treatment.

See also COMPLETE BLOOD TEST.

blood vessel cancer   See ANGIOSARCOMA.

blood vessel sarcoma   See SOFT-TISSUE SARCOMA.

BMS-354825   a novel, oral, multitargeted anticancer agent undergoing clinical trials ("BMS" stands for the compound's manufacturer, Bristol-Myers Squibb).

BMT   See BONE MARROW TRANSPLANTATION.

BNCT   See BORON NEUTRON CAPTURE THERAPY.

board certification   a status physicians attain by passing tests before peers in their field of specialization. When doctors finish their residency in their field, they become eligible for board certification. This involves taking rigorous written and oral exams before doctors who practice in that specialty. Some boards require that doctors recertify after a certain number of years. The specialty boards are private, voluntary, and nonprofit organizations founded to conduct exams, issue certificates of qualification, and improve and broaden opportunities for additional training. Doctors who have board certification are listed in the *Directory of Medical Specialists*. To find out if a doctor is board-certified call the American Board of Certified Specialities at 1-800-776-CERT or go to its Web site at www.certifieddoctor.org.

bone cancer   a sarcoma (malignant tumor) in the skeletal system. Primary bone cancer, cancer originating in the bone, is relatively rare. (It should not be confused with secondary tumors in the bone that have metastasized (spread) from other cancers in the body, most commonly the breast, lung, thyroid, prostate, or kidney.)

A great deal of progress has been made in the treatment of bone cancer. In 1972, only about 20% of the people diagnosed with osteosarcoma survived for more than five years, and amputation was the only effective treatment. Today, as many as 80% of those diagnosed with localized bone cancer survive for five years or longer.

In the United States in 1999 there were about 2,600 new cases of primary bone cancer and about 1,400 deaths related to the disease. The most common type is OSTEOSARCOMA (also called osteogenic sarcoma), which originates in newly forming tissue, most often in the long bones of the arms and legs. CHONDROSARCOMA, tumors made of abnormal cartilage, is the second most common bone cancer. EWING'S SARCOMA is the third most frequently diagnosed bone cancer, believed to originate in immature nerve tissue. Although Ewing's sarcoma causes less bone destruction, it is more likely to enter the bloodstream and metastasize than other forms of bone cancer. Ewing's sarcoma is the most common form of bone cancer in children, affecting primarily

BONE CANCERS—MOST COMMON FORMS

Type of Cancer	Tissue of Origin	Location in Body	Most Common Ages
Osteosarcoma (osteogenic sarcoma)	Osteoid (bone)	Knee, upper leg, upper arm	10–25
Chondro-sarcoma	Cartilage	Pelvis, upper leg, shoulder	30–60
Ewing's sarcoma	Immature nerve tissue, usually in bone marrow	Leg, hip, arm	10–20
Malignant giant cell tumor	Connective tissue of bone marrow	Knee, vertebra	40–55
Fibrosarcoma of bone	Connective tissue within bone marrow cavity	Leg, arm, hip	30–40
Chordoma	Cellular remnants of fetal spinal cord	Upper/lower end of spinal column or skull	55–65

teenagers. Other types of bone cancer include FIBROSARCOMA OF THE BONE, CHORDOMA, MALIGNANT GIANT CELL tumor, ADAMANTINOMA, and reticulum cell sarcoma juxtacortical osteosarcoma.

The most common bone cancers by type, tissue of origin, body location, and ages affected are listed above.

The cause of bone cancer is not known. Some researchers speculate that osteosarcoma may be triggered by overactivity of bone cells. Medical treatments may also be a contributing factor. Studies of children treated with radiation therapy have shown that some of those children later developed bone cancer. Children treated with an ALKYLATING anticancer drug may also be at a greater risk. A very small number of families have been found in which siblings developed bone cancers, which may indicate a very rare genetic defect.

Early symptoms of bone cancer can vary considerably; the most common may be "dull and

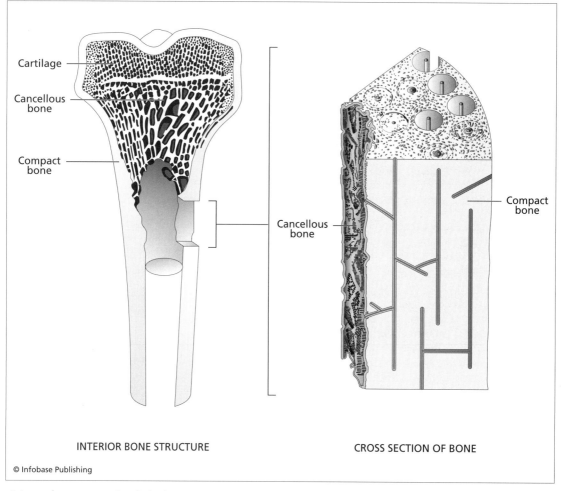

Cartilage

Cancellous bone

Compact bone

Cancellous bone

Compact bone

INTERIOR BONE STRUCTURE

CROSS SECTION OF BONE

© Infobase Publishing

Primary bone cancer is relatively rare. Courtesy NCI.

aching" pain and swelling. Tumors in or near joints may cause stiffness or tenderness. Tumors in the pelvic bones and at the base of the spine can affect bladder or bowel function. Malignant giant cell tumor can cause bone fractures, as can other bone cancers.

Procedures in the diagnosis and evaluation of bone cancer may include an ALKALINE PHOSPHATASE TEST of the blood, X-rays, BONE SCAN, a CT SCAN, FLUOROSCOPY, and a bone BIOPSY.

Bone tumors can be grouped into five categories based on where they develop, how they grow, and how they look on X-rays or scans. Following is a brief description of the five categories:

- benign/latent—tumor grows slowly with normal growth of person and then stops; frequently disappears spontaneously and never becomes malignant (cancerous); when surgically removed, the bone heals quickly; does not grow back
- benign/active—tumor grows continuously; surgical removal includes a margin of healthy bone tissue to prevent the tumor's return
- benign/aggressive—tumor grows rapidly and extends into adjacent bone tissue but does not spread to another part of the body; is likely to recur unless a margin of healthy tissue is removed along with the tumor

- malignant/low-grade—a cancerous tumor that is likely to spread outward from the original site but not likely to spread to other parts of the body; removal of the tumor and a margin of healthy tissue may be the only treatment necessary
- malignant/high-grade—a cancerous tumor that grows rapidly and spreads to surrounding tissue and to other parts of the body; in addition to removal of the tumor and surrounding tissue, radiation therapy and chemotherapy may be needed.

In determining treatment, the type of bone cancer is not as important as the site, size, and extent of spread from the original site.

The primary treatment for bone cancer is surgery. Adjuvant chemotherapy may also be given (see ADJUVANT THERAPY). For specific information on the latest state-of-the-art treatment, call the National Cancer Institute's Cancer Information Service at 1-800-4-CANCER (1-800-422-6237), or for a TTY: 1-800-332-8615.

bone graft   using bone from another part of the body to replace bone that has been removed during surgery.

bone marrow   the inner, spongy substance in the center of the bone that produces all of the red blood cells (erythrocytes), most of the white blood cells (leukocytes), and all of the platelets (thrombocytes). All blood cells derive from primitive stem cells in the bone marrow. Stem cells are primitive precursor cells in the bone marrow that give rise to all blood elements. Functionally, bone marrow should be considered an organ system living inside the bone. The bone marrow system is located throughout the body in the inner portion of the skeletal system.

Bone marrow plays a significant role in the development, diagnosis, and treatment of cancer. For example, leukemia is a condition in which there is an abnormal production, by the bone marrow, of white blood cells and sometimes red blood cells, although that is much less common. The bone marrow may produce too many blood cells that may function poorly or not at all. Those cells eventually crowd out the existing healthy cells and prevent the bone marrow from producing properly functioning blood cells that the body needs. The abnormal blood cells also can infiltrate vital organs and glands, causing them to enlarge and/or malfunction.

Testing the bone marrow for malignant (cancerous) cells is performed in the diagnosis of leukemia and many other cancers. The procedure—a BONE MARROW ASPIRATION or BONE MARROW BIOPSY—can be done on an outpatient basis or in a doctor's office.

Bone marrow transplantation (BMT) is recognized as a treatment for some cancers, such as leukemia and lymphoma. The patient's bone marrow is replaced with healthy bone marrow. BMT is being investigated for its use as a supportive treatment as well. Removing and storing a patient's bone marrow allows the patient to be given a much higher dose of chemotherapy or radiation, which ordinarily could severely damage or destroy the marrow. Higher doses are potentially more effective treatment. After the chemotherapy or radiation treatment is completed, the healthy bone marrow can be transplanted back into the body.

bone marrow aspiration   [sternal tap, bone tap] extraction by suction of a small amount of bone marrow for microscopic examination.

After a topical anesthetic has been applied, a long, hollow needle is inserted into a bone (usually the back of the hip, a rib, or breastbone). The procedure usually takes about 15 or 20 minutes and can be done in a doctor's office. The marrow that is collected is biopsied (microscopically examined for cancer cells).

Bone marrow aspiration may be used in the diagnosis of leukemia and other cancers as well as many other disorders such as anemia. Bone marrow aspiration is also used to harvest (remove) bone marrow for a BONE MARROW TRANSPLANTATION, although that procedure is done under general anesthesia. Bone marrow aspiration may also be performed to determine how effective a bone marrow transplant has been.

See also BONE MARROW BIOPSY.

bone marrow biopsy   microscopic examination of a piece of bone and bone marrow for cancer. It is virtually the same as a BONE MARROW ASPIRATION, only the needle is inserted more deeply to get a larger sample of the marrow. The most commonly used site for a bone marrow biopsy is a protuberant accessible part of the hip. An actual core of bone with marrow inside is removed for analysis. The patient is given local anesthesia for this procedure so as to cause as little discomfort as possible.

bone marrow depression [bone marrow suppression]   a condition characterized by the decreased ability or inability of the BONE MARROW to make red and white blood cells and platelets. This is a common side effect of chemotherapy (anticancer drugs). The three types of chemotherapy drugs that usually have this side effect are the ALKYLATING agents, ANTIMETABOLITES, and antitumor ANTIBIOTICS.

Bone marrow depression is a major factor in determining the frequency of treatment and amount of drug given to a patient. Persons with below-normal blood levels are at greater risk for infections, anemia, and serious bleeding. If the blood counts are low, the chemotherapy dose may be reduced or postponed to allow the bone marrow to recover and the blood count to return to normal.

Because of the much greater susceptibility to infections resulting from bone marrow depression, patients are advised to take the following preventive measures:

- Wash hands frequently, always before eating and after using the bathroom.
- Avoid crowds and people who have infectious diseases such as chicken pox or the flu.
- Do not tear or cut nail cuticles; use a cuticle cream remover instead.
- Avoid using a hard toothbrush or dental floss.
- Use an electric shaver rather than a razor to prevent cuts.
- Do not squeeze or scratch pimples.
- Take a daily warm shower and pat dry your body rather than rubbing it briskly.
- Clean any cuts or scrapes immediately with warm water and soap.
- After bowel movements, clean the rectal area gently but thoroughly.

Bone marrow depression is usually reversible.

bone marrow donor   a person who donates some of the substance from the center of the bone, which produces blood cells, to be withdrawn for infusion into another person. The donor is chosen whose marrow most closely matches that of the recipient. The procedure is usually performed under general anesthesia, although a local may be used. In most instances, the donor is admitted to the hospital the day before the procedure. Generally, two units of blood are drawn and stored to be used after the procedure if necessary. The marrow is removed primarily from the pelvic bones; the breastbone may also be used when necessary. Usually four to eight small incisions are made. As many as 30 extractions of marrow are taken from the incisions. In all, about 3 to 5% of the donor's marrow and blood cells are removed (one to two pints). The procedure usually takes less than an hour. After the marrow has been removed, it is processed to remove blood and bone fragments.

The bone marrow replenishes itself in the donor in a relatively short period of time, within a few weeks. The only side effect may be some soreness around the sites of the incisions, usually lasting a short time.

Although donating bone marrow is virtually a risk-free procedure, there can occasionally be complications such as infection that can occur at the site of the incisions.

The National Marrow Donor Program (NMDP) can facilitate transplantation. It maintains a registry of bone marrow donors and can be reached at 1-800-526-7809 or 1-800-627-7692.

bone marrow harvest   removal by needle of some of the BONE MARROW from the center of the bone, which produces blood cells, from a donor or from the patient (autologous) for use in BONE MARROW TRANSPLANTATION. It is generally performed under general anesthesia. The marrow is removed from several locations on the front and back of the hips and/or breastbone. Bone marrow that is removed from the patient is purged of any cancer cells and then kept frozen until it is ready to be transplanted. Bone marrow from a donor is processed to remove any blood and bone fragments.

bone marrow suppression   See BONE MARROW DEPRESSION.

bone marrow test   a general term referring to the removal of BONE MARROW by a needle, and microscopic examination of it to evaluate abnormal blood conditions. The tests may include BONE MAR-ROW ASPIRATION, BONE MARROW BIOPSY, and BONE MARROW TREPHINE.

bone marrow transplantation (BMT) a procedure developed in the 1950s (in the era of organ transplantation) by which a patient with a major disease of the bone marrow, such as leukemia or aplastic anemia, received the donated marrow of a healthy person (allogeneic or syngeneic).

The main purpose of BMT in the treatment of most cancers is to enable the patient to be given very large, and potentially more effective, doses of chemotherapy and/or radiation that cause severe damage to the bone marrow, making a patient far more susceptible to infections that can be life-threatening. As a treatment for other nonhemato-logic (blood) cancers, it became obvious that a person's own healthy marrow could be removed, stored, and reinfused as a rescue after the administration high-dose chemotherapy, enabling the patient to regain the ability to fight off infections. A patient with breast cancer, for whom a transplant is suggested, would most likely be involved in this kind of procedure, for example.

As technology developed it became clear that the most vital cell needed to restore bone marrow function—the primative progenitor cell known as the stem cell—could also be isolated from peripheral blood, thereby simplifying the procedure.

The choice of which form of transplant is best for which candidate is being clarified. Following are the ways in which a transplant can be performed:

- *the patient's own bone marrow or peripheral blood (source of stem cells) is used.* After it is harvested, it is frozen and stored. To make sure there are no cancer cells in the marrow or blood a process called purging—using—chemotherapy to wipe out any cancer cells—may be employed.
- *allogeneic*—The marrow comes from a sibling, parent, or an unrelated donor. It must be as closely matched to the patient's marrow as possible. To find a match, scientists look at six markers called HUMAN LEUKOCYTE ANTIGENS (HLA), which are found on white blood cells. The more markers that match, the better the chance of success.
- *syngeneic*—The perfectly matched marrow that comes from an identical twin. While this type of

transplant has the highest success rate, it is also relatively rare.
- *cord blood*—Blood found in the umbilical cords that in the past was considered medical waste and discarded. It is a valuable source of stem cells that can be used in transplantation procedures.

The way BMT is performed can vary from one medical center to another, and new methods are introduced as research advances are made.

Before the transplantation is performed, the patient undergoes a series of different tests. A catheter is usually inserted into a large vein in the chest for transplanting the marrow as well as giving blood, antibiotics, and other drugs, administering nutritional support, and drawing blood. The patient is given high doses of anticancer drugs and/or radiation therapy. When the cancer cells and healthy cells are destroyed, the new, healthy marrow can be given. The healthy marrow is delivered through the catheter and travels through the blood-stream to the bone marrow where it starts to make red and white blood cells and platelets.

Side effects, usually short term, of the high doses of anticancer drugs and/or radiation therapy can include nausea, vomiting, irritation of the lining of the mouth and gastrointestinal tract, lowered blood count, damage to vital organs, hair loss, and a loss of appetite. Long-term side effects, which are usually a result of the anticancer drug and radiation treatment, can include infertility, early menopause, cataracts, and secondary cancers.

During the treatment and after the bone marrow transplant, patients are very susceptible to infection. They are put into protective isolation (a hospital room that is kept as free as possible from infectious agents) until the transplanted marrow produces enough white blood cells to fight infection. That process, called engraftment, usually takes between 14 and 30 days. In peripheral blood stem cell transplants the period of time is substantially shorter.

A patient may experience any of several complications as a result of the BMT, including infections, GRAFT VERSUS HOST DISEASE, and bleeding, most often from the nose or mouth, under the skin, or in the intestinal tract. Liver disease may also develop in the weeks and months following the BMT.

Although bone marrow transplantation has become standard therapy for some cancers, investigations into other applications continue. It is estimated that as many as four times the number of patients now undergoing allogeneic BMTs a year could benefit from the procedure if more compatible donors could be found. INTERFERON, COLONY-STIMULATING FACTORS, RADIOACTIVE substances, and MONOCLONAL ANTIBODIES are being investigated for their role in aiding the BMT process.

See PERIPHERAL BLOOD STEM CELL TRANSPLANTATION.

bone marrow trephine   extraction of a tiny piece of BONE MARROW for microscopic examination for cancer cells. This is similar to a BONE MARROW ASPIRATION or biopsy but a larger needle is used. It is done much less frequently than in the past.

bone metastasis   cancer in the bone that has spread from another part of the body. Virtually any cancer can metastasize (spread) to the bone. Breast, lung, and prostate cancer account for more than 80% of bone METASTASES, and 50% of people with those cancers will develop bone metastases. Bone metastases can cause debilitating pain, bone fractures, impaired walking, and severe neurological impairment.

Procedures used to diagnose bone metastasis may include bone scan, CT SCAN, MRI, and MYELOGRAPHY.

Treatment depends on a number of factors—the location and extent of bony destruction, the severity of morbidity, the availability of effective anticancer therapy, and the overall status of the patient. RADIATION THERAPY is commonly used. CHEMOTHERAPY and HORMONE THERAPY may also be used. Some bone metastases, particularly in lymphomas, may be cured with chemotherapy or radiation therapy, but for most patients, only palliative treatment to improve quality of life is appropriate. For the latest state-of-the-art treatment information, call the National Cancer Institute's Cancer Information Service at 1-800-4-CANCER (1-800-422-6237), or for a TTY: 1-800-332-8615.

bone scan   an image taken of the entire body skeleton or specific area after the injection of a tracer radioactive substance into the blood, which carries it to the bones. Areas in the bone with cancer where cells are dividing rapidly will pick up more of the radioactive substance, resulting in "hot spots" on the developed film image of the body. The hot spots may be an indication of cancer. A bone scan may be performed to check for other cancers that have spread to the bone such as prostate or breast cancer. Other abnormal conditions can also show up as hot spots on a bone scan, including arthritis, infection, or a bone that has been injured, making the scan difficult to interpret.

See also NUCLEAR SCAN.

bone tap   See BONE MARROW ASPIRATION.

booster radiation therapy   a second phase of intensive RADIATION THERAPY after completion of the original treatment to the original site of the cancer. It may be administered externally or internally.

boron neutron capture therapy (BNCT)   A form of radiotherapy using an isotope of boron proposed in 1936 for the localized treatment of human malignancy. Although clinical trials of this method have been disappointing, because of poor results in other treatments of gliomas there is still some investigative interest in this therapy; there are also centers that offer BNCT therapy.

Bortezomid [Velcade; PS341]   the first proteosome inhibitor introduced into clinical trials. This agent was granted accelerated FDA approval in 2003 for treatment of advanced MYELOMA. Side effects include THROMBOCYTOPENIA (low platelet count) and painful peripheral neuropathy (pain along the course of the small nerves). Its use in other hematolgoic malignances is being explored.

bowel   See INTESTINES.

bowel cancer   See COLON/RECTAL CANCER.

bowel resection   in cancer treatment, surgical removal of the cancer in the bowel (intestine) along with a small amount of healthy tissue on either side. The healthy parts of the bowel are then sewn together.

Bowen's disease (bo'enz)   a rare form of SKIN CANCER that usually occurs on areas of the skin unexposed to the sun. It is a raised reddish pink growth with scaling. Some doctors consider it a PRECANCEROUS condition.

BPH   See BENIGN PROSTATIC HYPERPLASIA.

brachytherapy (brak"e-ther'ah-pe) one type of INTERNAL RADIATION in which the radioactive source, which is sealed in a container, is placed on the surface of the body near the tumor or a short distance from the affected area. The term "brachytherapy" is sometimes used to describe all types of internal RADIATION; however, it is only one form of internal radiation.

brain cancer   a primary cancerous TUMOR in the brain. Brain cancer is relatively rare. Eighty-five percent of cases occur in adults over the age of 40; the remaining 15% occur primarily in children and young adults up to the age of 20. More men than women are affected. In 1999 there were about 16,800 new cases of brain cancer diagnosed in the United States and approximately 13,100 deaths from the disease.

There are many different types of brain tumors, only some of which are cancerous. A malignant (cancerous) tumor can spread to other parts of the brain.

While a BENIGN (noncancerous) brain tumor does not spread, it can be just as devastating because the skull cannot expand to accommodate the MASS growing inside. Also, some benign tumors become MALIGNANT.

The symptoms of a brain tumor can vary depending on what part of the brain is affected. The most frequent signs of a brain tumor are subtle changes in personality, memory, and intellectual performance that may go unnoticed. A common symptom is a headache; however, it is not necessarily persistent or severe. Nausea and vomiting unrelated to food consumption occur in about a quarter of the people with a brain tumor.

Some of the procedures used in the diagnosis of brain cancer are X-RAYS, CT SCAN, EEG, MRI, CEREBRAL ANGIOGRAPHY, PNEUMOENCEPHALOGRAPHY, and SPINAL TAP (lumbar punctures).

Brain cancer is classified according to the type of cell in the tumor and its HISTOLOGIC GRADE (how different the tumor cells are from the cells that are near it). Following is the National Cancer Institute's (NCI) classifications for adult brain tumors:

Astrocytomas

- noninfiltrating astrocytoma—a relatively slow growing tumor that usually does not grow into the tissues around it
- well-differentiated mild and moderately anaplastic astrocytoma—slow growing but not as slow growing as noninfiltrating astrocytomas; the tumor starts to grow into other tissues around it
- anaplastic astrocytoma—the cells of this tumor look very different from normal cells and grow more rapidly
- glioblastoma multiforme (also called astrocytoma grade IV)—tumors that have cells that look very different from normal cells and grow very quickly

Brain Stem Gliomas   tumors located in the bottom part of the brain that connects to the spinal cord (the brain stem).

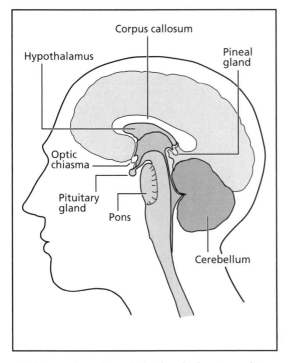

Median section through the head, showing relative size and position of the brain and its components.
Infobase Publishing.

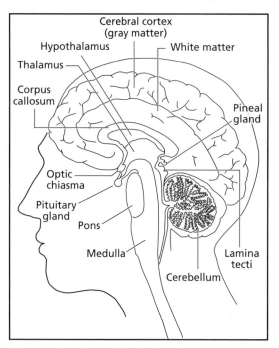

Cerebral cortex
(gray matter)

Hypothalamus   White matter

Thalamus

Corpus
callosum

Pineal
gland

Optic
chiasma

Pituitary
gland

Pons

Medulla

Lamina
tecti

Cerebellum

Cross section through the brain. Infobase Publishing.

Ependymal Tumors   tumors that begin in the ependyma, the cells that line the passageways in the brain where special fluid that protects the brain and spinal cord (called cerebrospinal fluid) is made and stored

- well-differentiated ependymoma—the cells look very much like normal cells and grow quite slowly
- anaplastic ependymoma—the tumors cells do not look like normal cells and grow more rapidly than well-differentiated ependymal tumors
- ependymoblastoma—rare cancers that usually occur in children; they may grow very quickly

Oligodendroglia Tumors   tumors that begin in the brain cells that provide support and nourishment for the cells that transmit nerve impulses.

- well-differentiated oligodendroglioma—slow-growing tumors with cells that look very much like normal cells
- anaplastic oligodendroglioma—faster-growing tumor with cancer cells that look very different from normal cells

Other Brain Tumors

- mixed gliomas—tumors that occur in more than one type of brain cell, including cells of astrocytes, ependymal cells, and/or oligodendrocytes
- medulloblastoma—tumors that begin in the lower part of the brain; almost always found in children or young adults; it may spread from the brain to the spine
- pineal parenchymal tumors—tumors found in or around the pineal gland, a tiny organ located near the center of the brain; they can be slow growing (pineocytomas) or fast growing (pineoblastomas); astrocytomas may start there
- germ cell tumors—tumors arising from the sex cells
- craniopharyngioma—tumors that occur near the pituitary gland (a small organ about the size of a pea just above the back of the nose that controls many of the body's functions)
- meningioma—tumors that occur in the membranes that cover and protect the brain and spinal cord (the meninges); they usually grow slowly
- malignant meningioma—a rare form of meningioma that grows more quickly than other meningiomas
- CNS lymphoma—tumors of the LYMPH SYSTEM that begin in the brain

Recurrent   cancer that has recurred (come back) after it has been treated; it may return to the brain or to another part of the body

Treatment depends on cell type, location of the tumor, the general state of health of the patient, and other factors. The three types of treatment being used are surgery, radiation therapy, and chemotherapy. Biological therapy is being studied in clinical trials. For specific information on the latest state-of-the-art treatment, call NCI's Cancer Information Service at 1-800-4-CANCER (1-800-422-6237), or for a TTY: 1-800-332-8615.

Childhood brain tumors are generally classified by their location within the brain rather than by stage. Following is NCI's classification system:

Infratentorial tumors   tumors found in the lower part of the brain, usually the cerebellum or brain stem; the cerebellum is the most common site of brain tumors in children; tumors found in this region are:

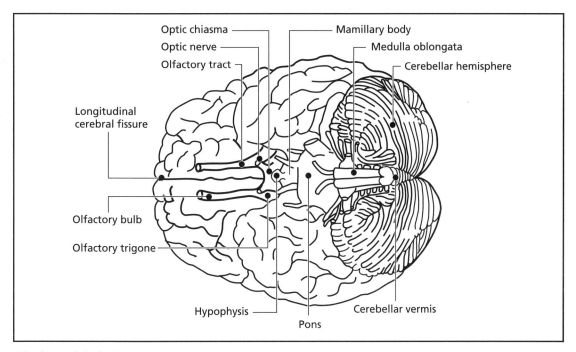

Optic chiasma
Optic nerve
Olfactory tract
Mamillary body
Medulla oblongata
Cerebellar hemisphere
Longitudinal cerebral fissure
Olfactory bulb
Olfactory trigone
Hypophysis
Pons
Cerebellar vermis

The base of the brain. Infobase Publishing.

- medulloblastoma—a rapidly growing tumor that can spread to other parts of the nervous system; depending on the size of the tumor after surgery and the presence or absence of spread to other areas, patients may be classified as standard risk or high risk
- cerebellar astrocytoma—generally a slow-growing tumor that usually does not spread to adjacent tissues or outside the region
- infratentorial ependymoma—a tumor arising from the lining of the lower part of the brain; it may spread to other areas of the brain and spinal cord
- brain stem glioma—astrocytomas arising in the lowest part of the brain; they may grow rapidly or slowly but rarely spread from their original location

Supratentorial tumors   tumors that are found in the upper part of the brain; tumors found in this region are:

- cerebral astrocytoma—a tumor found in the upper part of the brain; it may grow slowly (low grade) or rapidly (high grade)

- supratentorial ependymoma—a tumor arising from the lining of the upper part of the brain; it may grow rapidly or slowly
- craniopharyngioma—a nonmalignant tumor in the pituitary region; it causes problems because of pressure on nearby structures
- intracranial germ cell tumor—tumors that may arise in the middle of the brain; they tend to be malignant and can spread
- optic nerve tract glioma—a slow-growing tumor that can arise from the optic nerve or other portions of the optic tract
- pineal parenchymal tumor—tumors that arise in the center of the brain near the pineal gland; they can spread to other parts of the CENTRAL NERVOUS SYSTEM
- primitive neuroectodermal tumor—tumors that arise in the upper part of the brain; they sometimes spread to other parts of the central nervous system.

Treatment depends on cell type, location of the tumor, the general state of health of the patient,

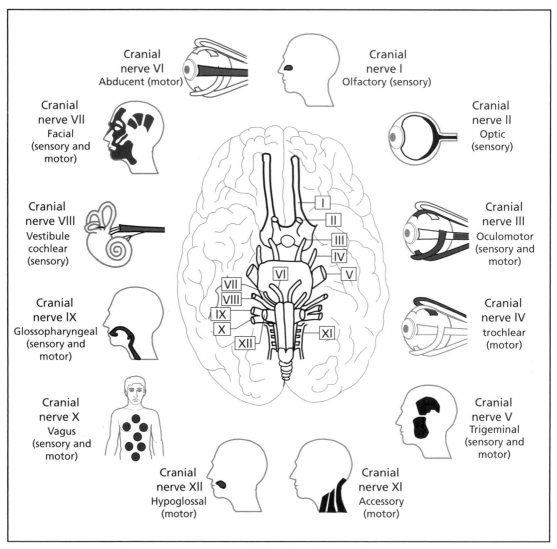

The base of the brain, showing cranial nerves and the bodily functions they control. Infobase Publishing.

and other factors. Surgery, a craniotomy, is the most common treatment for adult brain tumors. Radiation therapy may also be performed. Chemotherapy is being used on a limited basis. Clinical trials are investigating new treatments. For specific information on the latest state-of-the-art treatment, call NCI's Cancer Information Service at 1-800-4-CANCER (1-800-422-6237), or for a TTY: 1-800-332-8615.

brain metastasis (mĕ-tas′tah-sis)   cancer that has spread to the brain from another site in the body, most commonly the lung or breast. Other primary tumors that metastasize to the brain include melanoma, sarcomas, and tumors arising in the kidney or colon. In addition, unknown primaries sometimes present with brain metastases. The incidence of brain metastasis is far more prevalent than primary BRAIN CANCER.

Symptoms of metastases to the brain may include headaches, vision problems, seizures, loss of sensation or difficulties walking and balancing, lethargy, emotional lability, or personality changes. The diagnosis of brain metastases may include, in addition to a NEUROLOGIC WORKUP or examination, a CT SCAN and MRI.

RADIATION THERAPY is the primary treatment for brain metastasis. Surgical removal of the tumor is limited to a few situations. Chemotherapy has a limited role in treatment.

brain scan   an examination of the brain after the administration of a small and relatively harmless amount of radioactive substance. The two-dimension picture taken by a gamma camera or retilinear scanner can show concentrations of the substance. Certain radioactive substances gather in areas of the body where cells are dividing rapidly; these "hot spots" may be an indication of cancer.

The brain scan procedure is relatively simple. After the administration of the radioactive substance, by IV (injected into a vein) or by mouth, the patient lies on a narrow table and the scanning machine takes pictures. A brain scan can take anywhere from 20 minutes to about an hour.

A brain scan may be used in the detection of brain tumors and other disorders and as a way of checking the progress of treatment.

See also NUCLEAR SCANS.

brain stem glioma   See BRAIN CANCER.

brain tumor   an abnormal growth of tissue in the brain. A brain tumor can be malignant (cancerous) or benign (noncancerous).

BRCA gene   associated with breast and/or ovarian syndromes. Of approximately 200,000 breast cancer cases per year in the United States, approximately 5–10% are associated with obvious hereditary predisposition and mutation in the gene such as BRCA1 & BRCA2. Approximately one in 150 to one in 800 people carry a genetic susceptibility in the general population. There is a higher prevalence in certain ethnic groups. For more information, go to: http://www.genome.gov/10000940

BRCA mutation   mutation of a gene, either BRCA1 or BRCA2, associated with a major (60–85%) increase in lifetime risk of developing INVASIVE BREAST CANCER by age 70. It is also associated with a 15–25% incidence of OVARIAN CANCER. For more information, go to: http://www.genome.gov/10000940

breast calcifications   deposits of calcium that can be seen on a mammogram of the breast. There are two types:

- macrocalcifications, which are large deposits and are usually not related to cancer
- microcalcifications, which are specks of calcium that may be found in an area of rapidly dividing cells

A cluster of microcalcifications (many in one area) may signal the presence of cancer.

See also MAMMOGRAPHY, MACROCALCIFICATIONS, and MICROCALCIFICATIONS.

breast cancer   the general term for a variety of different types of cancer that can occur in the breast. It is the cancer that affects most women in the United States. As of 1999, one in eight women in the United States would get breast cancer at some point in her lifetime; there were an estimated 176,300 new cases and 43,700 deaths from breast cancer in 1999. About two-thirds of all breast cancers occur in women over the age of 50. Men may get breast cancer, though rarely, accounting for less than 1% of all breast cancer cases.

Breast cancer can develop in the milk ducts, between DUCTS, in fat, in LYMPH or blood vessels, in the nipple, and in the LOBES where the milk is produced. Each breast has 15–20 sections called lobes, which have many smaller sections called LOBULES. The lobes and lobules are connected by thin tubes called ducts. The most common type of breast cancer is DUCTAL CANCER. It is found in the cells of the ducts. Cancer that begins in the lobes or lobules is called LOBULAR CARCINOMA. Lobular carcinoma is more often found in both breasts than other types of breast cancer. When it is NONINVASIVE, confined to the inside of a duct or lobule (small lobe), it is, in most instances 100% curable by surgical removal.

People at a greater risk of getting breast cancer are women who are 50 or older; have a family history of breast cancer (mothers and/or sisters); have never had children or have had a child after the age of 40; and/or have had breast cancer in the past. Other possible risk factors include diet (fat intake has been linked to breast cancer), obesity, race or national origin (breast cancer is more common in North American and European women than Asian and African women), and early onset of menstruation and late menopause.

There are many types of breast cancer. The most common type is INVASIVE DUCTAL CANCER, Which accounts for 70 to 80% of the breast cancers. Following are brief descriptions of the different kinds of breast cancers:

Noninvasive (in situ)

• DUCTAL CARCINOMA IN SITU (also called DCIS, intraductal carcinoma, and noninfiltrating ductal papillary carcinoma)—cancer that arises in the ducts of the breast and that has not invaded adjacent tissue. It accounts for about 1% of all breast cancers. Surgical removal of the cancer is usually a cure
• LOBULAR CARCINOMA IN SITU (also called LCIS and lobular neoplasia)—cancer that arises in the lobules of the breast and has not invaded adjacent tissue. It occurs less frequently than ductal carcinomas. Over time, it is associated with a higher incidence of invasive cancer in either breast. Management choices include observation for life, tamoxifen, and not radical surgery.
• PAGET'S DISEASE of the nipple—arises in the nipple as a slowly progressive reddening and thickening of the nipple. It accounts for about 3% of all breast cancer. An INTRADUCTAL CARCINOMA (above), which cannot be felt, is generally found under the nipple. Paget's disease is usually noninvasive

Invasive

• INFILTRATING DUCTAL CARCINOMA—tumors that feel hard, which may be "fixed" to the skin or chest wall. The nipple may be retracted. It is the most frequently diagnosed breast cancer (70–80%). It often spreads to the AXILLARY LYMPH NODES
• INFILTRATING LOBULAR CARCINOMA—tumors that arise in the small end ducts or lobules, similar in appearance and behavior to infiltrating ductal carcinoma. It accounts for about 5% of all breast cancers.
• MEDULLARY CARCINOMA—a ductal tumor that may grow quite large but with a generally good prognosis. It accounts for about 3% of all breast cancers.

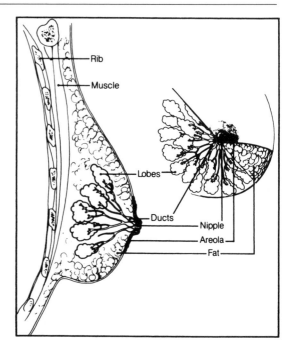

Cross section and cutaway front view of the breast.
Courtesy NCI.

• MUCINOUS (COLLOID) CARCINOMA—a ductal tumor that contains mucus-producing cells, giving the tumor a glistening appearance. It accounts for about 2% of all breast cancers and has a highly favorable prognosis
• tubular carcinoma (also called orderly carcinoma)—it displays tubular structures and accounts for about 1% of breast cancers. It has a favorable prognosis
• COMEDOCARCINOMA—ductal tumor that begins in the lining and grows into the duct itself until it is completely filled. It accounts for about 5% of all breast cancers. Although it may grow quite large, it is not likely to spread beyond the breast or invade the skin, giving it a favorable prognosis
• INFLAMMATORY—the breast looks inflamed, red; ridges may appear on the breast; the breast may have a "pitted" appearance like an orange peel. It represents between 1 and 2% of all breast cancers. It is a highly malignant cancer with a poor prognosis
• secretory—extremely rare, it occurs in girls before puberty. It has an excellent prognosis

- ADENOID CYSTIC CARCINOMA—a very rare, slow-growing version of ductal carcinoma accounting for less than 1% of all breast cancers. It has a favorable prognosis

The cause of breast cancer is not fully understood. It is known, however, that there are many different factors, both hereditary and environmental, that may "interact" in its development.

Studies show that heredity does play a role in breast cancer. How great a role is not known, but it does not appear to be as important as many people think. A small number of breast cancer cases are genetically linked. About 5% to 7% of breast cancers develop in women who have inherited a dominant cancer gene. (Inheriting that gene in no way guarantees that the woman will develop cancer, but it puts her at a higher risk.) In 70% of the women who develop breast cancer, there is no known family history of breast cancer. The rest of the breast cancer cases, about 25%, occur in women where other family members have had breast cancer, but it is not passed on directly through a dominant gene. Thus, it appears that breast cancer that is "inherited" is quite rare, and when there is a "history" of breast cancer in a family, other factors, such as environment and lifestyle, may play a role.

Epidemiological studies have shown a hormonal link to breast cancer. Women who get their period at an early age—and those who are older when they stop menstruating—are at a higher risk of developing breast cancer. Women who have never been pregnant are at a greater risk, as are women who have their first child in their mid-30s or later. In addition, some breast cancers are clearly ESTROGEN DEPENDENT. However, there is no convincing evidence that estrogen supplements or birth control pills, which contain estrogen, actually cause breast cancer.

Epidemiological studies have suggested high levels of fat in the diet as a risk factor in breast cancer as well as other cancers. For example, women in Japan, whose diets contain much less fat than those of women in the United States, are much less likely to develop breast cancer. The daughters of Japanese women who have immigrated to this country have a greatly increased risk of breast cancer compared with Japanese women still living in Japan. Obesity also appears to be a risk factor and may be related to fat consumption.

Exposure to high levels of radiation can cause breast cancer, as well as other cancers. A study of women exposed to radiation from the atomic bombing of Hiroshima and Nagasaki showed a higher rate of breast cancer. It was highest among the women who were the youngest when exposed. Epidemiological studies have also suggested that alcohol consumption may play a role in the development of breast cancer.

The most common symptom of breast cancer is a lump or thickening in the breast or armpit. Other symptoms may be a change in the size or shape of the breast, discharge from the nipple, and/or a change in the color or texture of the skin of the breast or areola such as dimpling, puckering, or scaliness. Most breast cancers are found by women themselves who discover a lump in a breast.

The most frequent diagnostic procedures include PALPATION (feeling the breast for lumps), MAMMOGRAPHY, BIOPSY, ULTRASOUND, THERMOGRAPHY, and TRANSILLUMINATION. A definitive diagnosis cannot be made without a biopsy. Eighty percent of the lumps that are biopsied are BENIGN (noncancerous).

The American Cancer Society recommends the following guidelines for the screening/detection of breast cancer in women without symptoms:

- *women 20 and older*—perform BREAST SELF-EXAMINATION every month
- *women 20–40*—perform breast self-exam every month; have a physical exam of the breasts by a doctor every three years
- *women 40 and over*—perform breast self-exam every month; have a physical exam of the breasts by a doctor every year; have a mammogram every year
- *women with personal or family histories of breast cancer*—consult a doctor about the need for more frequent examinations.

Following is the National Cancer Institute's (NCI) staging for breast cancer:

- Stage 0—in situ (also called noninvasive carcinoma, intra ductal carcinoma, ductal carcinoma in situ, and lobular carcinoma in situ)—very early breast cancer
- Stage I—the tumor is no bigger than two CENTIMETER (cm); has not spread beyond the breast

- Stage II
  - the tumor is no bigger than 2 cm but has spread to the lymph nodes under the arm (axillary lymph nodes) or
  - the tumor is between 2 and 5 cm and may or may not have spread to the lymph nodes under the arm or
  - the tumor is bigger than 5 cm but has not spread to the lymph nodes under the arm
- Stage IIIA
  - the tumor is smaller than 5 cm and has spread to the lymph nodes under the arm, which have grown into each other or into other structures and are attached to them or
  - the tumor is bigger than 5 cm and has spread to the lymph nodes under the arm
- Stage IIIB
  - the tumor has spread to tissues near the breast (chest wall, including the ribs and muscles in the chest) or
  - the tumor has spread to lymph nodes near the collarbone
- Stage IV—the tumor has spread to other organs of the body, most often the bone, lungs, liver, or brain
- Inflammatory breast cancer—usually spreads quickly
- Recurrent—cancer has returned to the same site or to another part of the body after treatment.

Treatment depends on the stage of the disease, the general state of health of the patient, and other factors. Surgery is a primary treatment in breast cancer. There are a number of different surgical procedures including MASTECTOMY (total, partial, modified, radical) and LUMPECTOMY. CHEMOTHERAPY (anticancer drugs), HORMONE THERAPY, and RADIATION THERAPY are also used. BIOLOGICAL THERAPY and BONE MARROW TRANSPLANTATION are being studied in clinical trials. For specific information on the latest state-of-the-art treatment, by stage, call NCI's Cancer Information Service at 1-800-CANCER (1-800-422-6237), or for a TTY: 1-800-332-8615.

See also BREAST CANCER GENES and TWO-STEP PROCEDURE.

breast cancer genes [BRCA1 and BRCA2 (*BR* for "breast," *CA* for "cancer")] genes which, when mutated, are thought to predispose women to breast

and ovarian cancer. BRCA1 was the first major breast cancer gene to be isolated and mapped to chromosome 17 in 1990. In 1994 scientists were able to pinpoint its exact location and make copies of it. The BRCA2 was found a short time later. BRCA1 and 2 are tumor-suppressor genes. When there is a mutation in either the BRCA1 or 2 gene, it can no longer control cell growth and division, thereby resulting in an increased risk of breast and ovarian cancer. Mutations have been found throughout the BRCA1 and BRCA2 genes, and new mutations are being reported. It is estimated that two-thirds of inherited breast cancer is caused by either the BRCA1 or BRCA2 gene. Relatives of breast cancer patients who carry this defective gene may be more likely to develop breast or ovarian cancer. Tests are available to determine who has the genetic defect long before any cancer appears.

The BRCA1 gene has been associated with a greater risk of colon, pancreatic, and, in men, prostate cancer. There are indications that the BRCA2 gene may increase the risk of cancers of the prostate and larynx.

See also BREAST CANCER.

Breast Cancer Prevention Trial (BCPT) a clinical trial conducted to assess whether the antiestrogen drug tamoxifen could prevent breast cancer. The study, started in 1992, was stopped 14 months before it was scheduled to end because of the promising results. It found that the incidence of breast cancer was cut almost in half in the women taking tamoxifen. Late in 1998 the FDA approved the use of tamoxifen for the prevention of breast cancer in women at high-risk, making it the first drug approved for the prevention of breast cancer.

See also TAMOXIFEN.

Breast Cancer Risk Assessment Tool a tool to help health care providers discuss the option of TAMOXIFEN with women who seek the drug as a preventive measure. It was developed after the Breast Cancer Prevention Trial (BCPT) showed that women at increased risk of breast cancer who took tamoxifen had approximately 49% fewer diagnoses of invasive breast cancer than women who were assigned to a placebo. Tamoxifen offered a prevention benefit along with no increased risk of serious side effects for younger women (ages 35 to 49) compared to the placebo, but the prevention benefit for women ages 50 and older came with a risk of serious side effects. With answers to some medical and personal questions, a woman's risk of developing breast cancer in the next five years and over her lifetime (to age 90) can be estimated enabling her to make the most appropriate choice as to whether or not to take tamoxifen to reduce that risk.

breast conservation   See LUMPECTOMY.

breast needle localization   a procedure used to locate calcifications or thickenings in the breast, which are detected by MAMMOGRAPHY but cannot be felt, in order to do a BIOPSY. The procedure involves injecting dye through a needle that has been placed in the area to be biopsied, thereby enabling the surgeon to locate it.

breast reconstruction [reconstructive mammoplasty, mammoplasty]   using plastic surgery to make a "new" breast after a MASTECTOMY (surgical removal of the breast). Plastic surgeons have been developing methods of breast reconstruction since the late 19th century, first used for women whose breasts had been damaged by a fire or other injury.

The reconstruction of the breast can frequently be done during the same operation when the breast is removed. There are several different procedures used in reconstruction of a breast. Which procedure is used depends on a number of factors, including the type of mastectomy, skin and muscle conditions, and the size of the breast.

In a simple breast reconstruction, a small incision is made along the lower part of the breast area, usually through the mastectomy scar. A saline or SILICONE IMPLANT is put in the pocket created under the chest muscle. This can be performed on an outpatient basis under local or general anesthesia. It can be done on women who have a healthy chest muscle and enough good-quality skin to cover the implant.

For women who have healthy chest muscle and skin, but do not have enough skin to cover an implant, a temporary "tissue expander" may be used. A deflated expander is implanted through an incision made in the mastectomy scar. Over a period of eight to 10 weeks, more and more fluid is injected into the expander, gradually enlarging the expander and stretching the skin over it. When the skin has stretched to the point where an implant of the desired size can be implanted, the tissue expander is removed and the permanent implant is inserted. This can be performed on an outpatient basis under local or general anesthesia.

There are three kinds of procedures that involve moving tissue from another part of the body to the breast area. The latissimus dorsi reconstruction is done when chest muscles have been removed and there is too little skin to hold and cover an implant. Skin, muscle, and other tissue from the back are transferred to the reconstruction site. The latissimus dorsi, a broad, flat muscle in the back below the shoulder blade, is transplanted to make a new muscle on the front of the chest. An implant is then placed under the new muscle. The operation takes several hours under general anesthesia. It leaves a scar on the back.

The abdominal advancement reconstruction is often used for women who are large breasted. Skin and fat from the chest and abdomen below the mastectomy site are moved to the breast area. This is a relatively simple procedure. There is a good match of skin texture and color and less scarring to other areas of the body.

Another procedure is the rectus abdominus reconstruction, or transverse abdominal island flap, which is used when much skin and muscle have been removed during the mastectomy. One of the two abdominal muscles, the rectus abdominus, is transferred upward under the abdominal skin to the mastectomy site along with skin and fat from the abdomen. The flap of muscle, skin, and fat are shaped into a breast. If there is enough tissue from the abdomen available, an implant may be unnecessary.

In the latest procedure, a free flap-skin, fat, and muscle are removed from the abdomen, buttock, or thigh and transplanted at the mastectomy site. An artery and vein are attached to existing blood vessels that had served the original breast. This procedure has several advantages. The blood supply is healthier, less muscle is transferred, there is a better match to the remaining breast, and the reconstructed breast loses or gains weight with the rest of the body. It is a longer, more complicated procedure and therefore is more expensive.

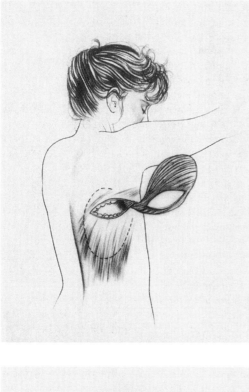

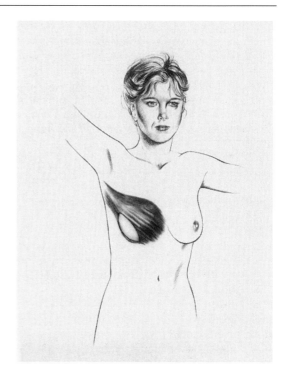

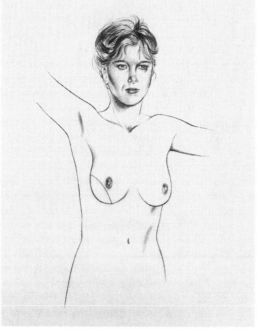

Latissimus dorsi breast reconstruction, where skin muscle and other tissue from the back are transferred to the reconstruction site. The first illustration shows the latissimus dorsi muscle, with skin flap raised. In the second, the flap is tunneled under the skin from the back to the front of the chest. The third illustration shows the flap in place, re-creating breast contour with reconstructed nipple and areola. Courtesy NCI.

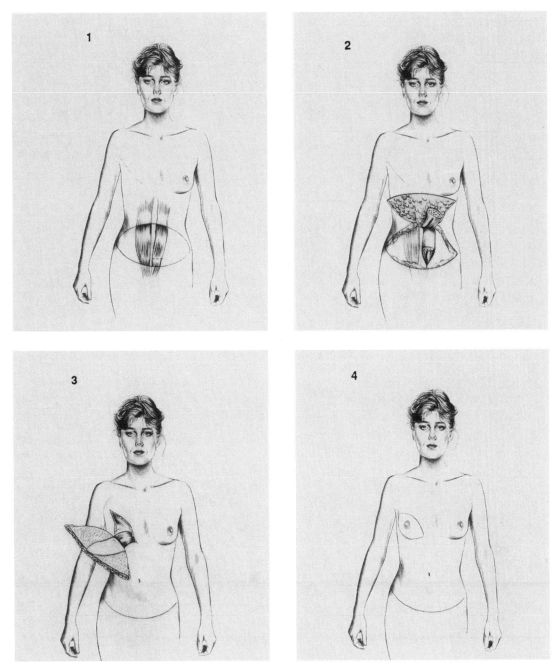

Rectus abdominus breast reconstruction, where one of the two abdominal muscles, the rectus abdominus, is transferred upward to the reconstruction site under the abdominal skin. The four steps shown here illustrate (1) the two parallel rectus abdominus muscles with flap outlined; (2) the flap of muscle, skin, and fat raised; (3) the flap tunneled under the skin to the reconstruction site; (4) flap in place, re-creating breast contour with reconstructed nipple and areola. Courtesy NCI.

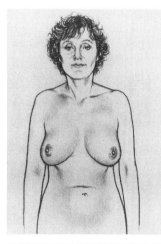
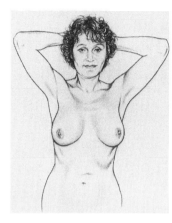
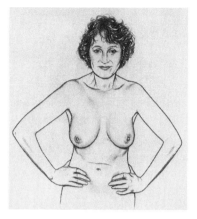
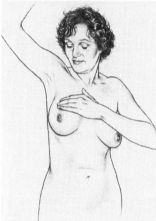
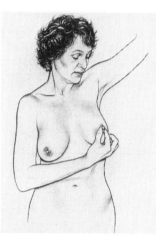

Breast self-examination. The American Cancer Society recommends that women do a breast self-exam every month. Check the six steps in the entry BREAST SELF-EXAMINATION *for guidelines on performing the exam.* Courtesy NCI.

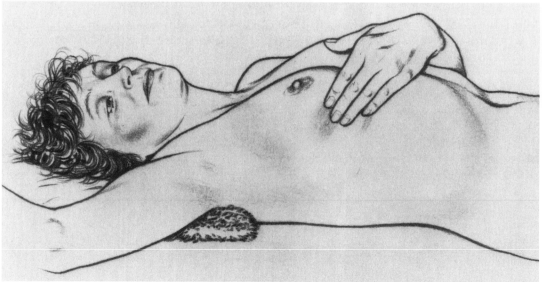

With any of these methods a nipple and areola can be added to the breast later, when the new breast has stabilized in shape and position. Sometimes the nipple of the diseased breast can be saved in a procedure called nipple banking. The nipple is removed and temporarily grafted to another part of the body until it can be attached to the new breast. Or a nipple and areola can be reconstructed using tissue from another part of the body.

Depending on the extent of the operation, a woman can usually resume normal activities in 2–3 weeks. She may have to wait a few weeks longer before doing strenuous exercises.

breast self-examination (BSE)   examination by a woman of her breasts, both by feeling for lumps or anything suspicious as well as by looking at them carefully in a mirror for any changes in contour, swelling, dimpling or puckering of the skin, or changes in the nipple. The American Cancer Society recommends that women perform breast self-examination every month. The best time to do it is two or three days after the end of menstruation. That is when the breasts are least likely to be tender or swollen. Postmenopausal women should choose a day that is easy to remember, such as the first day of the month.

By examining her breasts regularly, a woman will be able to tell when she feels something unusual. There are two parts to the BSE—looking and feeling. Following are some guidelines on how to do breast self-examination:

1. standing before a mirror, look for anything unusual, such as a discharge from the nipples or puckering, dimpling, or scaling of the skin
2. still looking in the mirror, clasp the arms behind the head and press them forward—look for any change or shape in the contour of the breasts
3. press the hands firmly on the hips and bow slightly toward the mirror; pull the shoulders and elbows forward—again, look for any change or shape in the contour of the breasts
4. with the left arm raised, use three or four fingers of the right hand to explore the left breast firmly, carefully, and thoroughly; begin at the outer edge and press the flat part of the fingers in small circles, moving the circles slowly around the breast gradually working toward the nip-ple—be sure to cover the entire breast; examine the area between the breast and underarm, including the underarm; feel for any unusual lump or mass
5. gently squeeze the nipple and look for any discharge; repeat steps 4 and 5 on the right breast
6. lying on the back with either the right or left arm extended over the head, examine the breasts the same way as in steps 4 and 5.

Any changes should be reported to your doctor. As many as 90% of breast cancers are found by a woman performing breast self-examination.

See also SCREENING.

Breslow's staging   a method of describing MELA-NOMA known as MICROSTAGING developed by Dr. Alexander Breslow.

Bricker's pouch   a procedure to divert urine after removal of the bladder. The urine goes into an external pouch that is emptied manually, about every two hours. It is named after the surgeon who devised the technique.

See also URINARY DIVERSION.

BRM   See BIOLOGICAL RESPONSE MODIFIERS.

bromfenac   sodium capsules
See DURACT.

Brompton cocktail [Brompton's solution, hospice mix]   a mixture of different doses of drugs such as morphine, heroin, and cocaine in a liquid of alcohol, syrup, and chloroform water, used to treat excessive pain. Originally used in the early 1900s, it came back into general use in the 1970s, when it was first used at a hospice in England to treat pain in cancer patients. It has since gone back into virtual disuse, with the multi-drug approach being replaced by contemporary ANALGESICS. This term is of historic interest.

bronchioloalveolar lung cancer (brong-ke-ōl″al-ve'o-lar) [alveolar cell lung cancer]   a type of ADENOCARCINOMA CANCER OF THE LUNG that is not associated with smoking, arising from the terminal bronchioles or alveolar walls of the lung. Some studies suggest it has a better prognosis than other

ADENOCARCINOMAS. It may be multicentric—arising spontaneously in several discrete locations. It is treated as a NON-SMALL CELL LUNG CANCER.

See also LUNG CANCER.

bronchofiberscope   See BRONCHOSCOPY.

bronchogenic   carcinoma (brong-ko-jen'ik) a type of LUNG CANCER originating in the bronchial tubes, the two large air tubes (called bronchi) that branch from the windpipe into the lungs.

bronchogram   See BRONCHOGRAPHY.

bronchography (brong-kog'rah-fe) an   X-RAY examination of the bronchial tubes (the large air tubes leading to the lungs) and the tubes leading to and forming branches in the lung using a contrast medium. After administration of a local anesthetic, a catheter about 20 inches long is inserted through the nose. The contrast medium is given through the catheter, and then the X-rays are taken. The procedure usually takes less than an hour and can be done in a doctor's office. It may be used in the diagnosis of LUNG CANCER and other disorders.

bronchoscope   See BRONCHOSCOPY.

bronchoscopy (brong-kos'ko-pe) [fiberoptic bronchoscopy, bronchofiberscope]   an examination of the bronchi (the large air tubes leading to the lungs), trachea (windpipe), and lungs. After the patient has been given a local or general anesthetic, a bronchoscope (a flexible tubular instrument with a light and a magnifying device) is inserted through the mouth or nose, down the throat, and then into the lung. A visual examination is done, and usually some cells or small pieces of tissue from the bronchial wall are obtained for a biopsy. A rigid bronchoscopy, performed with a metal tube, is still used by thoracic surgeons to complement, or provide additional information to, the bronchoscopy performed with the newer, flexible scope. Bronchoscopy is performed in a hospital setting. It takes about an hour, but some physicians recommend that a patient stay overnight. A bronchoscopy may be used in the diagnosis of LUNG CANCER as well as other disorders.

See also ENDOSCOPY.

Broviac catheter (bro've-ak kath'ĕ-ter)   the same as a HICKMAN CATHETER except the catheter has a smaller diameter.

BSE   See BREAST SELF-EXAMINATION.

BSF-1   See INTERLEUKIN-4.

BSF-2   See INTERLEUKIN-6.

BSO   See BILATERAL SALPINGO OOPHORECTOMY.

BU   See BUSULFAN.

buccal mucosa (buk'al mu-ko'sah)   the tissue lining the inside of the mouth.

Burkitt cell acute lymphocytic leukemia   See B-CELL ACUTE LYMPHOCYTIC LEUKEMIA.

Burkitt's lymphoma   a fast-growing form of NON-HODGKIN'S LYMPHOMA that was first described in Africa by David Burkitt in 1958 and is very common in children there. In the United States, Burkitt's lymphoma makes up a significant portion of the undifferentiated B-CELL LYMPHOMAS in children. The most common sites of occurrence in Americans are the neck and digestive system. It is often associated with the EPSTEIN-BARR VIRUS (a herpes-like virus) and a specific chromosomal abnormality. Burkitt's lymphoma is also seen as one of the forms of aggressive lymphomas in AIDS patients.

See also LYMPHOMA.

Burton, Lawrence   See   IMMUNOAUGMENTATIVE THERAPY.

Burzyncki, Stanislaw   a doctor in Texas who has developed his own treatment for cancer using substances present in human urine. He calls the substances antineoplastons. According to the National Cancer Institute, no information has been supplied to support claims for its effectiveness. The NCI evaluated two of the "antineoplastons" used by Dr. Burzyncki and found no activity that would warrant further investigation.

busulfan [Myleran, BU] an ALKYLATING anti-cancer drug, used to treat chronic myelogenous leukemia (CLM). It is taken by mouth. Common side effects may include nausea, vomiting, and diarrhea. Occasional or rare side effects may include BONE MARROW DEPRESSION, skin darkening, hair loss, breast enlargement, impotence, sterility, chronic lung problems, and eye problems. It is one of the more commonly used anticancer drugs. Because busulfan contains butanediol dimethylsulfonate, it is listed by the U.S. National Toxicology Program as a known carcinogen.

butanediol dimethylsulfonate See CARCINOGENS.

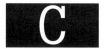

CA 15-3 a TUMOR MARKER that may be measurable in some patients with recurrent BREAST CANCER. Approximately 70% of the patients with metastatic breast cancer will have an elevated CA 15-3 blood level. Cancers of the ovary, lung, and prostate may also raise CA 15-3 levels. Elevated levels of CA 15-3 may be associated with noncancerous conditions, such as benign breast or ovarian disease, endometriosis, pelvic inflammatory disease, and hepatitis. Pregnancy and lactation can also cause CA 15-3 levels to rise. It may be used with other diagnostic procedures to monitor breast cancer patients.

CA 19-9 [carbohydrate antigen] a TUMOR MARKER that is measurable in the blood. It appears in certain patients with cancers of the pancreas, stomach, bileduct, and colorectal has become known as the "pancreatic cancer antigen." It also may be used with other procedures such as CEA, a test performed on the blood, to monitor cancer patients.Noncancerous conditions that may elevate CA 19-9 levels include gallstones, pancreatitis, cirrhosis of the liver, and cholecystitis.

CA 27-29 a tumor marker, similar to the CA 15-3 antigen, found in the blood of most breast cancer patients. CA 27-29 levels may be used in conjunction with other procedures to check for recurrence in women previously treated for stage II and stage III breast cancer. Levels can also be elevated by can-cers of the colon, stomach, kidney, lung, ovary, pancreas, uterus, and liver. Elevated levels can be found in noncancerous conditions such as first trimester pregnancy, endometriosis, ovarian cysts, benign breast disease, kidney disease, and liver disease.

CA 125 a protein that can be measured in the blood and an important TUMOR MARKER in OVARIAN CANCER. Elevated levels of CA 125 are found in 80% of the patients with epithelial ovarian cancer. It is highly predictive of cancer recurrence, and it is widely used in decisions regarding the treatment of patients with ovarian cancer. However, CA 125 is not recommended as a general screening test for ovarian cancer. A normal level does not exclude the presence of cancer. CA 125 levels may also be elevated by cancers of the uterus, cervix, pancreas, liver, colon, breast, lung, and digestive tract. Noncancerous conditions that can cause elevated CA 125 levels include endometriosis, pelvic inflammatory disease, peritonitis, pancreatitis, liver disease, and any condition that inflames the pleura (the tissue that surrounds the lungs and lines the chest cavity). Menstruation and pregnancy can also cause an increase in CA 125.

cachectin See TUMOR NECROSIS FACTOR.

cachexia (kah-kek'se-ah) [wasting syndrome] severe protein loss in the body leading to emaciation, weakness, fatigue, weight loss, impaired wound healing, an increased loss of appetite, and a decrease in tolerance for aggressive cancer treatment. This condition can lead to apathy, anxiety, and restlessness. Cachexia can occur in a cancer patient who has difficulty eating because of the treatments he or she is undergoing—common side effects of chemotherapy (anticancer drugs) are nausea and vomiting, a change in taste, and mouth sores. However, the most severe forms of cachexia are secondary to the cancer itself. Although cachexia can be treated by PARENTERAL NUTRITION, the administration of various nutrients intravenously, its use to reverse cancer-related cachexia has been very disappointing and is generally discouraged. In this setting, quality of life has not been improved and patients may die sooner. MEGACE (megestrol acetate) is useful in some patients as an appetite stimulant.

See also ENTERAL FEEDING and HYPERALIMENTATION.

CAF a combination of the anticancer drugs CYTOXAN, ADRIAMYCIN, and 5-FU sometimes used in the treatment of breast cancer. See individual drug listings for side effects.

See also COMBINATION CHEMOTHERAPY.

caffeine a chemical found in coffee, tea, chocolate, and other foods. Once thought to be a possible risk factor in pancreatic cancer, it is no longer considered a carcinogen.

calcifications See BREAST CALCIFICATIONS.

calcitonin (kal″sĭ-to′nin) a hormone produced by special cells in the thyroid that may help regulate levels of calcium in the blood. Calcitonin may be used as a TUMOR MARKER in some cancers. Abnormal levels of calcitonin may be an indication of familial MEDULLARY CARCINOMA OF THE THYROID (MTC), MULTIPLE ENDOCRINE NEOPLASIA (associated with medullary thyroid carcinoma), and MYELOMA.

calcium a mineral found in the body that is important in the body's skeleton and function. The regulation of calcium metabolism is carefully maintained in the body normally by the interaction of the parathyroid, vitamin D, and CALCITONIN. Higher-than normal levels of calcium in the blood (HYPERCALCEMIA) may be an indication of cancer as well as other disorders.

calcium leucovorin See LEUCOVORIN CALCIUM.

calusterone [Methosarb] See ANDROGEN.

CAM (complementary and alternative medicine) CAM is a group of diverse medical and health care systems, practices, and products that are not presently considered to be part of conventional (traditional) medicine. Conventional or traditional medicine is medicine as practiced by holders of M.D. (medical doctor) or D.O. (doctor of osteopathy) degrees and by their allied health professionals, such as nurses, physical therapists, and dietitians. Some practitioners of conventional medicine are also practitioners of CAM.

See NATIONAL CENTER FOR COMPLEMENTARY AND ALTERNATIVE MEDICINE.

Camey procedure an internal method of URINARY DIVERSION for people who have had their bladder removed but do not require a STOMA. A section of the ileum (lower part of the small intestine) is removed during surgery; one end is attached to the URETERS and the other is connected to the remainder of the urethra, forming a canal for the urine. To avoid leakage, the person must urinate frequently.

CAMP a combination of the anticancer drugs CYTOXAN, ADRIAMYCIN, METHOTREXATE, and PROCARBAZINE sometimes used in the treatment of NON-SMALL CELL LUNG CANCER. See individual drug listings for side effects.

See also COMBINATION CHEMOTHERAPY.

Campath See ALEMTUZMAB.

Camptosar [irinotecan] In metastatic colorectal cancer, this drug is FDA-approved (in combination with 5-FU and Leucovorin) as first-line therapy. It is also approved as a single agent in the treatment of colorectal cancer in the event of failure of 5-FU-based chemotherapy. It is also used in treatment of lung cancer. Camptosar is given via an intravenous (IV) line and is a moderate VESICANT. Side effects include EMESIS; in addition Camptosar can cause diarrhea, early or late, and may be dose-limiting.

cancer a general term for more than 100 diseases characterized by the uncontrolled, abnormal growth of cells in different parts of the body that can spread to other parts of the body. Different cancers have "unique" characteristics requiring different treatments. Cancer is frequently a chronic—that is, recurring—disease.

Cancer has been around for centuries. Evidence of cancer has been found in skeletons of prehistoric animals and in Etruscan, Peruvian, and Egyptian mummies. A link between the environment and a tumor was first observed in England in 1775 by Percival Pott, who found that cancer of the scrotum appeared frequently in chimney sweeps in London.

Today, cancer is classified into five major groups:

- CARCINOMA—a cancerous tumor or lump, originating in the surface tissue of body organs. It is the most common form of cancer, accounting for 80% to 90% of cases
- SARCOMA—a cancerous tumor originating in the bone, cartilage, muscle, fibrous connective tissue, or fatty tissue
- MYELOMA—a cancerous tumor originating in the plasma cells of the BONE MARROW
- LYMPHOMA—a cancerous tumor originating in the lymph system
- LEUKEMIA—cancer originating in the blood-forming tissue

Cancer cells cause harm in a number of different ways. They deprive normal cells of nourishment or space. They can form a mass, or tumor, which may eventually invade and destroy normal tissues. They can also spread (metastasize) by traveling through the bloodstream or lymphatic system to other parts of the body.

Most cancers take years to develop. For example, lung cancer used to be fairly rare among women. After World War II, millions of women started smoking when it became "socially acceptable." About 40 years later, lung cancer replaced breast cancer as the leading cause of death from cancer among women. Cancer that is detected and treated before it has invaded adjacent organs or metastasized has the greatest possibility of being cured.

The risk of cancer increases as one ages. However, it can affect males and females of any age, any social class, and any nationality.

In the early 1900s most people who got cancer died within a few years. By the 1930s one person in five lived five or more years after being treated. That changed to one in four in the 1940s, and one in three in the 1950s. In 1990 it was four in ten, or 40%. However, when normal life expectancy is taken into account, the relative five-year survival rate is 50%.

Different cancers have different symptoms. The American Cancer Society has a general list of seven basic symptoms that could be warning signs of cancer:

1. unusual bleeding or discharge
2. a lump that does not go away
3. a sore that does not heal within two weeks
4. change in bowel or bladder habits
5. persistent hoarseness or cough
6. indigestion or difficulty in swallowing
7. change in a wart or mole

These symptoms can also occur in many other conditions. If they persist, medical attention should be sought.

There are four types of treatment for cancer. In the early 1900s, SURGERY was the only known treatment for cancer. In the 1930s, radium (RADIATION THERAPY) was recognized as an effective treatment for cancer. CHEMOTHERAPY (anticancer drugs) was first used in the 1950s, when it successfully treated choriocarcinoma, a gynecological cancer. Treatment became increasingly more effective as combinations of surgery, radiation, and chemotherapy became more common in the treatment of different cancers. The 1970s and 1980s saw the increasing development of immunotherapy or BIOLOGICAL THERAPY. Although this type of treatment is still in its earliest stage, many researchers are optimistic that the continuing investigation of biological therapy will find ways for the body's own IMMUNE SYSTEM to fight successfully the cancer battle within it.

Another focus of continuing research is the development of new diagnostic tests, and the refinement of tests already in use, that detect cancer in its earliest stage and accurately show where in the body it has spread and that can assess the possibility that the cancer will recur, or return, after it has been treated. Some of the newer techniques and tests being studied include using high-frequency sound waves to produce detailed pictures of structures in the body; measuring minute differences of heat in the body to locate cancer; and using TUMOR MARKERS, biological substances in the body that can indicate the presence of cancer.

Finally, scientists continue to search for the causes of cancer and ways to prevent it. Some researchers theorize that cancer cells are always present in the body and that the immune system is always fighting them off until something goes wrong, and one area being heavily researched is the role that genes play in the development of cancer (and in its treatment). Scientists are also trying to identify additional CARCINOGENS, agents that cause cancer. One carcinogen that has been known about for years is cigarette smoke. It is well documented that smoking puts a person at a much greater risk of getting lung cancer as well as other cancers. Some foods and vitamins, such as beta-carotene and fiber, are being investigated for their role in preventing cancer. However, beta-carotene is not recommended for use by smokers.

See subject index for types of cancers, symptoms, side effects, drug treatments, and other major topics included in this volume.

cancer genes   See ONCOGENE.

Cancer Genetics Network   a national network of eight centers created in 1998 by the National Cancer Institute (NCI) specializing in the study of inherited predisposition to cancer. The network supports collaborative investigations into the genetic basis of cancer susceptibility, explores mechanisms to integrate this new knowledge into medical practice, and identifies means of addressing the associated psychosocial, ethical, legal, and public health issues. The network also facilitates the exchange of information on cancer genetics and research resources within the larger cancer and cancer genetics communities. (See Appendix 1 under NATIONAL CANCER GENETICS NETWORK for additional information; see also: http://epi.grants.cancer.gov/CGN/enrollment.html)

cancer prevention trial   a clinical trial done for the purpose of finding ways of reducing the risk of developing certain types of cancer. Prevention trials are conducted with healthy people who have not previously had cancer as well as with people who have had cancer and are trying to reduce the chance of either developing a new type of cancer or reappearance of cancer (recurrence).

The two kinds of cancer prevention clinical trials are: action studies—to find out whether actions people take, such as exercising more or quitting smoking, can prevent cancer, and agent studies—to evaluate whether taking certain medicines, vitamins, minerals, or food supplements (or a combination of them) can prevent cancer.

Prevention clinical trials are conducted in phases. Phase I attempts to identify how best to give the study agent (e.g., by mouth), the dose, and side effects. Phase II focuses on learning whether the agent has an effect in preventing cancer. In Phase III people are randomly assigned to groups; an intervention group or a control group. The intervention group receives the promising preventive agent, and the control group receives a different agent or a placebo.

For more information on clinical trials conducted by the National Cancer Institute (NCI), which is part of the National Institutes of Health (NIH), see: http://www.cancer.gov/clinicaltrials. To speak with an information specialist from the NCI's Cancer Information Service—within the United States, Monday through Friday 9:00 A.M. to 4:30 P.M. local time, call 1-800-4-CANCER (1-800-422-6237), or for a TTY: 1-800-332-8615.

cancer registry   See TUMOR REGISTRY.

CAP   a combination of the anticancer drugs CIS-PLATIN, ADRIAMYCIN, and CYCLOPHOSPHAMIDE (CYTO-XAN) sometimes used in the treatment of ovarian cancer, NON-SMALL CELL LUNG CANCER, and cancer of the kidney, bladder, and prostate. See individual listings for side effects.

See also COMBINATION CHEMOTHERAPY.

capecitabine   See XELODA.

carbohydrate antigen   See CA 19-9.

carbon dioxide laser   a laser that uses carbon dioxide to produce a powerful light beam. In LASER

THERAPY for cancer, the carbon dioxide laser is primarily used as a surgical tool. The carbon dioxide laser is used to shrink or destroy tumors. The light energy changes to heat and cuts or vaporizes cancerous tissue with relatively little bleeding. When it is used with an ENDOSCOPE, the laser's light is transmitted through the flexible endoscope, enabling the surgeon to see and work, with great precision, in parts of the body that otherwise could only be reached with traditional surgery.

carboplatin (kar″bo-pla′tin) [CBDCA, JM-8, Paraplatin, cyclobutan dicarboxylate platinum] an ALKYLATING anticancer drug, which by the early 1990s was considered the drug of choice in the treatment of OVARIAN CANCER. It is also used in a variety of other cancers, including cancer of the lung, head, and neck. It was designed to be as effective as CISPLATIN, the parent compound, with less toxicity. It is given by IV (injection into a vein). Possible side effects are severe nausea and vomiting, BONE MARROW DEPRESSION, ANEMIA, kidney problems, and neurological damage.

carboxamide   See DTIC.

carcinoembryonic antigen   See CEA.

carcinogens (kar-sin′o-jenz) substances known to cause and/or promote cancer. Carcinogens can be created byhumans, such as cigarette smoke, or simply be present naturally in the environment, as is ULTRAVIOLET RADIATION from the sun, both of which are known to play a major role in the development of cancer. X-RAYS and VIRUSES are also known carcinogens.

Carcinogens can work to cause cancer in different ways. Some cause changes that turn a normal cell in the body into a cancer cell. Others can set up conditions that help the action of other factors that cause the cancer.

Many cancers develop slowly. It can take from five to 40 years for cancer todevelop after exposure to a cancer-causing agent, making it difficult to identify carcinogens. The number of exposures and the length of time exposed to acarcinogen are two of the factors that play a role in when and if cancer will develop. However, many people exposed to carcinogens never get cancer.

Controversy continues over what substances and environmental factors do cause cancer. Researchers continue to conduct epidemiological and laboratory studies to find more answers. There is no evidence that there is a "safe" level for any carcinogen. Following is a list of substances that the federal government's National Toxicology Program identified as carcinogenic in its 1998 annual report. Its findings are based on evidence from human studies that indicate a causal relationship between exposure to the substance and human cancer:

- aflatoxins—toxic metabolites produced by fungi, associated with the development of liver cancer
- 4-aminobiphenyl (aminodiphenyl)—a chemical linked with bladder cancer
- arsenic and certain arsenic compounds—chemical(s) used in pesticides, wood preservatives, and other products, associated with cancer of the lung, skin, liver, and other cancers
- asbestos—people exposed to asbestos may be at a greater risk of developing lung cancer, mesothelioma, and other cancers as well as asbestosis, a noncancerous disease of the lungs
- azathioprine—used medically, it has been linked with increasing the risk of developing non-Hodgkin's lymphomas, skin cancer, and other tumors in various organs
- benzene—used as a solvent and gasoline additive; may increase a person's risk of developing leukemia
- benzidine—used in dyes in textiles and paper; exposure has been linked to bladder cancer
- bis(chloromethyl) ether—chemicals linked to a greater risk of lung cancer, mainly oat cell carcinomas
- butanediol dimethylsulfonate (Myleran, Busulfan)—an anticancer drug used to treat some forms of leukemia and polycythemia that may lead to the development of leukemia and other blood disorders
- chlorambucil (Leukeran)—an anticancer drug that may be used in the treatment of leukemia, lymphomas, and other cancers that may put people at a greater risk for developing leukemia
- 1-(2-chloroethyl)-3-4-methylcyclohexyl)-1-nitrosourea (MeCCNU)—an anticancer drug used to treat gastrointestinal cancers that may cause acute nonlymphocytic leukemia

- chromium hexavalent, chromium and certain chromium compounds, lead chromate, strontium chromate—studies have shown an increased risk for developing lung cancer among some workers. There is also a suggestion of increased risk of other cancers
- coal tar, creosote (coal and wood)
- coke oven emissions
- conjugated estrogens (a mixture principally of piperazine estrone sulfate, sodium equilin sulfate, sodium estrone sulfate)—a mixture of naturally occurring forms of estrogen that is associated with endometriosis as well as other possible cancers, including liver, testicular, embryonal cell carcinomas, teratomas, choriocarcinomas, and interestitial cell carcinomas
- cyclophosphamide (CYTOXAN, CTX, endoxan, neosar)—an anticancer drug sometimes used in the treatment of malignant melanoma, multiple myeloma, leukemias, lymphoma, neuroblastoma, EWING'S SARCOMA, mycosis fungoides, rabdomyosarcoma, cancers of the breast, ovary, lung, testis and endometrius which may cause bladder cancer, leukemia, and other cancers
- cyclosporin A (cyclosporine A; ciclosporin)—an immunosuppression agent associated with lymphoma or skin cancer
- diethylstilbestrol (DES)—a synthetic hormone once taken during pregnancy that may cause adenocarcinoma of the vagina or cervix and vaginal adenosis in daughters exposed in utero
- erionite—a naturally occurring fiber which may cause malignant mesothelioma
- melphalan (Alkeran, L-PAM, phenylalanine mustard, L-phenylalanine mustard, and L-sarcolysin)—an anticancer drug used in the treatment of breast and ovarian cancer and myeloma which may cause second primary cancers, mainly leukemias
- methoxsalen with ultraviolet A therapy (PUVA)—methoxsalen is a naturally occurring substance produced by several plants and a fungus used, along with ultraviolet A (radiation) to treat mycosis fungoides and is associated with an increased risk of squamous cell skin cancer. See METHOXSALEN
- mineral oils
- mustard gas—associated with respiratory tract cancer. See MUSTARD GAS
- phenacetin—ANALGESIC mixtures containing phenacetin—prescription and over the counter analgesics with phenacetin have been linked to several different cancers, including renal, transitional cell, and bladder
- 2-naphthylamine—an industrial chemical associated with bladder cancer
- radon—a naturally occurring radioactive gas that can cause lung cancer
- thioTEPA (tris(1-aziridinyl)phosphine sulfide)—an anticancer drug used in the treatment of HODGKIN'S DISEASE, cancers of the breast, ovary, and bladder
- thorium dioxide—a radioactive substance associated with a number of different cancers, including liver cancers, kidney, and hematologic disorders
- vinyl chloride—a colorless, flammable gas associated with an increased INCIDENCE of various cancers, including lung, liver, brain, lymphomas, and other cancers among people working with vinyl chloride

However, there is no evidence that there is any exposure level that is safe.

See also SMOKING and ULTRAVIOLET RADIATION and SUSPECTED CARCINOGENS and the subject index for additional carcinogens.

carcinoid syndrome (kar′sĭ-noid) a clinical picture of variable manifestation due to release into the bloodstream of active endocrine proteins by CARCINOID TUMORS. The classic triad consists of intense flushing, diarrhea, and valvular heart disease. A variable set of commonly used diagnostic tests is a urine collection for 5-HIAA, a metabolic product. A search for the origin of the tumor product (serotonin) may involve imaging (CT SCAN or MRI), the OCTREOTIDE SCAN, or urinary 5-HIAA.

carcinoid tumor a slow-growing gastrointestinal endocrine TUMOR that may produce highly active hormones and cause symptoms. It arises from neuroendocrine cells most prevalent in the gastrointestinal tract, pancreas, or bronchi. These cells can METASTASIZE and may cause bleeding or intestinal obstruction as well as the CARCINOID SYNDROME. Diagnosis may be difficult and includes the use of CT SCAN or MRI, as well as OCTREOTIDE SCAN, and urinary 5-HIAA collection, a metabolic product of the tumor. Treatment options include surgery, OCTREOTIDE, and CHEMOTHERAPY.

See also SMALL INTESTINE CANCER.

carcinoma (kar″sĭ-no′mah)   one of the five basic kinds of CANCER. It is a cancerous tumor that arises in the epithelial tissues (tissues lining a surface or cavity) of the skin and mucous membrane in glands, lungs, urinary bladder, nerves, etc. Carcinomas are the most common form of cancer, accounting for about 80 to 90% of all cancers. There are several types of carcinomas affecting SQUAMOUS CELL, BASAL CELL, transitional cell and glandular epithelium. The term *carcinoma* is frequently used synonymously with cancer.

carcinoma in situ (kar″sĭ-no′mah in si′tu) [cancer in situ]   cancer confined to its original position site; the earliest stage of cancer, staged as "0." Surgical removal of carcinoma in situ is usually a cure. Among the cancers that have an insitu stage are anal, bladder, breast, cervical, colon, endometrial, esophageal, lung, rectal, and stomach.
  See STAGING.

carcinoma in situ of the breast   See BREAST CANCER and DUCTAL BREAST CARCINOMA IN SITU.

carcinoma of unknown primary (CUP)   See UNKNOWN PRIMARY.

carcinosarcoma (kar″sĭ-no-sar-ko′mah)   a very malignant (cancerous) tumor containing two different types of cancer cells—the first resembling TRANSITIONAL CELL CARCINOMA cells and the second resembling SARCOMA cells. This may occur in many different sites.

care giver   a designated individual (family member, spouse, neighbor, friend, etc.) identified as the person who will be responsible for an individual at home. Many available programs that deal with the terminal ill person at home require such a person to ensure proper care for the patient. The lack of such a person may be used to deny care in some settings.

CARET (Beta-)Carotene and Retinol Efficacy Trial   a NUTRITIONAL INTERVENTIONAL STUDY launched in 1985 in the United States to evaluate potential dietary causes of LUNG CANCER. Lung cancer rates, however, increased in both groups.

carmustine   See BCNU.

cartilage (kar′tĭ-lij)   the tough, firm flexible tissue that covers portions of the bones of the freely moving joints.

case control study   an observational study in which researchers compare factors found in people with a certain disease to factors among people without that disease.

Casodex [bicalutamide]   an antiandrogen used in combination therapy with a luteinizing hormone-releasing hormone (LHRH) analogue for the treatment of advanced prostate cancer. The most common side effects of this drug combination may include hot flashes, pain, or weakness and loss of strength. Casodex is taken orally.

CAT scan   See CT SCAN.

cathartic (kah-thar′tik)   a drug or compound to treat or prevent serious CONSTIPATION. It may be given orally or rectally.

cathepsin D (kah-the′sin)   an enzyme produced in the body. Its presence, at high levels, may indicate which women who have had early stage node-negative breast cancer are at the greatest risk of having a recurrence. Early in 1990 researchers called cathepsin D the single most important factor in predicting whether a woman with breast cancer that had not spread to the lymph nodes would have a recurrence. It is currently being used by some cancer centers along with DNA analysis and HORMONE RECEPTOR STATUS to characterize a woman's risk of recurrence of breast cancer, when she is diagnosed. Tissue from the original breast cancer is used for the test.

catheter (kath′ĕ-ter)   a flexible tube inserted into the body for drainage, for injection of fluid, such as chemotherapy (anticancer drugs), and for removal of substances such as blood or urine. Some catheters can remain in the body for a period of time. A Foley catheter is a type widely used to drain urine from the bladder to outside the body.
  See also HICKMAN CATHETER, INDWELLING CATHETER, and BROVIAC CATHETER.

caudal   anesthesia (kaw′del   an″es-the′ze-ah)   injection of a numbing agent into an area outside the spinal canal. It is not as complete an anesthetic as when the agent is injected into the fluid surrounding the spinal cord. It also requires someone very skilled in performing this procedure. The major advantage of caudal anesthesia is that it avoids the headaches that frequently accompany SPINAL ANESTHESIA.

cauterization (kaw″ter-ĭ-za′shun) [cautery] the use of heat to destroy abnormal cells. It may be used to treat DYSPLASIA, abnormal cervical cells that may be precancerous. To perform the procedure, a cautery probe, which has a high-frequency electric current at its tip, is touched to the affected area for just a few seconds. The heat kills only the surface cells.

cautery See CAUTERIZATION.

CBC See COMPLETE BLOOD COUNT.

CBDCA See CARBOPLATIN.

CBI (cetuxamab, bevacizumab, and Irinotecan) an investigational combination of new agents (in 2005) being studied the the treatment of colorectal cancer.

C-cell carcinoma of the thyroid See MEDULLARY CARCINOMA OF THE THYROID.

CCNU [CeeNU, lomustine] an ALKYLATING anticancer agent sometimes used in the treatment of cancers of the kidney, lung, and brain and lymphomas and melanomas. It is taken by mouth. Common side effects may include nausea and vomiting. Occasional or rare side effects may include low blood count, mouth sores, hair loss, and liver, kidney, and eye problems. CCNA has been implicated as as a cause of secondary leukemia.

CCOP See COMMUNITY CLINICAL ONCOLOGY PROGRAM.

CD a combination of the anticancer drugs cytarabine (ARA-C) and daunorubicin (DAUNOMYCIN [CERUBIDINE]) sometimes used in the treatment of ANLL. See individual drug listings for side effects.
    See also COMBINATION CHEMOTHERAPY.

CD (Cluster of differentiation) a term developed in 1982 using ANTIBODIES to detect ANTIGENS of particular types on the surface of white blood cells (LEUKOCYTES). One uses FLOW CYTOMETRY to detect a specific sub-population of cells expressed as "CD + suffix" (e.g., CD-20).

CDC a combination of the anticancer drugs CARBOPLATIN, doxorubicin (ADRIAMYCIN), and CYTOXAN sometimes used in the treatment of ovarian cancer. See individual drug listings for side effects.
    See also COMBINATION CHEMOTHERAPY.

CDDP See CISPLATIN.

CEA (carcinoembryonic antigen) a substance normally found in a fetus, which, when found at elevated levels in the blood of adults, may indicate the presence of COLON/RECTAL CANCER or other types of cancer. It has been used to monitor patients for recurrence of a number of different cancers, including breast, lung, ovarian, pancreatic, stomach, and colon/rectal. It is referred to as an "oncofetal antigen" because of its similarity to fetal tissue.
    CEA is a TUMOR MARKER that may be found in increased amounts in some cancer patients. Elevated CEA levels may also be found in people who do not have cancer—smokers, for example. For that reason it is not considered useful as a screening device. It also has questionable value as a diagnostic tool, although elevated levels in people with symptoms can strongly suggest cancer. CEA levels may also be an indication of the effectiveness of treatment. It has been used to monitor patients for the recurrence of a number of different cancers, including breast, lung, stomach, and ovarian.

cecostomy (se-kos′to-me) making a hole in the cecum, the part of the intestine between the last part of the small bowel (ileum) and the beginning of the colon. Because surgical access to the cecum is relatively easy, this procedure is used to create a temporary diversion of fecal waste in cases where there is bowel obstruction. It is done in two steps— first, the malignant (cancerous) tumor is surgically removed and the artificial opening for body waste is created; at a later time, the colon is rejoined so that the device outside the body is no longer needed and normal functioning is resumed.
    See also COLOSTOMY.

CeeNU   See CCNU.

celioscopy   See LAPAROSCOPY.

cell cycle   the phases that a cell goes through in dividing. Methods of describing events taking place at the level of the individual cell have been helpful in cancer research. For many years scientists have been studying the patterns of growth of normal tissue as compared with that of cancerous tissue. Both normal tissue and cancer tissue are composed of billions of individual cells. A malignant (cancerous) tumor may be described as a population of cancer cells that increases continually, where cell birth exceeds cell death; whereas in normal tissue, during steady periods, cell birth equals cell death.

In both normal and cancer cells a cell growth cycle can be divided into discrete phases. These are best portrayed by a diagram called the cell cycle.

S is the phase of cell cycle during which DNA is synthesized or manufactured. M is the phase of actual mitosis (cell division). Both of these points can be measured or marked on an individual cell. The mitotic phase can be seen under a regular light microscope, and the synthetic phase can be marked by a technique known as "thymidine incorporation" (labeling the cell with the radioactive substance tritium).

The other points in the diagram are:

- $G0$ phase—thought to be made of a population of cells resting or not in cycle

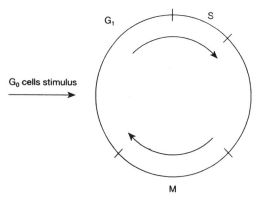

The cell cycle.

- $G1$ phase—a variable time during which the cell makes RNA prior to its synthesis of DNA during the S phase
- $G2$ phase—a brief period before the cell actually divides (undergoes mitosis)

Active cells, then, may be seen constantly in a dynamic fashion, and cancer may be thought of as a disorder of cells that are constantly increasing.

While it was thought that these concepts may be useful in the treatment of cancer, until recently, using these concepts in planning the treatment of cancer has been extremely laborious and impractical. The recent development of FLOW CYTOMETRY has made this data far more accessible and its use more practical and likely.

CHEMOTHERAPY is thought to be effective only against cells when they are dividing, and certain drugs may target one area of this cell cycle (e.g., the S phase) in a specific way. On a very basic, cell level, that is how anticancer drugs work.

cell differentiation   the process whereby young immature" cells take on individual characteristics and reach their "adult" form and function. Differentiated cancer cells resemble normal cells and have a better prognosis than undifferentiated cells.

See DIFFERENTIATION.

cell-mediated immunity   one type, or part, of the body's IMMUNE SYSTEM, protecting the body from fungus infections, TB, and tumors. The protection is provided by the cells themselves rather than a soluble ANTIBODY. Cell-mediated immunity involves two types of lymphocytes (white blood cells), the B CELL and the T CELL (derived in different ways), which play major roles in the immune system. Immunologists divide the human immune response into humoral (performed by soluble antibodies secreted by B cells into the body fluids) or cellular (directed by cells especially T cells and their secretions). T cells regulate cell-mediated immunity, the cellular part of the immune response, which includes marrow rejection and delayed skin hypersensitivity.

centimeter (cm)   a way to measure size in the metric system. In cancer, the size of many tumors is measured in centimeters. One cm is less than half inch. Following are the equivalents of inches to centimeters for six inches.

inch	cm
1	2.52
2	5.07
3	7.62
4	10.16
5	12.70
6	15.24

central nervous system (CNS) the portion of the nervous system consisting of the brain, spinal cord, and cranial (head) nerves. The CNS controls intelligence and emotion. The other part of the nervous system is the peripheral nervous system, consisting of the peripheral nerves that run from the spinal cord to all other parts of the body. It controls conscious activities and automatically maintains posture and muscle tone.

central nervous system preventive therapy See CNS PREVENTIVE THERAPY.

cerebellar astrocytoma classified as an INFRATENTORIAL TUMOR—tumors found in the lower part of the brain, usually the cerebellum or brain stem; the cerebellum is the most common site of brain tumors in children; generally a slow-growing tumor that usually does not spread to adjacent tissues or outside the region

cerebellum (sair-uh-bell′um) the portion of the brain in the back of the head between the cerebrum and the brain stem.

cerebral angiography (sĕ-re′bral an″je-og′rah-fe) [cerebral anteriography] an examination by X-RAY of arteries of the brain using a medium contrast or dye. The dye is injected into the carotid and/or vertebral arteries in the neck through a tube or catheter. The resulting X-ray, called an angiogram, shows the extent of the mass or tumor in the brain. This procedure may be used in the diagnosis of BRAIN CANCER and other disorders.

cerebral arteriography See CEREBRAL ANGIOGRAPHY.

cerebrospinal fluid (CSF) (sĕ-re′bro) the liquid that flows around the brain and through the spinal cord. It bathes and cushions the CENTRAL NERVOUS SYSTEM. A small sample of this fluid is extracted during a SPINAL TAP. The fluid is analyzed for cancer cells or evidence of other disorders such as infections.

cerebrum (sĕ-ree-brum) the largest part of the brain, divided into two hemispheres, or halves.

Cerubidine See DAUNOMYCIN.

cervical cancer cancer of the cervix, or neck of the uterus. It is one of the most common cancers, accounting for 6% of all cancers in women. The number of cases of invasive cervical cancer has been decreasing. The average age for "preinvasive," or very early, cervical cancer is 38; for invasive cervical cancer that has spread deeper into the cervix and/or nearby tissues and organs, 45 to 55.

Women at a greater risk of getting cervical cancer have had sexual intercourse at an early age, multiple partners, more than five pregnancies, and a history of syphilis or gonorrhea, as well as women whose mothers took DES while pregnant. Epidemiologic studies convincingly demonstrate that the major risk factor for development of preinvasive or invasive carcinoma of the cervix is HPV (human papillomavirus) infection, which far outweighs other known risk factors. It is estimated that more than 6 million women in the United States have HPV infection. A study of over 2,200 Latin American women found that those with the virus were eight times more likely to develop cervical cancer.

There are usually no symptoms for cervical cancer in its earliest stages. It could be present for 10 years before the onset of symptoms. The most common symptom, when the cancer is in an invasive, more advanced stage, is abnormal bleeding (which can be a symptom of other conditions as well).

The major screening procedure for cervical cancer is the PAP SMEAR. Other procedures that may be used in diagnosis include the SCHILLER TEST, COLPOSCOPY, CONIZATION (taking a cone-shaped piece of tissue from the cervix), and dilation and curettage (D & C).

Following are the NATIONAL CANCER INSTITUTE's (NCI) STAGING for cervical cancer.

- Stage 0 or CARCINOMA IN SITU—very early cancer found only in the first layer of cells of the lining of the cervix. This is the most curable stage.
- Stage I—cancer is throughout the cervix but has not spread nearby
  IA—a very small amount of cancer is deeper in the tissues of the cervix
  IB—a larger amount of cancer is in the deeper tissues of the cervix
- Stage II—cancer has spread to nearby areas but is still inside the pelvic area
  IIA—cancer has spread beyond the cervix to the upper two-thirds of the vagina
  IIB—cancer has spread to the tissue around the cervix
- Stage III—cancer has spread throughout the pelvic area; it may have spread to the bones of the pelvis and/or gone into the lower part of the vagina; it also may have spread to block the tubes that connect the kidneys to the bladder (the ureters)
- Stage IV—cancer has spread to other parts of the body
  IVA—cancer has spread to the bladder or rectum (organs close to the cervix)
  IVB—cancer has spread to faraway organs such as the lungs.

Treatment depends on the stage of the cancer, general state of health of the patient, and other factors. Treatment is frequently surgery, including CRYOSURGERY, conization, HYSTERECTOMY, and other procedures. RADIATION THERAPY and CHEMOTHERAPY may also be used.

The U.S. Food and Drug Administration approved the first vaccine for cervical cancer in June 2006. The FDA approved the vaccine for women between the ages of nine and 26. The vaccine protects against four of the 70 different types of human papillomavirus, or HPV, which can develop into cervical cancer. These four are considered the most significant.

For specific information on the latest state-of-the-art treatment, by stage, call NCI's Cancer Information Service at 1-800-4-CANCER (1-800-422-6237), or for a TTY: 1-800-332-8615.

cervical dysplasia   See CERVICAL INTRAEPITHELIAL NEOPLASM.

cervical intraepithelial neoplasm (CIN) [cervical dysplasia]   abnormal tissue in the CERVIX. CIN is DYSPLASIA that is found in the cervix. When it is severe it may be known as cervical cancer IN SITU, which is cancer in its earliest stage. CIN is considered a precursor of cervical cancer. When it is diagnosed as cancer in situ, its removal is considered a cure.

cervix [uterine cervix]   the neck or lower part of the uterus. It connects with the vagina.
See also CERVICAL CANCER.

CF   See LEUCOVORIN CALCIUM.

CF   a combination of the anticancer drugs CIS-PLATIN and 5-FU sometimes used in the treatment of GESTATIONAL TROPHOBLASTIC TUMOR. See individual drug listings for side effects.
See also COMBINATION CHEMOTHERAPY.

CFL   a combination of the anticancer drugs CIS-PLATIN, 5-FU, and LEUCOVORIN CALCIUM sometimes used in the treatment of GESTATIONAL TROPHOBLASTIC TUMOR. See individual drug listings for side effects.
See also COMBINATION CHEMOTHERAPY.

CFM   a combination of the anticancer drugs CYTOXAN, 5-FU, and METHOTREXATE sometimes used in the treatment of breast cancer. See individual drug listings for side effects.
See also COMBINATION CHEMOTHERAPY.

CFPT   a combination of the anticancer drugs CYTOXAN, 5-FU, PREDNISONE, and METHOTREXATE sometimes used in the treatment of breast cancer. See individual drug listings for side effects.
See also COMBINATION CHEMOTHERAPY.

CGL   See CML.

CHAD   a combination of the anticancer drugs CYTOXAN, HEXAMETHYLMELAMINE, ADRIAMYCIN, and CISPLATIN sometimes used in the treatment of ovarian cancer. See individual drug listings for side effects.
See also COMBINATION CHEMOTHERAPY.

CHAP   See CHAD.

cheek cancer See MOUTH CANCER.

chemo (ke′mo) a slang or informal way of referring to CHEMOTHERAPY.

chemoembolization (ke″mo-em″bo-lĭ-za′shun) technique of delivering anticancer drugs directly to cancer tissue (e.g., a liver tumor) through a CATHETER along with an agent that causes the blood flow to slow down. The goal is twofold: to prolong the time that the tumor is exposed to the chemotherapy and, at the same time, to diminish the blood supply going to the tumor, thereby debilitating the cancer cells and making them more vulnerable to the drugs. Chemoembolization is one form of REGIONAL CHEMOTHERAPY.

See also EMBOLIZATION.

chemoprevention using anticancer drugs, chemicals, vitamins, and/or minerals to prevent cancer. In 1980, the National Cancer Institute established the Chemoprevention Program after growing evidence indicated that various agents could stop or reverse cancer progression in animals, and reduce the incidence or risk of cancer in humans. Chemoprevention research included clinical trials of possible preventive agents in people considered to be at high risk for certain types of cancer. The development of synthetic compounds for clinical trials is also being investigated. From lab and epidemiologic studies more than 500 potential agents have been identified. For example, a major study successfully completed found that TAMOXIFEN, taken by women without cancer, could prevent the development of breast cancer in some high-risk women. Studies are being done with various agents to find out if they play any role in preventing or inhibiting cancer.

chemoprevention trial See CANCER PREVENTION TRIAL.

chemoprophylaxis (ke″mo-pro″fĭ-lak′sis) See CHEMOPREVENTION.

chemoradiotherapy a combination of CHEMOTHERAPY plus RADIOTHERAPY.

chemorads a colloquial term for CHEMORADIOTHERAPY, which is chemotherapy plus radiotherapy.

chemoreceptor trigger zone (CTZ) a distinct part of the brain that, when stimulated by noxious agents such as anticancer drugs, can activate another part of the brain called the vomiting center, possibly producing nausea and vomiting.

chemosensitivity assay a test performed on cancerous tissue removed from a patient to assess its vulnerability to a variety of CHEMOTHERAPY drugs. The assay attempts to predict response to treatment or suggest to the doctor which drugs are likely to be useful. Although in theory this seems of great benefit, the practicality of this test remains somewhat uncertain. There are several techniques that have been available for several years, and there are strong proponents of its use. However, many ONCOLOGISTS are not yet convinced. Another problem is that the patient's medical insurance may be unwilling to pay for this procedure, which can cost more than $1,000.

chemosurgery (ke″mo-sur′jer-e) the use of anticancer drugs to remove or shrink a tumor before, or instead of, SURGERY.

chemotherapist (ke″mo-ther′ah-pist) a trained cancer specialist such as a MEDICAL ONCOLOGIST or hematologist, who directs the administration of CHEMOTHERAPY, anticancer drugs.

chemotherapy (ke″mo-ther′ah-pe) [chemo] the treatment or control of cancer using anticancer drugs, highly toxic medications that destroy cancer cells by interfering with their growth or preventing their reproduction. Chemotherapy may also be used to prolong life when a cure is improbable and to provide palliation (relief of symptoms).

The first anticancer drug was serendipitously discovered during World War II. The chemical mustard gas, to which some American seamen were accidentally exposed, proved to be effective against lymphomas. The first cure using only chemotherapy was in the treatment of a case of choriocarcinoma (a cancer of the placenta) with METHOTREXATE in 1950. Chemotherapy became a major form of cancer treatment in the 1970s when CLINICAL TRIALS proved the effectiveness of chemotherapy in treating various forms of cancer. In 1980, more than 46,000 cancer patients were cured by anticancer drugs alone, or in combination with other treatments such as RADIATION THERAPY and/or SURGERY. Of the thousands of drugs that have been tested, fewer than three dozen have been found to be effective and have been approved for use. New ways to alleviate or reduce some of the common side effects of chemotherapy have been found. There are also new and increased ways to enhance the effectiveness of the treatment.

Chemotherapy works by interrupting the CELL CYCLE, a series of phases all cells go through, and preventing cells from reproducing. The final phase is when the cell reproduces by splitting in half. At each phase, the cell is performing a specific function such as making proteins or enzymes or DNA. Different chemotherapy drugs are effective at interrupting different cell phases; in other words, the cell must be in a specific phase for the chemotherapy to affect it. Therefore, chemotherapy is effective only against the cells it comes in contact with that are in their vulnerable phase for that particular anticancer drug.

Generally, the smaller the tumor is when diagnosed, the more effective the chemotherapy is. The larger the tumor, the greater the number of cancer cells, the greater the possibility that some of the cells will become resistant to the chemotherapy.

There are a number of different types, or classes, of chemotherapy drugs. The different types, which are effective against different cell phases, include ALKYLATING agents, ANTIMETABOLITES, anticancer ANTIBIOTICS, plant ALKALOIDS, HORMONES, and others. To be as effective as possible, different types of chemotherapy drugs are frequently used together (COMBINATION CHEMOTHERAPY). In that way, as many cell phases as possible will be vulnerable at the same time. In addition, chemotherapy can be used alone or along with other treatments such as radiation therapy, surgery, and/or BIOLOGICAL THERAPY. When chemotherapy is used with other treatments, it may be given before surgery to reduce the size of the tumor so that the surgery can be more effective. Chemotherapy may also be given after the PRIMARY TREATMENT, as ADJUVANT THERAPY, to destroy any remaining cancer cells.

The type of chemotherapy given a patient, and the dose, is determined by a number of different factors, including the kind of cancer, its STAGE, the objective of the treatment (cure, extending survival, or palliative), and the medical condition of the patient. All chemotherapy drugs approved by the Food and Drug Administration for use in cancer patients have gone through rigorous clinical trials to determine which particular cancer or cancers they are most effective in treating, what the most effective dose is, and the side effects. Because chemotheraphy does not distinguish between "good" and "bad" cells, the dose that is given must be enough to kill as many cancer cells as possible and at the same time not put the patient at the risk of life-threatening side effects.

Whereas surgery and radiation therapy generally treat one specific site in the body, chemotherapy can treat cancer throughout the body, systemically. (Chemotherapy is commonly referred to as "systemic treatment.") To treat the cancer systemically, chemotherapy is most frequently administered by IV, an injection into the vein, enabling the drug to enter the bloodstream rapidly and circulate through the body. In many patients, an INDWELLING CATHETER is implanted in the vein. The drug can be given through the catheter, eliminating the need for repeated injections. Other ways that chemotherapy can be given are:

- intraperitoneal—injected into the membrane lining the abdomen
- intramuscularly—injected into the muscle; it enters the bloodstream more slowly
- intra-arterially—injected into an artery; the artery chosen can deliver the drug to a specific site in the body
- orally—in pill or capsule form; it enters the bloodstream through the lining of the stomach or upper intestines
- intracavitarily—injected into body cavities such as the chest or abdomen
- intrathecally—injected into spinal fluid
- topically—applied to the cancer site, such as in skin cancer

Chemotherapy may be given daily, weekly, biweekly, monthly, or by continuous infusion—or on any schedule that has proved to be effective. This is generally determined by the MEDICAL ONCOLOGIST.

Chemotherapy is most effective against rapidly reproducing cells—again, both good and bad cells. Therefore, healthy cells in the body that divide rapidly will be the most affected. Some of those cells that normally divide rapidly are hair cells, bone marrow cells, and the cells lining the mouth and other parts of the intestinal tract. Thus, people on chemotherapy may develop BONE MARROW DEPRESSION, lose their hair, and get mouth sores—some of the more common and unpleasant side effects of chemotherapy.

Chemotherapy can have many different other side effects—ranging from unpleasant to life threatening—depending upon, among other things, the degree of toxicity of the particular drug. Different people frequently have different reactions to the same chemotherapy. Some people seem to get through it with few and/or minor side effects, while others are completely debilitated by the drugs. There is no relationship between the severity of the side effects experienced by the person and how well the chemotherapy is working.

Some side effects are immediate, occurring right after or shortly after administration of the drug. Others may appear long after the chemotherapy is over. Most side effects are temporary, lasting only as long as the chemotherapy, eventually disappearing after the chemotherapy is stopped.

One of the most dreaded side effects is nausea and vomiting. The chemotherapy drugs most likely to induce nausea and vomiting are CISPLATIN, DTIC, STREPTOZOCIN, MUSTARGEN, and a high dose of ARA-C. Drugs with a high potential to induce nausea and vomiting but not quite as likely as those already mentioned include SEMUSTINE, BCNU, CCNU, CYTOXAN, COSMEGEN, MITHRACIN, PROCARBAZINE, and a high dose of methotrexate. Drugs that induce nausea and vomiting about 50% of the time include 5-FU, ADRIAMYCIN, DAUNORUBICIN, L-ASPARAGINASE, and MUTAMYCIN. Most drugs have a very low potential for inducing nausea and vomiting. And even with the drugs that are very likely to, not every patient has this side effect. In action, the administration of ANTIEMETIC (antinausea) drugs can eliminate or reduce nausea and vomiting.

There are a number of other ways a patient can alleviate or reduce many of the side effects. Following are some common side effects with suggested steps for dealing with them:

- *nausea and vomiting*
  - eat many small meals throughout the day
  - avoid sweets and fried and fatty foods
  - eat foods at room temperature
  - eat slowly and chew well
  - eat dry foods like toast, dry cereal, or crackers
  - avoid a heavy meal right after treatment
  - drink clear, unsweetened beverages such as apple juice or light sodas
  - avoid offensive odors
  - stay out of the kitchen while food is being prepared
  - rest after eating
  - breath through the mouth when feeling nausea
- *diarrhea*
  - try a clear liquid diet to give bowels a time to rest
  - drink fluids to replace those lost
  - eat smaller amounts of food more often
  - avoid foods that cause cramps, such as coffee, beans, nuts, cabbage, broccoli, and cauliflower
  - avoid highly spiced foods and sweets
  - avoid milk and milk products
  - increase lost potassium by eating bananas, oranges, potatoes
- *constipation*
  - drink a lot of fluid
  - eat high-fiber foods (bran, raw fruits, whole grain breads, nuts, vegetables)
  - keep up normal level of activity; if possible, exercise

Other common side effects may include ANTICIPATORY NAUSEA AND VOMITING, ALOPECIA (hair loss), ANOREXIA, bone marrow depression, DRY MOUTH, FATIGUE, INFECTION, STOMATITIS (mouth sores).

Various techniques used to eliminate or reduce the side effects of chemotherapy include HYPNOSIS, IMAGERY, and RELAXATION TECHNIQUES.

See also Subject Index for drugs included in this volume.

chewing tobacco   See SMOKELESS TOBACCO.

CHEX-UP   a combination of the anticancer drugs CYTOXAN, HEXAMETHYLMELAMINE, 5-FU, and CISPLATIN sometimes used in the treatment of ovarian cancer. See individual drug listings for side effects.

See also COMBINATION CHEMOTHERAPY.

childhood cancers [pediatric cancers]   the cancers that most commonly affect children. Although childhood cancer is relatively rare, about 8,000 new cases are diagnosed each year. It is surpassed only by accidents as the most common cause of death among children 15 and younger. Advances in treatment have improved the prognosis for many children with cancer: 65% of the children will survive at least five years. That is a 40% increase over the survival rate in the early 1960s.

The most common childhood cancers are the LEUKEMIAS and the LYMPHOMAS which account for close to 50% of pediatric cancers. Other cancers which are common in children are WILMS' TUMOR, BRAIN CANCER, EWING'S SARCOMA, RETINOBLASTOMA, RHABDOMYOSARCOMA, NEUROBLASTOMA, OSTEOGENIC SARCOMA, and OSTEOSARCOMA.

childhood Hodgkin's disease   See HODGKIN'S DISEASE.

childhood leukemia   See ALL.

childhood nephroblastoma   See WILMS' TUMOR.

childhood non-Hodgkin's lymphoma   See NON-HODGKIN'S LYMPHOMA/CHILDHOOD.

childhood rhabdomyosarcoma   See RHABDOMYO-SARCOMA.

chimeric antibody (ki-me′rik an′tĭ-bod″e) a hybrid substance (still in an early stage of development) made by combining ANTIBODIES and parts of antibodies, from different organisms—usually human and mouse. It has the specificity of a MONO-CLONAL ANTIBODY, but is expected to be more effective than the ordinary monoclonal because it is less easily rejected by the body's IMMUNE SYSTEM. Chimeric antibodies to fight lymphoma are now available as Rituxan. Efforts are under way to produce chimeric antibodies for use in diagnosis. They appear to have the potential to track down and illuminate remote and microscopic tumors when they are armed with ten times more radioactive material than the usual monoclonal antibody.

chlorambucil   See LEUKERAN and CARCINOGENS.

chlorodeoxyadenosine   See LEUSTATIN.

chloroma (klo-ro′mah) [myeloblastomas] a mass of white blood cells that can form as a result of leukemia. Chloromas can cause obstructions in the intestines and other problems.

chlorotrianisene [Tace]   See ESTROGEN.

CHOEP   a combination of CHOP plus etoposide used in the treatment of DLBCL (diffuse large B-cell lymphoma).

cholangiocarcinoma (ko-lan″je-o-kar″sĭ-no′mah) cancer of the bile ducts in the liver. It is extremely rare.
  See BILE DUCT CANCER.

cholangiogram   See CHOLANGIOGRAPHY.

cholangiography (ko-lan″je-og′-rah-fe) an X-RAY of the bile ducts in the liver used in the diagnosis of BILE DUCT CANCER. A substance is given by IV (injected into a vein) or taken by mouth before the procedure, which makes the ducts more visible on the X-ray.

cholecystectomy (ko″lĕ-sis-tek′to-me) a surgical procedure in which the gallbladder is removed. This may be performed in the treatment of GALL-BLADDER CANCER. Part of the liver around the gallbladder and LYMPH NODES in the ABDOMEN may also be removed.

cholecystogram   See CHOLECYSTOGRAPHY.

cholecystography (ko″lĕ-sis-tog′rah-fe) [oral gallbladder test] an X-ray of the gallbladder and bile ducts. The patient is given a contrast dye, in the form of pills, 12 hours before the procedure to increase the visibility of the gallbladder and bile ducts on the X-ray pictures.

cholesteatoma   See CONGENITAL BRAIN TUMOR.

chondrosarcoma (kon″dro-sar-ko′mah) cancer of the cartilage and bone-forming tissue. It occurs most often in middle-aged and older people, most frequently in the hips and legs. It is extremely rare in children. The most common symptom is a lump or mass in the pelvic area followed by pain. It can be low grade and slow growing or high grade and fast growing. Treatment depends on the type and stage of the disease. Chondrosarcoma is usually treated with surgery, sometimes amputation, and sometimes CHEMOTHERAPY, anticancer drugs. For specific information on the latest state-of-the-art treatment by stage, call the National Cancer Institute's Cancer Information Service at 1-800-4-CANCER (1-800-422-6237), or for a TTY: 1-800-332-8615.

See also BONE CANCER and SOFT TISSUE SARCOMA.

CHOP a combination of the anticancer drugs CYTOXAN, hydroxydoxorubicin (ADRIAMYCIN), Oncovin (VINCRISTINE), and PREDNISONE sometimes used in the treatment of non-Hodgkin's lymphoma. See individual drug listings for side effects.

See also COMBINATION CHEMOTHERAPY.

CHOP-BLEO a combination of the anticancer drugs CYTOXAN, hydroxydoxorubicin (ADRIAMYCIN), VINCRISTINE, PREDNISONE, and BLEOMYCIN sometimes used in the treatment of NON-HODGKIN'S LYMPHOMA. See individual drug listings of side effects.

See also COMBINATION CHEMOTHERAPY.

chordoma (kor-do'mah) cancer of the spinal column or skull. It affects primarily middle-aged and older people. It is a rare cancer.

See also BONE CANCER and SOFT TISSUE SARCOMA.

chordotomy See CORDOTOMY.

choriocarcinoma (ko″re-o-kar″sĭ-no'mah) a cancer of the placenta or, rarely, a germ cell cancer in the testes or ovaries. Choriocarcinoma was the first cancer to be cured by chemotherapy (anticancer drugs). In the mid-1950s METHOTREXATE was tested in women with choriocarcinoma. A significant number of women were cured of a disease that, until then, was always fatal.

Choriocarcinoma occurs most often in Asian women and women over 40. Symptoms may include abnormal vaginal bleeding following abortion or childbirth or uterus size out of proportion for pregnancy stage Diagnostic procedures may include a BIOPSY, ULTRASOUND, NUCLEAR SCAN, and HUMAN CHORIONIC GONADOTROPIN test (HCG).

The tumor may have formed from a HYDATIDIFORM MOLE or from tissue that remains in the uterus following abortion or the birth of a baby.

See also GESTATIONAL TROPHOBLASTIC TUMOR.

choroidectomy (ko″roi-dek'to-me) surgical removal of parts of the eye. It may be done as a treatment of INTRAOCULAR MELANOMA.

chromium See CARCINOGENS.

chromosome (cro'mo-sōm) a rod-shaped structure in the nucleus of a cell. Chromosomes contain the genes that are composed of DNA—which encodes all the genetic information.

chromosome abnormalities a group of identified CHROMOSOME rearrangements or aberrations that are consistently associated with certain cancers.

chromosome markers specific characteristics on a CHROMOSOME that indicate a predisposition to a particular kind of cancer. This is under active, intense investigation.

chronic (kron'ik) of long duration, of frequent recurrence; a condition that lasts a long time. In cancer, the leukemias are diagnosed as ACUTE or chronic. A chronic form of the disease follows a different course than an acute form and may be treated differently.

chronic atrophic gastritis (kron'ik ah-trof'ik gastri'tis) [gastric atrophy] a noncancerous condition that destroys stomach glands, changes gastric juice secretions, and causes the stomach lining to become inflamed. It has been linked to STOMACH CANCER. A causal relationship has not been established. However, gastritis is known to occur before stomach cancer. It may not cause any symptoms, or it may cause vague stomach discomfort, nausea, and vomiting.

chronic cystic mastitis See FIBROCYSTIC CHANGES.

chronic granulocytic leukemia (CGL) See CML.

chronic lymphatic leukemia See CLL.

chronic lymphocytic leukemia See CLL.

chronic lymphogenous leukemia See CLL.

chronic lymphoid leukemia   See CLL.

chronic myelocytic leukemia   See CML.

chronic myelogenous leukemia   See CML.

chronic myeloid leukemia   See CML.

chronic myeloproliferative disorders (MPD)
See MYELOPROLIFERATIVE DISORDERS.

chronic myelosis leukemia   See CML.

chronic ulcerative colitis   See CROHN'S DISEASE.

chronic vulvar dystrophy   a condition in which there is a thickened, whitish area in the vulva. This may precede VULVAR CANCER. Many patients who develop vulvar cancer have a history of chronic vulvar dystrophy.

cigar smoking   Cigar smoke contains most of the same carcinogens and cancer-producing chemicals found in cigarettes, including the human carcinogens (benzene, vinyl chloride, ethylene oxide, arsenic, cadmium, nitrosamines, and polynuclear aromatic hydrocarbons), but at higher levels. Smoking cigars daily can cause cancers of the lung, larynx, esophagus, lip, tongue, mouth, throat, and pancreas. Cancer deaths among men who smoke cigars are 34% higher than nonsmokers. Cigar smokers have four to 10 times the risk of nonsmokers of dying from laryngeal, oral, or esophageal cancers. Since 1993, cigar sales in the United States have increased by about 50%.

cigarettes   See SMOKING.

CIN   See CERVICAL INTRAEPITHELIAL NEOPLASM.

cine esophagography   See ESOPHAGOGRAPHY.

CINV   CHEMOTHERAPY-induced nausea and vomiting

circadian stage dependence (ser"kah-de'an) [circadian rhythm]   using the rhythmic biologic cycle that takes place in people (about every 24 hours) in cancer treatment planning and adminis-tration. These daily rhythmic changes in physiological function and behavior are called circadian. Researchers theorize that chemotherapy may be most effective if administered during certain parts of the circadian rhythm. Programmable pumps are being used that can deliver the bulk of a 24-hour infusion during a preset time (e.g., between 3:00 P.M. and 9:00 P.M.). Studies on the value of this practice are ongoing.

CISCA   a combination of the anticancer drugs CISPLATIN, Cytoxan, and Adriamycin sometimes used in the treatment of cancer of the kidney, bladder, and prostate. See individual drug listings for side effects.
See also COMBINATION CHEMOTHERAPY.

cis-diamminedichloroplatinum   See CISPLATIN.

cisplatin (sis'plah-tin) [cis-platinum,   Platinol, platinum, cis-diamminedichloroplatinum, CDDP] an ALKYLATING agent (anticancer drug) sometimes used in the treatment of cancer of the testes, ovary, head and neck, bladder, prostate, lung, breast, esophagus, and cervix and lymphomas, myeloma, melanoma, and osteogenic sarcoma. It is given by IV (injection into a vein). Common side effects include severe nausea and vomiting. Occasional and rare side effects include bone marrow depression, kidney damage, and hearing and eye problems. Cisplatin is a very commonly used anticancer drug and plays an important role in the treatment of cancer.

cis-platinum   See CISPLATIN.

c-kit   this protein is a tyrosine kinase receptor, a member of the PDGFR family, that is found on GIST and provides the molecular target for the use of Gleevic in this entity. It is detectable clinically by staining of the tumor for CD 117. In theory, other tumors expressing c-kit would also respond to Gleevic.

cladribine   See LEUSTATIN.

Clark's classification system   a way of describing MELANOMA devised by Dr. Wallace Clark, Jr., at the University of Pennsylvania. It classifies the melanoma by how deeply it penetrates the skin. The Clark level correlates with prognosis of cure.

CLB   See LEUKERAN.

clear cell adenocarcinoma (ad"ĕ-no-kar"sĭ-no'mah) a very rare type of VAGINAL CANCER seen in women whose mothers took DES (diethylstilbestrol) during pregnancy.

clinical cancer centers   a network of medical centers that have support from the National Cancer Institute (NCI) for programs to investigate new treatments or for research programs. They are located throughout the United States. See Appendix II for a list of clinical cancer centers.

clinical staging of cancer   See STAGING.

clinical trials [investigational trials]   a systematic evaluation of a possible new cancer treatment conducted with cancer patients after the treatment has had some benefits in animal testing or laboratory testing. The treatment is evaluated for its effectiveness in reducing or eliminating disease and to determine its role in the overall treatment of one or more particular cancers. A clinical trial may be done by the National Cancer Institute, a drug company, or a hospital to determine the most effective dose of a drug, to compare different combinations of treatments, or to determine the effect of the drug on a tumor.

Before a patient takes part in a clinical trial, he or she must sign a form giving his or her INFORMED CONSENT. Participation is completely voluntary, and a patient can leave the trial at any time. Clinical trials are performed progressively in four phases. Following is a brief description of each phase:

- Phase I—the first use of the treatment in humans after studies done on animals have shown the treatment to have an effect on tumors. A phase I trial attempts to find a safe and tolerable dose for humans and to determine whether the treatment is effective against tumors. It is generally appropriate only for patients with a specific widespread disease that has not responded to standard therapies.
- Phase II—attempts to determine which other cancers the treatment may be effective against.
- Phase III—compares the new treatment with the standard treatment for results and SIDE EFFECTS in order to determine whether the new treatment is as good as, or better than, the standard treat-

ment. Patients participating in a phase III trial may be getting a treatment that will replace the current standard treatment.
- Phase IV—refines the integration of the new treatment and determines its place in the PRIMARY TREATMENT plan.

Not everyone is eligible to take part in a clinical trial. Each study requires patients with certain types and stages of cancer and certain health standards. Someone considering taking part in a clinical trial may want to ask the following questions:

— What is the purpose of the study?
— Who has reviewed and approved it?
— Who is sponsoring it?
— What does the study involve? What kinds of tests and treatments?
— What is likely to happen with or without treatment?
— What are other choices and their advantages and disadvantages? (What are the standard treatment for this type of cancer and how do they compare with the treatment used in the study?)
— How could the treatment affect daily life?
— What side effects are expected?
— How long will the study last?
— Is hospitalization required? If so, for how long and how often?
— What are the costs? Will any of the treatments be free?
— If the treatment proves harmful, then what treatment will be done?
— What type of follow-up care is part of the study?

Clinical trials play an important role in cancer, producing new and more effective treatments.

CLL (chronic lymphocytic leukemia) [chronic lymphatic leukemia, chronic lymphogenous leukemia, chronic lymphoid leukemia]   the most common type of leukemia, and the major type of a group of diseases known as "lymphoproliferative disorders." CLL is a disorder in which too many white blood cells are produced in the BONE MARROW, LYMPH SYSTEM, and blood system.

CLL   accounts for about 30% of the leukemias reported in the United States. It progresses slowly and is most often seen in people over the age of 60. It affects two to three times the number of men as women.

The onset of symptoms is slow, with about a quarter of newly diagnosed patients having no symptoms. It is not uncommon for the disease to be discovered during an examination for some other complaint. When symptoms are present, they can include a general feeling of ill health, fatigue, lack of energy, fever, loss of appetite and weight, or night sweats. Diagnostic procedures include blood tests and BONE MARROW BIOPSY.

Following is the NATIONAL CANCER INSTITUTE'S (NCI) STAGING for chronic lymphocytic leukemia:

- Stage 0—a lymphocyte (a type of white blood cell) count greater than 15,000/cubic millimeter
- Stage I—a lymphocyte count greater than 15,000/cubic millimeter and enlargement of lymph nodes
- Stage II—a lymphocyte count greater than 15,000/cubic millimeter, enlargement of lymph nodes, and enlargement of the liver or spleen
- Stage III—a lymphocyte count greater than 15,000/cubic millimeter, anemia with or without lymph node enlargement, or enlargement of the liver or spleen
- Stage IV—a lymphocyte count greater than 15,000/cubic millimeter and a low platelet count with or without enlargement of lymph nodes, liver, or spleen or anemia
- Recurrence—cancer returns after treatment

Treatment depends on the stage of the disease as well as on other factors; measurement of ZAP-70 and a genetic profile may provide prognostic information. LCC is treated with chemotherapy and/or monoclonal antibodfies, less frequently radiation. For specific information on the latest stage-of-the-art treatment, by stage, call NCI's Cancer Information Service at 1-800-4-CANCER (1-800-422-6237), or for a TTY: 1-800-332-8615 (1-800-422-6237).

See also LEUKEMIA.

cloacogenic cancer (klo″ah-ko-jen′ik) [basaloid carcinoma]   a rare type of ANAL CANCER.

clomiphene (klo′mĭ-fēn)   an experimental ANTI-ESTROGEN drug once used in the treatment of some patients with breast cancer.

cm   See CENTIMETER.

CMF   a combination of the anticancer drugs CYTOXAN, METHOTREXATE, and 5-FU used in the treatment of breast cancer. CMF was the first proven ADJUVANT THERAPY. See individual drug listings for side effects.

See also COMBINATION CHEMOTHERAPY.

CMFP   a combination of the anticancer drugs CYTOXAN, METHOTREXATE, 5-FU, and PREDNISONE sometimes used in the treatment of breast cancer. See individual drug listings for side effects.

See also COMBINATION CHEMOTHERAPY.

CMFVP [Cooper regimen]   a combination of the anticancer drugs CYTOXAN, METHOTREXATE, 5-FU, VINCRISTINE, and PREDNISONE sometimes used in the treatment of breast cancer. See individual drug listings for side effects.

See also COMBINATION CHEMOTHERAPY.

CML (chronic myelogenous leukemia) (mi″ĕ-loj′ĕ-nus)   one of the four main types of LEUKEMIA (chronic myelocytic, chronic myelosis, chronic granulocytic, GGL, chronic myeloid), accounting for 20% of all leukemia cases in Western countries. It usually affects adults between the ages of 30 and 50. In 1999 there were approximately 4,500 new cases diagnosed and 2,300 deaths attributed to the disease. In CML an overproduction of white cells results in too many white cells in both the bloodstream and the BONE MARROW.

There are no obvious symptoms early in the disease. CML is frequently discovered during a routine examination. Diagnostic procedures include a COMPLETE BLOOD COUNT and a BONE MARROW BIOPSY.

CML is associated with a unique CHROMOSOMAL ABNORMALITY called the PHILADELPHIA CHROMOSOME or Ph chromosome. It was the first human cancer with a consistent CHROMOSOME MARKER. Ph represents translocation of a small part of one chromosome for another. The cure of CML requires a treatment that results in the disappearance of this marker.

The National Cancer Institute (NCI) has broken down chronic myelogenous leukemia into the following phases:

- chronic phase—less than 5% BLAST CELLS (immature cells) and PROMYELOCYTES (cells not fully developed) in the bone marrow

- accelerated phase—5 to 30% blasts in the bone marrow
- blastic phase—greater than 30% blasts in the peripheral blood or bone marrow
- meningeal—involvement of the CENTRAL NERVOUS SYSTEM; this is rare.

Treatment depends on the phase (stage) of the disease as well as other factors. The major forms of treatment for CML are chemotherapy, biological treatment (INTERFERON), BONE MARROW TRANSPLANTATION (ALLOGENEIC or SYNGENEIC). For specific information on the latest state-of-the art treatment, by phase or stage of CML, call NCI's Cancer Information Service at 1-800-4-CANCER (1-800-422-6237), or for a TTY: 1-800-332-8615.

CMPD (chronic myeloproliferative disorders) See MYELOPROLIFERATIVE DISORDERS.

CMV See CYTOMEGALOVIRUS.

CNS See CENTRAL NERVOUS SYSTEM.

CNS preventive therapy [CNS prophylaxis] a procedure that may be used in the treatment of leukemia, primarily acute lymphocytic leukemia. It generally consists of WHOLE BRAIN IRRADIATION combined with the injection of anticancer drugs. It is done to prevent a recurrence of leukemia in the CENTRAL NERVOUS SYSTEM.

CNS prophylaxis See CNS PREVENTIVE THERAPY.

COAP a combination of the anticancer drugs CYTOXAN, Oncovin (VINCRISTINE), ARA-C, and PREDNISONE sometimes used in the treatment of AML. See individual drug listings for side effects.
See also COMBINATION CHEMOTHERAPY.

COB a combination of the anticancer drugs CISPLATIN, Oncovin (VINCRISTINE), and BLEOMYCIN sometimes used in the treatment of head and neck cancers. See individual drug listings for side effects.
See also COMBINATION CHEMOTHERAPY.

cobalt-60 a radioactive isotope of the element cobalt that is widely used in EXTERNAL RADIATION THERAPY.
See also COBALT TREATMENT and NUCLEAR SCAN.

cobalt machine See COBALT TREATMENT.

cobalt treatment a type of EXTERNAL RADIATION THERAPY using the metal cobalt that has been made radioactive. The radioactive cobalt (isotope) is enclosed in the cobalt machine. The radioactive beam is emitted when a window in the machine is opened. The penetration of the radioactive beams into the body is a factor of how fast the electrons are programmed to hit the body.
See also RADIATION THERAPY.

codeine (ko'dēn) a NARCOTIC drug used to relieve or control pain. It is given by injection into a muscle or taken by mouth. It is available by prescription only.
See also ANALGESIC.

coffee See CAFFEINE.

cohort study large groups of people are followed over a long period of time. Researchers try to identify factors associated with illnesses that develop in some of the people in the group. One of the most well-known studies is the 45-year-old Framingham Heart study, sponsored by the National Heart, Lung and Blood Institute (NHLBI), part of the National Institutes of Health (NIH). (See also http://www.framingham.com/heart)

cold knife conization See CONIZATION.

cold spot a possible indication of a malignant (cancerous) tumor in the thyroid that shows up on a thyroid scan. After a small dose of radioactive material is swallowed, an instrument evaluates the absorption of the material by the tumor. If there is little absorption, the lump is called "cold," indicating that the lump may be cancerous.

colectomy (ko-lek'to-me) surgical removal of part of the colon or the whole colon. It is a treatment of choice for colon cancer and other disorders.

Coley's toxin [Coley's fluid] a preparation of bacterial toxins once used in the therapy of cancer. It is currently not recognized as a useful treatment. It is named after the surgeon W. B. Coley.

colon (kō-lin) the middle section of the large bowel, the last five or six feet of the large intestine.

The colon is part of the body's digestive system. It is divided into the ascending portion (the right side) and the descending or sigmoid portion (the left side). See COLON CANCER.

colon cancer   cancer of the large bowel or colon, which is the last six feet of the intestine.

People at the greatest risk are those who are over 40, have a family history of cancer of the colon, rectum, or the female organs, have polyps in the colon, or have a history of ulcerative colitis (ulcers in the lining of the large intestines).

Symptoms may include rectal bleeding, blood in the stool, jet-black stool, a change in bowel habits, alternating between constipation and diarrhea, crampy abdominal pain, weakness, loss of weight, and loss of appetite. (These symptoms can also be caused by other, noncancerous conditions.)

Diagnostic procedures may include DIGITAL RECTAL EXAM, SIGMOIDOSCOPY, LOWER GI SERIES, COLONOSCOPY, CEA, and BIOPSY.

Testing the tumor for a genetic profile (MSI) has provided a new method of assessing prognoses.

There is more than one way of staging colon cancer. One method is DUKES STAGING SYSTEM; another is the modified ASTLER COLLER STAGING system. Following are the three most common methods of staging used by the National Cancer Institute (NCI):

- Stage 0 or carcinoma in situ—cancer that is found only in the top lining of the colon
- Stage I, or Dukes A, or MAC A or B1—cancer that has spread beyond the top lining of the colon to the second and third layers and involves the inside wall of the colon, but has not spread to the outer wall of the colon or outside the colon
- Stage II, or Dukes B, or MAC B2 or B3—cancer that has spread outside the colon to nearby tissue but has not gone into the LYMPH NODES
- Stage III, or Dukes C, or MAC C1–C3—cancer that has spread to nearby lymph nodes but has not spread to other parts of the body
- Stage IV, or Dukes D—cancer that has spread to other parts of the body
- Recurrent—cancer has returned to the same site or another part of the body after treatment.

Treatment of colon cancer depends on the stage of the disease, the general health of the patient, and other factors. SURGERY is the most common treatment. There are a number of different surgical procedures used, depending on the extent of disease. If the cancer is found in a small bulging piece of tissue (polyp) it will be removed in a POLYPECTOMY. If the cancer is larger, the cancer and some tissue around it will be surgically removed in a WEDGE RESECTION. If more cancer is present, a BOWEL RESECTION will be performed, during which nearby lymph nodes will be removed. If the cancer is more extensive, a COLOSTOMY may be performed. Other treatments include RADIATION THERAPY, CHEMOTHERAPY, and CLINICAL TRIALS. For specific information on the latest state-of-the-art treatment by stage, call NCI's Cancer Information Service at 1-800-4-CANCER (1-800-422-6237), or for a TTY: 1-800-332-8615.

See also COLON/RECTAL CANCER.

colon/rectal cancer [colorectal cancer]   the presence of cancerous cells in the colon (the last six feet of the large intestine), the rectum (the last eight to ten inches of the colon), or cecum (a pouch in the lower right side of the abdomen; the first part of the large intestine). Because the rectum is part of the colon, COLON CANCER and RECTAL CANCER are often referred to as one. Colon/rectal cancer is the second most common cancer in the United States. Colon/rectal cancer is more prevalent in densely populated, industrialized regions than in rural areas. There are high rates in North America and northern and western Europe. Rates are lower in less developed areas such as Africa, Latin America, and most of Asia.

Colon cancer occurs in more than twice as many people as rectal cancer. Less than 6% of the cases occur in people under 50; incidence increases until age 75, when it tapers off. The average age at the time of diagnosis is 60. Those at risk include people with chronic ulcerative colitis (ulcers in the lining of the large intestines) and CROHN'S DISEASE, women with a history of breast cancer, and people with a family history of colon/rectal cancer (FAMILIAL MULTIPLE POLYPOSIS OF THE COLON.)

Animal experiments and population studies suggest that diet plays a role in the development of colon/rectal cancer. It appears that increased FIBER in the diet can reduce the risk, and that lowering the amount of fat in the diet also reduces the risk of colon/rectal cancer. Scientists think that dietary fat increases the amount of bile acids in the colon. The bile fats may damage the lining or may be converted to secondary bile acids, which are known to cause tumors in animals. Fat in the diet may also increase the amount of damaging chemicals in the bowel, which may result in changes in the cell membrane and/or affect hormone regulation. Other dietary factors are also being investigated for a possible role in the development of colon/rectal cancer. Although a proven link with cancer has not been established, studies are being pursued with chemicals produced by frying, smoking, or grilling meat and fish and certain nitrogen-containing compounds. Another area of investigation is dietary factors that can inhibit the development of cancer. For example, it has been shown that certain increased levels of vitamins and minerals can reduce the number of colon cancers in animals. The National Cancer Institute (NCI) is investigating what role, if any, vitamins A, C, and E, BETA-CAROTENE, CALCIUM, and NSAIDS may play in preventing colon cancer in humans.

The role of heredity is not fully understood. It appears that roughly 5 to 7% of colon/rectal cancer may be affected by heredity. However, in families where it appears at an unusually early age, children are at a much greater risk of developing the disease. Abnormal genes have been found in patients with some forms of colon/rectal cancer. Tests are being developed to determine who carries these genes long before cancer appears.

Symptoms of colon/rectal cancer may include

- diarrhea or constipation
- blood in or on the stool (either bright red or very dark in color)
- stools that are narrower than usual
- general stomach discomfort (bloating, fullness, cramps)
- frequent gas pains
- a feeling that the bowel doesn't empty completely
- loss of weight with no reason
- constant tiredness

These symptoms can be caused by many other problems. If any persist for two weeks, a physician should be seen.

Diagnostic procedures may include a digital RECTAL EXAM, SIGMOIDOSCOPY, OCCULT BLOOD STOOL TEST, COLONOSCOPY, a LOWER GI SERIES, and BIOPSY.

For staging and treatment options see COLON CANCER and RECTAL CANCER.

colonoscope See COLONOSCOPY.

colonoscopy (ko″lon-os′ko-pe) a procedure used for the examination of the colon (the lower part of the large intestine). A lighted, tubular instrument with a viewing device called a colonoscope is inserted through the rectum. The patient is usually under a local anesthetic. Tiny samples of tissue can be taken for BIOPSY.

colony-stimulating factors (CSF) [growth factors, hematopoietic growth factors] naturally occurring substances that stimulate the BONE MARROW to produce white and red blood cells and PLATELETS. They can be artificially reproduced by new technology. They were first discovered in the mid 1960s. Colony-stimulating factors are a prominent part of cancer's newest form of treatment—BIOLOGICAL THERAPY.

Researchers have high hopes for CSFs. Many are optimistic that they will eventually play a major role in the treatment of cancer and are investigating their use in a number of different roles. Because CSFs stimulate the bone marrow to produce more blood cells, they may be used to enable patients on chemotherapy (anticancer drugs) to tolerate larger doses that are more effective in fighting cancer. As chemotherapy kills "good" cells along with the "bad" cells, the CSFs could foster a faster recovery of the bone marrow and its ability to produce blood cells. CSFs may also be useful in helping people with compromised or weakened IMMUNE SYSTEMS recover from infections by boosting the production of white blood cells that fight infections. CSFs may be a drug enhancer, increasing the effectiveness of anticancer drugs, and they may be used in helping to separate cancer cells from bone marrow that has been removed from a patient's body. Among the CSFs being developed are:

- interleukin-1 (IL-1) (hematopoietin-1)—stimulates the growth of early, immature forms of bone marrow cells;

- interleukin-2 (IL-2) (adesleukin, Proleukin, Teceleukin, recombinant, and rlL-2)—stimulates the growth and activities of a wide range of cells
- interleukin-3 (IL-3) (multi-CSF)—stimulates the growth of many bone marrow elements
- interleukin-4 (IL-4) (B-cell stimulatory factor-1)—enhances B cell growth and antibody production
- interleukin-5 (IL-5) (eosinophil CSF)—stimulates the production of the blood cells known as eosinophils
- interleukin-6 (IL-6) (thrombopoietin)—stimulates the production of platelets
- interleukin-11 (IL-11) (Neumega, Oprelvekin)—used to prevent thrombocytopenia
- GM-CSF (granulocyte/macrophage CSF, sargramostim, Leukine, Prokine) supports the growth of bone marrow elements known as GRANULOCYTES and MACROPHAGES
- G-CSF (granulocyte CSF, Neupogen, filgrastim) stimulates the growth of granulocytes and serves as a growth factor for peripheral blood stem cell mobilization
- erythropoietin (EPO, Epogen Procrit, epoetin alpha, Eprex)—stimulates the production of red blood cells

colostomate (ko-los′to-māt) term used for a person who has had a COLOSTOMY.

colostomy (ko-los′to-me) a surgical procedure that may be used in the treatment of COLON/RECTAL CANCER if the tumor is low in the rectum. The tumor and tissue around it are removed. A new opening in the body is made for the elimination of waste. A section of the colon is attached to the abdominal wall to create the artificial opening (stoma) through which waste material from the body can pass into a bag. The colostomy may be permanent—if the lower part of the rectum has to be removed; or temporary—to give the colon a chance to heal. Only 10 to 15% of colostomies are permanent. See Appendix for support organizations.

colposcope See COLPOSCOPY.

colposcopy (kol-pos′ko-pe) [vaginoscopy] examination of the vagina and cervix with a colposcope (a magnifying instrument that contains a light). The doctor uses a speculum to separate the walls of the vagina to expose the surface. The doctor may then swab the area with a brown liquid (this is called a SCHILLER TEST), after which he or she views the area through the colposcope. The brown liquid makes any abnormal area show up as white or yellow spots. The doctor can also remove tissue for a BIOPSY, which may cause some minor discomfort like a menstrual cramp. The procedure takes 10 or 15 minutes and can be done in a doctor's office. There may be a brown vaginal discharge for a few days, but there are no long-term effects.

combination chemotherapy (ke″mo-ther′ah-pe) the use of a number (generally between two and four) of different anticancer drugs together to treat cancer. This is done for a number of reasons. By using several different drugs, cells in the different phases in the cancer CELL CYCLE are attacked by the specific drug to which they are vulnerable during that phase, thereby killing off as many cancer cells as possible. Using a combination of drugs decreases the possibility that some cancer cells will "escape" because they have, or have built up, resistance to the one chemotherapy agent. In addition, when several drugs are used together, the cancer cells' ability to repair damage is decreased and the cancer cells' ability to develop a resistance to the drugs is delayed or prevented. Combination chemotherapy is the most effective treatment for most cancers.

See also CHEMOTHERAPY.

combination therapy [combined modality therapy] using more than one therapy—chemotherapy, surgery, radiation, immunotherapy, etc.—for the most effective response.

combined modality therapy See COMBINATION THERAPY.

comedocarcinoma (kŏ-me″do-kar″sĭ-no′mah) a type of BREAST CANCER that starts in the lining of the duct and grows into the duct until it is filled. It is not likely to spread beyond the breast.

COMLA a combination of the anticancer drugs CYTOXAN, Oncovin (VINCRISTINE), METHOTREXATE, LEUCOVORIN RESCUE, and ARA-C sometimes used in the treatment of non-Hodgkin's lymphoma. See individual drug listings for side effects.

See also COMBINATION CHEMOTHERAPY.

Community Clinical Oncology Program (CCOP) a program funded by the NATIONAL CANCER INSTITUTE (NCI) to link community-based doctors with the CLINICAL TRIALS COOPERATIVE GROUP PROGRAM, cancer centers, and public health departments for participation in NCI-approved treatment and CLINICAL TRIALS. The program, which has been funded by the NCI since 1983, promotes greater participation by patients in clinical trials and disperses the latest research findings to the community level.

compassionate drug certain experimental agents under investigation, not yet released to the public, that may be provided to individuals on a "compassionate" basis. A qualified physician must make the request, usually through the drug company. The drug company is not allowed to charge for the drug, and special permission must be obtained from the Food and Drug Administration. This is usually done in cases where all other standard treatments for the patient have been exhausted. Detailed records are kept about the use and response of the agent.

Compazine See ANTIEMETIC.

complement system a series of about 25 proteins in the body that work to help antibodies destroy antigens. The proteins either puncture the cell membrane of the bacteria or facilitate PHAGOCYTOSIS. The complement system also helps rid the body of antigen/antibody complexes.

See also ANTIGEN and ANTIBODY.

complementary and alternative medicine (CAM) See NATIONAL CENTER FOR COMPLEMENTARY AND ALTERNATIVE MEDICINE.

complementary medicine a therapy that is generally called complementary when it is used in addition to conventional treatments. Some examples are mind/body control interventions such as visualization or relaxation; manual healing, including acupressure and massage; vitamins or herbal products; and acupuncture. When the treatment is used instead of the convention treatment it is known as alternative medicine.

See NATIONAL CENTER FOR COMPLEMENTARY AND ALTERNATIVE MEDICINE.

complete blood count (CBC) a test to check the number of red cells, white cells, and platelets in a sample of blood. The blood may be taken from a fingertip or vein. Other factors monitored in the blood count are the hemoglobin (the amount of oxygen-carrying protein) and the hematocrit (percentage of red blood cells). A retic or reticulocyte count (percentage of young red cells) may be requested separately but can be performed on the same blood sample. The results of a CBC can supply a wealth of information helpful in the detection of ANEMIA, an infection, or a blood-clotting problem. Since CHEMOTHERAPY (anticancer drugs) can cause a drop in the number of blood cells being produced by the bone marrow, a BONE MARROW DEPRESSION, a blood count is usually done before every chemotherapy treatment. If the doctor decides that the counts are too low, he or she may postpone the treatment.

complete mastectomy See SIMPLE MASTECTOMY.

complete remission See REMISSION.

Comprehensive Cancer Center a medical center designated as such by the National Cancer Institute (NCI). NCI-designated Comprehensive Cancer Centers conduct research and provide services directly to cancer patients. These facilities must demonstrate expertise in each of three areas: laboratory, clinical, and behavioral and population-based research. Comprehensive Cancer Centers are expected to initiate and conduct early phase, innovative clinical trials and to participate in the NCI's cooperative groups by providing leadership and recruiting patients for trials. Comprehensive Cancer Centers must also conduct activities in outreach and education, and provide information on advances in health care for both health care professionals and the public. (See Appendix II for a listing of NCI Comprehensive Cancer Centers, and Appendix III for a listing of NCI's Clinical Cancer Centers.)

To be so designated, an institution must first secure a peer-reviewed cancer center support grant from NCI. Then a review committee made up of nonfederal scientists determines if the centers meet set criteria. The latest criteria, revised in 1989, require that the centers:

1. have a strong core of basic laboratory research in several fields;
2. find ways to transfer research findings into clinical practice;
3. conduct clinical studies, especially ones of importance to the community served by the center;
4. participate in high-priority CLINICAL TRIALS;
5. conduct research in the areas of cancer prevention and control;
6. provide research training and continuing education for health care professionals;
7. offer a wide range of cancer information services for patients, health professionals, and the surrounding community;
8. provide community service and outreach activities related to cancer prevention and control.

There are 394 comprehensive cancer centers, and 22 cancer centers in the United States (for a total of 61 centers). The comprehensive cancer center program evolved during the 1960s when there was an emphasis on expanding the cancer research base at various institutions throughout the United States. The program was formally authorized by Congress in the National Cancer Act of 1971. There are a growing number of freestanding comprehensive cancer centers that have been established independent of the NCI generally following the same criteria such as Salick Health Care Network and others.

See Appendix II for a list of Comprehensive Cancer Centers.

computed tomography   See CT SCAN.

computerized axial tomography   See CT SCAN.

computerized mammography   See DIGITAL MAMMOGRAPHY.

computerized transaxial tomography   See CT SCAN.

cone biopsy   See CONIZATION.

congenital (kon-jen′ĭ-tal) a condition in the body existing at or before birth.

congenital brain tumor (kon-jen′ĭ-tal) a tumor that has existed in the brain since birth. These include dermoids (sometimes called dermoid cysts or cystic teratomas), teratomas, cholesteatomas, and craniopharyngiomas.

conization (kon″ĭ-za′shun) [cone biopsy, cold knife conization, surgical conization] microscopic examination of a small, wedge-shaped tissue sample surgically obtained from the CERVIX for cancer cells. The amount of tissue removed depends on the extent of abnormal cells. This surgical procedure may be performed for the diagnosis (and sometimes treatment) of CERVICAL CANCER. It is usually performed in a hospital since it requires general anesthesia. Complications after the surgery may include heavy bleeding up to a week or so later. Conization generally has been replaced by the noninvasive COLPOSCOPY.

conjugated equine estrogen [Premarin] See ESTROGEN and CARCINOGENS.

conjugated estrogens a mixture of naturally occurring forms of estrogen. They are used as a prescription drug for treating a number of different conditions, including treatment following oophorectomy and treatment for breast and prostate cancer. The Federal Drug Administration has ruled that estrogens for general use must carry patient and physician warning labels concerning use, risks and contraindications.

See also ESTROGEN REPLACEMENT THERAPY.

connective tissue cancer   See SOFT-TISSUE SARCOMA.

consolidation therapy a way of treating LEUKEMIA. After the patient is initially treated with INDUCTION THERAPY and is in REMISSION for several weeks, a second phase of treatment (consolidation therapy) is started to destroy any remaining cancer cells, thereby preventing a relapse. Patients receive repeated cycles of the same, or different, combinations of drugs. The dose is not as high as during induction therapy, and the drugs are usually given over a shorter period of time.

constipation   a condition in which evacuation of feces from the bowel (intestines) is difficult and infrequent; and/or the passage of dry, hard stool. In cancer patients, this can be a side effect of chemotherapy. It can also be a result of a tumor causing blockage, HYPERCALCEMIA, pain medication, or an insufficient amount of fiber, bulk, or fluid in the diet.

To avoid constipation, or alleviate the condition, patients are advised to eat a high FIBER diet and drink about three quarts of liquids a day. Prunes can also be added to the diet. Patients are also advised to maintain physical activity to keep up muscle tone and promote the motility of the GASTROINTESTINAL TRACT. Medical agents can also be used in the treatment of constipation.

contact thermography   See THERMOGRAPHY.

continent ileal reservoir (il'e-al) [Kock pouch] a URINARY DIVERSION that is entirely contained within the body for patients who have had their bladder removed. A piece of the ileum and/or colon is used to create an artificial urine reservoir. The ureters drain into the new, internal storage area. The patient then drains the internal storage area by inserting a CATHETER through a stoma, an opening made in the abdominal wall during the surgery. It must be drained about every six hours.

continuation therapy   See MAINTENANCE THERAPY.

continuous infusion chemotherapy (ke"mother'ah-pe)   delivery of lower doses of CHEMOTHERAPY (anticancer drugs) over a long time using a portable battery-operated pump. One example is the treatment of METASTATIC colon cancer with 5-FU over a period of weeks. Many of the standard chemotherapy agents may be used in this way, although there are few standardized regimens. Continuous infusion is based on the concept that some drugs may perform best if the tumor being treated is exposed to the agent for many days or weeks. Because of better technology with CATHETER placement and pump design, this is an area of active investigation. Side effects of the drug are often different than those commonly seen when the same drug is given by IV (injection into the vein) over a short period of time.

contrast dye   See CONTRAST MEDIUM.

contrast film   a special film used for an X-RAY when a foreign substance is put into the body to obtain a better picture of an organ.

contrast medium [contrast dye]   a substance used during some diagnostic procedures to enable parts of the body to show up better on X-RAYS. In most cases, the contrast medium is injected into the body. For example, in an IVP a small amount of a special iodine-containing solution is injected into a vein before the test is performed. Contrast mediums may be administered in other ways, as well, depending on the procedure. For example, in a LOWER GI SERIES barium goes into the body through a tube inserted into the rectum. In an UPPER GI SERIES the barium is swallowed.

contrast X-ray   a picture of the body taken using electromagnetic waves (X-RAY) in conjunction with a CONTRAST MEDIUM. A contrast medium used in an X-ray can enhance visualization.

Cooper regimen   See CMFVP.

COP   a combination of the anticancer drugs CYTOXAN, Oncovin (VINCRISTINE), and PREDNISONE sometimes used in the treatment of NON-HODGKIN'S LYMPHOMA. See individual drug listings for side effects.

See also COMBINATION CHEMOTHERAPY.

COP-BLAM   a combination of the anticancer drugs CYTOXAN, Oncovin (VINCRISTINE), PREDNISONE, BLEOMYCIN, ADRIAMYCIN, and PROCARBAZINE sometimes used in the treatment of NON-HODGKIN'S LYMPHOMA. See individual drug listings for side effects.

See also COMBINATION CHEMOTHERAPY.

COPE   a combination of the anticancer drugs CYTOXAN, Oncovin (VINCRISTINE), Platinol (CISPLATIN), and ETOPOSIDE sometimes used in the treatment of LEUKEMIA. See individual drug listings for side effects.

See also COMBINATION CHEMOTHERAPY.

COPP   a combination of the anticancer drugs CYTOXAN, Oncovin (VINCRISTINE), PROCARBAZINE, and PREDNISONE sometimes used in the treatment of NON-HODGKIN'S LYMPHOMA. See individual drug listings for side effects.

See also COMBINATION CHEMOTHERAPY.

cord blood transplantation   cord blood is found in the umbilical cords. It is a valuable source of stem cells that can be used in transplantation procedures. In the past cord blood was considered medical waste and discarded. Then it was discovered that the fetal cells are a rich source of active stem cells for transplantation to other people. They are now harvested, characterized, and stored in select blood banks. Cord cell transplantations are being evaluated for when they would be most appropriate as well as their effectiveness.

cordectomy (kor-dek′to-me) [also called cordotomy, not to be confused with the cordotomy that is used to relieve pain]   surgical removal of the vocal cord. This is one treatment for laryngeal cancer.

cordotomy (kor-dot′o-me)   a surgical procedure to relieve pain by "interrupting" its transmission through nerve pathways by cutting the bundles of nerves in the spinal cord that transmit the pain. It may be done by open surgery or percutaneously (through the skin) by STEREOTACTIC SURGERY. The procedure can have a serious side effect, as the nerves that are cut also transmit other sensations such as pressure and temperature; no longer having those sensations puts a patient at a greater risk of injury to the affected area. In 7% to 10% of the patients, pain develops in the side opposite the cordotomy. And in some patients, while pain is relieved in the initial site, pain at another site becomes as severe as the original pain that was alleviated.

The pain-relieving effects of a cordotomy are sometimes temporary. When the procedure is first done, it is successful in about 90% of the patients. That figure drops to 80% after three months. At the end of a year, about 40% of the patients report the return of pain.

Cordotomy also refers to a CORDECTOMY, surgical removal of a vocal chord.

core needle biopsy [needle biopsy, wide-core needle biopsy]   removal of tissue for microscopic examination for cancer cells. A special needle is used through which a minuscule cutting instrument can be inserted to cut and extract the tissue sample. This procedure may be used in the diagnosis of a number of different cancers, including prostate, liver, breast, and bone marrow. In the diagnosis of PROSTATE CANCER, the needle is inserted either through the area between the scrotum and anus or through the rectum.

CORT   See ADRENOCORTICOIDS.

corticosteroid   an important hormone commonly used in the treatment of cancer. See ADRENOCORTICOIDS.

cortisone   an important hormone commonly used in the treatment of cancer. See ADRENOCORTICOIDS.

Cosmegen (kos′mĕ-jen) [DACT, actinomycin D, dactinomycin]   an ANTIBIOTIC anticancer drug sometimes used in the treatment of testicular cancer, melanoma, CHORIOCARCINOMA, WILMS' TUMOR, NEUROBLASTOMA, RHABDOMYOSARCOMA, EWING'S SARCOMA, RETINOBLASTOMA, and KAPOSI'S SARCOMA. It is given by IV (injection into a vein). Common side effects may include nausea and vomiting, swelling of the vein, and hair loss. Occasional or rare side effects may include mouth sores, BONE MARROW DEPRESSION, skin rash, acne, loss of appetite, diarrhea, fever, and fatigue. Rare second malignancies have been reported after this treatment.

Cowden syndrome   a hereditary cancer predisposition syndrome characterized by multiple HAMARTOMAS with a high risk of benign and malignant tumors of the thyroid, breast, and endometrium.

CP   a combination of the anticancer drugs CYTOXAN and Platinol (CISPLATIN) sometimes used in the treatment of ovarian cancer. See individual drug listings for side effects.

See also COMBINATION CHEMOTHERAPY.

CPT-11   See CAMPTOSAR.

CPT (current procedural terminology) code   a listing of descriptive terms and identifying codes for reporting medical services and procedures performed by doctors. This "uniform language" provides an effective way for physicians, patients, and third parties to communicate with one another. The CPT code was initiated in 1966.

The CPT code serves a wide variety of functions. It is the most widely accepted terminology for the reporting of physician procedures and services under government and private health insurance programs. It is used administratively for processing claims and developing guidelines for medical care review. And it can be used in medical education and research by providing a basis for local, regional, and national comparisons. Because the medical field changes so rapidly, with some terms becoming obsolete and others being added, the American Medical Association updates the CPT code annually.

CR (complete remission)   See REMISSION.

cranial   pertaining to the head.

craniopharyngioma (kra″ne-o-fah-rin″je-o′mah) a noncancerous tumor of the brain that can occur in the area of the pituitary, usually in children.
See also CONGENITAL BRAIN TUMOR.

craniopharynglioma   See   CONGENITAL   BRAIN TUMOR.

craniotomy (kra″ne-ot′o-me)   a surgical procedure in which the skull is cut open and a piece is removed so that the brain is exposed and a benign (noncancerous) or malignant (cancerous) tumor is removed. The piece of skull is then put back in place or a metal or fabric covering is used to close the opening. A craniotomy may also be performed in the treatment of pituitary cancer as well as a number of other conditions.

Crohn's disease (krōnz) [chronic ulcerative colitis, regional enteritis, regional ileitis]   a chronic, or long-term, inflammation of part of the digestive tract. It usually occurs in the final section of the small intestine. Symptoms of Crohn's disease may be periodic cramps, diarrhea, a general sense of feeling ill, and a slight fever. People with Crohn's disease are at a higher risk of developing intestinal or COLON RECTAL CANCER.

cross resistance   See DRUG RESISTANCE.

crossover chemotherapy   a change in the drugs being used in the treatment of a patient's cancer. The second set of drugs uses different cancer inhibiting mechanisms from the first. This may be done to prevent a building up of resistance to the first set of drugs and/or when the cancer has not responded to the initial therapy.

cryosurgery (kri″o-sur′jer-e) [cryotherapy, freezing surgery]   a surgical procedure using liquid nitrogen or carbon dioxide to destroy a tumor by freezing. The substance is placed in a hollow metal probe that is inserted into the tumor or applied to its surface. The procedure may be repeated several times, during the same operation, to make sure it has destroyed the tumor. Cryosurgery may be used in the treatment of LIVER CANCER, PROSTATE CANCER, CERVICAL CANCER, and skin cancer. It can be done in a doctor's office, but it does require special training and skill.

cryotherapy   See CRYOSURGERY.

cryptorchidism (krip-tor′kĭ-dizm)   undescended testicles. This is a risk factor in TESTICULAR CANCER.

CSF   See COLONY-STIMULATING FACTOR.

CSRA (Chemo-Sensitivity and Resistance Assay) an in vitro laboratory assay done to evaluate the most appropriate chemotherapy or combination of therapies. It is done by exposing a portion of tumor tissue removed from the patient by biopsy to a panel of chemotherapeutic agents. The goal of this test is to be more predictive than the traditional methods of choice. However, these tests remain controversial, not universally accepted, and expensive; an insurance reimbursement is not assured.

CT   a combination of the anticancer drugs cytarabine (ARA-C) and thioguanine (6-TG) sometimes used in the treatment of childhood ANLL. See individual drug listings for side effects.
See also COMBINATION CHEMOTHERAPY.

CT scan [CAT (computerized axial tomography) scan, computerized transaxial tomography, computed tomography, ACTA (automatic computerized transverse axial)]   a diagnostic procedure combining an X-RAY with a computer to produce highly detailed cross-sectional pictures (slices) of the entire body and/or brain. The pictures have a three-dimensional quality and show very small differences that are present in soft tissue, as well as bone, in the body. It is generally 100 times more sensitive than X-rays. It was first used in 1972.

An IV (injection into the vein) or oral contrast may also be required for optimal results in certain circumstances. The CT scan uses a minimal amount of radiation (an amount comparable to that used in a dental exam) and is a painless procedure with no after effects. Frequently the patient can take the test without undressing.

During the test, the patient lies very still on a stretcher-like table. The scanner moves around the patient's body taking X-rays from different angles (the table can be moved as well). As with traditional X-rays, the patient is told to hold his or her breath while each picture is taken. The pictures are processed by a computer. The final image, called a composite picture, appears on a cathode-ray tube, a device similar to a television picture tube and screen. The image can be printed on paper and can be stored on magnetic tape or disc, and it can also be transmitted digitally.

The CT scan is very useful in the diagnosis of brain disorders and in the detection of cancers that began in or have spread to internal organs. It is used in the diagnostic and METASTATIC WORKUP of many cancers, including those of the lung, brain, breast, bladder, prostate, liver, adrenal glands, lymph nodes, spine, spleen, uterus, ovaries, and pancreas.

CTL [cytoxic T cell]   See KILLER CELLS.

CTX   See CYTOXAN.

CTZ   See CHEMORECEPTOR TRIGGER ZONE.

culdocentesis (kul″do-sen-te′sis)   a procedure in which a doctor inserts a needle through the vaginal wall and removes fluid from the space surrounding the ovaries. The fluid is then studied for the presence of abnormal or malignant cells. This procedure is not considered appropriate for routine screening.

culdoscope   See CULDOSCOPY.

culdoscopy (kul-dos′-ko-pe)   a visual examination of female genital organs and pelvic tissue by a lighted, tubular instrument (culdoscope) that is inserted through an incision in the wall of the vagina. This may be used in the diagnosis of ovarian cancer, endometrial cancer, and fallopian tubes cancer.

CUP (carcinoma of undetermined primary origin)
See UNKNOWN PRIMARY.

cure   the successful treatment of a disease. With cancer, the use of the word *cure* can be somewhat ambiguous. Generally, it is a state in which the cancer has been successfully treated and will never return. However, in practical terms, the absence of symptoms (being cancer free) for five years after treatment is considered a cure for many different kinds of cancers. The rationale is that the cancer will usually become symptomatic within five years if it has spread to other areas. There are exceptions. In some cases a person may not be considered cured until he or she has been cancer free for a substantially longer period of time. IN SITU cancer, cancer in its earliest stage that has not spread into adjacent tissue, is usually considered cured after treatment. Basal cell and squamous cell skin cancers are also usually considered cured after treatment. Hodgkin's disease and testicular cancer are also examples of adult cancers curable with treatment now available, even when in an advanced stage.

curet   See CURETTE.

curettage (ku″rĕ-tahzh′)   surgical scraping or cleaning of a body cavity or organ. Curettage is the procedure used most often to treat basal cell carcinoma. It may also be used in the diagnosis of CERVICAL CANCER, when the lining of the uterus is scraped to obtain cells for a BIOPSY.

See also D & C.

curette (ku-ret′) [curet]   a spoon-shaped surgical instrument used to scrape and remove material from the wall of a body cavity or the skin in a CURETTAGE. In cancer this may be done to obtain tissue for a BIOPSY or to remove a cancerous tumor (usually on the skin).

current procedural terminology See CPT CODE.

Cushing's syndrome See PITUITARY TUMOR.

cutaneous melanoma See MELANOMA.

cutaneous metastases (ku-ta′ne-us mĕ-tas′tah-sēz) the spread of cancer from another site to the skin. Occasionally, cutaneous metastases are the first sign of cancer. They are not common, occurring in 2.7 to 4.4% of cancer patients, most frequently in women with advanced breast cancer and men with advanced bronchogenic carcinoma. Cutaneous metastases can also metastasize from melanoma and cancer of the ovaries, the oral cavity, the colon/rectal area, and stomach as well as other primary sites. The lesions on the skin develop as hard, immovable nodules, plaque formations, and ulcerating wounds. Most occur on the front of the trunk of the body. The arms and legs are rarely affected.

The treatment of the cutaneous metastases depends on the PRIMARY CANCER and the extent of the metastases. Systemic CHEMOTHERAPY (anticancer drugs) may be used. Solitary lesions may be surgically removed or treated with RADIATION THERAPY, CHEMOTHERAPY, HORMONE THERAPY, or BIOLOGICAL THERAPY.

cutaneous T-cell lymphoma See MYCOSIS FUNGOIDES.

CV a combination of the anticancer drugs CISPLATIN and VePesid (ETOPOSIDE) sometimes used in the treatment of SMALL CELL LUNG CANCER. See individual drug listings for side effects.
See also COMBINATION CHEMOTHERAPY.

CVEB a combination of the anticancer drugs CISPLATIN, VINBLASTINE, ETOPOSIDE, and BLEOMYCIN sometimes used in the treatment of kidney, bladder, and prostate cancer. See individual drug listings for side effects.
See also COMBINATION CHEMOTHERAPY.

CVI a combination of the anticancer drugs CISPLATIN, VePesid (ETOPOSIDE), and IFOSFAMIDE WITH MESNA sometimes used in the treatment of nonsmall cell lung cancer. See individual drug listings for side effects.
See also COMBINATION CHEMOTHERAPY.

CVP a combination of the anticancer drugs CYTOXAN, VINCRISTINE, and PREDNISONE sometimes used in the treatment of NON-HODGKIN'S LYMPHOMA. See individual drug listings for side effects.
See also COMBINATION CHEMOTHERAPY.

CVPP a combination of the anticancer drugs CCNU, VINBLASTINE, PROCARBAZINE, and PREDNISONE sometimes used in the treatment of HODGKIN'S DISEASE. See individual drug listings for side effects.
See also COMBINATION CHEMOTHERAPY.

CYADIC a combination of the anticancer drugs CYTOXAN, ADRIAMYCIN, and DTIC sometimes used in the treatment of SOFT TISSUE SARCOMA. See individual drug listings for side effects.
See also COMBINATION CHEMOTHERAPY.

cyclamate See ARTIFICIAL SWEETENERS.

cyclobutane dicarboxylate platinum See CARBOPLATIN.

cyclophosphamide See CYTOXAN and CARCINOGENS.

cyst (sist) an irregular sac in the body containing fluid or semisolid material. It used to be thought that women who developed many cysts in the breast were at a greater risk of developing breast cancer. It is now believed that only certain lesions put a woman at a small, increased risk. Cysts in the breast (unlike cancerous lumps) are movable, spherically shaped, fairly soft, and subject to rapid changes in size. However, a doctor cannot always tell if a lump in a breast is a cyst, and for that reason a NEEDLE ASPIRATION BIOPSY may be performed.
See also FIBROCYSTIC CHANGES.

cystectomy (sis-tek′to-me) surgical removal of the bladder. The cystectomy may involve additional surgery depending on whether the cancer has spread. In women, this may include removal of the ovaries, fallopian tubes, uterus, and urethra. In men the prostate and seminal vesicles may be removed.

cystic disease See FIBROCYSTIC CHANGES.

cystogram See CYSTOGRAPHY.

cystography (sis-tog'rah-fe) an examination of the bladder by X-RAY using a contrast dye or some other CONTRAST MEDIUM to allow a finer definition of the organ. A urinary CATHETER is inserted through the urethra. The contrast medium is administered through the catheter into the bladder. When the bladder is full, the catheter is removed and the X-rays are taken. The procedure takes about half an hour. A cystography may be used in the diagnosis of bladder cancer.

cystoprostatectomy (sis''to-prah-stah-tek'to-me) surgical removal of the bladder and prostate in men. This may be performed in the treatment of URETHRAL CANCER.
See also CYSTOURETHRECTOMY.

cystoscope See CYTOSCOPY.

cystoscopy (sis-tos'ko-pe) [cystourethroscopy] a visual examination of the bladder using a lighted, tubular instrument (a cystoscope). The cystoscope is inserted through the urethra and up into the bladder. Air or water may be inserted into the bladder so that the doctor can get a better view of the bladder walls. Cystoscopic brushes can be inserted through the tubular instrument to pick up cells for microscopic examination. Small tumors can sometimes be removed through the tube. A cystoscopy is performed under general or local anesthesia, usually in a hospital. After the procedure, there may be a swelling of the urethra, which could result in difficulty in urinating. Besides cancer, this test may be used in the diagnosis of diverticula, fistulas, or stones.
See also ENDOSCOPY.

cystourethrectomy (sis''to-u-reth-rek'to-me) surgical removal of the bladder and urethra. This may be used in the treatment of URETHRAL CANCER.
See also CYSTOPROSTATECTOMY.

cystourethroscopy See CYSTOSCOPY.

Cytadren [aminoglutethimide, Elipten] an anticancer drug that may be used in the treatment of BREAST, PROSTATE, and ADRENAL CANCER. It works by blocking production of ESTROGEN and other adrenal cortical hormones. Because of its function

it may be referred to as a "medical ADRENALECTOMY." It is taken by mouth. Occasional or rare side effects may include lethargy, dizziness, skin rashes, facial bloating, BONE MARROW DEPRESSION, fever, loss of appetite, nausea, and vomiting.

cytarabine See ARA-C.

cytokines (si'to-kīnz) proteins secreted in small amounts by cells. They can also be made by RECOMBINANT DNA technology. Cytokines help regulate a variety of cell processes, including the immune process. They work along with lymphokines, another protein secreted by cells.
See also T CELL and BIOLOGICAL RESPONSE MODIFIERS.

cytology (si-tol'o-je) the study of cells, their origin, structure, and function.

cytomegalovirus (CMV) a specific type of herpes virus that causes infected cells to enlarge (megalo). In people who are immunodepressed because of AIDS or CANCER THERAPY, for example, this virus can cause major illness and disability. CMV retinitis is a major cause of blindness in such patients. Therapy is available to suppress the growth but not reverse the damage. The drug Foscarnet is used in the treatment of CMV.

Cytosar-U See ARA-C.

cytosine arabinoside See ARA-C.

cytotoxic drug (si''to-tok'sik) a drug that kills or harms specific cells in the body. The cytotoxicity of a drug is often used to indicate the negative side effects that anticancer drugs have on healthy cells.

Cytovene See GALLIUM NITRATE.

Cytoxan (si-tok'san) [cyclophosphamide, CTX, Endoxan, Neosar] an ALKYLATING anticancer drug sometimes used in the treatment of cancer of the BREAST, OVARY, LUNG, testis, and endometrium and LYMPHOMA, LEUKEMIA, MYELOMA, NEUROBLASTOMA, Ewing's sarcoma, MYCOSIS FUNGOIDES, and RHABDOMYOSARCOMA. It is given by IV (injection into a vein) or can be taken by mouth. Common side effects may include nausea and vomiting. Occasional or rare effects may include BONE MARROW DEPRESSION, hair loss, bloody urine, sterility, chronic lung problems, skin darkening, nasal stuffiness, second cancers, and eye problems. Cytoxan plays a major role in the treatment of cancer. It is one of the most commonly used anticancer drugs. Cytoxan has been listed by the federal government's National Toxicity Program as a known CARCINOGEN.

cytoxic T cells   See KILLER CELLS.

CYVADIC   a combination of the anticancer drugs CYTOXAN, VINCRISTINE, ADRIAMYCIN, and dacarbazine (DTIC) sometimes used in the treatment of sarcomas.

See also COMBINATION CHEMOTHERAPY.

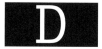

D

D & C (dilation and curettage) (ku″rĕ-tahzh′) a minor surgical procedure in which the uterus is scraped with an instrument known as a curette. After administration of a general or local anesthetic, the lining of the cervix is expanded (dilation) allowing the insertion of the curette, which is used to scrape the cervical canal and the uterine lining (endometrium). The cells obtained are biopsied (microscopically examined for cancer). After effects of a D & C may include some bleeding and staining for about two weeks and mild cramps or backache for a day or two. A D & C may be used in the diagnosis of CERVICAL CANCER. In addition to diagnosing cancer, a D & C may be performed to discover the cause of heavy or frequent periods, to remove tissue after a pregnancy, to terminate a pregnancy, or to treat an incomplete miscarriage.

dacarbazine See DTIC.

DACT See COSMEGEN.

dactinomycin See COSMEGEN.

DAN See DANOCRINE.

danazol See DANOCRINE.

Danocrine [DACT, danazoldan] an ANDROGEN used in the treatment of some cancer patients whose platelet count has dropped to below-normal levels.

Datril See ANALGESIC and ACETAMINOPHEN.

daunomycin (daw-no-mi′sin) [Rubidomycin, Cerubidine, daunorubicin (DNR)] an ANTIBIOTIC anticancer drug used in the treatment of some forms of acute leukemia. It is given by IV (injection into a vein). Common side effects may include nausea, vomiting, fever, red urine, hair loss, and severe BONE MARROW DEPRESSION that can last several weeks. Occasional or rare side effects may include heart problems, mouth sores, and liver problems.

daunorubicin (DNR) See DAUNOMYCIN.

DaunoXome See LIPOSOMAL DAUNORUBICIN.

DAVA See VINDESINE.

DBD See DIBROMODULCITOL.

DC a combination of the anticancer drugs DAUNOMYCIN and cytarabine (ARA-C) sometimes used in the treatment of childhood AML. See individual drug listings for side effects.
    See also COMBINATION CHEMOTHERAPY.

DCF [deoxycoformycin, Nipent] See PENTO-STATIN.

DCIS See DUCTAL BREAST CARCINOMA IN SITU.

DCPM a combination of the anticancer drugs DAUNOMYCIN, cytarabine (ARA-C), prednisolone, and mercaptopurine (6-MP) sometimes used in the treatment of childhood AML. See individual drug listings for side effects.

See also COMBINATION CHEMOTHERAPY.

DCT a combination of the anticancer drugs DAUNOMYCIN, cytarabine (ARA-C), and thioguanine (6-TG) sometimes used in the treatment of AML. See individual drug listings for side effects.

See also COMBINATION CHEMOTHERAPY.

DDD Lysodren See MITOTANE.

DDP See CISPLATIN.

debulking See TUMOR DEBULKING.

Decadron (dek'ah-dron) [DM, dexamethasone, Hexadrol] a synthetic ADRENOCORTICOID sometimes used in the treatment of leukemias, lymphomas, and brain cancer. It is widely used to reduce swelling of brain tissue in cases of primary and metastatic (cancer that has spread)-stage brain cancer. It has been found to be useful as an antiemetic (remedy to prevent vomiting) in combination with other agents. Decadron is widely used and plays an important role in cancer treatment.

Deca-Durabolin See ANDROGEN.

decompensation failure of the heart to maintain adequate blood circulation, marked by labored breathing, engorged blood vessels, and edema

Decytadine a more potent agent than Vidaza being evaluated in MDS (myelodysplastic syndrome; 2005).

See also AZACYTADINE

deep venous thrombosis See DVT.

Delalutin See HYDROXYPROGESTERONE CAPROATE and PROGESTERONE.

Deltasone See PREDNISONE.

Demerol (dem'er-ol) [meperidine] a strong NARCOTIC ANALGESIC drug used to treat pain. It is admin-istered by an injection into the muscle or taken by mouth. It relieves pain for a short period of time, two to three hours. For that reason it is usually given for intermittent episodes of intense pain, for example, after surgery. It is not the drug of choice for use in patients with severe chronic pain. Demerol is available by prescription only.

deoxycoformycin [pentostatin] a CHEMOTHERAPY drug given via IV (intravenous) used in treatment of HAIRY CELL LEUKEMIA.

deoxyribonucleic acid See DNA.

Depocyt [lipid encapsulated cytarabine] a CHEMOTHERAPY drug, approved by the FDA for treatment of LEPTOMENINGIAL METASTASIS. The lipid releases the drug more slowly and thus needs to be administered less frequently. Depocyt is given INTRATHECALLY (into the cerebrospinal fluid) by lumbar puncture or via an OMMAYA RESERVOIR into the lateral ventricles. It is limited by arachnoiditis (inflammation) and by its high cost.

Depo-Provera See PROGESTERONE.

depot (de'po) a site in the body where a drug may be accumulated, deposited, or stored, and from which it can be distributed. Some medications may be given with a delayed-release capability, such as ZOLADEX, which may be used in the treatment of prostrate cancer. For example, Zoladex is adminis-tered monthly so that the therapeutic effect is sustained for a month.

Depo-Testosterone (dep'o tes-tos'ter-ōn) an androgenic (male) hormonal drug used in the treatment of breast cancer. This is a long-acting agent, acting over a period of weeks. It is given intramuscularly (injected into a muscle).

See also ANDROGEN.

depression a feeling of melancholy, hopelessness, and dejection. Numerous theories indicate that depression may increase the risk of developing cancer. But in 1990 a 10-year study involving more than 1,000 people reported that depression is not a factor in the development of cancer. Reactive depression as a *result* of cancer is not an uncommon occurrence in cancer patients and their families. It is sometimes assumed that all patients with cancer must be depressed. Because of this assumption, major depression often is neither diagnosed nor treated when it could be. There are various forms of therapy for depression, depending on a number of different factors, including the degree of depression and its duration. In general, depressed patients are treated with supportive psychotherapy and antidepressant medication.

dermis (der'mis)   the lower or inner layer of the two main layers that make up the skin.

dermoid   See CONGENITAL BRAIN TUMOR.

DES (diethylstilbestrol) (di-eth"il-stil-bes'trol)   a synthetic HORMONE that acts like ESTROGEN. It was one of the first synthetic estrogen-like hormones that was inexpensive and could be taken orally. DES was developed in 1938 and prescribed for women from 1945 to 1971 to prevent miscarriage. In 1971 a link between DES and cancers of the female reproductive system was discovered, and the U.S. Food and Drug Administration issued a warning that it should not be used during pregnancy. A small number of adolescent girls, whose mothers had taken DES-type drugs during pregnancy, developed a very rare cancer—CLEAR CELL ADENOCARCINOMA of the vagina. There is an indication that daughters of women who took DES may have a higher risk of developing CERVICAL CANCER as well, since they are twice as likely to develop early cellular changes that might lead to cervical cancer. It has also been suggested that their sons may be more prone to be born with undescended testicles and to develop testicular cancer.

DES had also been a mainstay in the HORMONE THERAPY of prostate cancer by suppressing production of ANDROGEN. In men its side effects include breast swelling, change in voice, feet swelling, and an increase in vascular accidents such as strokes, heart attacks, etc. It has been listed by the federal government's National Toxicology Program as a known CARCINOGEN.

DESP   See ESTROGEN and CARCINOGENS.

dexamethasone   See DECADRON.

dexrazoxane   See ZINECARD.

detection   See SCREENING.

DHAD   See MITOXANTRONE.

DHL   See DIFFUSE HISTIOCYTIC LYMPHOMA.

diagnosis   a process or procedure by which a disease or illness is identified. In cancer, diagnosis is followed by STAGING in order to ascertain the extent of the cancer in the body. Generally, cancer can be definitively diagnosed only after a biopsy.
See also DIAGNOSIS/EVALUATION INDEX.

diagnostic radiologist   a radiologist who specializes in administering and interpreting X-RAYS used in the diagnosis of various cancers and other diseases.

diaphanography   See TRANSILLUMINATION.

diaphragm (di'ah-fram)   the thin muscle below the lungs and heart that separates the chest from the abdomen. A spasm of the diaphragm results in hiccups.

diarrhea   frequent or loose stool; one side effect of CHEMOTHERAPY.

dibromodulcitol [DBD, mitolactol, Elobromol]   a drug used in the treatment of recurrent invasive of metastatic squamous carcinoma of the cervix. It is taken by mouth. A common side effect may be BONE MARROW DEPRESSION. Occasional and rare side effects may include nausea, vomiting, loss of appetite, diarrhea, shortness of breath, skin darkening, itching, hair loss, difficulty in urinating, and an allergic reaction.

dideoxyinosine   See DDI.

Didronel   See ETIDRONATE.

diet   what a person habitually eats and drinks. There is evidence that what a person consumes can affect his or her risk of getting cancer. As many as one-third of all cancer deaths may be related to the food a person eats. Breast cancer and colon cancer seem to be most associated with diet; prostate and uterine cancer may be related as well. The biggest culprit in the diet is fat; the most beneficial food is FIBER.

A number of different studies—epidemiological and laboratory-based—have linked fat intake with breast and colon cancer. One study, reported in May, 2005, suggested that a low-fat diet given to women with early stage BREAST CANCER after completion of standard ADJUVANT THERAPY decreases the rate of recurrence.

In Argentina, where the population consumes a greater amount of beef (a major source of fat) than in the United States, the mortality rate for both breast and colon cancer is greater than in the United States. In Asian countries, where meat and fatty foods are consumed on a very limited basis, there is a much lower incidence of breast and colon cancer than in the United States. Studies have shown that when Japanese people move to the United States, their rate of breast and colon cancer increases. Second-generation Japanese Americans have virtually the same rate of breast and colon cancer as other Americans. Studies of vegetarians have found a lower rate of breast and colon cancer. And in animal studies, increasing the fat intake increases the development of the disease.

Fiber in the diet is believed to *reduce* the risk of COLON/RECTAL CANCER. In some studies, dietary fiber has inhibited chemically induced cancer of the colon and small intestine. Most studies examining a correlation between available food and cancer rates have found that countries where there was greater fiber-rich food intake, the rate of colon cancer mortality and incidence was lower. Studies on fat and fiber are not conclusive, but they do suggest very strongly that both play a role in cancer. Studies are also being done on the role different vitamins play in cancer prevention, including vitamins A, C, and E and beta carotene. Minerals such as iron and selenium are also being studied. Epidemiological research has indicated that a high consumption of alcohol may increase the risk for a number of cancers, including colon/rectal, breast, esophagus, pharynx, and mouth. The International Agency for Research on Cancer has categorized alcohol as a carcinogen.

The NATIONAL CANCER INSTITUTE has issued the following guidelines:

- Eat a variety of foods including fruits and vegetables; whole cereals; lean meats, poultry without skin; fish; dry peas and beans; and low-fat dairy products.
- Maintain a healthy weight.
- Choose a diet low in saturated fat and cholesterol—total fat should provide 30% or less of total calories, and saturated fat no more than 10% of total calories.
- Choose a diet with plenty of vegetables, fruit, and grain products—adults should eat at least three servings of vegetables and two servings of fruit a day.
- Use sugars in moderation.
- Use salt and sodium in moderation.
- If you drink alcoholic beverages, do so in moderation—two or fewer drinks a day.
- eat 20 to 30 grams of fiber a day, with an upper limit of 35 grams—fiber can be found in the following foods: bread, pastas, and cereals made with whole-grain flours such as rye, wheat, corn, oats, and all their bran; fruits and vegetables, especially apples, peaches, pears, potatoes, peas, and beans.

The American Cancer Society (ACS) and the National Academy of Science have come out with similar guidelines. They recommend including foods rich in vitamins A, C, and E, such as dark green and yellow vegetables, carrots, tomatoes, spinach, apricots, peaches, and cantaloupes for vitamin A and carotene; leafy vegetables, whole-grain cereals, nuts, and beans for vitamin E; and citrus fruits as well as other red, yellow, and orange fruits and vegetables for vitamin C. The ACS also recommends avoiding obesity and moderation in the consumption of salt-cured, smoked, and nitrate-cured foods.

Many cancer patients have difficulty with their appetite and with eating. This can be a result of the disease itself or its treatment. Anticancer drugs can alter the person's taste or cause mouth sores. Surgical procedures can make it difficult—and sometimes impossible—to eat normally. And the cancer itself can create a blockage, making eating difficult or impossible. A dietician may be called on to plan a diet that is both nutritious and palatable for a patient.

See also STOMATITIS.

diethylstilbestrol   See DES and ESTROGEN.

diethylstilbestrol diphosphate [DESP, Stilphostrol, stilbestrol diphosphate] See ESTROGEN and CARCINOGENS.

dietician   a person trained in foods and nutrition. See DIET.

differentiated cell   refers to the degree of maturity of the cell. The more mature or differentiated the cell, the more it resembles a normal cell.

differentiated tumor   a cancerous tumor with cells that resemble normal cells. The more differentiated the tumor, the better the chance that it will respond to treatment. It may also have a slower growth rate. The more abnormal, or undifferentiated, the more active and uncontrollable the cancer is likely to be.

See also UNDIFFERENTIATED CELLS.

differentiation   in cancer, it refers to how mature (developed) the cancer cells in a tumor are. Generally, the greater the differentiation

- the more like normal cells they are
- the less aggressive they are (they grow more slowly)
- the better the prognosis (the more likely it is that treatment will be effective)

Many types of cancer are graded by how differentiated the cells are. The grade may be one of the factors considered when planning treatment. In some cancers, well-differentiated tumors are assigned a grade of 1 or 2 and poorly differentiated tumors are graded a 3 or 4. In other cancers, the grading differentiation may assign different values on numbers.

differentiation therapy   the use of chemical agents to stop cancer cells from reproducing by causing them to mature and resemble normal cells. While they do not perform the functions that the normal cells perform, they do live and die as normal cells do. The same agents may also be able to make the existing cancer cells more responsive to radiation and chemotherapy. The more differentiated or mature the cancer cell is, the more suscepti-

ble, and responsive, it is to treatment. This therapy is under investigation.

diffuse histiocytic lymphoma (DHL) (his"te-o-sit'ik lim-fo'mah) [diffuse large cell lymphoma] a lymphoma once considered one of the most aggressive and difficult to control that now has a much higher rate of complete remission and long-term survival as a result of COMBINATION CHEMOTHERAPY.

See NON-HODGKIN'S LYMPHOMA.

diffuse large cell lymphoma   See DIFFUSE HISTIOCYTIC LYMPHOMA.

Diflucan   See FLUCONAZOLE.

digestive tract   the intestines and accessory glands where food is processed and digested. It includes the mouth, PHARYNX, ESOPHAGUS, STOMACH, and INTESTINES.

digital breast radiography   See DIGITAL MAMMOGRAPHY.

digital mammography (dij'ĭ-tal mam-og'rah-fe) [digital breast radiology, computerized mammography]   examination of the breast by using a computer along with the X-RAY to get a finer resolution. The computer element permits extraction of more information. It can compensate for underexposed and overexposed images, eliminating the need for repeated exposure of the woman. This is a very new, expensive procedure, with limited availability. Its high cost generally precludes its use for routine evaluation.

digital radiography (dij'ĭ-tal ra-de-og'rah-fe)   using a computer monitor to view regular X-RAYS. Standard X-rays are converted to digital signals, electronic data that can be stored and examined by a computer. That enables doctors to zoom in on a specific part of the X-ray and adjust the contrast.

digital rectal exam (dij'ĭ-tal rek'tal) [DRE]   an examination of the rectum. The digital rectal exam is a screening procedure for COLON/RECTAL CANCER and PROSTATE CANCER. The doctor gently inserts a rubbergloved and lubricated finger into the lowest four inches of the rectum and examines the smoothness of the rectal wall surface for lesions. In men the doctor will also examine the size and characteristics of the prostate. During the digital rectal exam, a stool sample may be taken for analysis for occult (hidden) blood. It is a quick painless exam, although it is not uncommon to find patients who feel embarrassed about taking it. The American Cancer Society recommends that everyone over the age of 40 have an annual digital rectal exam.

See also SCREENING.

DiGugliemo's syndrome   See ERYTHROLEUKEMIA.

Dilantin (di-lan'tin) [phenytoin]   an anticonvulsant drug that may be used in the treatment of brain cancer to prevent seizures. It acts on the central nervous system and must only be taken in controlled doses. It is taken by mouth and available by prescription only. Possible side effects include acne, excessive hairiness, and gum growth.

dilation and curettage   See D & C.

dilaudid (di-law'did) [hydromorphone]   a NARCOTIC, ANALGESIC painkiller available by prescription only. Dilaudid is more potent than heroin, starts working more quickly, and lasts longer, for three to six hours. It may be prescribed for cancer patients with severe pain. It can be given by IM (injection into the muscle), orally, or by rectal preparation.

dioxin [di-ox'in]   a general term that describes a group of hundreds of chemicals that are highly persistent in the environment, and found to be a "known human carcinogen" by the EPA, and the World Health Organization (among many others). Dioxin is formed as an unintentional by-product of many industrial processes involving chlorine such as waste incineration, chemical and pesticide manufacturing, and pulp and paper bleaching. Dioxin was the primary toxic component of AGENT ORANGE, was found at Love Canal in Niagara Falls, New York, and was the basis for evacuations at Times Beach, Missouri, and Seveso, Italy. A 2002 study shows dioxin to be related to increased incidence of breast cancer. (For more information, see http://www.ejnet.org/dioxin.)

diploid (dip'loid)   of cancer cells that contain the normal amount of DNA. Diploid tumors may be less aggressive than aneuploid tumors, which contain an abnormal amount of DNA.

See also PLOIDY.

dipping snuff   See SMOKELESS TOBACCO.

distal pancreatectomy (dis'tal pan"kre-ah-tek'to-me)   surgical removal of the tail (narrow part) of the pancreas. This may be performed in the treatment of PANCREATIC CANCER.

distraction   See RELAXATION TECHNIQUES.

diuretic [di"u-ret'ik]   a class of drug that causes an increase in urine flow by acting on the kidneys. Some are very potent. Diuretics are often used to control EFFUSIONS (accumulation of fluid) and reduce EDEMA (swelling) in cancer patients. They are also widely used in conditions other than cancer.

dizziness   may be a symptom of cancer (e.g., a brain tumor) or a side effect of cancer therapy. In general it is not a specific symptom and further testing may be needed to clarify its meaning.

DLBCL   See DIFFUSE LARGE B-CELL LYMPHOMA

DM   See DECADRON.

DMC   a combination of the anticancer drugs dactinomycin (COSMOGEN), METHOTREXATE, and CYTOXAN sometimes used in the treatment of GESTATIONAL TROPHOBLASTIC TUMOR. See individual drug listings for side effects.

See also COMBINATION CHEMOTHERAPY.

DNA (deoxyribonucleic acid)   one of the two nucleic acids found in all cells, the other being ribonucleic acid, RNA. DNA is found in the nuclei of CELLS. Chromosomes consist of long chains of double-stranded DNA. DNA is subdivided into GENES, which make up chromosomes. Thus DNA consists of all the GENETIC information of a living entity—the genome—and is essential for reproduction. Genes are the functional units of heredity and occupy a specific location on a chromosome. Genes are capable of autoreproduction at each cell division.

Genes direct the production of ENZYMES or other PROTEINS. The genes determine the unique characteristics of a person. They are responsible for passing on traits from generation to generation. Among all those genes there appears to be a very small subset that has the potential to undergo (genetic) alterations that lead to cancer. When those genes, called ONCOGENES, are switched on, or altered by mutations so that they produce an abnormal gene product, cancer may develop. Some chemotherapy (anticancer drugs) destroys cancer cells by interfering with the function or structure of DNA.

DNR   See DAUNOMYCIN.

DNR (do not resuscitate)   a specific order on a patient's chart specifying that cardiopulmonary resuscitation should *not* be used in the event of cessation of vital functions. DNR is, in effect, recognition of the futility of attempting to keep a person with terminal illness alive with advanced life support systems. In many states, physicians may issue the order. However, a DNR order is always discussed with the patient, family, and doctor before it is formalized. DNR also acknowledges that "death with dignity" may be best served in some people by not using extraordinary means to keep them alive.
    See also "Concern for the Dying" in the Index under supportive organizations. See ADVANCE DIRECTIVE.

docetaxel   See TAXOTERE.

dolasetron   See ANZEMET.

Dolophine   See METHADONE.

Donabinol   See ANTIEMETIC.

dosimetrist   (do"sim-ĕ'trist)   a person who plans and calculates the proper radiation dose for treatment, the number of treatments, and how long each should last. See RADIATION THERAPY.

dose density   a pharmacologic concept used in the adjuvant setting. It is based on models of the growth of cancer cells and essentially implies delivery of more drug in a shorter time than with traditional schedules, to increase effectiveness.

double-barrel colostomy   (ko-los'to-me)   a two-step surgical procedure involving removal of a malignant (cancerous) tumor in the colon and creating an artificial opening through which body wastes are collected outside the body, then after a period of time, rejoining the colon so that the device outside the body is no longer needed and normal functioning is resumed.
    See also COLOSTOMY.

double-blind   a CLINICAL TRIAL in which neither the doctor nor the patient knows which drug and/or dose is being administered and tested. The treatment can be quickly identified, if necessary, by a special code. In a single blind study the doctor knows which treatment the patient is getting, but the patient does not. Blind studies are performed to prevent personal bias from influencing reaction to the treatment and study results.

Down's syndrome   a congenital disease characterized by an extra chromosome. People with Down's syndrome area at an increased risk of developing leukemia.

DOX   See ADRIAMYCIN.

Doxil [Doxorubicin Liposome]   An IV ANTINEO-PLASTIC that takes advantage of the formulation that targets more drug to the tumor tissue. It is indicated in AIDS-related KAPOSI'S SARCOMA, and in recurrent or metastatic OVARIAN CANCER when both paclitaxel and platinum-based chemotherapy regimens are no longer effective. Its major toxicities include suppression of bone marrow, nausea, vomiting, and cardiotoxicity (destruction of the heart muscle). It may cause HAND-FOOT SYNDROME and reversible ALOPECIA. It causes a red-orange discoloration of the urine.

doxorubicin   See ADRIAMYCIN.

drain   in medical treatment, tubes or suction devices inserted in the body after some surgeries to drain fluids that may accumulate. Drains stay in place as long as necessary, generally only for several days, and are easily removed.

DRE   See DIGITAL RECTAL EXAM.

drinking water   water that is consumed from a tap or a bottle. The Environmental Protection Agency has set standards for drinking water in the United States. Some contaminants that may be found in water and that may be linked to cancer are arsenic, benzene, chromium, carbon tetrachloride (CTC), p-dichlorobenzene, 1,2-dichloroethane, 1,1,1,-trichloroethane, total trihalomethanes, vinyl chloride, and radon.

If you are concerned about your water (e.g., it does not smell right, it does not taste right) there are several courses of action you can take. The easiest is to call your local health department and ask about having your water tested. Someone from the health department may come out and test the water; or you will be told how to get it tested. If your water is bad, and it is well water, obtaining clean water is your responsibility. If your water is from a public utility or private supplier, providing drinkable water is their responsibility. You can call the Environmental Protection Agency (202-554-1404) and ask for a list of contaminants, including their official minimum levels. This agency can also supply you with information on what you can do if your water contains unacceptable levels of contaminants.

See also CARCINOGENS.

Drolban [dromostanolone propionate]   See ANDROGEN.

dromostanolone propionate [Drolban, Masteril, Macleron, Permastril]   See ANDROGEN.

Dronabinol   See MARIJUANA.

drug resistance   a condition in which a person's cancer cells no longer respond to the chemotherapy (anticancer drugs) that was chosen to treat him or her. The cancer cells become insensitive to the drug, making it no longer useful as a treatment. The cells have developed what is called an "R factor." Frequently, when another drug is tried the presence of the R factor will lead to resistance of the new drug as well. This condition is called cross resistance. Efforts are under way to identify drugs to overcome drug resistance.

See PSC-833.

drug tolerance   a condition in which greater and greater amounts of a drug are needed to be effec-

tive. This can occur in patients being treated with painkillers and patients being treated with CHEMOTHERAPY (anticancer drugs). In the case of drug tolerance to painkillers, a larger dose of the drug may be given or a different, more potent drug can be tried. In the case of chemotherapy the cancer cells may respond to an alternate drug.

dry heaves   See RETCHING.

dry mouth   See XEROSTOMIA.

dry orgasm   See RETROGRADE EJACULATION.

DTIC [dacarbazine, DTIC-Dome, imidazole carboxamide]   an ALKYLATING anticancer drug sometimes used in the treatment of MELANOMA, HODGKIN'S DISEASE, and SARCOMA. It is given by IV (injection into a vein). Common side effects may include nausea and vomiting. Occasional or rare side effects may include BONE MARROW DEPRESSION, flu-like symptoms, metallic taste, sensitivity to sun, liver damage, flushing of face, and skin rash.

DTIC-ACTD   a combination of the anticancer drugs dacarbazine (DTIC) and dactinomycin (COSMEGEN) sometimes used in the treatment of MELANOMA. See individual drug listings for side effects.

See also COMBINATION CHEMOTHERAPY.

DTIC-Dome   See DTIC.

duct   a tube or channel in the body that conducts fluid, especially the secretions of glands. For example, in the breasts, milk travels through the ducts. The ducts in the breast are the most common site of BREAST CANCER. Other cancers can develop in ducts.

See also DUCTAL BREAST CARCINOMA IN SITU.

ductal breast carcinoma in situ (DCIS) [noninfiltrating ductal papillary carcinoma, carcinoma in situ, intraductal carcinoma]   a type of BREAST CANCER made up of tiny cancers that are confined to the ducts. Because of improvements of mammography many new cases are being diagnosed, generally in women under the age of 50.

Although DCIS is considered a stage 0 breast cancer, it can nonetheless develop into an invasive cancer. Treatment options include mastectomy, excision (lumptectomy) plus radiation treatment, or excision alone. Chemotherapy is not used and in most cases lymph node dissection is not necessary since only 1 to 3% of women have position nodes.

Treatment of DCIS is generally considered a cure if done while the DCIS is still noninvasive.

Dukes' staging system   one of the ways of STAGING colon/rectal cancer. It is named for Cuthbert Dukes, a London pathologist who developed the staging system in 1932.

See also COLON/RECTAL CANCER.

dumping syndrome   a possible side effect of stomach surgery after removal of part or all of the stomach. After eating, the person may experience dizziness, weakness, sweating, nausea, vomiting, and/or palpitations when the remaining part of the stomach is emptied too quickly. It can usually be controlled by small, frequent feedings and a high-protein diet with dry foods and fluids in between meals.

duodenal carcinoma   (du"o-de'nal kar"sĭ-no'mah) a very rare cancerous tumor in the upper part of the small intestine known as the duodenum. This tumor is usually an ADENOCARCINOMA. Its primary treatment is surgery.

See also SMALL INTESTINE CANCER.

duodenogram   See DUODENOGRAPHY.

duodenography   (du"od-ĕ-nog'rah-fe) [hypotonic]   a diagnostic CONTRAST X-RAY of the duodenum (the uppermost eight or ten inches of the small intestine into which the stomach empties) and the pancreas, an adjacent organ. Medications and a CONTRAST MEDIUM are put into the stomach through a flexible CATHETER that is inserted through the nose, the pharynx, the esophagus (tube connecting stomach to throat), the stomach, and then the duodenum. Barium sulfate is administered through the catheter for contrast X-rays. Air is introduced for AIR-CONTRAST X-RAYS. The test can be done in a hospital, on an outpatient basis, or in a radiology suite. It takes about half an hour. One possible side effect of the test may be urinary retention in men with prostate problems. In addition, some people may experience irritation, caused by

the catheter, or the nasal passages, pharynx, and esophagus.

duodenoscope   See DUODENOSCOPY.

duodenoscopy   (du"od-ĕ-nos'ko-pe)   examination of the duodenum (the uppermost eight or 10 inches of the small intestine) and pancreas. It is a diagnostic procedure using a duodenoscope, a flexible fiberoptic instrument. The duodenoscope is passed through the mouth and esophagus (tube connecting the stomach and throat) and into the stomach and/or pancreas. Some anesthesia is used, especially in the throat to allow the tube to be inserted. Instruments can be inserted into the duodenoscope to take pictures or to get a tissue sample for a BIOPSY.

See also ENDOSCOPY.

Durabolin   [nandrolone]   See ANDROGEN.

Duract   (bromfenac sodium capsules) a long-lasting nonnarcotic pain medication indicated for the relief and management of acute pain. It is a nonsteroidal anti-inflammatory drug (NSAID).

DVP   a combination of the anticancer drugs daunorubicin (DAUNOMYCIN), VINCRISTINE, and PREDNISONE that may be used in the treatment of adult and childhood ALL. See individual drug listings for side effects.

See also COMBINATION CHEMOTHERAPY.

DVT (deep vein thrombosis)   a blood clot in the vein of a leg or the pelvis. DVT can occur in anyone. The usual initial treatment is anticoagulation with HEPARIN. There is an increased incidence of DVT in people with cancer or on CHEMOTHERAPY.

dye   See CONTRAST MEDIUM.

dysarthria   (dis-ar'thre-ah)   stammering and difficulty in pronouncing words distinctly. This phenomenon is caused by a disturbance in muscle control resulting from damage to the central or peripheral nervous system. It may be a symptom of brain cancer (or other disorders).

dysphagia (dis-fa′je-ah) difficulty or pain in swallowing. It is one of the main symptoms of cancer of the esophagus (tube connecting the stomach and throat) but of course may be a symptom of many other disorders.

See also ESOPHAGEAL CANCER.

dysphasia (dis-fa′ze-ah) impairment of speech characterized by the inability to coordinate speech and arrange words in a meaningful way. This may be a symptom of a brain tumor or other disorders.

dysplasia (dis-pla′ze-ah) abnormal development of size, shape, and organization of cells or tissue. It occurs most often in cells that reproduce rapidly. In some situations it may precede the development of cancer.

dysplasia of cervical cells (dis-pla′ze-ah sir′vǐ-kal) the earliest possible precancerous stage of abnormal cells on the surface of the cervix. Though the cells may eventually become cancerous, they often revert to normal without any treatment.

See also CERVICAL CANCER.

dysplastic nevi (dis-plas′tik ne′vi) certain types of unusual moles (nevus is a mole) that are more likely to become cancerous than ordinary moles. They have been seen in 20 to 35% of primary melanoma biopsies. They are usually larger than ordinary moles and have irregular borders that fade into the surrounding skin. They may be flat or raised above the skin surface. They are usually not a uniform color and may be brown with pink or red areas.

Dysplastic nevi tend to appear in members of the same family, although they are also seen in the general population. The inheritance of dysplastic nevi is called familial dysplastic nevus syndrome. People with the syndrome are at a greater risk of developing MELANOMA, especially if there are multiple cases of melanoma in the family. Family members who have had melanoma are also at risk of developing new melanomas. A definitive diagnosis of dysplastic nevi requires a BIOPSY, which can be done on moles removed by the doctor.

The dysplastic nevi seem normal when they first appear in early childhood, but they may increase in size dramatically when the body goes through hor-monal changes such as occur in puberty or pregnancy. At those times the appearance of the moles may change as well. A small number of the moles may progress to melanoma. (Most dysplastic nevi do not become cancerous.)

ORDINARY MOLES V. DYSPLASTIC NEVI (MOLES)

Characteristic	Ordinary Moles	Dysplastic Moles
Color	Uniformly tan, brown; one mole looks much like all others	Variable mixture of tan, brown, black, red/pink within a single mole; moles may look very different from each other
Shape	Round; sharp, clear-cut border between mole and surrounding skin; may be flat or elevated (bump)	Irregular border; may have notches; may fade off into surrounding skin; always a flat portion level with the skin, often occurring at edge of mole
Size	Usually less than 5 millimeters in diameter	Usually more than 5 millimeters; may be more than 10 millimeters
Number	Typical adult has 10–40 scattered over body	Usually more than 100, although some patients may not have an increased number of moles
Location	Generally on sun-exposed surfaces, above waist; scalp, breasts, buttocks rarely involved	Back most common site; may occur below waist and on scalp, breast, buttocks

Because people with familial dysplastic nevus syndrome are at greater risk of developing melanoma, they should check regularly for any changes in the moles' size, color, shape or outline, surface, or sensation and the surrounding skin as well as the development of new moles. Although changes in a mole do not necessarily mean that it is cancerous, it should be checked by a doctor. Melanoma caught early is usually curable by simple surgical removal.

See also MELANOMA.

dysplastic nevus syndrome   See DYSPLASTIC NEVI.

dyspnea (disp'ne-ah) difficulty or pain when breathing; shortness of breath. This symptom may occur in many clinical conditions including LUNG CANCER. Many cancers may spread to the lung or the lining of the lung from other sites in the body. This can also be a side effect of some anticancer drugs.

dysuria (dis-u're-ah) pain experienced during urination. This could be a symptom of cancer in the lower urinary tract as well as a symptom of other, noncancerous conditions, e.g., infection or stones.

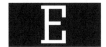

Eaton Lambert syndrome an uncommon MYAS-THENIA-like condition, associated with SMALL CELL LUNG CANCER. It is a PARANEOPLASTIC SYNDROME.

See also MYASTHENIC SYNDROME.

EBV See EPSTEIN-BARR VIRUS.

ECAT (emission computerized axial tomograph) scan a diagnostic test similar to the CT SCAN. After radioactive material is administered to the patient, the ECAT scanner records the charged particles given off from deep within the body. The picture that is taken is of the inside of the organ that is being studied.

See PET SCAN.

ECF combination of EPIRUBICIN, CISPLATIN, and 5-FU used to treat gastric carcinoma.

See STOMACH CANCER.

ECG See ELECTROCARDIOGRAPHY.

echoencephalogram See ECHOENCEPHALOGRAPHY.

echoencephalography (ek″o-en-sef″ah-log′rah-fe) an examination of the brain using ultrasound. A special machine projects high-frequency sound waves into the head. "Echoes" of the sound waves are then recorded as graphic tracings on a roll of paper attached to the machine. It is a noninvasive, painless procedure. Abnormal readings may be used in the diagnosis of a brain tumor or other irregularities in the brain.

EDAM See EDATREXATE.

edatrexate [10-EDAM, EDAM] a new drug being investigated in the treatment of NON-SMALL CELL LUNG CANCER. Its major side effect appears to be stomatitis (skin breakdown and ulcerations in and around the mouth).

edema (ĕ-de′mah) a swelling of tissue caused by an accumulation of fluid, which may cause discomfort and pain. Cancer patients may develop edema in many different ways, either directly or indirectly. For example, it may be a result of surgery. A woman with breast cancer may develop LYMPHEDEMA, a swollen arm in which the lymph passages are blocked or disrupted as a result of breast surgery. Patients with CACHEXIA can also develop edema. Edema can occur as a result of many other conditions, including heart failure, lung failure, liver failure, and kidney failure. Treatment is generally directed at reversing the condition or improving the underlying condition that caused it. A DIURETIC may be used to control edema.

EEG (electroencephalogram, electroencephalography) (e-lek″tro-en-sef″ah-log′rah-fe) an examination of the brain waves, a procedure that may be used in the diagnosis of brain cancer as well as other diseases. Electrodes (electrical conductors through which current enters or leaves a body) are secured to the skull either with glue or small needles. Brain waves are recorded while the patient is subjected to different stimuli. This can be performed on an outpatient basis or in a doctor's office and takes about an hour. It is a noninvasive, painless procedure. Although an electroencephalography will not show the presence of a tumor itself, it can show abnormal brain functioning that may be caused by the presence of a tumor.

effusion (ĕ-fu'zhun)   an accumulation of fluid in body tissue or cavities. It can be seen in benign or malignant conditions. A BIOPSY of the fluid will show whether malignant (cancerous) cells are present. The biopsy may also give clues as to the primary site of the cancer.

Malignant effusions are a result of cancer. Effusions in the pleura, the tissue covering the lungs and lining the inside of the chest cavity, are most commonly caused by cancers of the lung, breast, gastrointestinal tract, pancreas, or ovary. Malignant effusions in the abdomenare usually caused by cancer of the ovary, pancreas, stomach, or colon. About 50% of effusions in cancer patients are malignant.

Effusions may cause symptoms by pressure and by occupying space. Ascites is an effusion in the abdominal cavity.

The treatment of effusions includes mechanical removal and treatment of the condition causing the effusion and instillation of drugs into the cavity of decrease the fluid production.

Efudex   See 5-FU.

EGFR (epithelial growth factor receptor)   a tyrosine kinase receptor (of the Erb-B family) commonly altered in EPITHELIAL TUMORS. Selective blockade of EGFR is a fertile area of research and drug development, especially in NON-SMALL CELL LUNG CANCER, for which two drugs, Iressa and TARCEVA, are currently approved for treatment.

EGFR Inhibitors   a class of agents that block the growth factor or its receptor and act as antiangiogenesis agents.

EHDP   See ETIDRONATE.

8-methoxypsoralen   See METHOXSALEN.

8-MOP   See METHOXSALEN.

EKG (electrocardiogram)   See ELECTROCARDIOGRAPHY.

Eldisine   See VINDESINE.

electric blanket   a possible risk factor for some cancers in children. According to one study, using an electric blanket during pregnancy could slightly increase the risk of childhood cancer, such as leukemia and brain cancer, because electric blankets are a source of ELECTROMAGNETIC FIELDS. It is suggested that people who use electric blankets turn them on before getting into bed, to warm the bed, and then turn them off when in bed.

electric needle   See ELECTROCAUTERY.

electrocardiogram (EKG)   See ELECTROCARDIOGRAPHY.

electrocardiography (ĕ-lek"tro-kar"de-og'rah-fe) [ECG, EKG]   an examination of the heart's rhythm and muscle function. Electrodes (electrical conductors through which current enters or leaves a body) are placed at various places on the body. Small electrical currents produced by the heartbeats are measured and recorded on a strip of paper. This noninvasive, painless procedure, donein a doctor's office, takes about 15 minutes. An EKG is also done in the hospital before surgery and has been used to monitor use of the drug ADRIAMYCIN, which may affect heart function.

electrocautery (ĕ-lek"tro-kaw'ter-e) [electrodesiccation]   using an electric probe or needle to cauterize (burn) and destroy tissue. This procedure may be used in the treatment of nonmelanoma skin cancers (basal cell and squamous cell). A needle with a point through which an electric current is flowing is used to remove the growth on the skin. The doctor regulates the amount of electricity with a foot pedal.

electrocoagulation (ĕ-lek"tro-ko-ag"u-la'shun)   use of an instrument with an electric charge to stop bleeding.

electrode implants See EPIDURAL DORSAL COL-UMN STIMULATOR.

electrodesiccation See ELECTROCAUTERY.

electroencephalogram, electroencephalography See EEG.

electrofulguration See FULGURATION.

electro-larynx (lar'inks) a battery-operated device used for speaking by people who have had their voice box removed. The small box is held against the neck. When a button is pushed, the vibrating sound travels through the neck into the mouth where the sound is formed into words.

See also ESOPHAGEAL SPEECH.

electromagnetic fields (EMF) a combination of electric fields and magnetic fields that radiate from electric cables, power lines, wires, fixtures, and appliances. For many years scientists believed that this type of radiation was harmless. However, in 1989, as the result of a number of studies, the Congressional Office of Technology Assessment concluded that it could not be assumed there are no risks from EMF. In late 1989 the National Cancer Institute and the Children's Cancer Study Group started a collaborative, four-year study on whether low-frequency EMF exposure contributes to the development of acute lymphocytic leukemia (ALL) in children. In 1990 the Environmental Protection Agency released a draft report in which it stated that there were epidemiological studies of children and work-site exposure that indicated an association between magnetic fields and certain types of cancer, mainly leukemia and cancer of the nervous system, and lymphomas to a lesser extent. At the same time it said that other studies did not support an association and called for further research. In 1998 a report by the National Institute of Environmental Health Services (NIEHS), in which meta-analysis was done on EMF studies worldwide, concluded that EMF exposure is possibly carcinogenic to adults. It found limited evidence of an increased risk for childhood leukemia. A comprehensive study by researchers from the National Cancer Institute (NCI) and the Children's Cancer Group (CCG) found no evidence that mag-netic fields (EMFs) in the home increase the risk for acute lymphoblastic leukemia (ALL), the most common form of childhood cancer. In 1999, a report by NIH indicated there was no relationship to cancer.

electromagnetic radiation See ELECTROMAGNETIC FIELDS.

electron the part of the atom that has a negative charge. When an electron strikes an object at high energy, an X-RAY is produced. Electrons are used in RADIATION THERAPY.

electron beam therapy a radiation treatment using subatomic particles with a negative electric charge to deliver radiation. The electrons are produced by a special machine such as a betatron. The maximum dose of radiation is delivered by the electrons to the first few centimeters of tissue, after which the dose decreases rapidly. Because it penetrates only shallow depths of tissue, electron beam therapy can be used in the treatment of cancers of the skin, nose, lips, and eyelids without the scarring that may occur from surgical treatment. By varying the electron energy, the high dose of radiation can be administered to the specific area where it is needed.

See also RADIATION THERAPY.

electrosurgery a surgical procedure using a high-frequency current to cut tissue and coagulate (clot; stop the bleeding) the blood. The process can be done using a needle, blade, or disk electrodes. It may be used in the treatment of some cancers, including cancer of the skin, mouth, kidney, ureter, and rectum.

Elipten See CYTADREN.

Elitek [rasburicase] an intravenous agent approved for the initial management of pediatric patients with LEUKEMIA, LYMPHOMA, and other malignancies where CHEMOTHERAPY is likely to cause TUMOR LYSIS SYNDROME with resulting elevation of plasma uric acid levels.

Elliot's B Solution a solution that is used to dilute methotrexate sodium and cytarabine when it is used for INTRATHECAL administration (chemotherapy drugs injected into the cerebrospinal fluid) in the treatment of meningeal LEUKEMIA, lymphocytic LEUKEMIA, acute lymphocytic leukemia, and lymphoblastic lymphomas.

Elobromol   See DIBROMODULCITOL.

Elspar   See L-ASPARAGINASE.

EM   See ESTRAMUSTINE PHOSPHATE.

embolization (em"bo-lĭ-za'shun)   a technique to block the flow of blood (nourishment) to an organ in the body. In cancer patients it is done to slow the growth of the malignant (cancerous) tumor in the organ by diminishing its supply of blood. A temporary or long-acting blocking agent is injected through a CATHETER into the main arteries that supply that organ with blood. Embolization is most commonly used with liver cancer. It has also been used in kidney cancer before a RADICAL NEPHRECTOMY is performed to reduce the size of the tumor. Embolization has been used on a limited basis to control pain in bone metastases and in the treatment of bony tumors of the spine and pelvis. Side effects may include pain, fever, nausea, and vomiting for about one to four days.
     See also CHEMOEMBOLIZATION, HEPATIC ARTERY LIGATION, and ARTERIAL EMBOLIZATION.

embryonal cell cancer (em'bre-o-nal)   a cancerous tumor composed of cells that are similar to those present in the developing fetus. Embryonal tumors occur mostly in very young children and are rarely seen in anyone over the age of 16. The three types are WILMS' TUMOR, NEUROBLASTOMA, and RHABDOMYOSARCOMA.

Emcyt   See ESTRAMUSTINE PHOSPATE.

Emend [Aprepitant]   a new ANTIEMETIC of a class known as Neurokinin 1 (NK^1) receptor antagonists. It is indicated in combination with other antiemetics for the prevention of acute and delayed nausea and vomiting associated with use of HEC (highly-emetogenic chemotherapy).

emesis (em'ĕ-sis)   vomiting. Emesis is a frequent side effect of CHEMOTHERAPY (anticancer drugs)

and may be a side effect of RADIATION THERAPY and the cancer itself. An ANTIEMETIC may be given to patients before or during the administration of the anticancer drugs to prevent nausea and vomiting.

EMF   See ELECTROMAGNETIC FIELDS.

emission computerized axial tomograph   See ECAT SCAN.

encephalopathy (en-sef"ah-lop'ah-the)   a general term to describe abnormal brain function. There are many causes, including direct effect on brain tissue (e.g., a virus) and other chemical, drug, and metabolic factors. One form, known as AIDS encephalopathy, is caused by the HTLV-III virus in AIDS patients, resulting in progressive and irreversible brain damage. People with encephalopathy often have major disturbances of thought, behavior, and mood, causing great discomfort both to the patient and to family members, friends, and caretakers.

endocrine cancers (en'do-krĭn)   cancers of the endocrine system, including adrenocortical cancer, gastrointestinal carcinoid tumor, islet cell carcinoma, and thyroid cancer.

endocrine pancreas (en'do-krĭn)   the part of the pancreas that produces insulin and glucagon, hormones that regulate the breakdown of starches in the body. It is distinguished from the EXOCRINE PANCREAS, which gives rise to 95% of the cancers of this gland.

endocrine system (en'do-krĭn)   the network of ductless glands in the body that secrete HORMONES directly into the bloodstream. The hormones control the digestive and reproductive systems, growth, metabolism, and other processes.

endocrine therapy (en'do-krĭn)   alternating the level of various hormones in the body. See HORMONE THERAPY.

endometrial   referring to the uterus.

endometrial aspiration (en"do-me'tre-al as"pĭra' shun) [vaginal pool aspiration, aspiration curettage, vacuum curettage, vacuum aspiration] extraction of tissue from the uterine lining, by suction, for examination. A speculum is inserted into the vagina and a slender plastic tube called an endometrial aspirator (or cannula or vacurette) is passed through the cervix into the uterus. The tube is attached to a syringe or special vacuum pump that uses suction to remove a small amount of tissue from the lining of the uterus (endometrium). The cells are microscopically examined for cancer or other abnormalities. The procedure can be done in a doctor's office and takes about five minutes. It is only useful when a small amount of tissue is required. If a larger tissue sample is needed, a D & C is generally performed. Endometrial spiration may be performed in the diagnosis of ENDOMETRIAL CANCER as well as other disorders.

endometrial cancer (en"do-me'tre-al) [endometrial carcinoma, uterus cancer, uterine cancer] cancer of the lining of the uterus, the hollow, pear-shaped organ where a baby grows. It accounts for 13% of all cancers in women, primarily affecting women during the postmenopause, with an average age of 60 at diagnosis. The NATIONAL CANCER INSTITUTE (NCI) projected some 40,880 new cases for 2005 in the United States, with approximately 7,310 deaths from endometrial cancer in the same year. The death rate from endometrial cancer has been declining. In 1973 about 5 of every 100,000 American women died of endometrial cancer. In 1986 that number was down to 3 in 100,000. Most endometrial cancer affects women between the ages of 60 and 74 and accounts for 13% of all cancers in women.

The most common type of endometrial cancer is ADENOCARCINOMA. Other, less common types include adenosquamous carcinoma, papillary serous carcinoma, and the very rare clear cell carcinoma.

The cause of endometrial cancer is not well defined. Women at a greater risk of getting endometrial cancer have gone through menopause, never been pregnant, have a family history of the disease, have hypertension, are diabetic, and/or are obese. In addition, the presence of ENDOMETRIAL HYPERPLASIA seems to be associated with its development. Endometrial hyperplasia is considered a precancerous condition that may develop into cancer. Studies suggest that the hyperplasia is strongly linked with hormones. For example, estrogen replacement therapy for menopausal symptoms has been shown to increase the risk for the disease by two to eight times. (Using progesterone along with the estrogen appears to lower the risk.) The antihormonal drug TAMOXIFEN, used primarily in the treatment of breast cancer, appears to increase the risk of endometrial cancer. Patients on tamoxifen need careful gynecologic follow-up.

Obesity is also considered to be a cause of endometrial cancer. Women who have excess amounts of fatty tissue are twice as likely to develop this cancer as women who are of normal weight. This may be due to the fact that fatty tissue converts certain hormones into estrone, a form of estrogen, and that an elevated estrogen level may play a role in the development of endometrial cancer.

The most common symptom of endometrial cancer is bleeding after menopause. The bleeding may begin as a watery, blood-streaked discharge, with the discharge containing more and more blood. (This can also be a symptom for other disorders.) Among the procedures that may be used in the diagnosis and evaluation of endometrial cancer are a PELVIC EXAM, ENDOMETRIAL ASPIRATION, D & C, BIOPSY, and PAP SMEAR. (The Pap smear is more useful and reliable in detection of CERVICAL CANCER and is not that reliable for endometrial cancer.)

Following is the National Cancer Institute's staging for endometrial cancer:

- Stage 0 and in situ—atypical hyperplasia of the endometrium
- Stage I—cancer confined to the body of the uterus; it can further be divided into substages A and B based on whether the length of the uterine cavity and cervix affected is eight centimeters (cm) or less
- Stage II—cancer extends into the cervix
- Stage III—cancer extends outside the uterus but is confined to the true pelvis
- Stage IV—cancer extends beyond the true pelvis or has invaded the bladder or rectum or has distant metastasis
- Recurrent—cancer has returned to the same site or to another area after treatment.

Treatment depends on the stage of the disease, the patient's general state of health, and other factors. The four types of treatment used for endometrial

Female Genital System

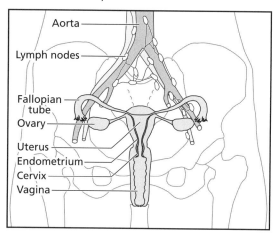

The endometrium is the lining of the uterus. Endometrial cancer accounts for 13% of all cancers in women. Courtesy NCI.

cancer are surgery, RADIATION THERAPY, CHEMOTHERAPY, and HORMONE THERAPY. Surgery is the most common treatment for endometrial cancer. The surgical options include a TOTAL ABDOMINAL HYSTERECTOMY AND BILATERAL SALPINGO-OOPHERECTOMY or a RADICAL HYSTERECTOMY. For the specific information on the latest state-of-the-art treatment, by stage, for endometrial cancer, call NCI's Cancer Information Service at 1-800-4-CANCER (1-800-422-6237), or for a TTY: 1-800-332-8615.

endometrial carcinoma   See ENDOMETRIAL CANCER.

endometrial hyperplasia (en″do-me′tre-al hi″per-pla′ze-ah)   an overabundance of cells lining the uterus. (A thickening in only one place is a polyp.) This is generally considered a precancerous condition, though not all cases of endometrial hyperplasia become malignant. However, endometrial cancer always begins with hyperplasia stage. When hyperplasia is severe, it is sometimes called IN SITU cancer of the endometrium. Symptoms of hyperplasia may include heavy bleeding during menstruation, erratic bleeding between periods, or abnormal or heavy bleeding during menopause. A D & C or ENDOMETRIAL ASPIRATION may be performed to

diagnose the cancer. Frequently, the removal of tissue in those procedures will serve as a cure. Under some conditions a HYSTERECTOMY may be performed, which eliminates any possibility of the development of endometrial cancer.

endometrium (en-do-me′tre-um)   the lining of the UTERUS. It is made up of several layers—surface epithelium, glands, blood vessels, and tissue spaces. The lining may develop ENDOMETRIAL CANCER.

endorectal ultrasound   a procedure in which a probe is inserted into the rectum to determine the size of a tumor and whether it has spread. The endorectal ultrasound may be used in the diagnosis of rectal cancer.
See also ULTRASOUND.

endorphins (en-dor′fins)   one of the natural substances produced by the brain to fight pain. Like NARCOTICS, they reduce the patient's perception of pain by binding to the "opiate receptors" on the surface of brain cells, though it is not known exactly how they work.
See also ENKEPHALINS.

endoscope (en′do-scōp) [fiber-optic instrument]   a thin, flexible instrument used to view the inside of an organ or body cavity. An endoscope can be equipped with light and an optical system; it may have the capacity to take pictures; and it may have a small tube through which air, chemical substances, or instruments like forceps can be inserted to obtain tissue samples for BIOPSY and remove small growths. The endoscope can be inserted through a body opening or through a small surgical incision while the patient is under anesthesia. It comes in various lengths for use in diagnostic procedures in different parts of the body, including the bronchial tubes in the lungs, colon, vagina, cervix, bladder, small intestine, esophagus, stomach, abdomen, mediastinum (the space between the lungs), surface of the lungs, and chest wall.
See also ENDOSCOPY.

endoscopic biopsy (en″do-skop′ik bi′ŏp-se)   a diagnostic procedure using an ENDOSCOPE to obtain cells or tissue for microscopic examination.
See also ENDOSCOPY.

endoscopic resection and fulguration   See TRANS-
URETHRAL RESECTION.

**endoscopic retrograde cholangiopancreatogra-
phy (ERCP)** (en″do-skop′ik ret′ro-grād ko-lan″jeo-
pan″cre-at-og′rah-fe)   an examination of the pancreas. A flexible fiber-optic tube is inserted down
the throat, through the stomach, and into the pancreas. A dye is then injected through the tube and
an X-ray is taken to show abnormalities in the
shape of the pancreas. The ERCP is also used to get
a sample of tissue for biopsy. Endoscopic retrograde cholangiopancreatography may be used in
the diagnosis of pancreatic cancer as well as other
disorders.
    See also ENDOSCOPY.

endoscopist (en-dos′ko-pist)   a doctor who specializes in examining internal organs using an
ENDOSCOPE.
    See also ENDOSCOPY.

endoscopy (en-dos′ko-pe) [fiber-optic endoscopy]
a diagnostic procedure using an ENDOSCOPE, a flexible instrument with a lighted tube and optical system, to examine the inside of many organs and structures in the body. Photographs can be taken or, if
necessary, small amounts of tissue can be removed
for BIOPSY during the procedure. Endoscopies can
generally be done in a doctor's office or on an outpatient basis. An assessment of the need for surgery can
be made, thereby eliminating the use of more radical
and potentially harmful diagnostic procedures.
Endoscopies are also less costly.
    The various endoscopies for diagnosing specific
cancers include: BRONCHOSCOPY, COLONOSCOPY,
COLPOSCOPY, CYSTOSCOPY, DUODENOSCOPY, ENDO-
SCOPIC RETROGRADE CHOLANGIOPANCREATOGRAPHY,
ESOPHAGOSCOPY, GASTROSCOPY, HYSTEROSCOPY,
LAPAROSCOPY, MEDIASTINOSCOPY, OTOSCOPY, PROTO-
SCOPY, SIGMOIDOSCOPY, and THORACOSCOPY.

Endostatin   the term, associated with the work of
Dr. Judah Folkman, for one of the novel ANTIAN-
GIOGENESIS agents. Because of difficulty with preparation and purification of this agent, clinical trials
are in the very early stage with conflicting results.

endothelioma (en″do-the-le-o′mah)   any tumor,
benign or cancerous, arising from the epithelial tissue (scale-like, flat cells) lining the blood or lymph
vessels.

Endoxan   See CYTOXAN and CARCINOGENS.

engraftment   the process in which transplanted
stem cells or bone marrow begin to manufacture
new red and white blood cells and platelets in the
recipient. It usually takes place between 14 and 30
days after a peripheral stem cell transplantation or
BONE MARROW TRANSPLANTATION.

enkephalins (en-kef′ah-lins)   one of the natural
substances produced by the brain to fight pain.
Like NARCOTICS, they reduce the patient's perception of pain by binding to the "opiate receptors" on
the surface of brain cells, though it is not known
exactly how enkephalins work.
    See also ENDORPHINS.

enteral feeding (en′ter-al)   a way of providing
nutritional support to malnourished patients, or
patients expected to become malnourished during
the course of their disease. Enteral feeding can be
given through a variety of tubes—the most commonly used are nasogastric tubes that go through
the nose. These can be used for a few days. For
patients who will need enteral feeding for anex-
tended period of time, or permanently, a STOMA may
be created in the stomach. Nutrients can be delivered into the stomach through the tube. Patients
who may require enteral feeding include those who
have had radical surgery in the oropharyngeal area
(mouth, throat), have partial obstruction in the gastrointestinal tract or short bowel syndrome (surgical
removal of a large amount of the small and large
intestines), or who are unconscious or ANOREXIC.

enterostomal therapist   See STOMAL THERAPIST.

enucleation (e-nu″kle-a′shun)   complete surgical
removal of an organ or tumor so that it comes out
clean and whole, like a nut from its shell. When
performed on the eye, for example, the eyeball is
removed after the eye muscles and optic nerve have
been severed. This may be performed in treatment
of INTRAOCULAR MELANOMA.

environmental tobacco smoke (ETS)   See PASSIVE
SMOKE.

enzyme (en′zīm)   a substance produced by cells in the body that can start or accelerate chemical transformations, such as burning up sugar to produce energy or breaking down food within the intestinal tract. Many enzymes are found in the digestive juices. The enzyme itself does not change during the chemical reaction. An enzyme can serve as a TUMOR MARKER. An elevated level can be an indication of cancer or a RECURRENCE of disease.

eosinophil (e″o-sin′o-fil)   one type of the white blood cell GRANULOCYTE. Normally it plays a role in allergic reactions, responding to foreign substances. Elevations of eosinophil cells may be seen in patients with asthma, drug reactions, etc. They may be elevated in EOSINOPHIL LEUKEMIA.

eosinophil colony-stimulating factor [eosinophil CSF]   See also INTERLEUKIN-5.

eosinophil CSF   See EOSINOPHIL COLONY-STIMU-LATING FACTOR.

eosinophilic leukemia (e″o-sin″o-fil′ik)   a form of LEUKEMIA affecting the eosinophils (a particular type of white blood cell, which contains granules that stain with acid dyes (eosin). The eosinophils increase during allergic reactions.)

EP-2101   a substance that is being studied as a treatment for cancer; in the family of drugs called cancer vaccines.

ependymal tumors   See BRAIN CANCER.

ependymoblastoma   See BRAIN CANCER.

ependymoma (ĕ-pen″dĭ-mo′mah)   a generally slow-growing tumor (GLIOMA) arising in the membranes lining the ventricles of the brain, the ependyma. It is most common in children and young adults. It may be either benign or malignant. See BRAIN CANCER.

EPI   See EPIRUBICIN.

epidemiology (ep″ĭ-de″me-ol′o-je)   a way of studying a disease by looking at the relationship between various factors such as where it has occurred and who is affected. An example of an epidemiological study might be the number of cases of lung cancer in a particular area compared with the number of people in that area who smoke. If there is a significantly higher incidence of lung cancer in that area than in the general population and there is also a greater proportion of people smoking than in the normal population, one might conclude that smoking was in some way linked to the development of lung cancer.

epidermis (ep″ĭ-der′mis)   the outer surface layer of the skin that contains both squamous and basal cells. See SKIN CANCER.

epidermoid cancer of mucous membranes (ep″ĭ-der′moid)   cancer arising in the lining of the upper air and food passages. Physicians commonly refer to this as aerodigestive tract cancer. Most of the tumors remain confined to the site where they originated, or to the lymph nodes in the neck, for relatively long periods of time. This cancer is strongly associated with tobacco (cigarette smoking, pipes, cigars, snuff, and chewing tobacco) and alcohol.

epidermoid carcinoma of the lung   See SQUA-MOUS CELL LUNG CANCER.

epidural anesthesia   See CAUDAL ANESTHESIA.

epidural catheter (ep″ĭ-du′ral kath′ĕ-ter)   a temporary or semipermanent tube that is placed in the epidural area (outermost part of brain and spinal cord) for administration of painkillers. It may be controlled by the patient. It may be used for short-term use, such as for the relief of pain after surgery, or for chronic administration in cases of serious cancer pain. One advantage of such a system is that it may allow the patient to control the amount of NARCOTIC required to achieve comfort. This is one form of patient controlled analgesia (PCA).

epidural dorsal column stimulator (ep″ĭ-du′ral dor′sal)   a surgical procedure to alleviate or lessen pain. Electrodes (electrical conductors through which current enters or leaves a body) are surgically implanted over the spinal cord. The patient can control the electrical impulses, which deaden pain.

epipodophyllotoxin   See ETOPOSIDE.

epirubicin (EPI)   an ANTIBIOTIC, anticancer drug in the treatment of breast, ovarian, stomach, colon/rectal, pancreatic, and head and neck cancer, soft tissue sarcoma, and NON-HODGKIN'S LYMPHOMA and leukemia. It is taken by IV (injected into a vein). Side effects may include hair loss, nausea, vomiting, myelosuppression, diarrhea, hives, and mouth sores.

epithelial   (ep-ĭ-the′le-ul)   refers to the cells that line the internal and external surfaces of the body.

epithelioma   (ep″ĭ-the″le-o′mah)   a cancer affecting mainly the EPITHELIUM, the tissue that covers the internal and external surfaces of the body, including the vessels and small cavities. Now more commonly called CARCINOMA, the type of cancer depends on the cell type of the epithelial tissue and where it is located in the body. Some of the common cell types are basal, squamous, and transitional. Carcinoma is the most common form of cancer.

epithelium   the tissue that forms the surface of the skin and lines hollow organs and all passages of the respiratory, digestive, genital, and urinary systems. See EPITHELIOMA and CARCINOMA.

EPO   See EPOGEN.

EPOCH   a combination chemotherapy regimen of ETOPOSIDE, PREDNISONE, ONCOVIN, CYTOXAN, and ADRIAMYCIN used in treatment of NHL. See individual drug listings for side effects.
   See also COMBINATION THERAPY.

epoetin alpha   See EPOGEN.

Epogen   [EPO, Procrit, epoetin, epoetin alpha, Eprex]   a COLONY-STIMULATING FACTOR that exclusively stimulates the production of red blood cells. It is used in the treatment of anemia in patients with nonmyeloid malignancies, kidney failure, and HIV. It is taken by IV (injected into a vein).

epothilone   a drug obtained from bacteria that interferes with cell division; some epothilones belong to the new class of chemotherapeutic agents undergoing CLINICAL TRIALS in 2005.

Eprex   See EPOGEN.

Epstein-Barr virus (EBV)   a common herpes-like virus known to cause infectious mononucleosis, and the first human tumor virus discovered. It was found by David Burkitt during studies of lymphoma in young children in East Africa in 1958. EBV appears to play a role in the development of BURKITT'S LYMPHOMA. There is also a link between this virus and NASOPHARYNGEAL CANCER. A possible association between EBV and HODGKIN'S DISEASE is less certain. Most adults have an antibody to EBV, indicating prior exposure, with no associated illness.

ER   See ESTROGEN RECEPTOR TEST.

ER positive   See ESTROGEN RECEPTOR POSITIVE.

Erbitux   [cetuximab]   a monoclonal antibody that acts as an ANTIANGIOGENESIS agent. Erbitux is FDA-indicated in combination with IRINOTECAN (CAMPTOSAR) for patients with EGFR-expressing metastatic COLORECTAL CANCER who are refractory to Irinotecan or as monotherapy (a single therapy) in patients who are intolerant of Irinotecan-based therapy. It is recommended that patients' tumors be screened for EGFR expression using IHC (immunohistochemistry) to determine appropriate use of this agent, which is very expensive. As with many monoclonal antibodies, there is danger of significant infusion reaction. Skin reactions are also common.

ERCP   See ENDOSCOPIC RETROGRADE CHOLANGIOPANCREATOGRAPHY.

Ergamisole   See LEVAMISOLE.

Erlotinib   See TARCEVA.

ERT   See ESTROGEN REPLACEMENT THERAPY.

erythema   (er″ĭ-the′mah)   red patches on the skin. Erythema of the skin may be a sign of underlying infection or inflammation. CHEMOTHERAPY (anticancer drugs) injections may also cause erythema of the skin. This usually disappears within several hours. Persistent redness of the skin at a chemotherapy injection site should be brought to the attention of a nurse or doctor.

erythrocyte   See RED BLOOD CELL.

erythrocyte sedimentation rate (ESR) (ĕ-rith″ro-sīt) a very old diagnostic test in which a special test tube is used to measure the rate of fall of red blood cells over time. An abnormal rate may be an indication of certain forms of cancer. In HODGKIN'S DISEASE, in its earliest stages, there is usually an abnormal rate when many other lab tests are normal. An elevated erythrocyte sedimentation rate may also be an early indication of multiple MYELOMA. Other causes of elevation of ESR include infections and inflammatory diseases, thus it is not cancer specific.

erythroleukemia (ĕ-rith″ro-lu-ke′me-ah) [Di-Gugliemo's syndrome]   a rare and difficult-to-treat form of acute nonlymphocytic leukemia affecting both red and white blood cells.

See also ANLL.

erythroplakia (ĕ-rith″ro-pla′ke-ah) [erythroplasia]   a condition in the mucous membrane of the mouth in which a reddened patch appears. As it progresses, it may appear as a sore or ulcer. In its early stages it may not be painful and may not be noticed by the person. A routine visit to the dentist may lead to its discovery. Although most ulcerations in the mouth are not cancerous, a doctor should be seen for any ulcer that lasts longer than two weeks. Erythroplakia is seen most often in heavy smokers and drinkers. It occurs equally in men and women and develops most often in people over the age of 60. Since it is considered a precancerous condition, it should be removed and biopsied.

See also MOUTH CANCER.

erythroplasia   See ERYTHROPLAKIA.

erythropoietin   See EPOGEN.

E-SHAP   a combination of the anticancer drugs ETOPOSIDE, CISPLATIN, ARA-C, and methylprednisolone (ADRENOCORTICOID) sometimes used in the treatment of NON-HODGKIN'S LYMPHOMA. See individual drug listings for side effects.

See also COMBINATION CHEMOTHERAPY.

esophageal cancer (ĕ-sof″ah-je′al)   cancer of the esophagus, the muscular tube that carries food from the throat to the stomach. In 2004, an estimated 14,250 people diagnosed with esophageal cancer have a form of esophageal cancer called ADENOCARCINOMA. It is one of the least curable and rapidly fatal cancers. It occurs much more commonly in men than women; and blacks develop it three to four times more often than whites. The average age at diagnosis is 68 to 70. Esophageal cancer occurs in approximately 13,500 Americans per year, causing about 12,500 deaths.

Smoking is the major cause of traditional SQUAMOUS CELL esophageal cancer. For example, people who smoke half a pack of cigarettes a day are four times more likely to develop esophageal cancer than a nonsmoker. The more a person smokes, the greater the risk of developing esophageal cancer. More than moderate consumption of alcohol also increases the risk of this type of cancer. People who smoke and drink may be 30 times more likely to develop esophageal cancer than people who do neither.

Over the past 20 years there has been a rising incidence of cancer of the lower third of the esophagus, where it meets the stomach (called the gastroesophageal [GE] junction). This cancer is an adenocarcinoma and is associated with Barrett's esophagus and with gastro-esophageal reflux disease (GERD).

The number of Americans diagnosed with the common form of esophageal cancer has increased sixfold over the last 25 years. About half of the estimated 14,250 people diagnosed with esophageal cancer in 2004 have adenocarcinoma. Although esophageal adenocarcinoma is relatively uncommon, researchers say it is now the fastest-growing form of cancer in the U.S., and its incidence is rising faster than BREAST CANCER, PROSTATE CANCER, or MELANOMA.

The most common symptom is dysphagia, a difficulty or pain when swallowing foods or liquids. Other symptoms may include sensations of pressure and burning or pain in the upper middle part of the throat, hoarseness, cough, fever, or choking. Because of the difficulty in swallowing food, weight loss can also be a common symptom.

Procedures used in the diagnosis and evaluation of esophageal cancer may include a BARIUM SWALLOW of the esophagus and chest, ESOPHAGOSCOPY, CT SCAN, and BLOOD TESTS.

Following is the National Cancer Institute's (NCI) staging for esophageal cancer:

- Stage 0 or carcinoma in situ—a very early cancer that has not spread below the lining of the first layer of esophageal tissue
- Stage I—cancer that involves a small portion of the esophagus, less than five CENTIMETERS (cm), and has not spread to adjacent structures, LYMPH NODES, or other organs
- Stage II—cancer has not spread to other organs but lymph nodes may be involved and:
  — a large portion of the esophagus is involved or
  — there are symptoms of blockage or
  — it has spread to involve the entire circumference of the esophageal area but has not spread to adjacent structures
- Stage III—cancer has spread to adjacent structures or there is extensive lymph node involvement; there is no spread to other organs
- Stage IV—cancer has spread to other organs
- Recurrent—cancer has returned to the same site or to another part of the body after treatment

Historically, most cancers were squamous cell. Recently, an increase in the number of adenocarcinomas has been noted.

Treatment depends on the stage of the disease, the general state of health of the patient and the cell type, and other factors. An ESOPHAGECTOMY, removal of the esophagus, may be performed. Esophageal cancer is also treated with RADIATION THERAPY and CHEMOTHERAPY (anticancer drugs). For specific information on the latest state-of-the-art treatment, by stage, call NCI's Cancer Information Service at 1-800-4-CANCER (1-800-422-6237), or for a TTY: 1-800-332-8615.

esophageal speech (ĕ-sof"ah-je'al) a type of speech used when the voice box has been removed. The tongue is used to force air into the very top part of the food pipe. The air is then forced out through the mouth enabling a sound to be made deep in the throat. That sound is used to make speech.

See also ELECTRO-LARYNX.

esophagectomy (ĕ-sof"ah-jek'to-me) surgical removal of the esophagus (tube that connects the stomach to the throat). The healthy part of the esophagus that remains is attached to the stomach so that swallowing is still possible. A plastic tube or part of the intestine may be used to make the connection. An esophagectomy may be performed in the treatment of ESOPHAGEAL CANCER.

esophagitis (ĕ-sof"ah-ji'tis) inflammation of the membrane of the esophagus (tube connecting the stomach and throat), which can be a side effect of RADIATION THERAPY or CHEMOTHERAPY. It causes a difficulty or pain in swallowing and can sometimes

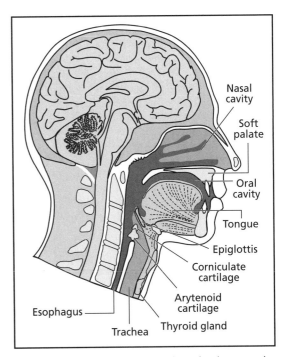

Cross section of the head and neck, showing the relative size and position of the esophagus. Smoking is the major cause of esophageal cancer.
Infobase Publishing.

progress to include painful ulceration, hemorrhage, and secondary infection.

esophagogastroduodenoscopy   See GASTROSCOPY.

esophagogram   See ESOPHAGOGRAPHY.

esophagography   an X-RAY examination of the esophagus (the tube connecting the throat to the stomach) using the CONTRAST MEDIUM barium, which is taken by mouth. An esophagography is usually done as part of a GI SERIES but can be done alone when the doctor wants to examine only the esophagus. It can be done in the doctor's office or at the hospital on an outpatient or inpatient basis and takes about half an hour. In a cine esophagography a video is taken during the esophagram to asses the swallowing mechanism.

esophagoscope   See ESOPHAGOSCOPY.

esophagoscopy (ĕ-sof″ah-gos′ko-pe)   a procedure used to examine the esophagus (the tube connecting the throat and stomach). An esophagoscopy may be used in the diagnosis of ESOPHAGEAL CANCER, as well as other disorders. An esophagoscope, a long thin tube with a light and lens at the end, is slid through the mouth into the esophagus. The inside of the esophagus can then be examined for a tumor. Sometimes the size of a tumor can be determined and cells and tissue can be obtained for a biopsy.

See also ENDOSCOPY.

esophagus   the muscular tube that runs from the back of the throat, through the neck and chest, and into the stomach. Food travels to the stomach through the esophagus.

essential thrombocythemia (ET)   a primary condition in which there is a sustained elevated level of platelets (thrombocytosis) in the absence of any other stimulation, such as infection or inflamation. This condition is one of the chronic myeloproliferative disorders (CMPD). Sustained thrombocytosis can result in serious bleeding or clotting. Treatment methods include the drug Anagrelide, approved for treatment of ET by the FDA, which may be useful in the other myeloproliferative disorders, as well as ASPIRIN or the biological agent INTERFERON.

Estinyl   See ESTROGEN.

Estracyt   See ESTRAMUSTINE PHOSPHATE.

Estracyte   See ESTRAMUSTINE PHOSPHATE.

estramustine phosphate (es″trah-mus′tēn fos′fāt) [EM, Estracyt, Estracyte, Emcyt]   an ALKYLATING anticancer drug sometimes used in the treatment of hormone refractory metastatic PROSTATE CANCER. It is taken by mouth. Common side effects may include nausea and vomiting. Occasional or rare side effects may include diarrhea, BONE MARROW DEPRESSION, heart problems, skin rashes, and the emergence of female characteristics. Its use is hampered by its cardiovascular side effects.

estrogen (es′tro-jen)   female sex hormones responsible for development of secondary sex characteristics, such as the growth of breasts. It is primarily produced in the ovarian follicle cells. A small amount is secreted by the adrenal gland. Synthetic estrogens are used in the treatment of cancer. Any hormone that affects the monthly cycle of changes taking place in the female genital tract is considered to be an estrogen. Estrogen has been linked with several cancers, including BREAST CANCER and ENDOMETRIAL CANCER. However, estrogen may be used in the treatment of PROSTATE CANCER.

Some of the estrogens that may be used in cancer treatment include:

- diethylstilbestrol (DES)
- diethylstilbestrol diphosphate (Stilphostrol, Stilbestrol diphosphate)
- chlorotrianisene (Tace)
- ethinyl estradiol (Estinyl)
- conjugated equine estrogen (Premarin)

Antiestrogen drugs, such as TAMOXIFEN, may be used in the treatment of cancers in which the tumor is dependent on estrogen, such as breast cancer.

See also CARCINOGENS.

estrogen cream (es′tro-jen)   a cream containing ESTROGEN, a female sex hormone. The estrogen in the cream can be absorbed into the body, the same way that an estrogen pill can. Its use is generally not advised for anyone who has had breast cancer.

estrogen dependent in breast cancer a tumor that is influenced by the presence of the hormone estrogen. Some breast tumors will not grow if deprived of estrogen.

estrogen receptor level (es'tro-jen) the amount of protein in a cancer cell to which ESTROGEN can attach. As determined by an ESTROGEN RECEPTOR TEST, the higher the level, the more likely the cancer is to be stimulated by estrogen (estrogen dependent) and the more likely that treatment with an ANTIESTROGEN drug will be an effective treatment.

estrogen receptor positive [ER positive] in breast cancer, a tumor that appears to be stimulated by the hormone estrogen and is dependent on estrogen for its growth. An ESTROGEN RECEPTOR TEST is performed to determine whether the tumor is wholly or partly dependent on estrogen.

estrogen receptor test (es'tro-jen) a test done during the biopsy of cancerous breast tissue to determine if its growth is dependent on the hormone ESTROGEN. The presence of the estrogen receptor on breast tissue correlates with prognosis and response to treatment. About two-thirds of breast cancers are estrogen receptor positive (estrogen dependent). In about half of those cancers, the tumor will shrink if the tumor is deprived of estrogen. The estrogen can be removed from the body by surgically removing the organs and glands that produce it (the ovaries, adrenal glands, and pituitary gland) or by the administration of an antiestrogen drug like TAMOXIFEN or other hormone to "block" the estrogen.

estrogen replacement therapy (ERT) (es'tro-jen) [hormonal replacement therapy] using natural or synthetic estrogen to replac eestrogen that is no longer being produced by the ovaries. ERT is primarily used to relieve symptoms caused by menopause or a HYSTERECTOMY, such as hot flashes, vaginal dryness, and osteoporosis (thinning of the bones). It is quite effective, though it can have some serious side effects.

Estrogen replacement therapy may increase a woman's risk of developing ENDOMETRIAL CANCER and BREAST CANCER as well as other disorders. Studies have shown that women taking replacement estrogens have a two to eight times higher risk of developing endometrial cancer than women who do not take the hormone. To prevent endometrial buildup, which can lead to endometrial cancer, progesterone may be given along with estrogen. (A woman who has undergone a total hysterectomy is in no danger of developing endometrial cancer.)

The association between ERT and breast cancer is less clear because studies have produced conflicting results. A study in 1989 of more than 23,000 women in Sweden who used replacement hormones found 10% more cancer that expected. The risk of breast cancer increased as the length of use increased. However, a study reported in 1991, of nearly 9,000 women in California, found no increased risk of breast cancer among women taking estrogen. It also found that women who had some estrogen therapy lived longer than those who did not. Many researchers feel the reduced risk of heart disease and osteoporosis that ERT provides outweighs the risk of breast cancer. The researchers concluded that the health benefits of ERT outweighed the risks associated with it. Women who have had breast cancer, however, are usually advised not to take estrogen replacement therapy.

It is recommended that women on ERT get a yearly checkup for any signs of cancer, and that they consult their doctor at any sign of vaginal bleeding (a possible symptom of endometrial cancer) or a lump in the breast (a possible sign of breast cancer). ERT remains controversial.

ethinyl estradiol [Estinyl] See ESTROGEN.

Ethyol [amifostine] used to reduce the cumulative renal toxicity associated with repeated administration of CISPLATIN in patients with advanced ovarian cancer and non-small cell lung cancer (NSCLC). It is being investigated in the treatment of myelodysplasia syndromes (MDS), and as a radioprotective agent. Possible side effects may include nausea and vomiting, drowsiness, sneezing, muscle and stomach cramps, flushing of the face. It is given by IV (injected into a vein).

etidronate [Didronel, EHDP] used in the treatment of PAGET'S DISEASE of the bone, a noncancerous condition, and hypercalcemia. It can be taken orally or by IV (injected into a vein).

Etopophos   See ETOPOSIDE.

etoposide (e-to′po-sīd) [VP-16213, Toposar, Etopophos, VePesid, epipodophyllotoxin]   an ANTI-BIOTIC anticancer drug which may be used in the treatment of cancers of the testes, lung, prostate, and uterus and lymphomas, acute nonlymphocytic leukemia, hepatoma, rhabdomyosarcoma, and Kaposi's sarcoma. It is given by IV (injection into a vein) or can be taken by mouth. Common side effects include nausea and vomiting. Occasional or rare side effects include BONE MARROW DEPRESSION, hair loss, lung problems, fever, chills, and loss of appetite. Etoposide is an important anticancer drug commonly used in the treatment of cancer.

ETS (environmental tobacco smoke)   See PASSIVE SMOKE.

Eulexin   See FLUTAMIDE.

euthanasia   the active step of the administration of a known lethal dose of medication to intentionally end the life of someone suffering from an incurable illness such as terminal cancer. This is not legal in the United States. As of 2005, Oregon is the only state that has in place legal protection for physician-assisted suicide. Some doctors and ethicists distinguish this from withholding or withdrawing life sustaining treatment, allowing death by the disease. That is referred to as "passive euthanasia" and is much more palatable to many caregivers. Euthanasia should also be distinguished from "assisted suicide," which is a complex legal/ethical issue at the time of publication of this book. In 1997, the Supreme Court unanimously ruled that there is no Constitutional right to physician-assisted suicide. In 1999, Dr. Jack Kevorkian was convicted of second-degree murder in the delivery of a controlled substance in the assisted suicide death of a man suffering from Lou Gehrig's disease.
See also LIVING WILL.

evidence-based medicine   the practice of basing treatment management decisions on published studies involving large numbers of patients that make the conclusions universally accepted. Not all questions in medicine have a large evidence base, thereby requiring reliance on experience or results of smaller studies.

Evista   See RALOXIFENE.

Ewing's sarcoma (u′ingz sar-ko′mah)   cancer in the marrow of the midshaft of the bone, most commonly in the thighbone, shinbone, and upper arm. It is a rare cancer that occurs most frequently in children and young adults. The first symptoms may be pain and swelling.
Procedures used in the diagnosis and evaluation of Ewing's sarcoma may include blood and urine tests. X-RAYS of the affected bone and the whole body and lungs, BONE MARROW ASPIRATIONS, CT SCANS, and occasionally FLUOROSCOPY.
Following is the National Cancer Institute's (NCI) staging for Ewing' sarcoma:

- Stage I (localized)—cancer below the elbow or knee, in the lower jawbone, skull, face, shoulder blade, vertebra (spinal column), or collarbone
- Stage II (localized)—cancer in the rib
- Stage III (localized)—cancer in the arm bone or thighbone
- Stage IV (localized)—cancer in the pelvis or sacrum (part of spinal cord)
- Metastatic—a tumor that has spread beyond the primary site to distant sites; the most common sites of spread are lung, bone, and BONE MARROW; LYMPH NODE and CENTRAL NERVOUS SYSTEM metastases are less common.

Treatment depends on the stage of the disease, the general state of health of the patient, and other factors. Treatments for Ewing's sarcoma include SURGERY, RADIATION THERAPY, and CHEMOTHERAPY. For specific information on the latest state-of-the-art treatment, by stage, call NCI's Cancer Information Service at 1-800-4-CANCER (1-800-422-6237), or for a TTY: 1-800-332-8615.
See also BONE CANCER.
Exatecan is an investigational (2005) chemotherapeutic agent being studied for the treatment of PANCREATIC CANCER.

excisional biopsy (ek-sizh′un-al bi′ŏp-se) [surgical biopsy, punch biopsy, shave biopsy] removal of a tumor or lesion for microscopic examination for cancer cells. This can also serve as treatment, for example in breast cancer when the entire lump is removed, the excisional biopsy is, effectively, a LUMPECTOMY; or in skin cancer, where the entire "suspicious" growth is removed. It implies removal of all abnormal tissue.

excretory urography See IVP.

exenteration (eks-en″ter-a′shun) surgical removal of the cervix, uterus, and vagina, and depending on the spread of cancer, the lower colon, rectum, or bladder. Plastic surgery may be needed. Exenteration may be used in the treatment of advanced CERVICAL CANCER and VAGINAL CANCER.

exfoliative cytology (eks-fo′le-a″tiv si-tol′ah-je) microscopic examination of cells that are "flaked off" interior surfaces of the body to determine if cancer is present. The most common and well-known application is the PAP SMEAR, in which exfoliated cells from the cervix are examined. Other uses include SPUTUM CYTOLOGY EXAM and URINE CYTOLOGY EXAM.

exocrine cancer See PANCREATIC CANCER.

exocrine pancreas (ek′so-krin) the part of the pancreas that produces juices consisting of salts, enzymes, and water that flow from small ducts into the main pancreatic duct. Those juices then enter the small intestine, where they aid in digestion. The exocrine pancreas is the site of 95% of all pancreatic cancers. This is distinguished from the ENDOCRINE PANCREAS, or hormone-producing portion of the gland.

exophthalmometer See EXOPHTHALMOMETRY.

exophthalmometry (ek″sof-thal-mom′ĕ-tre) examination of the eye by an exophthalmometer, a noninvasive device used to measure the protrusion of the eyeball. This may be used in the diagnosis of EYE CANCER.

experimental drug an agent being investigated for its efficacy in the treatment of cancer. See CLINICAL TRIALS.

experimental treatments See CLINICAL TRIALS.

exploratory laparotomy See LAPAROTOMY.

extended radical mastectomy surgical removal of the breast, the fat under the skin surrounding the breast, the muscles on the front of the chest that support the breasts, all the fat and lymph nodes that are in the armpit, the internal mammary nodes, and possibly the thoracic nerve. This operation, now rarely used, was an attempt to encompass all surrounding tissue in order to cure BREAST CANCER. It resulted in significant disfigurement and frequently discomfort for the patient.
See also MASTECTOMY and BREAST CANCER.

external radiation therapy [teletherapy] the use of radiation from a machine, usually at some distance from the body, to treat a cancer patient. Approximately 50% of all cancer patients will receive some type of RADIATION THERAPY. Most of them will receive "external" radiation as opposed to INTERNAL RADIATION.

The type of radiation used depends on a number of factors, including the type of cancer and its location. The different types include X-RAYS, ELECTRON BEAM THERAPY, and COBALT-60 gamma rays. High-energy radiation is used to treat many kinds of cancers that are located deep in the body. Low-energy X-rays are used to treat some kinds of skin diseases. The radiation is directed to a specific part of the body.

When radiation therapy is being given as a cure for cancer, such as in Hodgkin's disease, it is usually given for five days a week for six or seven weeks. PALLIATIVE TREATMENT, to alleviate the symptoms (pain), is given for a shorter period of time, two to three weeks. The total dose of the treatment is based on a number of different factors, including the general state of health of the patient, the size and location of the cancer, and the type of tumor. The treatment itself takes from one to five minutes.

Before treatment is started, an X-ray machine is used to define the patient's "treatment port," the exact place on the body where the radiation will be aimed. The area is marked on the skin with semi-permanent ink. This is called "simulation" and can take up to two hours.

Side effects of external radiation usually relate to the part of the body being treated. Most side effects, though not pleasant, are not serious and can be controlled with medication or diet. Most go away within a few weeks after treatment. The most common side effects are fatigue, changes to the skin, and loss of appetite.

To minimize side effects patients are advised to:

- get plenty of rest
- eat a balanced diet to prevent weight loss
- wear loose, soft cotton clothing over the treated area
- not rub or scrub treated skin
- not use harsh soaps, lotions, deodorants, medicines, perfumes, cosmetics, talcum powder, or other substances in the treated area without consulting a doctor
- not use adhesive tape on treated skin
- not apply heat (heating pad) or cold (ice pack) on treated skin
- protect the treated area from the sun; if possible, cover the area with clothing or a hat before going out; check with the doctor about using a sun block; use a sunscreen with at least 15 sun protection factor even after conclusion of the treatment and recovery of the skin for at least one year.

extrahepatic bile duct cancer   See BILE DUCT CANCER.

extralymphatic [extranodal] a condition in which lymphoma (HODGKIN'S DISEASE or NON-HODGKIN'S LYMPHOMA) is found in organs outside of the LYMPH SYSTEM such as the skin, lung, brain, etc.

extranodal   See EXTRALYMPHATIC.

extrapleural pneumonectomy   See PLEUROPNEU-MONECTOMY.

eye cancer   a rare cancer affecting men and women at equal rates. Estimates indicate that about 2,120 new cases of all primary intraocular cancers (eye and orbit) would be diagnosed in the United States in 2005, with 230 deaths related to the disease. Most, but not all of these will be MELANOMAS, with LYMPHOMAS being the next most common. Both of these cancers more often start in other parts of the body. Over 90% of melanomas start in the skin, while lymphomas are more likely to begin in lymph nodes.

The two most common forms of eye cancer are INTRAOCULAR MELANOMA (also called ocular melanoma) in adults and RETINOBLASTOMA in children under the age of two. Other, more rare cancers affecting the eye are tumors of the orbit (eye socket), muscle (RHABDOMYOSARCOMA), which occurs most frequently in children under 10, and FIBROUS HISTIOCYTOMA. Other cancers, most commonly breast cancer and lung cancer, may metastasize (spread) to the eye.

Symptoms of cancer in the eye may include protrusion of the eyeball, double vision, pain, and/or drooping of the eyelid. Eye cancer is rare and these symptoms are usually related to other disorders; but if they occur, a doctor should be consulted.

Procedures used in the diagnosis and evaluation of eye cancer may include examination by an exophthalmometer (instrument that measures the protrusion of the eyeball) or a slit lamp (which allows viewing of the anterior portions of the eye including the cornea and iris), OPTHALMOSCOPY (to see into the eye), FLOURESCEIN ANGIOGRAPHY (which uses dye injected into a vein in the arm to make a tumor more visible), CT SCAN, ULTRASOUND, NUCLEAR SCAN (where radioactive material is injected into the circulation and then followed by scanning devices), and a NEEDLE BIOPSY. For staging and treatment information, see INTRAOCULAR MELANOMA and RETINOBLASTOMA.

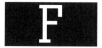

FAB See FRENCH-AMERICAN-BRITISH (FAB) CLASSIFICATION.

FAC a combination of the anticancer drugs 5-FU, ADRIAMYCIN, and CYTOXAN sometimes used in the treatment of breast cancer. See individual drug listings for side effects.

See also COMBINATION CHEMOTHERAPY.

fallopian tubes two slender ducts that connect the ovaries with the uterus.

fallopian tubes cancer (fal-lo'pe-an) an extremely rare cancer of the fallopian tubes, which run from the ovaries to the uterus. Most tumors in the fallopian tubes are metastases from other genital organs. It accounts for between 0.5 and 1.1% of all gynecological malignancies (cancers). The women most affected are between 40 and 60 years of age. Symptoms may include vaginal bleeding or discharge or pains in the abdomen or pelvis. A positive PAP SMEAR may be an indication of fallopian tubes cancer, but generally a definitive diagnosis requires surgery.

There are several ways of staging fallopian tubes cancer. Following is a modified version of the staging for OVARIAN CANCER that was devised by M. G. Dodson and others for fallopian tubes cancer:

- Stage I—growth limited to the tube
  IA—one tube, no ASCITES
  IB—both tubes, no ascites
  IC—one or both tubes with ascites with malignant cells
- Stage II—growth limited to the pelvis
  IIA—extension to uterus or ovary
  IIB—extension to other pelvic tissues
- Stage III—growth involving one or more ovaries with intraperitoneal metastases
- Stage IV—growth involving one or both tubes with distant metastases outside the peritoneal cavity
- Recurrent—cancer has returned to the original site or to another part of the body after treatment.

Treatment depends on the stage of the disease, the general state of health of the patient, and other factors. Treatments include SURGERY, RADIATION THERAPY, and CHEMOTHERAPY (anticancer drugs). For specific information on the latest state-of-the-art treatment, by stage, call the National Cancer Institute's Cancer Information Service at 1-800-4-CANCER (1-800-422-6237), or for a TTY: 1-800-332-8615.

FAM a combination of the anticancer drugs 5-FU, ADRIAMYCIN, and mitomycin-C (MUTAMYCIN) used in the treatment of STOMACH CANCER and NON-SMALL CELL LUNG CANCER. See individual drug listings for side effects.

See also COMBINED CHEMOTHERAPY.

familial atypical multiple mole melanoma (FAMMM) syndrome   FAMMM syndrome is a family tendency for developing the skin cancer MELANOMA. It was first recognized as a hereditary cancer in 1820 when an English surgeon diagnosed this disease in several members of the same family.

familial dysplastic nevus syndrome   See DYSPLASTIC NEVI.

familial medullary cancer (med′u-lār″e)   a cancer of the thyroid that runs in families. Fifty percent of the patient's brothers or sisters may have it. It usually always involves both lobes of the thyroid glands.

See also MEDULLARY CARCINOMA OF THE THYROID and THYROID CANCER.

familial multiple polyposis of the colon (FPC) (pol″e-po′sis) [familial adenomatous polyposis coli (FAPC), hereditary polyposis of the colon, familial polyposis, Gardner's syndrome]   a family tendency to develop hundreds to thousands of polyps (abnormal, mushroom-like growths) throughout the colon at a young age, usually as a teenager or young adult. People with FPC are at a much greater risk of developing COLON CANCER. It will occur in virtually 100% of the people with FPC by the time they are 50. It is recommended that people with a family history of FPC start regular screening for colon cancer at an early age. Although many people develop polyps without any symptoms, following are some symptoms that may occur and should be followed up by a physical exam: bright red blood in the stool; diarrhea that is not the result of diet or the flu; a long period of constipation; crampy pain in the stomach region; persistent decrease in size of stool; frequent feeling of distention (or bloating) in the abdominal or bowel region; weight loss; and/or unusual and continuing lack of energy. These may also be symptoms for other disorders but should be seen by a doctor if they persist.

Diagnostic tests for the presence of FPC may include flexible SIGMOIDOSCOPY, COLONOSCOPY, and barium enema (see LOWER GI SERIES). These tests are also used in the diagnosis of colon cancer.

Familial Ovarian Cancer Registry   See GILDA RADNER FAMILIAL REGISTER.

familial polyposis   See FAMILIAL MULTIPLE POLYPOSIS OF THE COLON.

FAMMM   See FAMILIAL ATYPICAL MULTIPLE MOLE MELANOMA (FAMMM) SYNDROME.

FAPC   See FAMILIAL MULTIPLE POLYPOSIS OF THE COLON.

Fareston   See TOREMIFENE.

fat   together with carbohydrate and protein, one of the three food categories. Both the National Cancer Institute and the American Cancer Society have recommended that Americans restrict their intake of fat to 30% or less of their total calories. While definitive data is not in, there is enough evidence to link fat to a number of cancers, including breast cancer and colon cancer.

See also DIET.

fatigue   a tremendous feeling of weariness; exhaustion. Fatigue is a common condition in cancer patients and is one of their most frequent complaints. Fatigue frequently increases as the cancer progresses. Fatigue may also be a symptom of the as-yet undiagnosed cancer and be a result of some therapies.

Following are brief descriptions of the factors that may contribute to fatigue in the cancer patient:

- tumors that enter the BONE MARROW and cause ANEMIA
- RADIATION THERAPY, CHEMOTHERAPY (anticancer drugs), and BIOLOGICAL THERAPY; in the case of radiation, increased energy is expended by the body in repairing damaged tissue
- other drugs such as analgesics for pain, antiemetics for nausea and vomiting, antidepressants, sleeping medication, and anticonvulsants
- not enough nutrients consumed to meet the energy requirements of the body, which may be a result of the body's inability to process nutrients efficiently; an increase in the body's energy requirements; or a decrease in the consumption of nutrients due to nausea and vomiting, anorexia, diarrhea or bowel obstruction
- depression and anxiety.

Fatigue in the cancer patient can be difficult to manage. In the healthy person suffering from fatigue, additional sleep is frequently all that is needed. In a person with cancer the solution is rarely that simple. Treatment of the cancer itself may eventually lessen the sense of fatigue as the tumor responds. However, until that happens, the treatment itself can be a major cause of fatigue.

In patients whose fatigue is a result, at least in part, from anemia, red blood cell transfusions may be administered. Nutritional support may also be useful in restoring some of the patient's energy. In patients whose fatigue is associated with DEPRESSION, therapy may be helpful and/or antidepressant medication. In cases where there are no real remedies for the fatigue, help may come in the form of planning the patient's activities with the patient to best use whatever energy he or she may have.

FCE a combination of the anticancer drugs 5-FU, CISPLATIN, and ETOPOSIDE sometimes used in the treatment of STOMACH CANCER. See individual drug listings for side effects.

See also COMBINATION CHEMOTHERAPY.

F-CL a combination of the anticancer drugs fluorouricil (5-FU) and LEUCOVORIN, sometimes used in the treatment of COLON CANCER. See individual drug listings for side effects.

See also COMBINATION CHEMOTHERAPY.

FCR Fludarabine, cyclophosphamide and Rituxin (Rituximab), being investigated for the treatment of chronic lymphocytic leukemia.

See CLL.

FDA (Food and Drug Administration) the federal agency established to protect the public health by regulating the availability of human and veterinary drugs, biologicals, medical devices, the country's food supply, cosmetics, and products that emit radiation. The FDA was established in 1938, when Congress passed legislation requiring proof of safety before a drug or device could be marketed. In 1962, the test of "efficacy" (meaning that the drug or device is effective at doing what it claims it can do) was added to "safety" as a requirement for approval by the FDA. The FDA is also responsible for bringing accurate, science-based information to the public to help people use medicines and foods to improve their health.

febrile neutropenia the occurrence of fever in a patient with NEUTROPENIA (either spontaneous or caused by side effects of CHEMOTHERAPY), which can be a life-threatening event. Because of the likelihood of infection as the cause of febrile neutropenia, the treatment of choice is urgent broad-spectrum antibiotics usually given by IV. In many cases, resolution may occur without a specific organism being identified, But prudent practice requires treatment as if the clinical condition could deteriorate if not addressed. Some chemotherapy regimens are expected to cause major neutropenia within a few days of administration, and patients are advised to seek care if fever develops.

fecal occult blood test See OCCULT BLOOD STOOL TEST.

feline leukemia a form of cancer caused by a retrovirus that occurs in cats. Cats can catch this leukemia from an infected cat. However, there is no indication that humans are in any way affected by this virus.

Femara [letrozole] an AROMATASE INHIBITOR (AI) drug used in the treatment of advanced breast cancer in postmenopausal women whose disease has progressed after antiestrogen therapy. Data generated in 2005 supports the preference of an AI class of drug over TAMOXIFEN as the preferred adjuvant hormonal agent for estrogen-receptor-positive (ER+) early stage breast cancer in postmenopausal women. Femara was approved for this use in December 2005. Possible side effects may include chest pain, shortness of breath, swelling of feet or lower legs, hypertension, and depression. It is taken orally.

femoral artery a major vessel that carries blood in the area of the groin or thigh from the aorta to the leg.

fentanyl citrate [Duragesic] a powerful narcotic that is contained in a patch and applied to the skin. It is very useful in managing chronic cancer pain. It is available by prescription only.

See also ANALGESIC and ACTIQ.

fiber [in food] material from plant cells that is nondigestible or only partially digestible in humans.

Fiber helps move food and by-products of digestion through the large intestine and out of the body. It helps prevent constipation and promotes a healthy digestive tract. In addition, there is strong evidence to suggest that including fiber in the diet may decrease the risk of COLON CANCER and other cancers.

Foods high in fiber

whole grain bakery products	cabbage
	celery
breakfast cereals and pasta	green beans
fruits	summer squash
apples	green peas
pears	parsnips
apricots	kale
bananas	spinach
berries	yams
cantaloupes	sweet potatoes
grapefruit	turnips and rutabagas
oranges	*all cooked dry beans*
pineapples	black
papaya	kidney
prunes and raisins	pinto
vegetables	navy
carrots	lima
broccoli	lentils
potatoes	split peas and black
corn	eyed
cauliflower	peas
brussels sprouts	popcorn

See also DIET.

fiber-optic bronchoscopy   See BRONCHOSCOPY.

fiber-optic endoscopy   See ENDOSCOPY.

fiber-optic instrument   See ENDOSCOPE.

fibrocystic changes (fi″bro-sis′tik) [formerly known as fibrocystic disease of the breast; also called fibrocystic condition, cystic disease, chronic cystic mastitis, mammary dysplasia, and lumpy breasts] a condition in the breast characterized by a combination of fibrous tissue and tiny cysts in one or both breasts. There is usually more than one cyst present. The cysts are movable, spherically shaped, fairly soft, and subject to rapid changes in size.

Fibrocystic changes is the most common benign (noncancerous) condition of the breast, affecting as many as 30% of women between the ages of 35 and 55. Women with cystic breasts were thought to be at a higher risk of BREAST CANCER. However, it now appears that women with fibrocystic changes are not at any greater risk of getting breast cancer, with a few exceptions. At times a doctor may feel a BIOPSY is indicated.

fibrocystic condition   See FIBROCYSTIC CHANGES.

fibrocystic disease of the breast   See FIBROCYSTIC CHANGES.

fibroid tumor (fi′broid) [benign uterine tumor, leiomyoma]   a very common benign (noncancerous) tumor of the uterus within the wall of the uterus or attached to the wall of the uterus by a stalk of tissue. Fibroid tumors are unlikely to spread or threaten life. They develop most often in women aged 35 to 45. About 20% of women over the age of 30 have fibroid tumors.

fibrosarcoma of soft tissue (fi″bro-sar-ko′mah)   a cancerous tumor originating in the fibrous tissue of the arms, legs, or trunk, often deep within the thigh. Fibrosarcomas occur most frequently in men in their 40s and 50s.

See SOFT TISSUE SARCOMA.

fibrosarcoma of the bone (fi″bro-sar-ko′-mah)   a type of BONE CANCER generally affecting the pelvis, leg, arm, or hip. It occurs most commonly in adults aged 30 to 40.

Filgrastim   See G-CSF.

finasteride   See PROSCAR.

fine needle aspiration   See NEEDLE ASPIRATION BIOPSY.

fine needle biopsy   See NEEDLE ASPIRATION BIOPSY.

5-fluoro-1-tetrahydro-2-furyluracil   See TEGAFUR.

5-fluorodeoxyuridine   See FUDR.

5-fluorouracil See 5-FU.

5-Fluracil See 5-FU.

5-FU [5-fluorouracil, fluorouracil, Adrucil, 5-Fluracil] an ANTIMETABOLITE anticancer drug sometimes used in the treatment of cancers of the colon, breast, ovary, prostate, stomach, liver, and pancreas. It is given most frequently by IV (injection into a vein). It may also be administered by infusion over days or months. Common side effects include nausea, vomiting, mouth sores, and diarrhea. Occasional or rare side effects may include black, tarry stools, stomach cramps, sensitivity to the sun, hair loss, skin rash, difficulty with balance, shortness of breath, heartburn, nail loss, and increase of tears. 5-FU is sometimes used in a cream form for basal cell skin cancer. 5-FU is a very widely used drug and is frequently used in combination with other drugs.

5-FU cream [fluorouracil, Efudex, Fluoroplex] used in the treatment of superficial basal cell carcinoma, as well as precancerous skin lesions. Side effects may include an inflammatory or allergic reaction, burning feeling where applied, skin rash, increased sensitivity of skin to sun, itching, oozing, soreness, or tenderness of skin.

5-FU modulation use of one of a variety of agents just before administration of 5-FU to enhance its anticancer activity. LEUCOVORIN CALCIUM, METHOTREXATE, and INTERFERON are among the drugs currently being used to modulate the effect of 5-FU.

5-FUDR See FUDR.

5 Q-minus syndrome a sub-type of myelodysplastic syndrome (MDS). Five to 10 percent of patients with MDS have a genetic feature (deletion of long arm of chromosome #5) as the sole genetic abnormality, which could mean a more favorable prognosis than for people with MDS who do not have 5 Q-minus syndrome.

five-year survival refers to the length of time a person must stay cancer free after treatment to be considered "cured." The "five-year survival" measurement applies to most cancers, but not all. In many IN SITU cancers, surgical removal is considered a cure.

See also CURE.

Fl a combination of the anticancer drugs FLUTAMIDE and LUPRON sometimes used in the treatment of kidney, bladder, and prostate cancers. See individual drug listings for side effects.

See also COMBINATION CHEMOTHERAPY.

flap surgery See BREAST RECONSTRUCTION.

FLe a combination of the drugs 5-FU and LEVAMISOLE sometimes used in the treatment of colon cancer. See individual drug listings for side effects.

See also COMBINATION CHEMOTHERAPY.

flexible sigmoidoscopy See SIGMOIDOSCOPY.

FLIPI (Follicular Lymphoma International Prognostic Index) a prognostic STAGING system involving nodal sites, LDH, age, stage and hemoglobin level assigning a risk group from "good" to "poor" based on a quantitative approach.

Florafur See TEGAFUR.

flow cytometry (si-tom′ĕ-tre) a diagnostic tool used in pathology, and performed on cancer cells that have been removed from the body, in which a suspension of cells flows through a beam of light allowing the simultaneous measurement of several predetermined parameters, including the amount of DNA in cells. Flow cytometry may be used to evaluate the risk of the recurrence of some cancers including breast, prostate, and bladder cancers. A fluorescent dye that attaches to DNA is added to the malignant (cancerous) cells. A flow cytometer, a laser-powered instrument with a computer system and terminal, measures the amount of DNA on the cells. An abnormal amount of DNA (too much or too little) may indicate a greater risk of recurrence of some cancers. Flow cytometry can also measure the percentage of cells in a particular phase (the synthesis phase) of dividing into "daughter" cells.

This sophisticated technology enables measurements to be made on thousands of cells in just a few minutes with a high degree of accuracy. Before flow cytometry those measurements would have to be made very carefully and very slowly by eye. It could take a skilled pathologist 30 minutes to count 2,000 to 3,000 cells, far fewer than flow cytometry can do in minutes. Flow cytometry can be used to complement other tests in order to get as much information as possible about the possibility of a cancer recurring.

See also S-PHASE FRACTION and ANEUPLOID.

FLOX a combination of bolus 5-FU, LEUCOVORIN, and oxaliplatin, used in treating metastatic colorectal cancer.

floxuridine See FUDR.

floxymesterone [Halotestin, Ora-Testryl] See ANDROGEN.

Fludara See FLUDARABINE.

fludarabine (flu-dar'ah-bēn) [Fludara] an anticancer drug used in the treatment of chronic lymphocytic leukemia (CLL). It is given by IV (injection into a vein). Major side effects may include bone marrow depression and immune suppression.

fludrocortisone See ADRENOCORTICOIDS.

fluorescein angiography (flu"o-res'e-in an"ge-og'rah-fe) a test used to examine the blood vessels of the retina of the eye. Dye is injected into a vein in the arm. When it reaches the eye, the doctor is able to see the blood vessels and whether a tumor or abnormality is present. It is a procedure that may be used in the diagnosis of EYE CANCER, such as INTRAOCULAR MELANOMA and other conditions.

Fluoroplex See 5-FU.

fluoroscope See FLUOROSCOPY.

fluoroscopy (flu"or-os'ko-pe) a diagnostic X-RAY procedure in which the X-ray is projected onto a screen much like a television. The X-ray is continuous, allowing the doctor to see the movement of internal organs. For example, the fluoro-scope (the machine used to take this X-ray) can show barium sulfate as it travels through the digestive tract during an X-ray examination. Because fluoroscopy is a continuous X-ray, there is greater exposure to radiation than in a conventional X-ray.

fluorouracil See 5-FU and 5-FU CREAM.

fluprednisole See ADRENOCORTICOIDS.

FLUT See FLUTAMIDE.

flutamide (flu'tah-mīd) [FLUT, Eulexin] a drug that may be used in the treatment of advanced PROSTATE CANCER. It is an ANTIANDROGEN drug, blocking the effects, on the cancer cell, of the small amounts of male hormones produced in the adrenal glands. In 1989 the Food and Drug Administration approved the use of flutamide in combination with LUPRON for the treatment of advanced prostate cancer.

FMS a combination of the anticancer drugs 5-FU, MUTAMYCIN, and STREPTOZOCIN sometimes used in the treatment of PANCREATIC CANCER. See individual drug listings for side effects.

See also COMBINATION CHEMOTHERAPY.

FNA (fine needle aspiration) See NEEDLE ASPIRATION BIOPSY.

FOFIRI 5-FU, LEUCOVORIN and Irinotecan, used in the treatment of metastatic colorectal cancer.

Folex See METHOTREXATE.

Foley catheter See CATHETER.

FOLFOX 5-FU, LEUCOVORIN, and oxaliplatin, used in the treatment of metastatic colorectal cancer.

follicular B-cell NHL (fo-lik'u-lar) those LYMPHOMAS in which the neoplastic (see NEOPLASM) cells form aggregates or NODULES that resemble normal artchitecture. The individual cells are MONOCLONAL B CELLS. PROGNOSIS varies depending on other details.

follicular cell thyroid cancer (fo-lik'u-lar) cancer of the follicular cell of the thyroid. This is one of the major cell types of THYROID CANCER. The follicular cell is the bulk of the gland. It performs the characteristic function of the thyroid gland, secreting the thyroid hormone. The cell is named for its appearance. It is arranged in thousands of microscopic sac-like structures called follicles.

FOMi/CAP a combination of the anticancer drugs 5-FU, Oncovin (VINCRISTINE), mitomycin-C (MUTAMYCIN), CYTOXAN, ADRIAMYCIN, and Platinol (CISPLATIN) sometimes used in the treatment of NON-SMALL CELL LUNG CANCER. See individual drug listings for side effects.
See also COMBINATION CHEMOTHERAPY.

food additives substances put into food to give it some desirable characteristic such as color, flavor, texture, stability, or resistance to spoilage. Food additives are regulated by the Food and Drug Administration. One group of additives that has come under considerable scrutiny for a role in causing cancer is food coloring. Red dye number 2 came under suspicion as a carcinogen in 1970 on the basis of two studies done in the Soviet Union. Its use in the United States was banned in 1976. However, it was never shown to cause cancer in any studies done in the United States.

Food and Drug Administration See FDA and Appendix I.

formaldehyde (for-mal'dĕ-hīd) a colorless, water-soluble gas with a pungent pickle-like smell used widely in manufacturing. The Environmental Protection Agency has classified formaldehyde as a "probable human carcinogen." People who work with formaldehyde include anatomists, embalmers, pathologists, and industrial workers who produce formaldehyde and products made with formaldehyde such as plywood, photographic film, and permanent press fabrics. Formaldehyde is also used in cosmetics, drug products, paper, textiles, and a variety of other products in the home, and urea formaldehyde

foam insulation has been used as insulation for homes and schools. Studies have shown that people exposed to formaldehyde in the workplace are at a greater risk of getting brain cancer, nasopharyngeal cancer, and leukemia. A controversial study by the National Cancer Institute in the 1980s found a 30% increase in lung cancer mortality among industrial workers.

4-aminobiphenyl See CARCINOGENS.

FPC See FAMILIAL MULTIPLE POLYPOSIS OF THE COLON.

freezing surgery See CRYOSURGERY.

French-American-British (FAB) classification a way of describing and reporting the two major subclasses of acute leukemia—acute lymphocytic leukemia (ALL) and acute nonlymphocytic leukemia (ANLL). This arose as a collaborative effort by pathologists from three countries, France, America, and Great Britain.

frozen section biopsy (bi'ŏp-se) a procedure used to make a fast diagnosis of suspicious tissue. A section of tissue obtained by BIOPSY is delivered immediately to the pathology laboratory where it is cut and quickly frozen in a machine called a cryostat. The tissue is then cut into very thin slices that are microscopically examined for cancer. The entire process can take just five minutes.

FUDR [floxuridine] an anticancer agent used primarily in the palliative management of colorectal cancer that has spread to the liver. It is given as a continuous regional intra-arterial infusion. FUDR may cause an injury to the bile duct system (sclerosing cholangitis) that may be fatal. It is also under investigation as an intraperitoneal agent in the treatment of stomach and ovarian cancer.

fulguration (ful"gu-ra'shun) [electrofulguration] a type of surgery using an electric current to destroy a tumor. This may be performed in the treatment of stomach, urethral, and rectal cancer.

fungus (fun′gus) a general term for a spore-bearing plant that lacks chlorophyll such as yeast, mold, mildew, and mushrooms. Some fungi cause infections, and several diseases of the lung are caused by fungus or mold. Fungus becomes more of a threat to a cancer patient whose IMMUNE SYSTEM is depressed as a result of the disease or its treatment. AIDS patients also are prone to infection by a variety of fungi because of their compromised immune system. Recently, powerful antifungal agents have been developed for treatment.

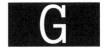

gadolinium (DTPA) (gad″o-lin′e-um) an IV (intravenous) contrast used to enhance MRI.

gallbladder a pear-shaped sac beneath the liver that stores bile (the substance used to break down fat) from the liver and secretes mucus. The gallbladder is a component of the digestive system. GALLBLADDER CANCER is fairly rare.

gallbladder cancer a fairly rare cancer arising in the gallbladder, a pear-shaped organ that lies just under the liver in the upper abdomen. It occurs in women three times as often as it does in men. It develops among elderly people more frequently than do other GASTROINTESTINAL CANCERS. In 1999 7,200 new cases were diagnosed and there were 3,600 deaths. Although most people who get gallstones will not get gallbladder cancer, 80 to 90% of the people diagnosed with gallbladder cancer in the United States also have gallstones.

One possible symptom of gallbladder cancer may be jaundice (yellowing of the skin, whites of the eyes) because of blockage to the adjacent bile duct system. Among the procedures that may be used in the diagnosis and evaluation of gallbladder cancer are X-RAYS, ULTRASOUND, CT SCANS, and possibly abdominal surgery. LAPAROSCOPY reemerged as a useful diagnostic test in the late 1980s.

The National Cancer Institute (NCI) stages gallbladder cancer as "localized" or "unresectable." If it is localized, the malignant (cancerous) tumor can

be completely removed by surgery. If it is unresectable, the tumor cannot be completely removed. Gallbladder cancer usually spreads by direct invasion into adjacent tissues, but metastases do occur.

Treatment depends on the stage of the disease, the general state of health of the patient, and other factors. Surgery and radiation may be used in the treatment of gallbladder cancer. For specific information on the latest state-of-the-art treatment, by stage, call NCI's Cancer Information Service at 1-800-4-CANCER (1-800-422-6237), or for a TTY: 1-800-332-8615.

gallium (gal′e-um) a rare, silvery metallic element that may be used in some NUCLEAR SCANS, including a GALLIUM SCAN, to show rapidly dividing cells.

gallium nitrate (gal′e-um ni′trāt) [Ganite, Cytovene] an anticancer drug used in the treatment of HYPERCALCEMIA, which has been associated with a number of different cancers. At high doses, nausea may be a side effect; however, nausea does not occur at the lower doses used in the treatment of hypercalcemia. Another side effect that has been observed is mild ANEMIA. The drug is given by IV (injected into a vein).

gallium scan (gal′e-um) a NUCLEAR SCAN that may be used to determine whether cancer has metastasized (spread) to other areas of the body.

The patient is scanned up to 72 hours after injection of GALLIUM, a radioactive tracer. It can take 48 hours for the gallium to localize to abnormal areas of the body. Usually the entire body is scanned. The gallium scan can show areas of rapidly dividing cells. It has been used with breast cancer, lung cancer, lymphoma, melanoma, head and neck cancers, metastases to the bone, brain, lung, and other cancers. It is also useful in identifying abnormal infections or inflammatory states involving the lungs. It is particularly helpful in the diagnosis of a pneumonia afflicting some patients with AIDS.

gamma camera   See NUCLEAR SCAN.

gamma interferon (in″ter-fēr′on) [immune interferon]   a type of INTERFERON produced by white blood cells (T CELLS) that have been stimulated by other agents. It activates MACROPHAGES (an immune cell) and has a much more potent effect on the IMMUNE SYSTEM than the two other interferons—alpha and beta. It appears that the maximum dose needed for the best effect is far below the maximum tolerated dose. Research is being conducted primarily in its usefulness in treating melanoma, as well as its use in combination with other BIOLOGICAL RESPONSE MODIFIERS.

gamma knife   a gamma knife is not a "knife" but a dedicated and very costly form of STEREOTACTIC RADIOSURGERY. It has been used to treat brain cancer in the United States since 1987.

gamma rays   radiation beams that are sometimes used in the treatment of cancer. They are similar to X-RAY beams but shorter. Emitted by a radioactive substance, gamma rays are used in high doses to treat cancer. See RADIATION THERAPY.

ganciclovir   See DHPG.

Ganite   See GALLIUM NITRATE.

Gardner's syndrome   See FAMILIAL MULTIPLE POLYPOSIS OF THE COLON.

gastrectomy (gas-trel′to-me)   a surgical removal of the stomach. When only part of the stomach is removed, it is called a "partial" gastrectomy. A gas-trectomy may be performed as a treatment for STOMACH CANCER as well as other disorders.

gastric   relating to or affecting the stomach.

gastric atrophy   See CHRONIC ATROPHIC GASTRITIS.

gastric cancer   See STOMACH CANCER.

gastric carcinoma   See STOMACH CANCER.

gastric polyps (gas′trik pol′ips)   a protruding growth occurring in the stomach. Their relationship to the development of cancer has not been determined. About 5% of the polyps in the stomach are ADENOMAS, which may become cancerous.

gastric tube   a CATHETER implanted in the stomach. This can be used to administer nutritional supplements to patients following surgery for STOMACH CANCER.

gastrointestinal (GI) cancers (gas″tro-in-tes′tĭ-nal)   a general term sometimes used for a group of different cancers that occur in the gastrointestinal tract.

gastrointestinal series   See GI SERIES.

gastrointestinal tract (gas″tro-in-tes′tĭ-nal)   the digestive system including the esophagus, stomach, small and large intestines, and the rectum. The chief function of the GI tract is to convert food into substances such as essential nutrients and fluids that can be absorbed into the bloodstream.
See also GASTROINTESTINAL CANCERS.

gastroscope   See GASTROSCOPY.

gastroscopy (gas-tros′ko-pe) [esophagogastro-duodenoscopy]   an examination of the stomach using a gastroscope, a thin lighted tube. The gastroscope is swallowed by the patient after the throat has been numbed with a local anesthetic. With the gastroscope, the doctor can see the inside of the stomach and collect tissue samples for biopsy. Gastroscopy may be used in the diagnosis of stomach cancer as well as other disorders.
See also ENDOSCOPY.

GBM   See GLIOBLASTOMA MULTIFORME.

G-CSF (granulocyte colony-stimulating factor) (gran'u-lo-sīt) [filgrastim, Neupogen] a natural substance in the body that helps control the production and proliferation of the immune and blood-forming cells in the bone marrow. Naturally occurring G-CSF regulates the production of white blood cells within the bone marrow. It may be given along with or after chemotherapy (toxic anticancer drugs) and/or radiation treatment to stimulate white blood cell production, thereby decreasing the risk of infection and the need for antibiotic treatment. It is indicated for peripheral blood stem cell mobilization in transplant programs.

G-CSF is one of the first of an exciting group of compounds known as hematopoietic growth factors to be approved. This material is commercially prepared using recombinant technology. In 1997 it was approved as a growth factor for peripheral blood stem cell mobilization. The only major side effect is bone pain, which occurs in about 20% of the patients receiving it. G-CSF is given by IV (injected into a vein) or subcutaneously (under the skin).

See also COLONY-STIMULATING FACTORS.

gefitinib   See IRESSA.

gemcitabine   See GEMZAR.

gemcitabine HCl   See GEMZAR.

Gemzar [gemcitaabine, gemcitabine HCl] used in the treatment of locally advanced or nonresectable pancreatic cancer, stage II, III, or IV. It may also be used for pancreatic cancer previously treated with 5-FU. It is primary palliative. It is also indicated for NON-SMALL CELL LUNG CANCER, BLADDER CANCER, SOFT-TISSUE SARCOMA, BREAST CANCER when given with paclitaxel as first-line after failure of prior ADJUVANT THERAPY.

Possible side effects include myelosuppression, nausea and vomiting, fever, rash, and flu-like symptoms. It is given by IV (injected into a vein).

Genasense   See AUGMEROSEN.

gene the biological unit of heredity that determines the traits we inherit from past generations. Genes occupy a specific place on a chromosome. A gene is capable of reproducing itself exactly at each cell division and works by directing the formation of an enzyme or other protein. A gene is a discrete segment of the DNA molecule. It is made of chemical sequences strung together in a certain order as part of the DNA double helix to make "words." Genes then manufacture proteins in their own image. The proteins carry out the cell's functions. There are thousands of genes on the chromosomes in each cell's nucleus. There are 23 matched pairs of chromosomes in the human nucleus. Minor changes in the genes can have a profound influence in the development of human disease. So far, nearly 800 specific genes have been linked to specific diseases. Some cause disease directly, as in the case of sickle-cell anemia. There are susceptibility genes that predispose a person to an illness if exposed to environmental toxins or other factors causing the gene to malfunction. Oncogenes are a family of genes that when mutated cause malignant accelerated growth. There are genes that are being investigated to correct certain diseases.

gene therapy the use of genes in the treatment of disorders or diseases in the body, including cancer. One major goal is to supply cells with healthy copies of missing or flawed genes. Scientists are working on ways to genetically alter immune cells that are naturally or deliberately targeted to cancers. They want to arm such cells with cancer-fighting genes and return them to the body, where they could more forcefully attack the cancer. Alternatively, cancer cells can be taken from the body and altered genetically so that they elicit a strong immune response. These cells can then be returned to the body in the hope that they will act as a cancer vaccine. Another possibility is to inject a tumor with a gene that makes the tumor cells vulnerable to an other drug so that treatment with the drug would kill only the cells that contain the foreign gene. Getting the gene into the tumor cell has been an area of intense ongoing research. The first use of gene therapy was in September 1990, on a severely immunodeficient four-year-old girl. She had been born without the ADA gene and as a result suffered from ADA deficiency disease, a rare, inherited disease that can result in death. To provide her with the ADA gene, her own white blood cells were removed and then altered, in a laboratory, by the addition of the human ADA gene. The white blood cells with the ADA genes were then reinfused into her body.

Cancer was first treated with gene therapy just months later, in January 1991. Two patients with advanced melanoma were treated at the National Institutes of Health (NIH). The patients were given transfusions of special cancer-killing cells, called TUMOR-INFILTRATING LYMPHOCYTES or TIL cells, taken from their cancerous tumors.

When cancer is present in the body, TIL cells occur naturally and migrate from other parts of the body to the site of the cancer, where they invade the tumor and kill cancer cells. While TIL cells may slow the progress of the cancer, the body generally cannot manufacture enough TIL cells to cure the cancer. TIL cells also have the ability to recognize and destroy cancer cells from the tumor that have spread to other parts of the body.

In gene therapy, TIL cells are extracted from the patient. In a laboratory, these TIL cells are given a gene capable of producing a potent antitumor substance called TUMOR NECROSIS FACTOR (TNF), a protein produced by the body in the course of bacterial infections. It was first recognized for its ability to kill cancer cells in mice. TNF also regulates inflammation and immunity by signaling the body to repair injuries and fight infections. The gene-altered TIL cells are transfused back into the patient, where they travel to the cancer site.

At a tumor site, TNF appears to work by cutting off the blood supply in that region. It is hoped that by using the TIL cells to carry the TNF-producing genes to the tumor site, the benefit of TNF will be maximized and its potential toxicity will be minimized. However, TNF can eventually harm the body if it is active for too long a period of time, or is in too high a concentration. It can cause shock or body wasting.

Gene therapy is in its infancy. It is possible that gene therapy will eventually be used to prevent or cure diseases. Researchers are hopeful that its development will become a major factor in the treatment of cancer as well as other disorders.

general anesthesia (an″es-the′ze-ah)   a state of unconsciousness induced by drugs, aesthesia. The entire body is free of the sensation of pain.

genetic markers   signs in the body that a person may have inherited a "predisposition" to a disease. Genetic markers can take two forms: physical signs that can be seen, or biochemical, physiological, or chromosomal irregularities that are only apparent in laboratory tests. Research into genetic markers is progressing rapidly. Certain physical signs can point to a predisposition for cancer. For example, people with NEUROFIBROMATOSIS have a high incidence of PHEOCHROMOCYTOMA.

Cancer is thought of by many as a disease of damaged or abnormal genes. Genetic predisposition includes inheritance of the BRCA and the colon cancer genes among the many genes that are rapidly being identified.

Two cancers known to be of genetic origin are RETINOBLASTOMA and WILMS' TUMOR in children.

genital herpes virus (her′pēz)   a sexually transmitted disease that causes sores on the genitals. Some research indicates that genital herpes may play a role in the development of CERVICAL CANCER. However, not every woman who has genital herpes virus develops cancer of the cervix.

genitourinary system (jen″i-to-u′ri-nar-e)   a single term for the genital and urinary system that recognizes their closeness during embryological development.

germ cell tumors   tumors that arise in reproductive tissue, such as some types of ovarian or testicular tumors. In men, germ cell tumors account for 95% of testicular cancer. In the late 1980s and early 1990s a small group of cancers known as nongonadal germ cell tumors have also been described, which occur in both men and women. In the past, these tumors were fatal. They are now very responsive to chemotherapy (anticancer drugs). Therefore, it is important that they be correctly diagnosed. There are certain blood tests—ALPHA-FETOPROTEIN and HUMAN CHORIONIC GONADOTROPIN—which can be used in diagnosis of germ cell tumors and in follow-up of therapy.

germ line   used in biology and genetics to describe cells that have genetic material that may passed along by offspring.

Gerson treatment an unconventional cancer treatment formulated by Dr. Max Gerson based on the consumption of "natural" foods that, he claimed, would restore the body's resistance and healing power lost through years of "artificial nutrition." His diet consisted of predominantly fruits and vegetables supplemented by such things as fresh calf liver juice, vitamins and minerals, and thyroid extract. Salt and spices and aluminum utensils could not be used. Enemas, including coffee enemas, were recommended on a regular basis. Dr. Gerson's methods were reviewed a number of times. There was no convincing evidence that the method worked, and it is not considered to be an effective cancer treatment. Dr. Gerson died in 1959.

See also UNCONVENTIONAL TREATMENT METHOD.

gestational trophoblastic tumor (jes-ta′shun-al trof″o-blas′tik) a rare cancer in women in which cancer cells grow in the uterus in the tissues that are formed after a woman conceives. This cancer accounts for less than 1% of the gynecological cancers in women.

There are two main types of gestational trophoblastic tumors: HYDATIDIFORM MOLE and CHORIOCARCINOMA. Hydatidiform mole (also called molar pregnancy) occurs when the sperm and egg cells join but there is no fetus developing in the uterus. The tissue that grows in the uterus resembles grapelike cysts and does not spread outside the uterus. Choriocarcinoma may develop from a hydatidiform mole or from tissue that remains in the uterus following an abortion or delivery of a baby. It can spread outside the uterus to other parts of the body. A third, very rare type of gestational trophoblastic tumor is known as uterine choriocarcinoma.

Symptoms may include constant vaginal bleeding; a uterus that remains enlarged or gets bigger after giving birth or having an abortion; or a pregnancy where there is no fetal movement. Procedures used in the diagnosis and evaluation of gestational trophoblastic tumor may include an internal exam, an ULTRASOUND, CT SCAN, and a BLOOD TEST for HUMAN CHORIONIC GONADOTROPIN, a TUMOR MARKER.

Following is the National Cancer Institute's (NCI) staging for gestational trophoblastic tumor:

• hydatidiform mole—cancer is found only in the space inside the uterus; if the cancer is found in the muscle of the uterus, it is called invasive mole (choriocarcinoma destruens)
• nonmetastatic—cancer cells have grown inside the uterus from tissue remaining following treatment of a hydatidiform mole or following an abortion or delivery of a baby; cancer has not spread outside the uterus
• metastatic—cancer cells have grown inside the uterus from tissue remaining following treatment of a hydatidiform mole or following an abortion or delivery of a baby; the cancer has spread from the uterus to other parts of the body

Metastatic gestational trophoblastic tumors are considered "good prognosis" or "poor prognosis":

• good prognosis:

1. the last pregnancy was less than four months earlier
2. the blood level of beta human chorionic gonadotropin (BHCG) is low
3. cancer has not spread to the liver or brain
4. chemotherapy (anticancer) drugs have not been given

• poor prognosis:

1. the last pregnancy was more than four months ago
2. the blood level of BHCG is high
3. cancer has spread to the liver or brain
4. chemotherapy has been given earlier and the tumor did not go away
5. the tumor started after completion of a normal pregnancy

Treatment depends on the stage of the disease, the general state of health of the patient, and other factors. The two most common treatments for gestational trophoblastic tumor are surgery and chemotherapy. Radiation therapy may be used in certain cases. For specific information on the latest state-of-the-art treatment, by stage, call NCI's Cancer Information Service at 1-800-4-CANCER (1-800-422-6237), or for a TTY: 1-800-332-8615.

GI series (gastrointestinal series) an examination of the upper and lower digestive tract by X-RAY after the administration of barium, a CONTRAST MEDIUM. The barium outlines or highlights irregularities that are present.

See LOWER GI SERIES and UPPER GI SERIES.

giant cell tumor of the bone   a benign (noncancerous) tumor in the bone that is aggressive and usually recurs after it is removed. It usually remains benign, although it can become cancerous. It occurs most frequently in young adults, over 20 years of age, near the end of a long bone such as the knee. Treatment is usually surgery. Occasionally RADIATION THERAPY is used.

See also MALIGNANT GIANT CELL and BONE CANCER.

Gilda Radner Familial Register   keeps track of and monitors families in which two or more members have had ovarian cancer. It is named after Gilda Radner, the comedienne who died of ovarian cancer in 1989, when she was 43 years old.

See Appendix I.

gingiva (jin′jĭ-vah)   the fleshy tissue covering the border of the teeth in the mouth.

GIST (gastrointestinal stomal tumors)   There are a group of NEOPLASMS that arise from precursors of the connective-tissue cells of the gastrointestinal tract. These are uncommon, occur primarily in middle age and older persons, and are found most often in stomach, small intestine, or other areas of the tract. The drug GLEEVIC has been able to induce complete remission, opening up the possibility of finding other difficult-to-treat tumors that may have a similar molecular target.

glands   groups of cells that secrete or excrete substances not related to their metabolic needs.

glandular epithelial   the lining and external surface of glands.

Gleason grading system   a system for describing PROSTATE CANCER that is based on the appearance of the cancer cells, and their degree of DIFFERENTIATION (how mature they are).

Gleevic [Imatinib]   is an oral chemotherapeutic primarily associated with the treatment of CML (chronic myelogenous leukemia). Its introduction in 2001 was a major advance and became a model for TARGETED THERAPY. This agent is a MONOCLONAL ANTIBODY designed to block a protein that produces a disease. Gleevic is considered a triumph of modern molecular biology. The FDA has approved Gleevic for use in FIRST-LINE treatment of adults with CHRONIC PHASE CML, and for chronic phase of CML patients who have failed INTERFERON. Gleevic is also used for CML in accelerated phase or BLAST CRISIS; CML in the pediatric population after STEM CELL TRANSPLANT failure or interferon resistance, and in some other scenarios as well. The major side effects are fluid retention, common to the monoclonal antibody drug class, and MYELOSUPPRESSION. Gleevic interferes with WARFARIN (COUMADIN) metabolism. It is generally well tolerated and in CML may induce a complete hematologic REMISSION in a matter of weeks, although cytologic remissions take longer.

Gliadel Wafer   See BCNU.

glioblastoma multiforme (GBM)   (gli″o-blas-to′ mah)   the most malignant (cancerous) and fastest-growing brain tumor. It accounts for more than half of all gliomas and 25% of all primary brain cancers. It affects mostly middle-aged people. Symptoms may include convulsions and signs of brain disturbance.

See GLIOMA and BRAIN CANCER.

glioma (gli-o′mah)   a form of BRAIN CANCER named for the type of cells or parts of the brain where it originates. Gliomas can also arise in structures attached to the brain, such as the pineal gland (small gland in the lower part of the brain), pituitary gland (small gland at the base of the brain), or retina (part of the eye connected to the brain by the optic nerve). The five major types of gliomas are:

- ASTROCYTOMA—a tumor in the brain that can be benign (noncancerous) or malignant (cancerous); astrocytomas account for 10% of all brain tumors
- GLIOBLASTOMA MULTIFORME—the most malignant and fastest-growing tumor in the brain; 25% of all primary brain cancers are this type
- EPENDYMOMA—a slow-growing tumor arising in the ventricles, the spaces in the brain that con-

tain the cerebrospinal fluid; children and young adults are most frequently affected

- MEDULLOBLASTOMA—a fast-growing tumor arising in the lower part of the brain, occurring most frequently in children
- OLIGODENDROGLIOMA—a very rare, slow-growing tumor in the brain that is frequently benign

Gliomas account for a majority of the primary cancers arising in the brain.

glomus tumor (glo'mus) [chemodectoma] a benign (noncancerous), rare, generally very small tumor of neural tissue usually occurring in the head and neck. More women than men develop glomus tumors. It is rare to see glomus tumors in people under the age of 20. Glomus tumors grow slowly and can be asymptomatic for several years, occasionally 20 years and longer. Treatment is usually surgical. RADIATION THERAPY may also be used.

Glossary of Molecular Biology See MOLECULAR BIOLOGY.

glucagonoma (glu"kah-gon-o'mah) a rare cancerous tumor of the ENDOCRINE PANCREAS.

See ISLET CELL CARCINOMA.

GM-CSF (granulocyte macrophage–colony-stimulating factor) (gran'u-lo-sīt mak'ro-fāj) [Leukine, Prokine, Sargramostim] a naturally occurring COLONY-STIMULATING FACTOR, or growth factor in the body that is known to stimulate the development of GRANULOCYTES and MACROPHAGES (two types of white blood cells) in the BONE MARROW. It was approved by the Food and Drug Administration, in 1991, for use in the treatment of patients with NON-HODGKIN'S LYMPHOMA, HODGKIN'S DISEASE, and acute lymphoblastic leukemia undergoing AUTOLOGOUS BONE MARROW TRANSPLANTS. It is indicated in bone marrow transplantation to reconstitute normal marrow function. GM-CSF is also indicated following induction CHEMOTHERAPY in ACUTE MYELOGENOUS LEUKEMIA (AML). It is used to mobilize peripheral blood stem cells for stem cell transplantation, and after transplant to hasten myeloid recovery. It is used in chemotherapy-induced NEUTROPENIA SOLID

TUMORS. It is given either intravenously (IV) or subcutaneously (SC).

See PERIPHERAL STEM CELL TRANSPLANTATION.

gonadal aplasia (go-nad'al ah-pla'zhe-ah) failure of the testes to develop during prenatal development. Studies have shown a link between this condition and the occurrence of TESTICULAR CANCER.

gonadotropin-hormone-releasing hormone See LUTEINIZING HORMONE-RELEASING HORMONE.

gonioscope See GONIOSCOPY.

gonioscopy (go"ne-os'co-pe) an examination of the front portion of the eye using a special lamp or an instrument called a gonioscope. Gonioscopy is used in the diagnosis of glaucoma and can also be useful in the detection of ocular melanoma.

goserelin acetate See ZOLADEX.

grading a way of describing cancer cells in terms of how malignant or aggressive they are (how quickly they spread). Cancer cells are microscopically examined for their HISTOLOGIC TUMOR GRADE or degree of DIFFERENTIATION. The more differentiated the cell is (more like a normal cell) the lower the grade and the better the prognosis. For example, NON-HODGKIN'S LYMPHOMA can be categorized as low grade (slow growing), intermediate grade, or high grade (rapidly growing). When non-Hodgkin's lymphoma is diagnosed it is staged and graded (the staging describes the extent of the disease in the body and the grading describes how aggressive it is). The grade of the tumor plays a role in decisions regarding treatment.

graft versus host disease (GVHD) a not uncommon side effect of BONE MARROW TRANSPLANTATION. When the new marrow is transplanted, it attacks the host (recipient). The new marrow, particularly its T CELLS, identifies the host as "foreign" and launches an attack against it. The most common sites of graft versus host disease are the skin, liver, and gastrointestinal tract. A patient can have GVHD in any one of those sites or all three. About half the patients receiving bone marrow that is not genetically identical to their own (ALLOGENEIC BONE MARROW

TRANSPLANT) develop acute GVHD. About 25% of allogeneic transplant patients develop chronic GVHD.

GVHD that occurs within nine days after the transplant is known as acute GVHD. GVHD can also occur up to a year later, at which time it is called chronic GVHD. Acute GVHD can cause a range of symptoms from mild to severe and even, on rare occasion, death. The most common symptoms are skin rashes, jaundice, liver disease, and diarrhea. Chronic GVHD can cause temporary darkening of the skin and hardening and thickening of patches of skin and the layers of tissue under the skin; dry mouth and eyes; bacterial infections; and weight loss. Occasionally the liver, esophagus, and other parts of the gastrointestinal tract are affected.

To prevent or reduce the likelihood of GVHD, drugs are given to the patient after the transplant to help suppress the T cells and reduce the risk of GVHD. Another method under investigation is eliminating the T cells from the donated marrow.

granisetron hydrochloride   See KYTRIL.

granulocyte (gran'u-lo-sīt) [myelocyte, polymorphonuclear cell]   one kind of WHITE BLOOD CELL produced in the bone marrow. Granulocytes fight bacteria by engulfing and destroying them. Granulocytes contain potent chemicals that enable them to digest microorganisms. Some of those potent chemicals can contribute to inflammatory reactions and are responsible for allergic reactions (an inappropriate and harmful response of the immune system). There are a number of different types of granulocytes: NEUTROPHILS, BASOPHILS, and EOSINOPHILS are found in the blood; mast cells are found in connective tissue.

granulocyte colony-stimulating factor   See G-CSF.

granulocyte macrophage–colony-stimulating factor   See GM-CSF.

granulocytic leukemia (gran'u-lo-sit"ik) [myelocytic leukemia]   one type of leukemia arising in the white blood cells that fight bacteria.
    See LEUKEMIA.

granulocytopenia   See NEUTROPENIA.

graphic stress telethermometry   See THERMOGRAPHY.

Grawitz's tumor   See KIDNEY CANCER.

gray (Gy)   a measurement used for the amount of radiation absorbed by the body. The term RAD had been used but has been replaced by gray. One hundred RADs equal one gray.

group-C status   a drug still under investigation but whose distribution has been permitted, by the National Cancer Institute, to patients for whom there is no other treatment.

growth factor   See COLONY-STIMULATING FACTORS.

guaiac test   See OCCULT BLOOD STOOL TEST.

gynecologic oncologist (gi"nĕ-ko-loj'ik on-kol'o-jist)   a doctor who specializes in cancers of the female reproductive system. He or she can perform surgery. To be certified by the American Board of Obstetrics and Gynecology the person must be a licensed doctor of medicine, have had three years of residency in obstetrics and gynecology, have successfully completed the written examination of the board, have had at least 12 months of independent practice, and have successfully completed an oral examination given by the board.

gynecological cancers   cancers of the female reproductive system including cancers of the CERVIX, UTERUS (ENDOMETRIAL), vagina, vulva, and fallopian tubes; breast cancers may be included.

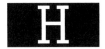

Habitrol See NICOTINE PATCH.

hair dye chemicals used to color hair. The chemicals in hair dyes can enter the circulatory system through the scalp. In tests performed on animals by the National Toxicology Program (NTP), some of the chemicals previously used in hair dyes caused cancer in the animals. According to the National Cancer Institute, current hair dyes do not contain carcinogens.

hair loss See ALOPECIA.

hairy cell leukemia (HCL) [leukemic reticuloendotheliosis] a fairly rare form of LEUKEMIA affecting mostly middle-aged and older men. It is called "hairy cell" because the cells have irregular hairlike projections. They also have a unique flow cytometry pattern, aiding in diagnosis. The cell of origin is a LYMPHOCYTE.

Symptoms of hairy cell leukemia may include fatigue and malaise (vague, generalized discomfort), infection, fever, and loss of appetite and weight. It is one cause of massive splenomegaly (a grossly enlarged spleen).

Treatment of hairy cell leukemia depends on a number of different factors. It is one of a number of different cancers that may go "untreated" indefinitely. Treatments include splenectomy (removal of the spleen), CHEMOTHERAPY (anticancer drugs), and BIOLOGICAL RESPONSE MODIFIERS. A purine analog, a chemotherapeutic, is widely used, and is associated with long remissions.

Rather than being staged, hairy cell leukemia is divided into two categories:

- untreated—a patient has had no prior treatment other than blood products, antibiotics, and allopurinol (a drug used to treat gout)
- progressive hairy cell leukemia, postsplenectomy—low blood counts (red, white, or platelets, or any combination) are unrelieved or worsening, and/or there is a progressive increase in the number of circulating hairy cells.

For specific information on the latest state-of-the-art treatment, call the National Cancer Institute's Cancer Information Service at 1-800-4-CANCER (1-800-422-6237), or for a TTY: 1-800-332-8615.

See also LEUKEMIA.

half-life the time it takes for half the amount of a drug or radioisotope (a substance used as a contrast medium in NUCLEAR SCANS) to leave the body through natural processes.

Halotestin [Ora-Testryl] See ANDROGEN.

Halsted mastectomy See RADICAL MASTECTOMY.

HAMA (human anti-mouse antibody) can develop in a person as a consequence of exposure to certain monoclonal antibodies and could cause a serious allergic response if the person were re-exposed to another product derived from mouse tissue in its production.

hamartoma   A benign (noncancerous) growth made up of an abnormal mixture of cells and tissues normally found in the area of the body where the growth occurs.

hand-and-foot syndrome   pain and discomfort in the hands and feet. It is a major side effect of infusional 5-FU, as well as XELODA, BAY43-9006, and DOXIL. There is a possibility that the vitamin B-6 may alleviate the discomfort.

HCG   See HUMAN CHORIONIC GONADOTROPIN.

HCI   See HYCAMTIN.

HCL   See HAIRY CELL LEUKEMIA.

HDMTX   See HIGH-DOSE METHOTREXATE WITH LEU-COVORIN RESCUE.

head and neck cancer   a term encompassing a variety of cancers that occur in the head and neck region including upper airway and food passages, nose, paranasal sinuses, nasopharynx, mouth, lips, tongue, gums, cheek, tonsils, pharynx, larynx, and esophagus. Almost all of these tumors arise from the surface EPITHELIUM and are known as either SQUAMOUS CELL type or epidermoid type cancers.

The area of the mouth and throat may be subdivided by ear, nose, and throat surgeons into very small anatomic subdivisions. However, to the layperson such breakdowns really have little practical consequence. And although some head and neck cancers may have a different microscopic appearance, they are usually treated in the same way.

See also EPIDERMOID CANCER OF MUCOUS MEMBRANES.

heartburn   a burning discomfort behind the lower part of the breastbone. It is most often associated with stomach acid irritating the lower esophagus (esophagitis). Heartburn may be an early symptom of stomach cancer.

heat treatment   See HYPERTHERMIA THERAPY.

heavy chain disease   a rare, LYMPHOPLASMACYTIC disorder characterized by a proliferation of cells that secrete a portion of an immunoglobulin (antibody) molecule. The normal immunoglobulin is made up of both "light" and "heavy" components or "chains." See MYELOMA.

HEC (highly emetogenic chemotherapy)   CHEMOTHERAPY that is likely to cause emesis (vomiting) in a majority of patients.

helper cells   cells that protect the body against infections and some cancers.

hemangioblastoma   (hĕ-man″je-o-blas-to′mah) a very rare and slow-growing brain tumor accounting for 2% of tumors in the brain. Symptoms may include imbalance and problems in walking.

See also BRAIN CANCER.

hemangiopericytoma   (hĕ-man″je-o-per″ĕ-si-to′mah)   a rare tumor arising in the cells that form part of the blood vessel walls of small capillaries. Hemangiopericytomas account for about 3% of all SOFT TISSUE SARCOMAS in children. They can be malignant (cancerous) or benign (noncancerous). They can occur in any part of the body, but most often occur in the lower extremities. They also occur in adults and, very rarely, in infants. They are treated with surgery, RADIATION THERAPY, and/or CHEMOTHERAPY (anticancer drugs).

hemangiosarcoma   (hĕ-man″je-o-sar-ko′mah)   a rare type of SOFT TISSUE SARCOMA originating in the blood vessels in the arms, legs, and trunk. They account for about 2% of all soft tissue sarcomas.

hematemesis   (hem″ah-tem′ĕ-sis)   vomiting of blood. The vomited material may be very bloody, which is very serious (and can be very frightening); or it may look like "coffee grounds," which is a result of small amounts of blood that are digested by the stomach. Hematemesis may be associated with several conditions, including benign ulcers, malignant ulcer of the stomach (cancer), esophageal cancer, and other disorders.

hematologist   (he″mah-tol′o-jist)   a medical doctor who specializes in diseases of the blood and blood-forming organs. The Board of Internal Medicine grants certification to doctors who complete a three-year residency in internal medicine followed by three additional years in a specialized training program.

hematopathologist (hem″ah-to-pah-thol′o-jist) a doctor who specializes in the microscopic examination of abnormal blood cells.

hematopoietic growth factors See COLONY-STIMULATING FACTORS.

hematopoietin-1 See INTERLEUKIN-1.

hematoporphyrin derivative (HPD) (hem″ah-to-por′fĭ-rin) a nontoxic dye that fluoresces under light and is attracted to cancer cells. It is used in PHOTODYNAMIC THERAPY.

hematuria (he″mah-tu′re-ah) the presence of blood in the urine. It may be visible to the eye or identified only under a microscope. Hematuria is the most common symptom of bladder cancer. It may also be a symptom of a tumor in the urinary tract. In a patient who has cancer, hematuria may be the result of a recurrent tumor in the urinary tract. Hematuria can be caused by other disorders as well, such as kidney stones or infections. When urinating is painful, it is more likely that the hematuria is caused by an infection that can be treated with medication. When there is no pain, it is less likely that it is being caused by an infection and may be more serious.

Hematuria can also be a side effect of cancer treatment, particularly the anticancer drug CYTOXAN, which is used in the treatment of leukemia, lymphoma, and other cancers. It may occur months after the drug has been given.

hemilaryngectomy See PARTIAL LARYNGECTOMY.

hemimastectomy See LUMPECTOMY.

hemolysis (he-mol′ĭ-sis) a condition in which red blood cells are prematurely destroyed. In cancer patients this may result in anemia because of the body's inability to compensate through increased bone marrow production. Many forms of cancer, as well as the treatments (e.g., the anticancer drug MUTAMYCIN), may be associated with significant hemolysis. Hemolysis can also occur in many noncancerous conditions.

hemoptysis (he-mop′tĭ-sis) coughing up of blood. Hemoptysis may be a warning sign of LUNG CANCER. The blood enters the sputum because of bursting small blood vessels in the lung. Many lung infections, such as TB and bacterial pneumonia, can also cause hemoptysis.

heparin (hep′ah-rin) an anticoagulant drug used to decrease blood clotting. It may be used to treat blood clots and to prevent clots from becoming dislodged. Small amounts of heparin are used to flush and keep open an INDWELLING CATHETER in a patient.

Heparin is given by IV (injection into a vein) or, when used to flush a catheter, injected directly into the catheter.

hepatoblastoma See LIVER CANCER/CHILDHOOD.

hepatocellular carcinoma See LIVER CANCER.

hepatoma (hep″ah-to′mah) a tumor arising in the liver that can be benign (noncancerous) but is most frequently malignant (cancerous). When people talk about hepatomas, they are usually referring to LIVER CANCER. Hepatomas are frequently referred to as hepatocellular carcinomas, which are actually one type of malignant hepatoma. Benign tumors in the liver are very rare and can usually be surgically removed. Another example of a malignant hepatoma is a hepatoblastoma.

Hepatomas, or hepatocellular carcinomas, are the most common primary liver cancer. There is an association with prior exposure to viruses causing hepatitis. In certain parts of the world (East Asia) it occurs in epidemic proportions related to the incidence of the virus.

Most tumors in the liver are malignant. And most of those tumors have originated in other parts of the body and metastasized (spread) to the liver. These metastasized cancers would not be called "hepatomas."

hepatomegaly (hep″ah-to-meg′ah-le) enlargement of the liver. This may be associated with a variety of cancers. Primary and secondary LIVER CANCER are commonly associated with hepatomegaly, which may be detected by physical exam and/or X-RAY tests such as the CT SCAN or ULTRASOUND. Hepatomegaly may also be caused by other, noncancerous conditions, such as heart failure.

HER-2/neu a gene that promotes the production of a protein that is believed to help cancer cells reproduce. Elevated levels in breast, prostate, and ovarian cancers can indicate a greater chance of recurrence. See ONCOR TEST.

herbal treatment the use of plants and plant products for medical therapy. This is one of the oldest medical practices and is still a major force in many forms of folk and traditional medicine around the world. It is used for the treatment of numerous disorders, including cancer.

In the treatment of cancer, it has been reported that as many as 3,000 different plant species have been used worldwide. Plant products are the source of some of the drugs used in CHEMOTHERAPY (anticancer drugs). One of the best known is ETOPOSIDE derived from the mayapple plant. It was approved by the Food and Drug Administration in 1983 for use in the treatment of patients with testicular cancer, small-cell lung cancer, nonlymphocytic leukemias, and non-Hodgkin's lymphomas. ALKALOIDS, including VINBLASTINE and VINCRISTINE, are other examples of anticancer drugs developed from plants.

Herbal products are also used in UNCONVENTIONAL TREATMENT METHODS in the United States.

herbicide (er′bĭ-sīd) an agent that is used to destroy weeds, commonly on pastureland and in growing wheat, corn, sorghum, and rice. Some herbicides have been associated with cancer. For example, a study in Kansas found that farmers who used herbicides had a higher risk for NON-HODGKIN'S LYMPHOMA than the general population. 2,4-D was the most frequently used herbicide in that study. In occupational studies, workers exposed to the herbicides phenoxyacetic acid or chlorophenol have a higher-than-expected incidence of lymphoma.

All herbicides sold in the United States must be approved by the Environmental Protection Agency.

Herceptin [trastuzumab] a monoclonol antibody genetically engineered to act against the protein generated by the HER-2/NEU gene, was approved late in 1998 for metastatic breast cancer patients expressing the gene. Herceptin has shown great promise in combination with taxol (an anticancer drug) in clinical trials for women with advanced breast cancer as well as advanced ovarian cancer. Patients whose breast camcers have an above normal level of the HER-2/neu gene may have increased tumor growth, accelerated disease progression, poor response to conventional chemotherapy, and earlier death. The potential patients for whom Herceptin would be appropriate are the 30% of breast cancer patients and 20% of ovarian patients whose tumors show high levels of the HER-2/neu gene. Possible side effects include chills and fever (usually with the first dose), diarrhea, low white blood cell count, and infections. Herceptin is given by IV (injected into a vein).

hereditary cancer predisposition syndromes many have been identified and are being studied as to incidence and possible prevention. Several of these include HEREDITARY RETINOBLASTOMA, BRCA-ASSOCIATED BREAST AND OVARIAN CANCER SYNDROMES, LI-FRAUMENI SYNDROME, and COWDEN SYNDROME.

hereditary nonpolyposis colorectal cancer See HNPCC.

hereditary pancreatic cancer pancreatic cancer thought to be related to a GERM LINE genetic mutation. For example, it was recognized that President Carter's family had a very high incidence of PANCREATIC CANCER.

hereditary pancreatitis (pan″kre-ah-ti′tis) inflammation of the pancreas, an organ in the body located deep in the abdomen that plays a major role in digestion and insulin secretion. People with this condition are at a greater risk of developing PANCREATIC CANCER.

hereditary polyposis of the colon See FAMILIAL MULTIPLE POLYPOSIS OF THE COLON.

hereditary retinoblastoma retinoblastoma is the most common primary malignant tumor of the eye in children. However, it represents only 1% of pediatric malignancies. There are approximately 200 cases per year in the United States with 50% linked to hereditary factors. The retinoblastoma gene (RBI) was cloned in 1986.

hermaphroditism (her-maf″ro-di′tizm) the development of both male and female sex characteristics in the same person. This condition has been linked to TESTICULAR CANCER.

heroin an ANALGESIC drug that has been used in the alleviation/control of pain. A NARCOTIC, heroin is a member of the MORPHINE family of drugs. Heroin is highly addictive. It is illegal in the United States (the only exception being its use in research) and its importation has been banned. Studies conducted in the United States have concluded that although heroin is a potent painkiller, it is no more effective than morphine when morphine is administered appropriately.

Heroin had been used as a painkiller in England. However, morphine is now being used more frequently in England as well because it has been shown to be just as effective as heroin.

herpes simplex (her′pēz) a very common virus that causes mouth and lip blisters called cold sores. Once someone has had herpes simplex, it can recur at any time. People are most vulnerable to it when their IMMUNE SYSTEM is lowered. Cancer patients, AIDS patients, and people who have undergone a BONE MARROW TRANSPLANTATION are at a higher risk of getting herpes simplex than the average person because of their lowered immune response. In cancer patients this can be a side effect of chemotherapy (anticancer drugs) or the disease. In AIDS patients it is a result of the disease itself.

herpes zoster See SHINGLES.

Hexadrol (hek′sah-drol) this is a brand of the drug dexamethasone. It is also sold under the brand name DECADRON.

Hexalen See HEXAMETHYLMELAMINE.

hexamethylene bisacetamide (HMBA) a drug being investigated in the United States for its role in the treatment of a number of different cancers including lung cancer and leukemia. HMBA is a new type of anticancer drug. Instead of destroying cancer cells, it appears to have the potential to convert cancer cells into normal cells, a cell-differentiating agent.

hexamethylmelamine [HMM, alteramine] an anticancer drug approved in late 1990. It may be used in the treatment of persistent or recurrent ovarian cancer after primary chemotherapy (anticancer drugs). It is taken by mouth. The major side effects may be nausea and BONE MARROW DEPRESSION. Occasional or rareside effects may include mental depression and confusion, hallucinations, diarrhea, abdominal cramps, cystitis, an impaired sense of touch, and hair loss.

Hickman catheter a hollow silicone (soft, rubber-like material) tube inserted and secured into a large vein in the chest for long-term use to administer drugs or nutrients. The catheter is inserted through a small incision made near the collarbone. A "tunnel" is made under the skin to another site where the catheter exits. The catheter is then pulled through the tunnel and into the vein leading to the heart. Medication, blood products, nutritional support, and new bone marrow can be delivered through the part of the catheter extending outside the body, and blood can be drawn from the body through the catheter. This device must be scrupulously cared for to prevent infection. The Hickman catheter may be left in the body for months. Removing it is a relatively simple procedure.

See also INDWELLING CATHETER and BROVIAC CATHETER.

high-dose chemotherapy the administration of extremely high and potentially lethal doses of chemotherapy (anticancer drugs) to select patients with select cancers. The development of techniques to harvest, store, and reinfuse the patient's own stem cells (autologous), and the availability of growth factors (colony stimulating factors [CSF]), has made it possible to use high-dose chemotherapy, thus enabling its evaluation as a treatment. The procedures that enable the use of high-dose chemotherapy are autologous bone marrow transplantation and peripheral blood stem cell transplantation. In 1998 80% of transplants used peripheral blood stem cells.

high-dose methotrexate (HDMTX) with leucovorin rescue (meth″o-trek′sāt lu″ko-vor′in)   administrating METHOTREXATE at a much higher dose than would be safe were it not for the LEUCOVORIN RESCUE given after. HDMTX may be used in the treatment of adult and childhood bone sarcoma and other cancers.

high LET   See PARTICLE BEAM RADIATION.

high linear energy transfer (high LET) radiation See PARTICLE BEAM THERAPY.

high risk   a person who has a greater chance of getting a particular form of cancer, or any disease, than the average person for any number of reasons. For example, a person who smokes is at a higher risk of getting lung cancer than a person who does not smoke. A woman whose mother, grandmother, and sister have had breast cancer is at a higher risk than a woman who has had no breast cancer in her family.

High risk may also be used to define differences in the chance of RECURRENCE of the disease after primary surgery. For example, in early-stage breast cancer, many patients are now described as high risk or low risk of eventual relapse based on a series of different factors.

von Hippel-Lindau's disease   an inherited disorder that puts a person at a greater risk of developing KIDNEY CANCER.

histiocyte   a type of MACROPHAGE.

histiocytic non-Hodgkin's lymphoma (his″te-o-sit′ik)   a type of NON-HODGKIN'S LYMPHOMA characterized by histiocytic cell types (large cancer cells that resemble MACROPHAGES or HISTIOCYTES). This lymphoma can occur in the chest, abdomen, pelvis, or neck.

histocompatibility testing (his″to-kom-pat″ĭ-bil′ĭ-te) [tissue testing]   examining and comparing the body tissue of a potential donor and recipient before an organ transplant. This procedure is performed to find people with similar combinations of HUMAN LEUKOCYTE ANTIGENS (HLA) in the body tissue. Histocompatibility testing precedes the transplantation of bone marrow and other organs such as the kidneys, heart, lungs, liver, and pancreas. It is done to find two people with the best tissue match. The closer the match is of the tissue between the organ donor and recipient, the better the chance that the transplanted bone marrow or organ will "take," and not be rejected. Finding a suitable match (only identical twins have a perfect match) can be very difficult because there are so many different combinations of HLAs. Generally, there is a greater possibility of finding suitable donors among family members, including siblings, parents, children, aunts, uncles, cousins, and grandparents. Acceptable donors are found in only 10% of the cases.

histologic tumor grade (his″to-log′ik)   the degree of DIFFERENTIATION of cancer cells determined by microscopic examination. There are four levels, which progress from Grade I (highly differentiated/nearly normal) to Grade IV (poorly differentiated/very abnormal). The greater the differentiation and the lower the grade, the better the PROGNOSIS. Tumors may be referred to as "high" grade or "low" grade. Determining the histologic tumor grade is known as GRADING.

HIV (human immunodeficiency virus) (im″u-no-dĕ-fish′en-se) [human T-cell lymphotropic virus III (HTLV-III)]   one of the HTLV viruses and the virus that causes AIDS. The virus can cause a tremendous weakening of the body's immune system by killing certain LYMPHOCYTES (a type of white blood cell). It is not the virus that directly causes illness; rather it is the eventual inability of the body to fight off infections. The virus was identified at virtually the same time in France and the United States in the early 1980s.

HIV positive   having the antibody to the HIV (human immunodeficiency virus) in the blood, the result of prior exposure to the virus. The HIV may be in the body for years before there are any symptoms of AIDS, the disease it causes. Many people, called carriers, are totally without symptoms. It is unclear whether all people who are HIV positive will eventually become ill with AIDS. Major efforts are being made to identify and counsel HIV positive people. See Appendix I for AIDs organizations.

hives   See URTICARIA.

HLA See HUMAN LEUKOCYTE ANTIGENS.

HMBA See HEXAMETHYLENE BISACETAMIDE.

HMM See HEXAMETHYLMELAMINE.

HN2 See MUSTARGEN.

HNPCC a hereditary syndrome that is caused when a person inherits a mutation in one of five different genes. If people born with HNPCC do not undergo early and regular SCREENING, they have a much higher risk of developing COLON CANCER than the general population.

Hodgkin's disease one of the two basic types of LYMPHOMA, Hodgkin's is a cancer that develops in the LYMPHATIC SYSTEM, the part of the body's circulatory system that helps fight disease and infection. Although it rarely does, it can start in almost any part of the body, including the liver, bone marrow, and spleen. Hodgkin's disease is relatively rare. It accounts for 1% of all cancer cases in the United States. In 2005, there were an estimated 7,350 new cases of Hodgkin's disease and 1,410 deaths related to the disease. Because of better treatment, death rates have fallen by more than 60% since the early 1970s. It is most commonly seen in young adults between the ages of 15 and 35 and in people over 55. It affects more men than women.

There are four different cell types of Hodgkin's disease: lymphocyte predominant, nodular sclerosis, mixed cellularity, and lymphocyte depleted.

The cause of Hodgkin's disease is not known. Some studies have found a higher incidence of Hodgkin's disease among the brothers and sisters of Hodgkin's patients. In Japan, there were a greater number of cases of Hodgkin's disease among survivors of the atomic bomb explosion at Hiroshima than would be expected in the general population. People with compromised IMMUNE SYSTEMS caused by immune disorders or immunosuppressive drugs are more likely to develop Hodgkin's disease. In addition, studies have shown a higher rate among woodworkers and chemists.

The most common symptom of Hodgkin's disease is a painless swelling in the LYMPH NODES under the arm or in the neck or groin. Other symptoms may include fevers, night sweats, feeling tired, weight loss, or itchy skin. Procedures used in the diagnosis and evaluation of Hodgkin's disease may include blood tests, X-RAYS of the chest, bones, liver, and spleen, and a BIOPSY of tissue from an enlarged lymph node. A major factor that distinguishes Hodgkin's disease from other lymphomas is the presence of the REED-STERNBERG CELL in the biopsy. The Reed-Sternberg cell (a giant cell with several nuclei) is almost always found in Hodgkin's disease. If Reed-Sternberg cells are not present, a diagnosis of Hodgkin's disease is rarely made. FLOW CYTOMETRY is also useful in diagnosis.

In Hodgkin's disease, prognosis and successful treatment are very dependent on accurate STAGING. Following is the National Cancer Institute's (NCI) staging for adult Hodgkin's disease:

- Stage I—the cancer is found in only one lymph node area or in only one area or organ outside of the lymph nodes in the same area
- Stage II
  — the cancer involves more than one group of lymph nodes on the same side of the diaphragm (the thin muscle under the lungs that helps in the breathing process) or
  — the cancer is found in only one area or organ outside of the lymph nodes and in the lymph nodes around it; other lymph node areas on the same side of the diaphragm may also have cancer cells
- Stage III—the cancer involves lymph node groups above and below the diaphragm, may or may not involve the spleen (which is considered part of the lymphatic system)
- Stage IV
  — the cancer has spread to organs in addition to the lymph nodes, including the liver, lung, bones, and BONE MARROW or
  — the cancer has spread to only one organ outside of the lymph system, but lymph nodes far away from that organ are involved
- Relapsed—the cancer has recurred (returned) after treatment, either in the area where it started or in another part of the body

Treatment depends on a number of factors, including the type and stage of the disease, the patient's age and general state of health, whether or not surgery was performed to determine disease stage and the presence of certain symptoms, and other factors. The two main treatments used for adult Hodgkin's disease are RADIATION THERAPY and CHEMOTHERAPY. Hodgkin's disease was one of the first cancers found that could be cured with either radiation therapy or chemotherapy. A newer treatment, which is becoming more widespread, is BONE MARROW TRANSPLANTATION.

Hodgkin's disease in children is quite rare and seen very infrequently in children under 10 years of age. It is virtually the same disease as adult Hodgkin's disease with a few exceptions. It is less likely to be found in the lungs, bones, or bone marrow than in adult Hodgkin's. Treatment of older children is similar to that of adults. The treatment approach for children under the age of 13, or who have not reached sexual maturity, may be adjusted, when possible, to preserve the integrity of bony and connective tissue structures. That may mean less radiation and a greater reliance on COMBINATION CHEMOTHERAPY.

For specific information on the latest state-of-the-art treatment, by stage, call NCI's Cancer Information Service at 1-800-4-CANCER (1-800-422-6237), or for a TTY: 1-800-332-8615.

See also NON-HODGKIN'S LYMPHOMA.

holistic medicine (ho-lis'tik) the treatment of the "whole" person, not just the disease, medically, emotionally, and spiritually. It is considered an alternative medicine. It has developed at least partly in response to the ever-increasing specialization by physicians.

Holistic medicine has been around since before the first century. One of the first promoters of a holistic approach was Plato (427–327 B.C.), who told doctors to respect the relationship between body and mind. Hippocrates cautioned physicians about using any treatment that could interfere with the body's "natural healing process." However, since the time of Plato and Hippocrates, research has generated effective therapies for many diseases that had been incurable. Rigorous scientific studies have proven the worth, or worthlessness, of different treatments.

There are many legitimate doctors, nurses, and others who practice holistic medicine. However, there are some practitioners who advocate treat-

ments for which there is no scientific basis. These approaches can be dangerous to a patient with a life-threatening illness who is not getting a treatment that has been proven to be effective. Valuable time can be lost in the treatment of the disease.

See also UNCONVENTIONAL TREATMENT METHOD.

hormonal replacement therapy See ESTROGEN REPLACEMENT THERAPY.

hormone (hor'mōn) a substance produced by the endocrine glands of the body. Hormones are released directly into the bloodstream and have a specific effect on cells and organs in the body, stimulating or turning off their growth. Along with the nervous system, hormones coordinate and control various organs and tissues so that the body runs smoothly.

Hormone levels respond to conditions in the body. An infection, a stressful situation, or a change in the chemical composition of the blood are some of the conditions that can raise or lower the amount of a particular hormone. Examples of some hormones are insulin, ESTROGEN, and TESTOSTERONE. Hormones have been associated with some cancers. For example, some breast cancers are estrogen dependent, i.e., the cancerous tumor is stimulated to grow by the estrogen. Hormones are also used in the treatment of some cancers in HORMONE THERAPY. Synthetic hormones produced in a laboratory are used in treatment.

hormone assay (hor'mōn as-sa') a test performed on BREAST CANCER cells to determine if they are affected by HORMONES. This information is important in planning the most effective treatment.

See also ESTROGEN RECEPTOR TEST and PROGESTERONE RECEPTOR TEST.

hormone receptor status (hor'mōn) the degree to which a tumor is dependent, or not dependent, on HORMONES for growth. In breast cancer, an ESTROGEN RECEPTOR TEST and a PROGESTERONE RECEPTOR TEST are performed on the cancerous cells at the time of biopsy or surgery.

hormone therapy (hor'mōn) [endocrine therapy] the use or manipulation of HORMONES, natural or synthetic, to treat disease. In the treatment of cancer, hormone therapy can be administered three ways: by hormonal medication by injection or orally (by mouth); surgical removal of the hormone-producing glands; or radiation treatment to destroy hormone-producing cells.

Among the earliest hormone treatment for cancer was the removal of the ovaries and adrenal glands in women with breast cancer. The use of surgery in hormonal treatment is fairly rare today, replaced by the administration of drugs such as TAMOXIFEN, which blocks the body's use of the hormone ESTROGEN. Among the hormones used in the treatment of cancer are ADRENOCORTICOIDS (prednisone, cortisone, and others); estrogen (female hormones); ANTIESTROGEN; ANDROGEN (male hormones); and PROGESTERONE.

Some cancers treated by hormones are breast, prostate, and uterine. Multiple myeloma, HODGKIN'S DISEASE, leukemias, and lymphomas also respond favorably to the use of adrenocorticoid hormones.

hospice   program for caring for patients who are terminally ill. The focus of hospice care is not to cure the patient but to improve the quality of life for whatever time the patient has left and to make the dying process as comfortable and pain free as possible.

A team of medical, social, psychological, and spiritual workers work together to control the patient's pain and other symptoms so that he or she can remain as alert and comfortable as possible. At the same time support is offered to family members. The hospice seeks to provide a cheerful open environment for both the patient and family. The hospice may be located in the hospital, in a separate facility (freestanding), or in the patient's home.

The term *hospice* dates from medieval times when a hospice was a way station for travelers. Today's hospice movement got its start in the mid-1960s in England, when St. Christopher's Hospice was opened specifically for the care of terminally ill patients.

At a certain time in many cancer patients' lives, hospice care may make a meaningful difference in quality of life. In the mid-1980s, specific legislation was dedicated to this issue, to define benefits that may be covered by Medicare and to set standards of care. See Appendix I for names and addresses of organizations that can provide more information on hospice care.

hot spot   an area on the film of a diagnostic scan where a radioactive substance, injected into the body, has accumulated. Commonly referred to as "hot spots," their presence may be an indication of a cancerous area, especially in the bone.

Hoxey's herbal tonic treatment   an unproven cancer treatment declared ineffective in the 1950s after 10 years of litigation. At that time a federal court issued an injunction to stop sales of the "ineffective cancer treatment." The "treatment" consisted of a combination of 10 different herbs that Hoxey claimed corrected a chemical imbalance in the body that he said caused cancer. The tonic was said to have originated with Hoxey's great-grandfather, whose horse was cured of a leg cancer after grazing in a field where the herbs were growing. No objective, scientific data were ever published supporting his claims.

See also UNCONVENTIONAL TREATMENT METHOD.

HPD   See HEMATOPORPHYRIN DERIVATIVE.

HPV   See HUMAN PAPILLOMAVIRUS.

HTLV (human T-cell lymphotropic virus)   a group of RETROVIRUSES that have been identified in human tissue. The most well known is HTLV-III, more commonly known as HIV, which causes the disease AIDS. HTLV-I has been implicated in T-CELL LEUKEMIA, while HTLV-III has been found in a patient with HAIRY CELL LEUKEMIA.

HTLV-I (human T-cell lymphotropic virus 1)   a virus that has been identified in human T-CELL LEUKEMIA. It is estimated that 1 in 80 patients with HTLV-I will develop cancer. Researchers believe the virus can only be spread by prolonged, intimate contact and is not contagious like influenza or other common viral diseases.

HTLV-III   See HIV.

HU   See HYDREA.

human chorionic gonadotropin (HCG) (ko″re-on′ik gon″ah-do-tro′pin) a sex HORMONE that is secreted normally during pregnancy. When it is found in the blood of someone who is not pregnant, it serves as a TUMOR MARKER and may be an indication of a number of different cancers, including CHORIOCARCINOMA, TESTICULAR CANCER, and GESTATIONAL TROPHOBLASTIC TUMOR. Pregnancy and marijuana use can also cause elevated HCG levels. HCG blood levels can also be used as a monitor of how well a person is responding to treatment.

human immunodeficiency virus See HIV.

human leukocyte antigens (HLA) (lu′ko-sīt an′tĭ-jens) a series of protein markers found on white blood cells. In a HISTOCOMPATIBILITY TEST, HLAs are used to assess the similarity of the tissue of different people.

human leukocyte interferon See ALPHA INTERFERON.

human papillomavirus (HPV) (pap″ĭ-lo′mah-) a general term for more than 80 similar viruses that tend to cause warts, such as the fairly common warts that grow on hands and feet, or papillomas (noncancerous tumors). Some HPVs are transmitted sexually, through sexual intercourse or oral or anal sex. There are more than 30 types that can infect the genital tract. HPVs are the major cause of CERVICAL CANCER and ANAL CANCER.

Some HPV viruses are referred to as "low-risk" because they rarely develop into cancer. Those that can lead to the development of cancer are referred to as "cancer-associated types."

Risk factors for developing an HPV infection—and eventually possibly cancer—include having sexual intercourse at an early age and having many sexual partners. Women who smoke or have a lowered immune response are at a greater risk of cancer if they come in contact with cancer-associated HPVs. Treatment methods include cold cautery (freezing that destroys tissue), laser (a high-intensity light surgery), LEEP (loop electrosurgical excision—removal of tissue with a hot wire loop), conventional surgery, and two powerful chemicals (podophyllin and trichloroacetic acid) to destroy external genital warts when applied to them. Imiquimod cream, approved in late 1998, is an effective drug treatment. Research is continuing to find new ways to treat HPV infections or to prevent HPV infections with the use of a vaccine.

human T-cell lymphotropic virus See HTLV.

hybridoma (hi″-brĭ-do′mah) synthetic cell created in a laboratory by fusing together a healthy antibody-producing white blood cell and a cancerous white blood cell (plasmacytoma). The hybridoma can be used to produce unlimited quantities of a single, specific antibody known as a MONOCLONAL ANTIBODY, which has the ability to seek out specific and unique proteins on cancer cells. Monoclonal antibodies can be useful in a number of ways:

- they can identify specific types of leukemias and lymphomas, enabling doctors to determine the most appropriate treatment for that specific type
- they can track cancer antigens
- Alone, or linked with anticancer drugs, they can attack cancer metastases

One monoclonal antibody, known as OKT3, is helpful in preventing GRAFT VERSUS HOST DISEASE in bone marrow transplants as well as preventing the rejection of organ transplants. Hybridoma technology is being used in the investigation of cancer itself—its prevention, diagnosis, and treatment.

Hycamtin [topotecan, TOPO TPT, HCl] an anticancer (chemotherapy) drug, administered by IV (injection in to the vein) that comes from the bark of a Chinese tree, *Camptotheca acuminata*. It is FDA-approved in the treatment of patients with advanced OVARIAN CANCER who have failed platinum-based therapy, or those with small-cell lung cancer (SCLC) that has failed first-line therapy, Hycamtin works by interfering with the functioning of an enzyme, which eventually results in tumor cell death. The most common side effect is NEUTROPENIA. Other side effects that may occur include hair loss, anemia, diarrhea, mouth sores, nausea and vomiting, a rash, and THROMBOCYTOPENIA.

hydatidiform mole (hi″dah-tid′ĭ-form) [hydatid mole] a rare complication of early pregnancy in which part of the placenta forms into a mass of grape-like cysts. This is frequently a precursor of the rare cancer CHORIOCARCINOMA.

hydrazine sulfate (hi'drah-zin sul'fāt) studies to see if this chemical is useful in the treatment of cachexia caused by cancer have not had positive results, and this drug has essentially been abandoned.

Hydrea (hi-dre'ah) [HU, Hydroxyurea] an ANTIMETABOLIC oral anticancer drug sometimes used in the treatment of cancers of the head, neck, ovary, and colon and chronic myelogenous leukemia and acute leukemia. It is also used in the treatment of p. vera (See MYELOPROLIFERATIVE DISORDERS) and in ESSENTIAL THROMBOCYTHEMIA. Common side effects may include mild nausea and vomiting. Occasional or rare side effects may include BONE MARROW DEPRESSION, skin rashes, mouth sores, diarrhea, hair loss, hepatitis, and itching.

hydrocortisone See ADRENOCORTICOIDS.

hydromorphone (hi"dro-mor'fōn) See DILAUDID.

hydroxyprogesterone caproate See PROGESTERONE.

hydroxyurea See HYDREA.

hyperalimentation (hi"per-al'ĭ-men-ta'shun) the act of giving or receiving additional nutrients. Nutritional therapy or support is an important component in the care of many cancer patients, who, for a variety of reasons, have difficulty eating and/or whose absorption of nutrients has been disrupted. The easiest and most obvious way of increasing the intake of nutrients is to adjust the diet. This is generally done with the assistance of a nutritionist. However, for the many patients who are unable to take in food by mouth, hyperalimentation can be performed in two ways—through tubes (ENTERAL FEEDING) and intravenously (total PARENTERAL NUTRITION [TNP]).

hypercalcemia (hi"per-kal-se'me-ah) a condition characterized by high blood levels of calcium. Many cancer patients develop this condition because of extensive bone loss resulting in excess calcium entering into the bloodstream. It occurs most frequently in patients with multiple MYELOMA and BREAST CANCER. It occurs less frequently in patients with LUNG CANCER. BONE METASTASIS, which can be caused by a wide variety of cancers, is also a cause of hypercalcemia. It can also be caused by hormonal effects acting on bone metabolism.

Symptoms of hypercalcemia can be severe and may include fatigue, muscle weakness, and lethargy—all of which may result in a comatose state. Hypercalcemia can also cause nausea, anorexia, and severe constipation. Hypercalcemia is the most common life-threatening metabolic disorder associated with cancer. The best treatment for hypercalcemia is treatment for the cancer that is causing it. However, since hypercalcemia often occurs in patients whose cancer is advanced or has not responded to treatment, that is frequently not successful. There is no standard, completely effective treatment for hypercalcemia. Treatment is generally individualized and is based on a number of different factors including the condition of the patient and the degree of severity of the hypercalcemia. Increasing hydration and use of diuretics has been standard practice. A class of drugs known as BISPHOSPHATES has been developed as effective calcium-lowering agents (see BISPHOSPHANATES for a list of agents).

HyperCVAD the chemotherapy combination of fractionated Cyclophosphamide (CYTOXAN), VINCRISTINE (Oncovin), ADRIAMYCIN (DOXORUBICIN) and dexamethasone (DECADRON) used in treatment of NON-HODGKIN'S LYMPHOMA (NHL). (See individual drug listings for side effects; see also COMBINATION CHEMOTHERAPY.)

hyperfractionated radiation therapy (hi"per-frak'shun-a"tid) RADIATION THERAPY that is given in small doses throughout the day rather than in one big dose.

hypernephroma (hi"-per-nĕ-fro'-mah) See KIDNEY CANCER.

hyperplasia (hi"per-pla'ze-ah) the abnormal growth of normal cells resulting in an increase in the size of a tissue or organ. This is not itself a cancerous condition although it may become cancerous in some cases.

See also DYSPLASIA and ENDOMETRIAL HYPERPLASIA.

hyperplastic mucosal tags See HYPERPLASTIC POLYPS.

hyperplastic polyps (hi″per-plas′tik pol′ips) [hyperplastic mucosal tags]   one type of POLYP that may be found in the intestines and stomach. Hyperplastic polyps, which are the most common colon/rectal polyps, are harmless and do not lead to cancer, as do many other polyps in the intestines.

hyperthermia (hi″per-ther′me-ah)   an increase in body temperature.

See HYPERTHERMIA THERAPY.

hyperthermia therapy (hi″per-ther′me-ah) [heat treatment]   an investigational procedure that uses heat to kill cancer cells or make them more sensitive to chemotherapy and/or radiation. The rationale behind this treatment is that cancer cells do not seem to tolerate heat as well as normal cells. CLINICAL TRIALS are in progress to determine if this technique is effective, especially in combination with other methods of treatment such as surgery, radiation, and chemotherapy. Lip and oral cancers are among those that may benefit from hyperthermia.

Hyperthermia can be administered locally or to the entire body. In localized hyperthermia, the temperature is raised in a specific part of the body with ultrasound (high-frequency sound waves), microwaves, radio frequency waves, profusion (heating the blood going to one particular organ), or in other ways.

In whole body hyperthermia the patients entire body is heated for various lengths of time either externally, from the outside, or internally, from the inside. When done externally, the patient may be put in a thermal suit (like a space suit). External heat is then applied that is absorbed through the skin. In internal hyperthermia the patients blood is removed from the body, heated, and then returned.

hyperviscosity syndrome (hi″per-vis-kos′ĭ-te)   a condition caused by an increase in the thickness or flow of the blood. The abnormal protein that is produced in WALDENSTROM'S MACROGLOBULINEMIA can increase viscosity in about 50% of patients with this disease. Hyperviscosity can cause bleeding disorders, fatigue, weakness, headache, vertigo, signs of heart failure, and other symptoms. To reduce the thickness of the blood, PLASMAPHERESIS may be performed.

hypnosis   a trancelike state resembling sleep in which a person may be more susceptible to suggestion. This can be induced by a person trained in hypnosis; or it can be self-induced by a person who has learned the technique. Hypnosis can be useful in reducing or alleviating anxiety before or during cancer treatment; it also can be helpful in the management of pain.

hypogammaglobulinemia (hi″po-gam″ah-gl ob″u-lĭ-ne′me-ah)   a condition in which there is a reduced level of a particular class of protein in the body resulting in immunodeficiency.

hypopharyngeal cancer (hi″po-fah-ring′je-al) cancer of the lower part of the pharynx, the part of the throat adjacent to the larynx (voice box) and joining the esophagus. It is one of the major HEAD AND NECK CANCER sites. This is a rare cancer that usually has no symptoms until the tumor is fairly large. Symptoms may include a sore throat, difficulty in swallowing, ear pain, blood in the saliva, and a voice change. It is not uncommon for a mass in the neck to be the first sign of hypopharyngeal cancer. As a result, it is frequently diagnosed when the tumor is quite large, which reduces its chances for successful treatment. Procedures used in the diagnosis and evaluation of hypopharyngeal cancer may include LARYNGOSCOPY, ESOPHAGOSCOPY, CT SCAN, and BIOPSY.

The NATIONAL CANCER INSTITUTE (NCI) stages hypopharyngeal cancer in the following way:

• Stage I—the tumor is confined to one site in the hypopharynx and there is no evidence of spread of the tumor to LYMPH NODES or to other parts of the body
• Stage II—the tumor extends to an adjacent region or site within the hypopharynx without fixation of (being attached to) that side of the larynx; there is no evidence of spread of the tumor to lymph nodes or to other parts of the body

- Stage III—there is no evidence that the tumor has spread to other areas of the body and
  — the primary tumor extends to an adjacent region or site and immobilizes that side of the larynx; there is no spread to the lymph nodes or
  — the primary tumor of any size (below the size described in stage IV) has spread to only a single lymph node on the same side of the neck as the tumor, with the greatest dimension of the lymph node three CEN-TIMETERS (cm) or less
- Stage IV
  — the primary tumor is massive and invades bone or soft tissues of the neck even if it has not spread to distant parts of the body; no more than one lymph node is involved by the tumor on the same side of the neck as the primary tumor of no more than 3 cm in greatest dimension or
  — there is one abnormal lymph node larger than 3 cm in its greatest dimension, or there are multiple abnormal nodes of any size on the same side of the neck as the primary tumor, or there are abnormal nodes of any size on both sides of the neck, or there is one or more abnormal nodes on the opposite side of the neck from the primary tumor or
  — there is evidence of spread of the tumor to distant parts of the body
- Recurrent—cancer has returned to the original site or to another part of the body after treatment

Treatment depends on the stage of the disease, the general state of health of the patient, and other factors. Treatment may consist of surgery and/or radiation. Surgery is a common treatment for this disease. CHEMOTHERAPY may be used prior to surgery or after surgery, or it may be combined with RADIATION. A LARYNGECTOMY may be performed. For specific information on the latest state-of-the-art treatment, by stage, call NCI's Cancer Information Service at 1-800-4-CANCER (1-800-422-6237), or for a TTY: 1-800-332-8615.

hypophysectomy (hi-pof″ĭ-sek′to-me) surgical removal of the pituitary gland, the small gland at the base of the brain that affects all the other glands of the body. The gland is usually removed through the roof of the mouth and nasal passages. It is one method of HORMONE THERAPY in the treatment of some cancers, though other forms of modern hormonal management have essentially eliminated its use for breast cancer. Hypophysectomy is also used to treat primary PITUITARY TUMOR.

hypotonic See DUODENOGRAPHY.

hysterectomy (his-ter-ek′to-me) surgical removal of the uterus. A hysterectomy may be performed in the treatment of cancer as well as other diseases. The different kinds of hysterectomies are:

- SUBTOTAL HYSTERECTOMY (also called supracervical hysterectomy)—surgical removal of only the uterus
- VAGINAL HYSTERECTOMY—surgical removal of the uterus and cervix through the vagina
- TOTAL HYSTERECTOMY—surgical removal of the cervix and uterus
- TOTAL ABDOMINAL HYSTERECTOMY—surgical removal of the uterus by way of an abdominal incision
- TOTAL ABDOMINAL HYSTERECTOMY AND BILATERAL SALPINGO-OOPHORECTOMY—surgical removal of the uterus, both ovaries, and the fallopian tubes by way of an abdominal incision
- RADICAL HYSTERECTOMY (also called Wertheim's operation)—surgical removal of the cervix, uterus, and part of the vagina

hysterogram See HYSTEROGRAPHY.

hysterography (his′tĕ-rog′rah-fe) [metrography, uterography] an examination of the uterus by X-RAY after the administration of a CONTRAST MEDIUM. The dye is inserted via a catheter through the vagina and into the uterus. The picture that results is called a hysterogram. This may be performed in the diagnosis of ENDOMETRIAL CANCER.

hystero-oophorectomy (his′ter-o-o″of-o-rek′to-me) surgical removal of the uterus and ovaries. This may be performed in the treatment of OVARIAN CANCER, ENDOMETRIAL CANCER, and FALLOPIAN TUBES CANCER.

hysteroscope   See HYSTEROSCOPY.

hysteroscopy (his″ter-os′ko-pe)   an examination of the uterine cavity and fallopian tubes, which connect the ovaries and uterus, to diagnose cancer as well as other disorders. A hysteroscope, a flexible instrument with a lighted tube and optical system, is inserted through the vagina and cervix into the uterus in order to see the uterine cavity and fallopian tubes. Tissue may be removed for BIOPSY, microscopic examination for cancer cells.

See also ENDOSCOPY.

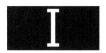

IAQ See INDOOR AIR QUALITY.

IAT See IMMUNOAUGMENTATIVE THERAPY.

ibuprofen See ANALGESIC and NONSTEROIDAL ANTI-INFLAMMATORY DRUGS.

ID a combination of the anticancer drugs IFOS-FAMIDE WITH MESNA and ADRIAMYCIN sometimes used in the treatment of soft tissue sarcoma. See individual drug listings for side effects.

See also COMBINATION CHEMOTHERAPY.

IDA See IDARUBICIN.

Idamycin See IDARUBICIN.

idarubicin [Idamycin] an antibiotic anticancer drug approved by the Food and Drug Administration in the fall of 1990 for use in the treatment of acute myelogenous leukemia (AML). It is given by IV (injection into a vein). Common side effects may include nausea, vomiting, fever, red urine, hair loss, and severe BONE MARROW DEPRESSION that can last several weeks. Occasional or rare side effects may include heart problems (rhythm distur-bances), mouth sores, and liver problems.

See also ANLL and ADRIAMYCIN.

Ifex See IFOSFAMIDE.

IFF See IFOSFAMIDE.

IFL the chemotherapy combination Irinotecan, 5-FU, and leucovirin used in therapy of METASTATIC COLORECTAL CANCER.

ifosfamide (i-fos′fahīd) [IFF, Ifex, isophosphamide] an anticancer drug that may be used in the treatment of NON-HODGKIN'S LYMPHOMA, SARCOMA, MELANOMA, acute lymphocytic leukemia (ALL), and cancers of the ovaries, pancreas, testes, and lung. It was approved by the Food and Drug Administration in 1991. It is given by IV (injection into a vein). Common side effects may include urinary tract prob-lems (bleeding from the bladder), nausea, vomiting, and hair loss. Occasional or rare side effects may include BONE MARROW DEPRESSION, confusion, seizures, drowsiness, liver damage, burning pain where the needle was inserted if the drug leaks dur-ing IV, stuffy nose, sterility, mouth sores, darkening of the skin, lung and heart problems, and anemia. Because of the irritating effect of this drug on the uri-nary bladder, it must be accompanied by an agent to protect the bladder, such as MESNA.

See also IFOSFAMIDE WITH MESNA.

ifosfamide with mesna (i-fos′fah-mīd) the use of MESNA along with IFOSFAMIDE in the treatment of some cancers. Mesna is a chemical compound that, when given with ifosfamide, appears to prevent, in most patients, hemorrhagic cystitis (bleeding from the bladder), a possible side effect of ifosfamide. This is sometimes referred to as a "mesna rescue."

IL-1   See INTERLEUKIN-1.

IL-2   See INTERLEUKIN-2.

IL-2/LAK   an investigational BIOLOGICAL THERAPY using INTERLEUKIN-2 with LAK CELL (lymphokine activated killer cells). This therapy seek to stimulate the body's IMMUNE SYSTEM to fight the cancer while sparing normal cells. It is being investigated in the treatment of many advanced cancers. Encouraging results have been reported in clinical trials with advanced melanoma and advanced kidney cancer. It is also being investigated in the treatment of AIDS.

IL-2/LAK treatment can have severe, but temporary, side effects, virtually all of them associated with the interleukin. The side effects may include:

• fever, chills, and headache
• nausea, vomiting, loss of appetite, and diarrhea
• low blood pressure
• weight gain from fluid retention
• irregular kidney of liver activity
• breathing difficulties (from fluid in the lungs)
• anemia
• skin rashes and itching.
• effects on the central nervous system (confusion, disorientation, combativeness, and increased anxiety).

See also IL-2/TIL and ADOPTIVE IMMUNOTHERAPY.

IL-2/TIL   an investigational BIOLOGICAL THERAPY using INTERLEUKIN-2 with TIL (tumor infiltrating lymphocytes) cells to stimulate the IMMUNE SYSTEM while, at the same time, sparing normal cells. It is being investigated in the treatment of many advanced cancers. This is a newer version of IL-2/LAK and appears to be more effective than the therapy with LAK cells. Since TIL cells appear to be far more potent than LAK cells, the treatment can be of a shorter duration. The side effects are similar to those for IL-2/LAK; however, they may be fewer or less severe since the patient is treated for a shorter period of time.

See also Adoptive immunotherapy.

IL-3   See INTERLEUKIN-3.

IL-4   See INTERLEUKIN-4.

IL-5   See INTERLEUKIN-5.

IL-6   See INTERLEUKIN-6.

IL-11   See INTERLEUKIN-11.

ileal bladder   (il'e-il) [ileal conduit, ileal loop]   a replacement for the urinary bladder. The ureters (the tubes from the kidneys to the bladder) are transplanted into a small segment of ileum (the lower part of the small intestine). The end of the ileum is then brought through the abdominal wall to form a stoma (an artificial opening) through which urine can be eliminated.

ileal conduit   See ILEAL BLADDER.

ileal loop   See ILEAL BLADDER.

ileostomy   (il"e-os'-to-me)   a surgical procedure to create an opening (stoma) in the ileum (the lower part of the small intestine) for the elimina-

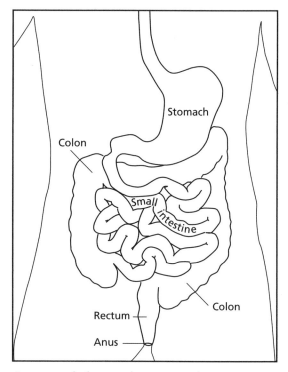

Anatomy before colon removal. Courtesy the American Cancer Society.

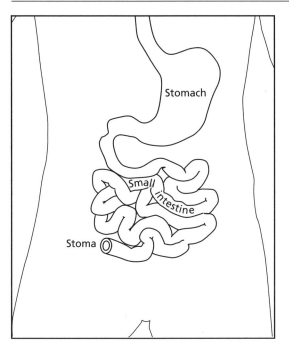

Anatomy after colon removal. Courtesy the American Cancer Society.

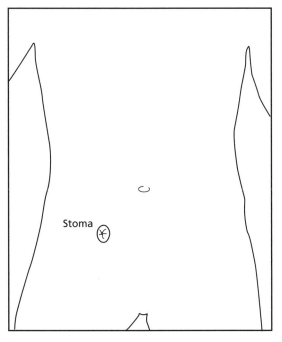

Ileostomy stoma. Courtesy the American Cancer Society.

tion of digestive wastes when the colon is removed. The wastes go through the abdominal wall into a bag outside the body. This is usually permanent. However, if the rectum does not have to be removed, it may be temporary. An ileostomy may be performed in the treatment of COLON/RECTAL CANCER as well as other, noncancerous disorders.

ileum the lower part of the small intestine.

IM See INTRAMUSCULAR.

IMAC a combination of the anticancer drugs IFOSFAMIDE WITH MESNA, ADRIAMYCIN, and CIS-PLATIN sometimes used in the treatment of bone cancer. See individual drug listings for side effects.
    See also COMBINATION CHEMOTHERAPY.

ImageChecker a device that analyzes mammograms and highlights suspicious areas following evaluation by the radiologist. A laser beam converts the image into a digital signal that is processed in a high-speed computer to identify possible signs of cancer. In the United States, for every 80 cancers detected through routine screening mammograms an estimated 20 more are missed. The ImageChecker improved the cancer-detection rate from 80 out of 100 to 88 out of 100.

imagery (im'ij-re) [virtually the same as visualization] a mind exercise in which the patient creates a picture in the mind, like a daydream. Depending on the image or visualization, it can be a way to reduce stress, control pain, and fight cancer. The person begins the exercise by getting into a comfortable position, taking some deep breaths, and relaxing. After achieving a relaxed state, the person imagines a particular situation. It may be a white light entering the body, bringing in energy, coursing through the body, then leaving the body and taking with it the "bad stuff"—pain, tension, discomfort, or cancer cells. Or it might be creating an image of the white blood cells as "knights on white horses" riding through the body attacking and destroying cancer cells. Practicing imagery can help some cancer patients deal better with their cancer by giving them a sense of some control in a situation in which they have virtually no control.
    Among those advocating imagery, or visualization, as an adjunct to conventional therapy (not a

replacement for conventional therapy) are Carl and Stephanie Simonton in their book *Getting Well Again* and Dr. Bernie Siegel in his book *Love, Medicine and Miracles.*

See also SIMONTON TECHNIQUE and UNCONVENTIONAL TREATMENT METHOD.

IMF a combination of the anticancer drugs IFOSFAMIDE WITH MESNA, METHOTREXATE, and 5-FU sometimes used in the treatment of breast cancer. See individual drug listings for side effects.

See also COMBINATION CHEMOTHERAPY.

imidazole carboximide See DTIC.

Imiquimod cream a treatment approved late in 1998 for human papillomavirus. See HUMAN PAPILLOMAVIRUS.

immune system a complex group of cells and substances, throughout the body, that interact to defend the body against foreign substances that might cause infection and disease. When the immune system is functioning successfully, it responds to those foreign agents quickly, appropriately, and effectively. When the immune system is not totally successful, the body can develop various ailments—from an allergy to arthritis to cancer and AIDS. (The HIV [AIDS virus] destroys specific cells, which results in the body's increased vulnerability to FUNGUS and other infections, as well as cancer.)

The immune system has several distinct and unique characteristics. It can "remember" certain previous experiences. For example, once a person has chicken pox, he or she builds up an immunity to it so that it will not recur. The immune system can recognize millions of different cells and can produce molecules or cells to counteract each one. It can also distinguish between "self" and "nonself," which enables it to fight and destroy nonself, or foreign, agents that are not part of the body. However, this important function can work against the body in an organ of bone marrow transplantation when the immune system can identify the new marrow as nonself, and reject it.

Immunologists divide the immune response into two parts that generally complement each other—the humoral system (pertaining to the fluids in the body) and the cellular system (pertaining

to the cells in the body). Humoral responses are performed by the antibodies, proteins that fight infections or harmful substances in the body. ANTIBODIES are produced by B CELLS (a WHITE BLOOD CELL) and secreted into the body fluid where they fight the foreign bodies. Cellular responses emanate from the cells themselves primarily T CELLS, white blood cells. T cells regulate cell-mediated immunity, which includes bone marrow rejection and delayed skin hypersensitivity. Other lymphocytes that play a role in the immune system include B cells and NATURAL KILLER (NK) cells. Other white blood cells involved in the immune system are granulocytes, which fight bacteria by engulfing and destroying them (there are three types: neutrophils, basophils, eosinophils), and monocytes, which produce macrophages, versatile cells that can engulf and destroy foreign substances in the body, rid the body of debris, and secrete chemical substances.

The main producer of the immune system cells is the body's BONE MARROW (the inner, spongy substance of bones). Other organs of the immune system, some of which may also produce white blood cells, include the tonsils (small, rounded mass composed primarily of lymphoid tissue located at the back of the throat), adenoids (glands located in the back of the nasal passage), LYMPH NODES (very small, beanshaped organs throughout the body), thymus (gland locatedhigh in the chest), spleen (small organ in the upper left side of the abdomen), appendix (small organ located in the intestine), Peyer's patches (collection of lymphoid tissues in the intestinal tract), and lymphatic vessels (system of narrow tubes through which immune cells travel).

The immune system provides the body's main defense against cancer and is the key part of the newest cancer treatment, BIOLOGICAL THERAPY.

immunoassay (im″u-no-as′sa) a test of body fluids such as blood or urine for specific ANTIGENS, ANTIBODIES, and other biological substances. The presence of a high or low level of one the substances could be a sign of cancer (or other diseases).

immunoaugmentative therapy (IAT) (im″u-no-awg-men′tah-tiv) a scientifically unsound and potentially hazardous treatment for cancer practiced at the Immunology Researching Center in the Bahamas. Lawrence Burton, a Ph.D. zoologist with no training in medicine, cancer research, or treating cancer patients, opened his clinic there in 1977 after the Food and Drug Administration refused to permit patients to receive the treatment in the United States.

The premise of IAT is that cancer is caused by IMMUNODEFICIENCY, which can be measured and corrected using a series of blood fractions extracted at the clinic.

In 1978 the Bahamian government asked the Pan American Health Organization to review the treatment. The health organization unanimously recommended that the center be closed. The clinic remained open, but only for the treatment of non-Bahamians.

See UNCONVENTIONAL TREATMENT METHOD.

immunodeficiency   a lowering of the body's ability to fight off infection and disease.

immunoenhancer   anything that increases the body's ability to fight off infections or disease.

immunoglobulins   See ANTIBODIES.

immunomodulation (im″u-no-mod″u-la′shun) a new emphasis on manipulating (modulating) the body's IMMUNE SYSTEM to fight cancer cells. On a practical level the recently introduced agent LEV-AMISOLE has been shown to augment the function of MACROPHAGES and T CELLS. Combined with the cytotoxic drug 5-FU, it is now a recommended, effectivetherapy for certain colon cancer patients at high risk of relapse after surgery.

immunosuppression (im″u-no-sŭ-presh′un)   the use of drugs or techniques to suppress, or interfere with, the body's IMMUNE SYSTEM and its ability to fight infections or disease. Powerful immunosuppressive drugs can inhibit the production of white blood cells or interfere with their actions in the immune system. For example, steroids suppress LYMPHOCYTE function, and the drug cyclosporine holds down the production of INTERLEUKIN-2, which is needed for T-CELL growth. Immunosuppression may be used during organ or BONE MARROW TRANSPLANTATION to prevent the body's own immune system from rejecting the new, foreign organ or bone marrow. Until their immune system is functioning normally, immunosuppressed patients are at a much higher risk of infections and developing LYMPHOMAS.

immunotherapy (ĭ-mu″no-ther′ah-pe)   a treatment that stimulates or boosts the body's IMMUNE SYSTEM so that it can fight the cancer.

See also BIOLOGICAL THERAPY.

implant   in INTERSTITIAL RADIATION, a small container of RADIOACTIVE material placed in the body in or near a cancer.

implant radiation   See INTERSTITIAL RADIATION.

impotence   the inability of a man to have an erection. Impotence can be a result of cancer or of cancer treatment. Some surgical procedures used in the treatment of prostate cancer (RADICAL PROSTATECTOMY) and bladder cancer (RADICAL CYSTECTOMY) may cause impotency. However, improvements in surgical techniques have reduced the likelihood of impotency.

See also SEXUAL ACTIVITY.

IMVP-16   a combination of the anticancer drugs IFOSFAMIDE WITH MESNA, METHOTREXATE, and ETOPOSIDE sometimes used in the treatment of NON-HODGKIN'S LYMPHOMA. See individual drug listings for side effects.

See also COMBINATION CHEMOTHERAPY.

in situ (in si′tu)   cancer in its earliest stage, that is confined to the place or site where it started. Some in situ cancers are considered precancerous. In situ cancers have a very good prognosis, and in most instances removal of the cancer is considered a cure. In situ is Latin for "in place" and is commonly referred to as "noninvasive."

in vitro   referring to a biological process or reaction taking place in an artificial environment, usually in a test tube in a laboratory. In vitro studies are usually the first step in the development of new treatments for cancer and other diseases. In vitro literally mean "in glass."

in vivo   referring to a biological process or reaction taking place in a living organism—e.g., an animal or human being. In cancer research, in vivo studies are conducted in CLINICAL TRIALS.

incidence   the total number of new cancers appearing in a population during a specific period of time such as a year. For example, in 1999 there were 176,300 new cases of breast cancer.

incidence rate   the number of new cancers per standard unit of population during a year. An incidence rate can be calculated for a specific cancer site, age, race, or sex. For example, in one year there were 6.0 cases of brain cancer per 100,000 people.

incisional biopsy (in-siz'shun-al bi'op-se)   removal of part of a tumor for microscopic examination for cancer cells. If cancer is diagnosed as a result of an incisional biopsy, some cancer has been left behind since only part of the tumor was removed. In an EXCISIONAL BIOPSY, the entire tumor is removed.

See also BIOPSY.

IND (investigational new drug)   a drug that is licensed by the Food and Drug Administration (FDA) for use in CLINICAL TRIALS but is not yet approved by that agency for commercial marketing. Drugs may be FDA-approved for one specific kind of cancer, or stage of cancer, and remain investigational for other cancers.

indication   a symptom, or condition that leads to the recommendation of a treatment, test, or procedure

indolent non-Hodgkin's lymphoma   a group of slow-growing NON-HODGKIN'S LYMPHOMA, including nodular or diffuse poorly differentiated lymphocytic, nodular mixed, diffuse well-differentiated lymphocytic lymphoma; or diffuse intermediate differentiated lymphocytic lymphoma. They primarily affect adults over the age of 40. The only symptom may be a painless swelling of the LYMPH NODES in the neck, under the arm, or in the groin.

indoor air quality (IAQ)   a term used in describing the degree of pollution in the air inside a building or home. The pollution level inside is usually greater than it is outside because it is in a confined space. The Environmental Protection Agency estimates that Americans spend as much as 90% of their time indoors. Therefore, indoor air pollution can be a much greater problem than the pollution out of doors. High concentrations of pollutants, some of which are CARCINOGENS, can pose a serious health threat. Some problems can be immediate and others long term, showing up many years after the initial exposure. Short-term problems may include dizziness, headaches, irritation of the eyes, nose, and throat, or simply fatigue. Long-term problems can be far more serious—and include cancer. Among the more common home pollutants are RADON and ASBESTOS, both known to cause lung cancer, and lead. The people most at risk from indoor air pollutants are young children, the elderly, the chronically ill, and people with respiratory problems. The degree of risk increases with the length of time of exposure and the concentration of a single pollutant, or a combination of pollutants, in the air.

induction therapy   the first phase of treatment with anticancer drugs of some types of leukemia. It is as aggressive as possible in order to destroy the highest number of abnormal white blood cells as quickly as possible. It usually lasts four to six weeks. COMBINATION CHEMOTHERAPY is commonly used.

The second phase is CONSOLIDATION THERAPY. MAINTENANCE THERAPY may be administered after consolidation treatment.

indwelling catheter   a thin tube implanted and anchored onto a large vein in the body with the rest of the tube extending through the skin. The indwelling catheter is used for the administration of anticancer drugs as well as other substances, including blood transfusions, nutrients, bone marrow, and other medications. Blood can also be drawn from the patient through the catheter. The indwelling catheter eliminates the need for repeated injections into the skin, which can be painful as well as stressful to a patient. Barring infection, it can stay in the body for months. One example is the HICKMAN CATHETER.

See also CATHETER, INFUSE-A-PORT, and VENOUS ACCESS DEVICE.

infantile   hemangiopericytoma (in'fan-tīl   hĕ-man"je-o-per"ĕ-si-to'mah)   a type of SOFT TISSUE SARCOMA originating in the blood vessels in the arms, legs, trunk, head, and neck in infants up to the age of one.

infection   a condition in which the body or an organ has been invaded by a disease-causing microorganism. Since infections occur more readily when the bone marrow's ability to produce white blood cells is decreased and the IMMUNE SYSTEM is lowered, they can be a dangerous side effect of CHEMOTHERAPY, which frequently affects the bone marrow. The body lacks sufficient defenses to fight infections, and an infection that ordinarily would be minor can be debilitating, even life threatening. For that reason, if a patient's white blood count in too low, chemotherapy will be postponed, or the dose lowered, to give the bone marrow time to restore the white blood cell count and the immune system. Infections are also a major problem in AIDS patients and can result in death. Symptoms of an infection include a fever, chills, sweating (especially at night), loose bowels, a burning feeling when urinating, a severe cough, and/or a sore throat. An infection with bacteria that invade the bloodstream is referred to as bacteremia. Bacteria that release by-products into the bloodstream may cause septicemia, which may progress to shock. A virus in the bloodstream is known as viremia. Fungus in the blood is known as fungemia.

infertility   the inability to produce offspring. In both men and women with cancer, infertility can be a result of their treatment. In men, undergoing the following procedures will always result in infertility:

- RADICAL PROSTATECTOMY
- RADICAL CYSTECTOMY
- ORCHIECTOMY (removal of both testicles)
- hormonal treatment for prostate cancer.

CHEMOTHERAPY, RADIATION THERAPY to the pelvis, a PENECTOMY or RETROPERITONEAL LYMPH NODE DISSECTION will frequently result in infertility. An ABDOMINOPERINEAL   RESECTION will   sometimes cause infertility. Removal of one testicle will rarely result in infertility.

In women, the following procedures will prevent a woman from bearing children:

- a RADICAL HYSTERECTOMY
- a radical cystectomy
- a PELVIC EXENTERATION
- an OOPHORECTOMY in which both tubes and ovaries are removed.

Other procedures which may affect a woman's fertility include chemotherapy, pelvic RADIATION THERAPY, and abdominoperineal resection. CONIZATION and the removal of one tube and ovary will, on rare occasions, result in infertility.

See also SEXUAL ACTIVITY.

infiltrating ductal carcinoma (duk'tal kar"sĭ-no'mah) [invasive ductal breast cancer]   the most common type of BREAST CANCER, accounting for about 70% of the breast cancer cases. It is in the cells in the ducts of the breast. The tumor feels hard and may be fixed to the skin or chest wall, or the nipple may be retracted. Invasive ductal cancers may not grow large, but they tend to spread rapidly to LYMPH NODES.

infiltrating lobular carcinoma (lob'u-lar kar"sĭ-no'mah) [invasive lobular breast carcinoma]   a type of BREAST CANCER that starts in the breast lobules, the small end ducts that branch off the lobes in the breast. These account for about 5% of all breast cancers. They are similar in appearance and behavior to INFILTRATING DUCTAL CARCINOMAS.

inflammation   a condition that occurs when a part of the body becomes red, swollen, or hot. It is usually accompanied by pain or tenderness, usually from irritation. In cancer, the area around a tumor can become inflamed, causing major discomfort. ANALGESIC drugs, specifically the NONSTEROIDAL ANTI-INFLAMMATORY DRUGS (NSAIDs), are used to treat inflammations. Through the early 1980s NSAIDs were available by prescription only. Many are now available over the counter.

inflammatory carcinoma of the breast (in-flam'ah-to"re kar"sĭ-no'mah)   a rare type of BREAST CANCER representing, at most, 4% of all breast cancers. There may be swelling, redness, and heat in a large part of the breast, and the skin may appear pitted or show signs of ridges. The redness and heat are caused by cancer cells blocking the lymph vessels in the skin of the breast. An aggressive cancer that can spread rapidly to other parts of the body, it appears abruptly and superficially appears like an infection or nflammation. Best results are usually from multimodality treatment combining CHEMOTHERAPY (anticancer drugs) RADIATION THERAPY, and surgery. For the latest state-of-the-art treatment for inflammatory carcinoma of the breast, call the National Cancer Institute's Cancer Information Service at 1-800-4-CANCER (1-800-422-6237), or for a TTY: 1-800-332-8615.

informed consent a legal standard for giving patients enough information about a medical treatment—its benefits and risks—so that he or she can decide whether to go ahead with the treatment or procedure. Informed consent is part of every CLINICAL TRIAL, as well as medical procedures that carry some risk. The written consent form is supposed to contain a clear statement of the purpose of the investigation as well as its possible benefits and risks so that the patient can make a clear choice as to whether to take part in the trial.

infratentorial tumors tumors found in the lower part of the brain, usually the cerebellum or brain stem; the cerebellum is the most common site of brain tumors in children; tumors found in this region are:

- MEDULLOBLASTOMA—a rapidly growing tumor that can spread to other parts of the nervous system; depending on the size of the tumor after surgery and the presence or absence of spread to other areas, patients may be classified as standard risk or high risk
- CEREBELLAR ASTROCYTOMA—generally a slow-growing tumor that usually does not spread to adjacent tissues or outside the region
- infratentorial ependymoma—a tumor arising from the lining of the lower part of the brain; it may spread to other areas of the brain and spinal cord
- BRAIN STEM GLIOMA—astrocytomas arising in the lowest part of the brain; they may grow rapidly or slowly but rarely spread from their original location

infuse-a-port [Mediport] a small device containing a thin CATHETER that is surgically implanted under the skin. The infuse-a-port is used for the administration of anticancer drugs as well as other substances including blood transfusions, nutrients, stem cells, and other medications. Blood can also be drawn from the patient by inserting a needle into the infuse-a-port reservoir. The infuse-a-port eliminates the constant need to search for a "good" vein, which can be a vexing problem, in some cases causing pain as well as anxiety, for a patient receiving regular treatments intravenously. It is similar in many ways to an INDWELLING CATHETER, but it is completely under the skin and does not need the regular care required by the indwelling catheter. It is also less prone to infections. Barring infection, it can remain in the body for months.

infusion pump a small battery-driven device used to deliver a constant or intermittent flow of anticancer drugs or pain medication to a patient. They are particularly useful for the administration of drugs that can be harmful if infused too rapidly. In many instances, the patient, or a family member, can be taught to replace the cartridge, bag, or syringe that holds the substance. Most patients with an infusion pump can be completely mobile.

See also INFUSION THERAPY.

infusion therapy use of an internal or external pump in CHEMOTHERAPY to deliver high concentrations of anticancer drugs directly to the cancer site over a long period of time. Because the chemotherapy is given over a period of days instead of minutes, the side effects are reduced. Most infusion chemotherapy is given into the venous system. It is also possible to direct therapy into the artery leading into an organ (called intra-arterial infusion). When an external pump is used for infusion therapy, the patient must carry it around. Although it may hamper some patients' ability to move, most patients adjust to it quickly and are not restricted in their movements. The internal pump is inserted into the body, where it delivers the drugs at an even rate over a period of time. When the supply is used up, the pump can be refilled by injecting it with another dose. Currently, the pump is being used for liver, colon, head and neck, and brain cancers, among others.

inguinal orchiectomy (ing′gwĭ-nal or″ke-ek′to-me) surgery to remove the testes through the groin.

Inosiplex See ISOPRINOSINE.

insufflation (in″sŭ-fla′shun) blowing powder, vapor, gas, or air into a body cavity in order to get a better picture. For example, air may be injected around the kidneys to get a better X-RAY of the adrenal glands.

See also AIR-CONTRAST X-RAYS.

interferon (in′ter-fēr′on) a class of protein produced in minuscule amounts by infected cells that appear to boost the body's IMMUNE SYSTEM. Interferon was discovered in 1975. It was the first CYTOKINE discovered. Since that time a tremendous amount has been learned about interferon, and its role in the treatment of cancer continues to be investigated. There are three major groups of interferons: alpha, beta, and gamma. The alpha interferon products (Intron A, Roferon-A, Wellferon, and Alferon N) have been found to be the most clinically useful. These are considered as a group to act as biological response modifiers (BRM) or antineoplastics. They are being used in the treatment of HAIRY CELL LEUKEMIA, AIDS-related KAPOSI'S SARCOMA, MELANOMA, MYELOMA, KIDNEY CANCER, CML, NON-HODGKIN'S LYMPHOMA, BLADDER CANCER, and other conditions.

The most common side effects include a flu-like syndrome that can be disabling, lowering of the white blood cells, or platelets. The drug is given either by IM (into the muscle) or SC (under the skin).

A significant role for the beta and gamma interferons is still being explored. Their use should be considered investigational.

interferon alpha-2A [Roferon-A] See ALPHA INTERFERON and INTERFERON.

interferon alpha-2b [Intron A] See ALPHA INTERFERON and INTERFERON.

interferon alpha-2c [Wellferon] See ALPHA INTERFERON and INTERFERON.

interferon alpha-2d [Alferon] See ALPHA INTERFERON and INTERFERON.

interferon beta [r-IFN-beta] An INTERFERON used in the treatment of primary BRAIN TUMORS, cutaneous T-CELL LYMPHOMA, MELANOMA, KIDNEY CANCER, AIDS-related KAPOSI'S SARCOMA.

interferon gamma 1-b [Actimmune] an INTERFERON used in the treatment of KIDNEY CANCER and chronic granulomatous disease.

interleukin (in″ter-lu′kin) a group of natural, hormone-like substances produced in the body by LYMPHOCYTES, white blood cells in the IMMUNE SYSTEM. Interleukins are one type of CYTOKINE and act as "messengers," carrying regulatory signals between blood-forming cells that are important in the immune system and stimulate the immune system to fight cancer. Interleukins are BIOLOGICAL RESPONSE MODIFIERS.

interleukin-1 (IL-1) (in″ter-lu′kin) [hematopoietin-1] a protein produced by a variety of different cells in the body including the natural KILLER CELLS, T-CELLS, and B CELLS. IL-1 triggers a wide range of processes involved in inflammation, a localized immune reaction. It activates T cells and stimulates bone marrow growth.

interleukin-2 (IL-2) (in″ter-lu′kin) [Proleukin, aldesleukin, Teceleukin, recombinant, and rIL-2] a protein produced by activated T cells in the body. It plays a central role in the regulation of the immune system. It was discovered in 1976 at the National Cancer Institute and was originally called T cell growth factor. IL-2 stimulates the growth and activities of a wide range of cells, including several types that can kill cancer cells such as LAK CELLS (lymphokine-activated killer cells), TIL cells (tumor-infiltrating lymphocytes), and CTL (cytotoxic T lymphocytes). Side effects of IL-2 may include chills, low blood pressure, rapid heartbeat, swelling, breathing difficulties, mental and emotional changes, itching, dry skin, rash, decreased urination, decreased appetite, diarrhea, nausea, vomiting, and dry or sore mouth. The side effects are generally temporary, going away when the treatment is over. IL-2 treatment has been most effective with advanced renal cell carcinoma and advanced melanoma. Some scientists believe that IL-2 therapy may help stop certain cancers from growing, which can improve the length and quality of life for some cancer patients. For high-dose IL-2 administration, the patient must either be in an ICU or in a specialized nursing unit.

interleukin-3 (IL-3) [multicolony-stimulating factor (multi-CSF)] another powerful interleukin that stimulates the growth of many precursor bone marrow cells. They are early cells with the potential to develop into mature blood cells.

interleukin-4 (IL-4) [B-cell stimulatory factor-1 (BSF-1)] enhances B-CELL growth and antibody production and stimulates the production of other immune system cells.

interleukin-5 (IL-5) [eosinophil-colony stimulating factor (eosinophil CSF)] stimulates the growth of the blood cells known as EOSINOPHILS, which kill bacteria.

interleukin-6 (IL-6) [B-cell stimulatory factor-2 (BSF-2), interferon beta-2] stimulates B-CELL growth.

interleukin-11 (IL-11) [Neumega, Oprelvekin] stimulates the production of platelets.

intermediate polyps (pol'ips) [tubulovillous polyps] POLYPS found in the intestines that are not associated with FAMILIAL MULTIPLE POLYPOSIS OF THE COLON, an inherited tendency to develop these growths. They occur in around 5 or 6% of the population. They will become cancerous in about 23% of the people who have them.

internal pump   See INFUSION PUMP and INFUSION THERAPY.

internal radiation therapy   insertion of a radioactive substance into the body, targeted to a specific cancerous site to destroy it from within. (Compare with EXTERNAL RADIATION.) Internal radiation places the high-energy rays as close to the cancer cells as possible. In that way, fewer normal cells are exposed to and damaged by the radiation and a higher dose of radiation over a shorter period of time can be given than with external radiation.

The three types of internal radiation are INTRA-CAVITARY RADIATION (radioactive sources are put into body cavities such as the mouth, anus, or vagina), INTERSTITIAL RADIATION (the radioactive sources are put into the tumor itself), and BRACHYTHERAPY (the radioactive sources are put on the surface of the body near the tumor). The term "brachytherapy" is frequently used to mean all internal radiation. It can also be implanted in a specific part of the body using radium needles, wires, iridium seeds, capsules, or a tube containing radium. Generally, when an implant is used, the patient receives general or local anesthesia.

Most implants stay in the body between one and seven days. Anesthesia is generally not needed to remove the implant. Once it is removed, there is no radioactivity in the body. Some implants are permanently inserted and not removed, most commonly for cancers of the prostate, mouth, and tongue. The radioactivity of the materials lessens each day so that after a few days there is little radiation emanating from the patient's body.

An implant in the body can give off radiation outside the body. Therefore, the container for the radiation source may be inserted, with the actual radiation inserted only when the patient is back in the room alone in order to limit the exposure of others to it. Some hospitals require a patient receiving implant radiation to stay in a private room. During the time the implant is in place, there may be restrictions on visitors limiting the length of time they can stay in the room and how close they can get to the patient. Visitors are usually advised to stay no longer than half an hour and sit at least six feet from the patient. Most hospitals do not allow pregnant women or children under the age of 18 to visit patients with implants.

There are usually no major side effects with implant radiation. There may be some discomfort from the device that is holding the implant in place.

Radiation implants are most commonly used for cancers of the head and neck, breast, uterus, and prostate. Some of the substances used in internal radiation are radium, cesium, and iridium.

See also RADIATION THERAPY.

International Union Against Cancer (IUAC)   an organization formed in the 1930s to consolidate efforts worldwide against cancer. It is comprised of multidisciplinary organizations and promotes international communication in cancer research, treatment and prevention. It is located in Geneva, Switzerland.

International Working Formulation for the histological classification of NON-HODGKIN'S LYMPHOMA. A way of describing non-Hodgkin's lymphoma. Developed by the National Cancer Institute and an international panel of pathologists in 1981 in order to standardize terms, the system classifies lymphomas as low grade, intermediate grade, or high grade.

interstitial implant   See INTERSTITIAL RADIATION.

interstitial radiation (in"ter-stish'al) [interstitial implant, implant radiation, needle implant]   a type of INTERNAL RADIATION treatment. Tiny bits of radioactive isotopes are inserted in hollow steel needles implanted in and around cancerous tissue in the body (as opposed to a body cavity). A higher dose of radiation can be administered to a specific site while sparing most of the normal tissue around it. The implant generally remains in the body from one to six days. It may be used in some cancers of the mouth, tongue, lip, breast, and prostate.

intestines (in-tes'tins) [bowel]   the last part of the DIGESTIVE TRACT, extending from the stomach to the anus. It has two main parts—the small intestine and the large intestine—which refers to the diameter of the tubes rather than the length. The colon is part of the large intestine. The intestines finish the digestive process started by the stomach and prepare the waste products for excretion from the body.

intra-arterial infusion   See INFUSION THERAPY.

intracavitary radiation (in"trah-kav'ĭ-tār"e)   a type of INTERNAL RADIATION treatment in which radioactive material is implanted in a body cavity such as the uterus, chest cavity, or vagina, as close to a tumor as possible. It can give a higher dose of radiation to a specific site while sparing most of the normal tissue around it. The implant may be removed after a period of time or put in permanently.

intraductal carcinoma   See DUCTAL BREAST CARCINOMA IN SITU.

intraluminal intubation and dilation (in"trah-lu'mĭ-nal in-tu-ba'shun)   insertion of a plastic tube into the esophagus to keep it open during radiation treatments. This procedure may be used in the treatment of ESOPHAGEAL CANCER.

intramuscular (IM) (in"trah-mus'ku-lar)   in cancer treatment, the delivery of anticancer or pain medication to the body by an injection into a muscle in the arm, buttocks, or thigh.

intraocular melanoma (in"trah-ok'u-lar mel"ahno'mah) [ocular melanoma]   cancer of the part of the eye called the uvea, which is composed of the iris (the colored part of the eye), the ciliary body (a muscle in the eye), and the choroid (a layer of tissue in the back of the eye). It is a type of MELANOMA and a very rare cancer, but the most common form of EYE CANCER in adults. If melanoma starts in the iris, there may be a dark spot on the iris. A symptom of melanoma in the ciliary body or choroid may be blurry vision. Intraocular melanoma is most frequently found during a routine eye examination.

Following is the National Cancer Institute's staging for intraocular melanoma:

- Iris—occurring in the front, colored part of the eye; it grows slowly and usually does not spread to other parts of the body
- Ciliary body/choroid—occurs in the back part of the eye
  - small size—up to 10 millimeters (mm) wide and up to 2 mm thick
  - medium/large size—more than 10 mm wide or more than 2 mm thick
- Extraocular extension—cancer has spread outside the eye, to the nerve behind the eye (the optic nerve) or to the eye socket
- Recurrent—the cancer has returned to the same site or to another part of the body after treatment

Treatment depends on the stage of the disease and other factors. The doctor may not recommend immediate treatment but rather watch carefully for any sign that the cancer is beginning to grow. The treatments used for intraocular melanoma include

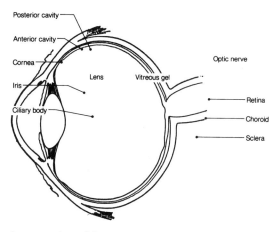

Labels: Posterior cavity, Anterior cavity, Cornea, Iris, Ciliary body, Lens, Vitreous gel, Optic nerve, Retina, Choroid, Sclera

Cross section of the eye. Courtesy NCI.

surgery, RADIATION THERAPY, and PHOTOCOAGULA-TION (killing the blood vessels that feed the tumor). For specific information on the latest state-of-the-art treatment, by stage, call NCI's Cancer Information Service at 1-800-4-CANCER (1-800-422-6237), or for a TTY: 1-800-332-8615.

intraoperative radiation therapy (IORT) (in"trah-op"er-a"tiv)   the delivery of a high dose of radiation to a cancerous tumor and surrounding tissue at the time of surgery. It may be the only form of RADI-ATION THERAPY given; or additional EXTERNAL RADIA-TION THERAPY may be delivered before or after the surgery.

intraperitoneal chemotherapy (in"trah-per"ĭ-to-ne'al)   a procedure used in the treatment of OVAR-IAN CANCER in which anticancer drugs are placed directly into the abdominal and pelvic cavity instead of being injected into a vein. The attraction of this procedure is the ability to place higher concentrations of the drugs to "bathe" the cancer areas. However, drug delivery deep into the tumor still remains a problem, with only a few layers of cancerous cells being affected. Drugs used in intraperitoneal chemotherapy include CISPLATIN, INTERFERON, and others.

intraperitoneal radiotherapy (in"trah-per"ĭ-to-ne'al)   a procedure that may be used in the treatment of OVARIAN CANCER. A radioactive liquid is placed directly into the pelvic and abdominal cavities. The liquid coats the area and kills cancer cells.

intrathecal chemotherapy (in"trah-the'kal)   a procedure in which anticancer drugs are injected into the cerebrospinal fluid. The drugs may be injected into the fluid through a lumbar SPINAL TAP or by use of a surgically placed device known as an Ommaya reservoir. Intrathecal chemotherapy and radiation treatment are the only useful treatments for LEPTO-MENINGEAL CARCINOMA, a very serious condition in which cancer cells spread directly into the spinal fluid. Intrathecal chemotherapy is also sometimes used with patients diagnosed with an aggressive NON-HODGKIN'S LYMPHOMA with bone marrow involvement in order to prevent a recurrence in the brain and spinal fluid.

intravenous (IV) (in"trah-ve'nus)   within a vein. In cancer treatment, it refers to the delivery of anti-cancer or pain medication into a vein. This can be done by injection or as a fluid drip in which the medication drips slowly into the vein through an IV needle, usually secured in the patient's hand or arm. Nutrients and anesthesia can also be administered through a vein.

intravenous anesthesia (in"trah-ve'nus an"es-the'ze-ah)   the injection of an anesthetic via vein into the bloodstream, putting the patient to sleep very quickly. After the initial dose, the anesthetic may continue to drip into the bloodstream at a controlled rate of speed.

intravenous immunoglobulin (IVIG) (in"trah-ve'nus im"u-no-glob'u-lin)   the administration of immunoglobulins (antibodies that fight infections or harmful substances in the body) by injection into a vein. Immunoglobulins have been used for injection in a muscle since 1952. In the last decade, preparations that can be given by IV into a vein have become available as well, and their use has grown widely over the past few years. IVIG is used in the treatment of immunodeficiency of many types. For example, in chronic lymphocytic leukemia, IVIG may be used as a treatment of immune thrombocytopenia (ITP).

intravenous pyelography   See IVP.

intravesical chemotherapy (in"trah-ves'ĕ-kal) insertion of anticancer drugs into the bladder, an ADJUVANT THERAPY sometimes used in early BLADDER CANCER. The anticancer drugs are inserted through a CATHETER into the urethra (tube which carries the urine from the bladder to the outside). The bladder is then washed with the drugs. This may be done before the primary treatment (surgery) or after surgery to kill off any remaining cancer cells.

intravesical immunotherapy (in"trah-ves'ĕ-kal ĭ-mu"no-ther'ah-pe) insertion of BCG (a vaccine) into the bladder. This form of ADJUVANT THERAPY is sometimes used in early bladder cancer. The BCG is inserted through a CATHETER into the urethra (tube that carries the urine from the bladder to the outside). The bladder is washed with the BCG, a substance that stimulates the IMMUNE SYSTEM. This may be performed before the primary treatment (surgery) or after surgery to kill off any remaining cancer cells.

Intron A See ALPHA INTERFERON and INTERFERON.

invasive cancer a stage of cancer in which cancer cells have spread to healthy tissue adjacent to the tumor. It may still be considered localized if it has not spread to other parts of the body. Compare with NONINVASIVE or IN SITU.

invasive ductal breast cancer See INFILTRATING DUCTAL CARCINOMA.

invasive lobular breast carcinoma See INFIL-TRATING LOBULAR CARCINOMA.

investigational new drug See IND.

investigational treatment or trials See CLINICAL TRIALS.

involuntary smoking See SECONDHAND SMOKING.

ionizing radiation (IR) a type of high-frequency radiation including X-RAYS and radon that can cause cancer. The greater the exposure the higher the risk. Although any part of the body can be affected, the thyroid gland and bone marrow are at the greatest risk.

IORT See INTRAOPERATIVE RADIATION THERAPY.

IPI (International Prognostic Index) the IPI is used to assess risk in patients with DLBCL. It contains three elements: age, LDH, and performance status.

IR See IONIZING RADIATION.

Iressa a new drug that is being investigated as a cancer treatment. It is sometimes called ZD 1839 or gefitinib. Iressa is a type of drug called a tyrosine kinase inhibitor. Iressa may block the cancer cell from growing and dividing. It is still in clinical trials.

iridectomy (ir"ĭ-dek'to-me) surgical removal of parts of the iris (the colored part of the eye).

iridium seeds (i-rid'e-um) small particles of the metallic element iridium, which can be implanted in the body at the site of the cancer to irradiate cancerous tissue from within. See INTERNAL RADIATION.

iridocyclectomy (ir"ĭ-do-si-klek'to-me) surgical removal of parts of the iris (the colored part of the eye) and the ciliary body (a muscle in the eye).

iridotrabulectomy (ir"ĭ-do-trah"bu-lek'to-me) surgical removal of parts of the iris (the colored part of the eye) and the supporting tissues around the cornea (the clear layer covering the front of the eye).

Irinotecan A chemotherapy drug given via IV (intravenous injection) used in colorectal cancer, approved in combination with 5-FU and leucovirin (IFL) as first-line treatment of patients with metastatic disease; also approved as a single agent as second-line therapy of patients with metastatic disease after failure of 5-FU-based chemotherapy. It is also active in NON-SMALL CELL LUNG CANCER (NSCLC) and SMALL CELL LUNG CANCER (SCLC). A major side effect is diarrhea, either early or late, and myelosuppression.
See CAMPTOSAR and CP-11.

irradiation See RADIATION THERAPY.

islet cell carcinoma (i'let kar"sĭ-no'mah) [endocrine cancer] a rare form of PANCREATIC CANCER that originates in the endocrine glands that produce hormones. Between 200 and 1,000 new cases are diagnosed each year in the United States. These tumors are usually soft and fleshy, slow growing, and with a more favorable PROGNOSIS than exocrine pancreatic cancer. The two major types of islet cell carcinoma, based on the type of hormone that is produced, are gastrinoma and insulinoma. Another, more rare form is glucagonoma. Insulinomas are more often benign (noncancerous) than malignant (cancerous). A common symptom is hypoglycemia (low blood sugar), which can cause restlessness, irritability, sweating, and flushing, because the tumor can interfere with insulin secretion and sugar regulation.

The tumor may be discovered by investigating conditions associated with excess production of the hormone insulin (low blood sugar) or gastrin (peptic ulcer). Diagnosis may require sophisticated tests that may reveal a small pancreatic tumor.

Although there is no formal staging of islet cell carcinoma, it is divided into three categories:

- cancers occurring in one site
- cancers occurring in several sites
- cancer that has spread to regional LYMPH NODES or distant sites

Islet cell carcinoma is highly treatable. Treatment depends on the extent of disease and other factors. Surgery and CHEMOTHERAPY are used in the treatment of islet cell carcinoma. For specific information on the latest state-of-the-art treatment, call the National Cancer Institute's Cancer Information Service at 1-800-4-CANCER (1-800-422-6237), or for a TTY: 1-800-332-8615.

isolation   perfusion [limb   perfusion] during CHEMOTHERAPY, the administration of anticancer drugs directly to the cancer site. This procedure is under investigation for its use in the treatment of MELANOMA occurring in the arm or leg. Chemo-therapy drugs are added to blood that is withdrawn from the patient. The blood is then pumped back into the major artery supplying the limb being treated. By administering chemotherapy directly to the affected area, higher doses can be given.

isophosphamide   See IFOSFAMIDE.

isoprinosine (i″so-prin′o-sīn) [Inosiplex]   an immuno enhancer. Previously promoted as one of many "wonder" drugs thought to be capable of treating AIDS, after careful study, it has proved to be of no benefit to AIDS patients or people with the AIDS virus.

isotope scan   See NUCLEAR SCAN.

isotretinoin   See ACCUTANE.

itching   See PRURITUS.

IUAC   See INTERNATIONAL UNION AGAINST CANCER.

IV   See INTRAVENOUS.

IVIG   See INTRAVENOUS IMMUNOGLOBULIN.

IVP   (intravenous   pyelography) (in″trah-ve′nus pi″log′rah-fe) [excretory   urography, KUB (kidneys, ureters, bladder]   an examination of the urinary system (kidneys, ureters, and bladder) by X-RAY. After an initial X-RAY of the abdomen is taken, a special iodine-containing solution is injected into a vein. The contrast solution goes into the kidney, and additional X-rays are taken. Another X-ray is taken after the patient urinates. An IVP is one of the tests that may be used in the diagnosis of kidney, testicular, endometrial, and prostate cancer. This is generally considered a safe procedure. However, a small number of patients are allergic to the CONTRAST MEDIUM used.

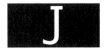

Jamshidi needle a standard instrument used to perform a BONE MARROW BIOPSY.

Janus gene The Janus kinase 2 (JAK) gene lying on chromosome 9p. A point mutation of this gene in 2005 was linked to several of the myeloproliferative disorders.

jaundice (jawn'dis) yellow coloration of the skin and whites of the eyes caused by an abnormal increase in bile pigment. Jaundice most frequently is the result of various liver diseases, including cancer of the liver, hepatitis, and cirrhosis. Another possible cause is obstruction of the bile ducts as a result of gallstones or a cancerous tumor in the pancreas. Jaundice can also be caused by a reaction to a drug or HEMOLYSIS, a blood disease.

Jewett & Strong staging a pathological staging BLADDER CANCER as superficial, deep, or metastatic.

JM-8 See CARBOPLATIN.

juxtacortical osteosarcoma See PAROSTEAL OSTEOSARCOMA and BONE CANCER.

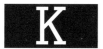

Kaposi's sarcoma (KS) (kap'o-sez sar-ko'mah) a rare cancer that causes slightly raised spots on the skin that range in color from purple to brown. It was first described by Moritz Kaposi, a European doctor, in 1872. It remained a very rare tumor until it started showing up in patients with acquired immunodeficiency syndrome (AIDS).

There are three types of Kaposi's sarcoma. The first, known as classic Kaposi's sarcoma, occurs most frequently in older men of Italian or eastern European Jewish origin. It also occurs in black African adult men and children who have not reached puberty. The second type can occur in patients who have undergone kidney transplant and other patients who are receiving therapy that suppresses the immune system. Immunosuppressive treatment–related Kaposi's sarcoma was first seen in 1969.

The third type, a recent, more aggressive form of the disease, is epidemic Kaposi's sarcoma, which primarily affects patients with AIDS. Approximately 15% of AIDS patients have it, which makes it 20,000 times more prevalent in the AIDS population than in the general population. First seen in 1981, this form can involve internal organs such as the lung, stomach, etc. People with epidemic Kaposi's sarcoma often die of complications resulting from their immunodeficiency rather than the cancer. The cause of Kaposi's sarcoma in AIDS patients appears to be infection with a separate virus in the herpes family.

Treatment for Kaposi's sarcoma depends on the type, the general state of health of the patient, and other factors. Indolent classic Kaposi's may not require immediate treatment. The traditional treatment for this disease is surgery to remove the lesions on the skin, ELECTRON BEAM THERAPY, and CHEMOTHERAPY. Several chemotherapeutic agents are active. HAART therapy to reduce viral load is considered first-line treatment in patients with HIV. BIOLOGICAL THERAPY is being investigated. For specific information on the latest state-of-the-art treatment, call the National Cancer Institute's Cancer Information Service at 1-800-4-CANCER (1-800-422-6237), or for a TTY: 1-800-332-8615.

See also SOFT TISSUE SARCOMA.

KCZ See KETOCONAZOLE.

keratosis (ker-ah-to'sis) a protruding overgrowth on the skin. Most are benign (noncancerous), but those caused by excessive sun exposure, known as actinic keratosis and solar keratosis, occasionally become cancerous.

ketoconazole (ke"to-kon'ah-zīl) [KCZ, Nizoral] an antifungal medication used to treat candida and other fungus infections that may infect patients with cancer and AIDS. It is taken by mouth.

kidney one of a matched pair of organs that regulate the composition of the body's internal fluids, manufacture urine, and excrete wastes. They lie in the small of the back on each side of the spine. The kidneys are essential to human life. Urine is drained from the kidneys to the bladder by the ureters.

kidney cancer [hypernephroma, renal cell carcinoma, Grawitz's tumor, renal adenocarcinoma] a fairly rare cancer of the lining of the tubules in the kidney through which urine passes. It accounts for about 2 to 3% of cancers in the United States. The American Cancer Society estimates there would be about 36,160 new cases of kidney cancer (22,490 in men and 13,670 in women) in the United States in the year 2005, and about 12,660 (8,020 men and 4,640 women) deaths from this disease. These statistics include both adults and children and include renal cell carcinomas and transitional cell carcinomas of the renal pelvis. Most people with this cancer are older. It is very uncommon under age 45, and its incidence is highest between the ages of 55 and 84. Kidney cancer typically. It affects twice as many males as females and is slightly more common in white men than black. It develops most frequently in men after the age of 65 and is more common in urban, industrial areas.

The causes of kidney cancer are not fully understood. It is known that smokers are twice as likely as nonsmokers to develop kidney cancer. Some researchers estimate that cigarette smoking is linked to 30% of kidney cancers in men and 24% in women. One researcher estimated that more than 80% of renal pelvis cancer in men and more than 60% in women would be prevented if people stopped smoking.

Another possible cause of kidney cancer is exposure to chemicals, both produced by the body and inhaled or digested. Because the kidneys filter waste, they are exposed to many chemical substances. Heavy, long-term use of the analgesic phenacetin is associated with renal pelvis cancer. The risk is 19 times greater for smokers who use phenacetin. The Food and Drug Administration banned phenacetin-containing products in 1983.

Occupational exposure is another possible cause. Some studies suggest that coke oven workers and insulation workers have an above-average rate of the disease. Reports show that workers in

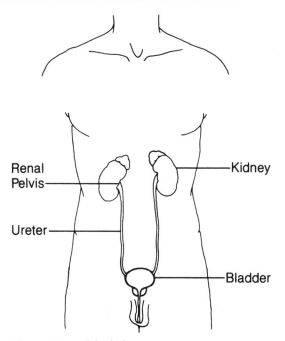

The position of the kidneys. Courtesy NCI.

the rubber, leather, petroleum, dye, textile, and plastics industries have an increased risk of kidney cancer.

There is also evidence that obesity may increase the risk of developing kidney cancer. Several studies show an increased risk among women, and at least one report says obese men may also be at risk.

Women treated with radiation therapy, particularly for problems in the uterus, are at a greater risk. Patients exposed to thorium dioxide, a radioactive substance used in the 1920s with certain X-RAYS (no longer used), have an increased rate of renal cell carcinoma.

Concerning familial cancers, there are several types of primary kidney cancer with different causes, different microscopic appearance (clear cell, papillary, etc), different courses, and different responses to therapy.

In the study of the hereditary forms, four main types have been identified. This has led to the finding of four kidney cancer genes. Teasing out the genetic cause of these may ultimately lead to a better

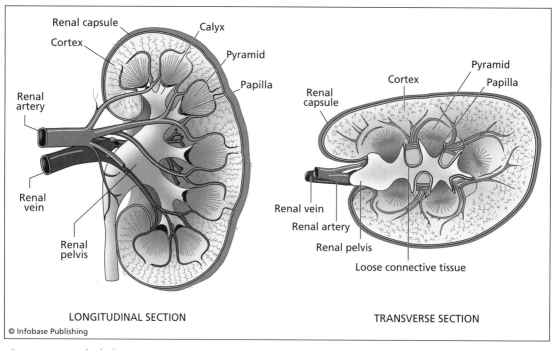

Cross section of a kidney.

understanding of the more common sporadic forms of kidney cancer.

One well-studied entity is clear cell carcinoma, associated with VON HIPPEL-LINDAU'S DISEASE (VHL). Affected individuals with VHL have a mutation of the VHL gene (a tumor suppressing gene on chromosome 3) which is the clear cell cancer gene, and the mutation causes the disease. People with a sporadic form of renal cell cancer have a mutation of this gene as well. Other inherited disorders include HEREDITARY PAPILLARY RENAL CELL CANCER and RENAL CELL CANCER ASSICIATED WITH BHD SYNDROME (BIRT-HOGG DUBÉ SYNDROME). Hopefully, disease-specific approaches to treatment based on targeting the genetic abnormalities will be available in the near future. TUBEROUS SCLEROSIS, STURGE-WEBER SYNDROME, NEUROFIBROMATOSIS, and ATAXIA TELANGIECTASIA put people at a greater risk for kidney tumors.

The most common type of kidney cancer is renal cell carcinoma, which arises in the lining of the renal tubules. About 85% of adult kidney cancers are this type. The next most common form of kidney cancer is TRANSITIONAL CELL CANCER OF THE RENAL PELVIS AND URETER, which resembles bladder cancer in many ways.

Among the symptoms that may be an indication of kidney cancer are pain on one side of the back, blood in the urine (hematuria), a mass in the flank or abdomen, high blood pressure, and fever. Occasionally patients with kidney cancer will have a loss of appetite, nausea and vomiting, constipation, weakness, and fatigue.

The diagnosis of kidney cancer can be difficult. Among the procedures that may be used in its diagnosis and evaluation are blood tests, IVP, ultrasound, URINALYSIS, SELECTIVE RENAL ARTERIOGRAPHY, CT SCAN, KIDNEY SCAN, and MRI. Although many tumors in the kidney are benign (noncancerous), sometimes surgery is necessary for a definitive diagnosis.

Following is the NATIONAL CANCER INSTITUTE'S (NCI) staging of kidney cancer:

- Stage I—cancer is confined to the kidney
- Stage II—cancer has spread into the fat surrounding the kidney, but has not spread beyond that to the capsule that contains the kidney
- Stage III—cancer has spread to the main blood vessel that carries clean blood from the kidney (renal vein) to the blood vessel that carries blood from the lower part of the body to the heart, or has spread to LYMPH NODES around the kidney.
- Stage IV—cancer has invaded surrounding organs such as the bowel or pancreas or has spread to distant sites such as the lungs, bones, opposite kidney, liver, or brain
- Recurrent—the cancer has returned after it was treated; it can return to the original area or occur in another part of the body

Treatment depends on the stage of the disease, the general state of health of the patient, and other factors. The treatments used for kidney cancer are surgery, CHEMOTHERAPY, RADIATION THERAPY, HORMONE THERAPY, ARTERIAL EMBOLIZATION, and BIOLOGICAL THERAPY. Surgery is the most common treatment for kidney cancer. There are four types of surgical procedures: a PARTIAL NEPHRECTOMY in which the cancer and part of the kidney around it are removed; a SIMPLE NEPHRECTOMY in which the entire kidney is removed; a RADICAL NEPHRECTOMY in which the kidney and the tissue around it are removed (some nearby lymph nodes may also be removed), and a BILATERAL NEPHRECTOMY in which both kidneys are removed. For specific information on the latest state-of-the-art treatment, by stage, call NCI's Cancer Information Service at 1-800-4-CANCER (1-800-422-6237), or for a TTY: 1-800-332-8615.

kidney scan [renal scan]   an examination of the structure of the kidneys after administration of a small, virtually harmless dose of a radioactive substance. A scanner starts taking pictures when the substance reaches the major arteries. Pictures are taken at about five-minute intervals for about half an hour. For additional information, if necessary, the pictures can be computer analyzed. It can be used to test for kidney function and possible kidney cancer. The kidney scan takes 30 to 45 minutes and can be done in a doctor's office or on an outpatient basis.

See also NUCLEAR SCAN.

killer cells [cytotoxic T cells]   one type of WHITE BLOOD CELL that can attack and destroy cells of a different type, such as cancer cells. Killer cells are also responsible for rejecting tissue, organ, and bone marrow transplants since they perceive the graft as foreign to the body. They are one type of T CELL.

See also NATURAL KILLER CELL and LAK CELLS.

Klinefelter's syndrome   a condition in which men have small testes and enlarged breasts and lack certain secondary sex characteristics, such as a low voice and beard growth. It is an inherited sex chromosome abnormality whereby the male has an extra "X" chromosome (XXY). This syndrome has been linked to TESTICULAR CANCER.

Kock pouch   See CONTINENT ILEAL RESERVOIR.

Krukenberg tumor   a cancer that originates in the stomach and spreads to an ovary, presenting as an ovarian mass.

KS   See KAPOSI'S SARCOMA.

KUB (kidneys, ureters, bladder)   See IVP.

Kupffer's cells (koop'ferz)   specialized MACROPHAGES that are found in the liver.

Kytril [granisetron hydrochloride]   an antiemetic drug to prevent or reduce nausea and vomiting. It is given by IV (injected into a vein).

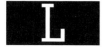

lacrimal gland tumor (lak′rĭ-mal) a swelling or growth in the lacrimal gland, the tear gland located in the upper outer quadrant of the eye socket. Less than 10% of the tumors found there are malignant (cancerous).

See also EYE CANCER.

lacrimation (lak′rĭ-ma′shun) a condition in which an excessive amount of tears are produced by the ducts. This may be an unpleasant side effect of CHEMOTHERAPY.

lactate dehydrogenase (LDH) (lak-tāt de-hi′dro-jen-ās) an enzyme found normally in the blood that is produced by many tissues, including the liver, red blood cells, and the brain. When it is found in the blood at higher-than-normal levels, it may be an indication of the presence of TESTICULAR CANCER, NON-HODGKIN′S LYMPHOMA, EWING′S SARCOMA, and some kinds of LEUKEMIA, and other cancers and may be considered a TUMOR MARKER. Above-normal levels of LDH may also be an indication of the recurrence of disease after treatment. LDH is found with increasing frequency as the disease progresses. In advanced testicular cancer, it has been found in as many as 68% of the cases. However, recurrence of disease may not be accompanied by elevated levels of LDH. Elevated levels of LDH may also be a sign of HEMOLYSIS of red blood cells.

Laetrile (la′ĕ-tril) a substance containing the poison cyanide, made from apricot pits, and touted as a cancer cure in the 1970s and 1980s.

Laetrile has been around for centuries. It was known as a poison in ancient Egypt, when the pharaohs' priests used it to execute their enemies. In 1840, it became a cancer "remedy" in France after a French country doctor reported that he had "cured" six patients with it, basing his conclusions on the fact that the six patients were still alive after two months of Laetrile. In 1980, cancer researchers conducted a study to determine whether Laetrile was effective against cancer and found that it killed just as many normal cells as cancer cell. After conducting a clinical study of Laetrile with patients, the National Cancer Institute concluded, in 1982, that Laetrile was ineffective as a cancer treatment and did not substantially improve symptoms in the patients studied. A year later, Laetrile was still a billion-dollar-a-year industry despite the multi-institution study that demonstrated that it was worthless.

See also UNCONVENTIONAL TREATMENT METHOD.

LAK (lymphokine-activated killer) cells cells in the immune system that have the potential to destroy cancer cells. They are generated when large doses of INTERLEUKIN-2 (IL-2) are injected into the patient's bloodstream. The IL-2 stimulates the production of lymphocytes (white blood cells that play a major role in the IMMUNE SYSTEM). The lymphocytes are then taken from the patient's blood and are bathed (exposed) to more IL-2, which causes them to reproduce at a faster rate than normal. They can be produced in great quantity. These stimulated cells, known as LAK cells, are then returned to the patient's bloodstream, where they have the potential of destroying cancer cells. Their possible usefulness is still being widely investigated.

See also IL-2/LAK.

laminar-air-flow unit (lam′ĭ-n ar) hospital rooms or other settings in which air is constantly circulated and filtered to remove any airborne particles. This is especially important for the protection of patients who are being treated with drugs that will suppress the IMMUNE SYSTEM, making them susceptible to infection. The laminar-air-flow unit protects the patient from contamination in the environment and from germs left by the people attending him or her. The created pattern of air flow sweeps infectious microbes away from the patient.

laminectomy (lam″ĭ-nek′to-me) a neurosurgical operation to remove a portion of bone from the spine to release compression on the delicate spinal cord. In cancer, as much of the tumor as possible is removed, but the main intent of the procedure is to remove pressure. Laminectomy may be performed from a posterior approach (the back, the traditional operation) or from the anterior (the front), which may be a more comprehensive undertaking.

laparoscope See LAPAROSCOPY.

laparoscopy (lap″ah-ros′ko-pe) [peritoneoscopy, celioscopy] examination of organs in the abdomen such as the uterus, ovaries, fallopian tubes, appendix, and liver with a laparoscope (a lighted tubular instrument) passed through a small incision in the abdominal wall. It is usually performed under general anesthesia in a hospital with the patient leaving on the same day. During the procedure, some tissue may be removed for a biopsy, a microscopic examination for cancer cells. Laparoscopy may be used as one of the procedures in the diagnosis of a number of different cancers, including ENDOMETRIAL CANCER, and ovarian, prostrate, and liver cancer as well as many other, noncancerous disorders. Many treatments and resections are now being done with a laparoscope as techniques and technology improve. A major advantage of this procedure is that it may eliminate the need for an exploratory LAPAROTOMY (abdominal surgery), and whenever possible, it is the procedure of choice. Indications and use of laparoscopic surgery are expanding rapidly with the popularity of the technique.

See also ENDOSCOPY. Large operations are now being done by laparoscopy.

laparotomy (lap-ah-rot′o-me) any surgical procedure in which the abdominal cavity is opened either to examine it (exploratory surgery) or to perform definitive surgery. Laparotomies may be performed in the diagnosis or treatment of HODGKIN'S DISEASE, OVARIAN CANCER, PANCREATIC CANCER, and other gastrointestinal cancers as well as other, noncancerous disorders.

See also EXPLORATORY LAPAROTOMY and SECOND LOOK SURGERY.

large bowel cancer See COLON/RECTAL CANCER.

large cell carcinoma See NON-SMALL CELL LUNG CANCER.

large cell lung cancer See NON-SMALL CELL LUNG CANCER.

large loop excision of the transformation zone See LEEP.

laryngeal cancer (lah-rin′je-al) [larynx cancer, cancer of the voice box] cancer of the larynx (voice box), one of the major HEAD AND NECK CANCER sites. The American Cancer Society estimated that in 2005, 9,880 men and women (7,920 men and 1,960 women) would be diagnosed with cancer of the larynx, with 3,770 deaths from the disease that year. There are three main sites where the cancer can occur:

- the glottis—the middle part of the larynx where the vocal cords are
- the supraglottis—the tissue above the glottis
- the subglottis—the tissue below the glottis.

Males over the age of 45 are more than four times as likely to be diagnosed with laryngeal cancer as women. People at the highest risk of developing laryngeal cancer are those who smoke and/or drink excessively. Symptoms appear early and may include a noticeable hoarseness, a lump in the throat, difficult or painful swallowing, pain in the throat, and shortness of breath.

Procedures used in the diagnosis and evaluation of laryngeal cancer may include direct examination and a biopsy of tissue removed through a LARYNGOSCOPY. Additional diagnostic procedures to determine the extent of the cancer may include LARYNGOGRAPHY (laryngeal tomography), chest X-RAYS, and CT SCAN.

Following is the NATIONAL CANCER INSTITUTE'S STAGING for laryngeal cancer:

- Stage I—tumor is confined to the site of origin with normal vocal cord mobility; there is no evidence of spread of the tumor to lymph nodes or to other parts of the body; the exact definition of Stage I depends on where the cancer started, as follows:
  — supraglottis—the cancer is only in one area of the supraglottis and vocal cord can move normally
  — glottis—the cancer is only in the vocal cords and the vocal cords can move normally
  — subglottis—the cancer has not spread outside the subglottis
- Stage II—the cancer is only in the larynx and has not spread to lymph nodes in the area or to other parts of the body
  — supraglottis—the cancer is in more than one area of the supraglottis, but the vocal cords can move normally
  — glottis—the cancer has spread to the supraglottis or the subglottis or both; the vocal cords may or may not be able to move normally
  — subglottis—the cancer has spread to the vocal cords, which may or may not be able to move normally
- Stage III—there are two ways in which the extent of the tumor is classified as stage III:
  — tumor is confined to the larynx and one or both vocal cords cannot move normally or
  — spread of the tumor to a single lymph node on the same side of the neck as the primary tumor, and the lymph node is three CENTIMETERS (cm) or less in its greatest dimension

- Stage IV—there are three ways in which the extent of disease can be classified as stage IV:
  — the cancer has spread to tissues around the larynx such as the pharynx or tissue in the neck; the lymph nodes in the area may or may not contain cancer or
  — there is one abnormal lymph node larger than 6 cm at its greatest dimension, or there are multiple abnormal nodes of any size on the same side of the neck as the primary tumor, or there is one abnormal node (or more) on the opposite side of the neck from the primary tumor or
  — there is evidence of spread to distant parts of the body
- Recurrent—cancer has returned to the original site or to another part of the body after treatment

Treatment depends on the stage of the disease, the general state of health of the patient, and other factors. The three types of treatment used are SURGERY, RADIATION THERAPY, and CHEMOTHERAPY. Surgery is a common treatment for laryngeal cancer. Following are the surgical procedures which may be used: CORDECTOMY, the removal of the vocal cord; SUPRAGLOTTIC LARYNGECTOMY, the removal of the supraglottis; PARTIAL LARYNGECTOMY or hemilaryngectomy, the removal of part of the larynx; and TOTAL LARYNGECTOMY, the removal of the entire larynx. LASER SURGERY is being investigated as a treatment for very early cancers of the larynx. For specific information on the latest state-of-the-art treatment, by stage, call NCI's Cancer Information Service at 1-800-4-CANCER (1-800-422-6237), or for a TTY: 1-800-332-8615.

laryngeal mirror (lah-rin′je-al)   a device used to examine the larynx (voice box). It resembles a dentist's mirror with a long handle. Doctors can see most tumors by using a laryngeal mirror.

laryngeal tomography   See LARYNGOGRAPHY.

laryngectomee (lar-in-jek′-to-me)   a term used to describe a person who has had his or her voice box removed via LARYNGECTOMY.

laryngectomy (lar-in-jek′to-me)   surgical removal of the larynx (voice box). A laryngectomy is one of the treatments for LARYNGEAL CANCER. In a partial laryngectomy, or hemilaryngectomy, only part of the voice box is removed. A tracheostomy (a hole in the front of the neck) is created for breathing.

laryngogram   See LARYNGOGRAPHY.

laryngography   (lar-rin-gog'rah-fe) [laryngeal tomography]   an X-RAY of the larynx (voice box) using a CONTRAST MEDIUM. A local anesthetic is used to enable the dye to be inserted into the larynx, after which the X-RAY is taken. The procedure takes about five to 10 minutes. A laryngography may be used, in addition to other tests, to evaluate the extent of LARYNGEAL CANCER.

laryngoscope   See LARYNGOSCOPY.

laryngoscopy   (lar-ring-gos'ko-pe) [larynx test]   an examination of the larynx (voice box). A laryngoscope (a hollow metal tube) is passed through the mouth into the throat to examine the voice box. Tissue samples may be removed for microscopic examination, a biopsy, for cancer cells. This procedure may be used in the diagnosis of LARYNGEAL CANCER.

larynx test   See LARYNGOSCOPY.

laser surgery   See LASER THERAPY.

laser therapy   (la'zer)   the use of extremely narrow, intense, and controlled light beams in the treatment of some forms of cancer. A laser beam can sever, fuse, or eliminate body tissue. Laser stands for light amplification by stimulated emission of radiation. The first working laser was developed in 1960. Lasers were first used medically in 1961 to treat a type of skin discoloration and to repair detached retinas.

Three kinds of lasers have gained wide use in medicine:

- carbon dioxide (CO_2)—used primarily in surgery; it can cut or vaporize tissue with relatively little bleeding as the light energy changes to heat
- argon—penetrates superficially and is useful in dermatology and eye surgery; used also with light-sensitive dye to treat tumors in PHOTODYNAMIC THERAPY
- neodymium:yttrium-aluminum-garnet (Nd:YAG) —can penetrate deeper into tissue than the other two lasers and cause blood to coagulate (clot) quickly; it can be carried through optical fibers to less accessible parts of the body

Lasers can be used in the diagnosis and treatment of cancer in a number of different ways. They may shrink or destroy a tumor with heat or activate a chemical that destroys tumor cells. Lasers can be used with endoscopes, flexible tubes that allow doctors to look into different parts of the body. They can be used with low-powered microscopes, giving physicians a clear view of the site being treated. They can also be used with a micromanipulator, which enables the doctor to make a cut that is less than the width of a very fine thread.

The ways lasers can be used in the treatment of a wide variety of different cancers include:

- removal of colon POLYPS that may become cancerous
- removal of tumors blocking the esophagus and colon
- removal of small tumors on the vocal cord
- treatment of in situ cancers of the cervix, vagina, and vulva
- treatment of cancers of the head and neck and respiratory system
- to control shrinkage of primary and secondary brain tumors
- breast cancer, which is becoming more common

Laser treatment has several advantages over traditional surgical treatment. It is more precise than a scalpel; the heat produced by the laser sterilizes the surgery site; there is less chance of infection; less operating time may be required; healing time is frequently reduced; there is less bleeding, swelling, and scarring; and more procedures can be done on an outpatient basis. The major disadvantages associated with laser treatment are the relatively small number of surgeons trained to use a laser, the high cost of the equipment, and the fact that strict safety precautions must be observed when using lasers.

New and better ways of using lasers in the treatment of cancer are being explored. As more doctors become trained in using lasers and the technology improves, lasers may play a larger role in the treatment of cancer.

L-asparaginase (el   as-par′ah-jin-ās) [asparaginase, Elspar] an anticancer drug typically used for acute lymphoblastic leukemia (ALL) and LYMPHOMA. It is given by IV (injection into a vein). Common side effects may include nausea, vomiting, swelling and burning of veins, fever, allergic response, abdominal pain, diabetes, and chills. Occasional or rare side effects may include liver damage, pancreatitis, drowsiness, weight loss, depression, clotting problems, seizures, and flu-like symptoms.

late intensification therapy the treatment with high dose chemotherapy of ALL patients who have been in REMISSION for six months or a year. The drugs that are used are different from those used during INDUCTION THERAPY and CONSOLIDATION THERAPY.

latissimus dorsi reconstruction (lah tis′ĭ-mus dor′si) a technique used in BREAST RECONSTRUCTION when there is little skin or muscle at the mastectomy site. Skin, muscle, and other tissue is transferred from the woman's back to the chest, where the breast is reconstructed. To create a new muscle on the chest a road, flat muscle from the back—the latissimus dorsi—is used.

LCIS See LOBULAR BREAST CARCINOMA IN SITU.

LDH See LACTATE DEHYDROGENASE.

LEEP (LOOP electrosurgical excision procedure) [LOOP diathermy, large loop excision of the transformation zone (LLETZ)] a surgical procedure used in the treatment of CERVICAL INTRAEPITHELIAL NEOPLASIA (abnormal, precancerous tissue in the cervix). After the cervix is anesthetized (numbed), an electrical wire loop is inserted into the vagina and all the precancerous tissue is sliced off and removed. It is then sent to a PATHOLOGIST for further analysis. This is a relatively new technique which is thought may be better than the traditional methods currently being used: CONIZATION, CRYOSURGERY, and LASER THERAPY. Studies have shown that when

LEEP is performed there is a greater likelihood of finding and removing all of the abnormal and/or cancerous cells. It is also a less costly procedure, can be done in a doctor's office, has a shorter recovery time and fewer complications.

leiomyoma (li-o-mi-o′-mah) a benign (noncancerous) tumor that develops in the smooth muscle tissue (muscles that control organs). This can occur in the stomach, uterus and other sites.
See also FIBROID TUMOR.

leiomyosarcoma (li-o-mi-o-sar-ko′mah) a cancer originating in the smooth muscle (muscles that control organs)—most often in the uterus and back part of the abdominal cavity (retroperitoneum). It can also arise in the walls of the blood vessels. It is a very rare cancer.
See also SOFT TISSUE SARCOMA.

Lenalidomide [Revlimed, Actimed] an analog of THALIDOMIDE that is more potent and that is less sedating, with no apparent teratogenicity (cause of fetal malformations). It is being evaluated primarily in the treatment of refractory MYELOMA and MDS (myelodysplastic syndrome, 2005).

lentigo maligna melanoma See MELANOMA.

leptomeningeal carcinoma (lep-to-mĕ-nin′je-al kar″sĭ-no′mah) cancer that has metastasized (spread) from another part of the body to the leptomeninges, the tissue lining the spinal canal (the meninges). Many cancers can metastasize to the leptomeninges, the most common being lymphoma and breast and lung cancer.

Solid tumors that may spread to the leptomeninges include breast cancer, SMALL CELL LUNG CANCER, melanoma, genitourinary cancer (of the genitals and urinary tract), HEAD AND NECK CANCER (usually by direct extension), and ADENOCARCINOMA of unknown primary. Lymphomas and leukemia can also metastasize to the leptomeninges. Signs that the cancer has spread include headache, mental change, uncoordinated movement, (cranial nerve palsies, facial distortions), and nausea and vomiting. There may also be seizures.

Procedures used in the diagnosis of leptomeningeal metastases may include a CT SCAN, MRI, and lumbar puncture (SPINAL TAP). Multiple lumbar punctures may be required to isolate malignant (cancerous) cells for a definitive diagnosis. Treatment for solid tumors and leukemia may be INTRATHECAL CHEMOTHERAPY, intraventrical chemotherapy, and RADIATION THERAPY. Treatment for lymphomas may be intrathecal chemotherapy and radiation therapy.

For the latest state-of-the-art treatment, call the National Cancer Institute's Cancer Information Service at 1-800-4-CANCER (1-800-422-6237), or for a TTY: 1-800-332-8615.

leptomeningeal metastasis   spread of malignant cells to the lining of the brain and spinal canal. Malignant cells floating in the spinal fluid and able to anchor and grow are responsible for the neurologic symptoms. The most common cancers doing this are LEUKEMIA, LYMPHOMA and cancers of the breast and lung, and MELANOMA. It is treated with either RADIATION or CHEMOTHERAPY injected into the spinal fluid. The drugs most commonly used are methotrexate, THIOtePa, and cytarabine. Systemic chemotherapy may also be used.

lesion (le′zhun)   any localized abnormal change in the structure of part of an organ or tissue as the result of an injury or disease. Although lesions can be benign (noncancerous) or malignant (cancerous). It is often a euphemism for "cancer."

letrozole   See FEMARA.

leucovorin calcium (lu″-ko-vor′in)   a form of the vitamin B folate (calcium leucovorin). Although by itself it has no anticancer effect, when given *before* the anticancer drug 5-FU it enhances 5-FU's activity within the cancer cell. It is also commonly given *after* methotrexate as a "rescue" from that drug's side effects.

See also LEUCOVORIN RESCUE and HIGH-DOSE METHOTREXATE WITH LEUCOVORIN RESCUE.

leucovorin rescue (lu″-ko-vor′in)   the use of the drug leucovorin calcium to counteract the life-threatening side effects of very high doses of the anticancer drug METHOTREXATE. Leucovorin is given in order to protect or "rescue" the patient after the deliverance of massive doses of methotrexate. It appears that the normal cells are more easily res-

cued, or saved, from the effects of the chemotherapy than the cancer cells. Leucovorin rescue is an important treatment in cancer.

See also HIGH-DOSE METHOTREXATE WITH LEUCOVORIN RESCUE.

leukapheresis (lu-kah-fĕ-re′sis) [leukopheresis]   a technique of harvesting GRANULOCYTES from donor whole blood. Granulocytes or leukocytes may then be transfused to patients undergoing intensive chemotherapy, which can lower the white blood count and make the patient more susceptible to infections. Leukapheresis can also be used to remove life-threatening white cells from a leukemia patient with LEUKOSTASIS. At excessively high levels, early leukemic cells may cause sludging and clotting in the small blood vessels. The patient's blood is drawn, a pint at a time, is separated into its components, and a large percentage of the white blood cells are removed until the white blood count is at a level that is not harmful to the patient.

leukemia   Rather than cancer "of the blood," as is commonly thought, leukemia is a cancer of the organs that make the blood: the BONE MARROW and LYMPH SYSTEM. Red and white blood cells, platelets, and lymph cells originate in the bone marrow and lymph system, where they "mature" before entering the bloodstream. While the same process takes place in a person with leukemia, the number of cells produced are abnormal, the rate at which they are produced, and their ability to function are altered.

The term *leukemia* comes from the Greek and means "white blood." An overabundance of abnormal white blood cells in the bloodstream can infiltrate vital organs and glands, causing them to enlarge and/or malfunction; or they can crowd out healthy cells and prevent the bone marrow from producing sufficient levels of normally functioning red, white, and clotting cells platelets.

Leukemia accounts for about 5% of all cancer cases in the United States. The American Cancer Society estimated that 34,810 men and women (19,640 men and 15,170 women) would be diagnosed with leukemia in 2005, with 22,570 deaths from the disease in that year.

Leukemia is the most common childhood cancer in the United States. The most common type of leukemia occurring in children is acute lymphocytic leukemia (ALL), accounting for 45%; it is most likely to occur in children aged six and younger. The second most common leukemia in children is acute nonlymphocytic leukemia (ANLL). However, leukemia is far more common in older adults. More than half of all leukemias occur in people over 60 years of age. Men are affected by leukemia about 30% more often than women. It occurs slightly more often in whites than blacks, and Jewish people have a slightly higher incidence than other whites.

About half the newly diagnosed leukemias are acute (immature cells still involved in the growth process are affected and the disease progresses rapidly), and half are chronic (cells in a more advanced stage of development are affected and the disease progresses slowly). Chronic leukemia can become acute in some circumstances.

The causes of leukemia are not fully understood, but mutations of a gene is the unifying concept. There are factors that are known to increase the risk of developing leukemia. There is evidence that radiation can induce leukemia; the greater the exposure, the higher the risk. There can be a delay of up to 20 years before leukemia develops in a person who has been exposed to excessive radiation. In Japan, among the people who survived the largest radiation doses from the atomic bombs, only one in 40 developed leukemia, which illustrates that susceptibility to radiation-induced leukemia varies from person to person. Since the potential hazard of excess exposure to X-RAYS has become widely known, exposure to it has declined.

Studies of families and twins with leukemia have shown a higher incidence than in the general population. It has also been found that leukemia occurs more often with certain congenital (present at birth) defects more often than can be attributed to chance. The role that viruses might play in the development of leukemia is still being investigated. In the middle 1980s, HTLV-1, a human T cell leukemia virus, was isolated and described by researchers at the National Cancer Institute. It is estimated that only one in every 80 people infected with HTLV-1 actually develops leukemia, and it appears that the virus can only be spread by prolonged, intimate contact.

Long-term exposure to certain chemicals like benzene, found in petroleum and coal-tar distil-lates, and some drugs have also been linked to leukemia. Some anticancer drugs are believed to be carcinogenic as well. For example, ALKYLATING agents have been associated with the later development of acute leukemia in some patients treated for Hodgkin's disease or ovarian cancer. People who have been treated with alkylating agents face a slightly higher risk of eventually developing leukemia (see TREATMENT-RELATED LEUKEMIA).

Four major types of leukemia and their subtypes are:

- lymphoproliferative disorders
  — chronic lymphocytic leukemia (CLL), which is also referred to as chronic lymphatic leukemia, chronic lymphogenous leukemia, or chronic lymphoid leukemia
  — HAIRY CELL LEUKEMIA (HCL)
  — PROLYMPHOCYTIC LEUKEMIA (PLL)
  — WALDENSTROM'S MACROGLOBULINEMIA
- chronic myelogenous leukemia (CML), which is also referred to as chronic myelocytic leukemia, chronic myelosis leukemia, or chronic myeloid leukemia
- acute lymphocytic leukemia (ALL), also referred to as acute lymphatic leukemia, acute lymphoblastic leukemia, or acute lymphogenous leukemia
- acute nonlymphocytic leukemia (ANLL), which encompasses a number of different types including:
  — acute myelogenous leukemia (AML), also known as acute myelocytic leukemia, acute myeloblastic leukemia, or acute granulocytic leukemia
  — acute monocytic leukemia
  — acute promyelocytic leukemia
  — acute erythroleukemia
  — acute myelomonocytic leukemia

The general symptoms of leukemia may include fever and flu-like symptoms; enlarged LYMPH NODES, spleen, and liver; bone pain, joint pain, paleness; weakness; tendency to bleed or bruise easily; and frequent infections.

The symptoms for CLL can be a general feeling of ill health, fatigue, lack of energy, fever, loss of appetite and weight, or night sweats. It is not uncommon for there to be no symptoms with the disease discovered during a routine examination, or an exam for some other complaint. The symptoms for CML may include fatigue, weight loss, or a sense of fullness or heaviness under the left ribs. The symptoms of ALL and ANLL are varied and can progress rapidly. The lymph nodes, spleen, and liver may be enlarged. There can be bone pain, paleness, tendency to bleed or bruise easily, and frequent infections.

Procedures used in the diagnosis and evaluation of leukemia may include blood tests, bone marrow biopsy, and spinal test. Leukemia can only be definitively diagnosed by microscopic examination of the blood and bone marrow. For staging and treatment information, see the four major types of leukemia—ALL, ANLL, CLL, and CML.

leukemic cells   See BLAST CELLS.

leukemic reticuloendotheliosis   See HAIRY CELL LEUKEMIA.

Leukeran (lu'ker-an) [chlorambucil] an ALKYLATING anticancer drug. It is now infrequently used in treatment of cancers of the breast, ovary, and testis, chronic lymphocytic leukemia (CLL), LYMPHOMAS, and CHORIOCARCINOMA. It is taken by mouth. Side effects may include fever, chills, sore throat, mouth and lip sores, unusual bleeding or bruising, side or stomach pain, joint pain, skin rash, swelling of feet or lower legs, convulsions, shortness of breath, and yellowing of eyes and skin. It is listed by the United States National Toxicology Program as being a known CARCINOGEN.

Leukerin   See 6-MP.

leukine   See GM-CSF.

leukocytes   See WHITE BLOOD CELLS.

leukopenia (lu″ko-pe′ne-ah)   a condition characterized by too few white blood cells. This may be a primary condition, a result of an illness (lymphoma or leukemia), or a consequence of cancer treatment.

leukopheresis   See LEUKAPHERESIS.

leukoplakia (lu″ko-pla′ke-ah)   a white, thickened patch that can appear in mucous membranes, such as in the mouth, lip, or tongue, the vulva, and the anal region. Cancer may develop in some of the whitened areas. When leukoplakia occurs in the mouth it is commonly associated with an injury to the mucous membranes and excessive use of tobacco, alcohol, and spicy food condiments. It may also appear in an area repeatedly injured by the sharp, projecting edge of a tooth. It is estimated that 5% of leukoplakia in the mouth eventually becomes cancerous.

leukostasis (lu″ko-sta′sis)   a clumping of immature blood cells in a patient who has LEUKEMIA. This can happen when the white blood cell count is 300,000 or higher, or 30 to 50 times normal. It is dangerous because it can cause heart attacks and strokes by blocking the arteries as well as smaller vessels (e.g. the retina). An urgent treatment is leukapheresis.

LEUP   See LUPRON.

leuprolide   See LUPRON.

Leustatin [cladribine, chlorodeoxyadenosine, 2CdA]   an anticancer drug used in the treatment of hairy cell leukemia (HCL). It can result in long remissions. Its primary and major possible side effect in immunosupression. It is given continuously by IV (injected into a vein) for seven days.

LEV   See LEVAMISOLE.

levamisole (lĕ-vam′ĭ-sol) [LEV, Ergamisol]   a drug once used in combination with 5-FU as ADJUVANT THERAPY for colon cancer. Its function as a cancer agent is thought to be due to stimulation or augmentation of the body's IMMUNE SYSTEM. Levamisole has been used as a treatment for intestinal worms in pets and people since the early 1970s. It is taken by mouth. Its side effects may include mild nausea, vomiting and diarrhea, skin rashes, and infrequent and temporary bone marrow damage, but as of 2005, it is used infrequently.

Levo-Dromoran [levorphanol]   a NARCOTIC drug used for the relief or control of pain. It is given by injection into a muscle or taken orally. It is available by prescription only.

levorphanol   See LEVO-DROMORAN.

LFS   See LI-FRAUMENI SYNDROME.

LHRH   See LUTEINIZING HORMONE-RELEASING HORMONE.

LHRH agonist leuprolide   See LUPRON.

lienography (li″ĕ-nog′rah-fe)   an X-RAY that outlines the spleen after an injection of a CONTRAST MEDIUM.

Li-Fraumeni syndrome (LFS)   a hereditary cancer predisposition syndrome originally defined in 1969. It was described as the association of rare pediatric sarcomas with early onset cancer in their parents. This is now associated with mutation of the P53 GENE.

light scanning   See TRANSILLUMINATION.

limb perfusion   See ISOLATION PERFUSION.

limb-sparing surgery   a surgical technique used in bone sarcomas to avoid amputation. This can be done with all spindle-cell sarcomas and can be used with as many as 80% of the patients with OSTEOSARCOMA.

Limb sparing surgery is done in three phases:

- the tumor is removed along with a margin of healthy tissue
- the limb is reconstructed using a PROSTHESIS or bone graft
- soft tissue and muscle transfers are made to cover and close the site and restore motor power.

Much progress has been made in limb salvage techniques. New knee prostheses allow some rotation, flexion, and extension. Efforts are under way to make a permanent prosthesis. Most of the devices can be custom made within a few weeks. To eliminate even that delay, modular systems that can be assembled in the operating room are now being developed and evaluated.

Linac   See LINEAR ACCELERATOR.

linear accelerator [megavoltage (MeV) linear accelerator, Linac]   a type of X-RAY machine used for EXTERNAL BEAM RADIATION THERAPY that employs high-energy beams. The linear accelerator can deliver high doses of radiation to deep-lying tumors. It administers a precise, intense beam directed to a particular site within the body where the cancer is located. This has the advantage of limiting, as much as possible, radiation damage to other parts of the body and to the skin. For that reason, it is now widely used and in most instances has replaced the cobalt machine used in COBALT TREATMENT for external radiation. See RADIATION THERAPY.

lip cancer   the presence of cancer cells in the lip. In 1992 there were approximately 3,600 new cases of lip cancer diagnosed in the United States and about 100 deaths. It occurs primarily on the lower lip of men over 40. Studies have indicated that smoking is a major cause of lip cancer. Chapping of the lips and sunburns are other factors thought to be related to the development of lip cancer. For diagnostic procedures, staging, and treatment see MOUTH CANCER.

liposarcoma (lip″o-sar-ko′mah)   cancer tumors that develop in fatty tissue, most often in the thigh. They are usually found in middle-aged men.
See also SOFT-TISSUE SARCOMA.

liposomal daunorubicin [DaunoXome]   a liposome encapsulated form of daunorubicin used in the treatment of advanced AIDS-related KAPOSI'S SARCOMA. It is given by IV (injected into a vein).

liposome   a fat globule matrix (inert) to which an active agent is physically attached (for example doxorubicin) to target delivery preferentially to tumor cells. It is a pharmaceutical effort to increase drug delivery for which there is evidence of efficacy. The final product may be more effect than the drug alone and may have slightly different side effects.

liver   an organ in the body that performs many functions, including digestion (converting food into energy), production of certain blood proteins, and elimination of many of the body's waste products. It is one of the largest organs in the body, located in the upper right side of the abdomen. The liver is essential to human life.

liver cancer/adult [hepatocellular carcinoma] a primary cancer that arises in the liver, as opposed to cancer that spreads to the liver from other parts of the body, known as LIVER METASTASES, which is quite common. Primary liver cancer is a relatively uncommon cancer in the United States, although in some parts of the world, such as developing countries in Africa and in East Asia, it is the most common cancer. The American Cancer Society estimated that 17,550 new cases (12,130 in men and 5,420 in women) of primary liver cancer and intrahepatic bile duct cancer would be diagnosed in the United States during 2005, with about 15,420 deaths from the disease (10,330 men and 5,090 women) in the United States during 2005. In contrast to many other cancers, the number of people who develop liver cancer had been increasing up to five years ago. This is no longer true, and the number of cases appears to be decreasing. As the statistics indicate, liver cancer occurs more frequently in men than in women.

The most common type of primary liver cancer is hepatocellular carcinoma, which arises in the liver cells. About 90% of the liver cancers in the United States are hepatocellular carcinoma. About 7% of the liver cancers start in the bile ducts of the liver (COLANGIOCARCINOMA). The rest are ANGIOSARCOMAS.

A number of factors have been identified that put people at a greater risk of developing primary liver cancer. People who have cirrhosis of the liver, either from alcoholism or other diseases, such as hepatitis B (a viral infection of the liver), are 40 times more likely to develop liver cancer. In addition, a number of environmental toxins are associated with liver cancer, including aflaxtoxin (derived from some molds), azo compounds (nitrogen compounds), and

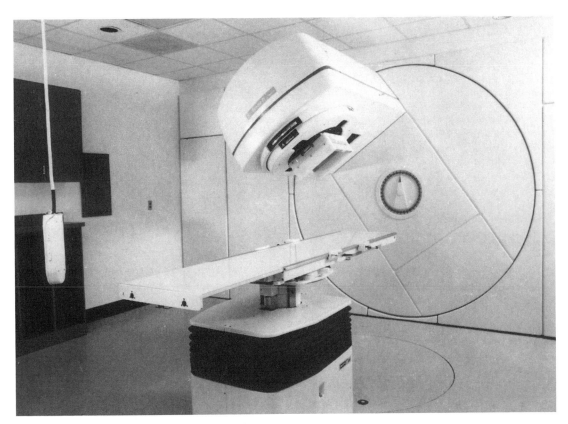

The "Saturne 41" medium-energy linear accelerator. Courtesy GE Medical Systems.

thorotrast (a CONTRAST MEDIUM that had been used in some X-ray exams and is no longer used.) Polyvinylchlorides (PVCs) have been linked with angiosarcomas.

Symptoms of liver cancer do not generally appear in its early stages. When symptoms do appear, they may include weight loss, malaise, loss of appetite, abdominal swelling, and pain. Other symptoms that may develop include jaundice (a yellow tinge to the skin), fever, and ascites (a buildup of fluid in the abdominal cavity). Sometimes liver cancer is diagnosed after it has metastasized (spread) to another part of the body. For example, if the cancer has gone to the bone, pain in the bone may eventually lead to a diagnosis of cancer that started in the liver.

Procedures that may be used in the diagnosis and evaluation of liver cancer may include liver function tests, a blood test for ALPHA-FETOPROTEIN, a LIVER SCAN, ANGIOGRAPHY, LAPAROSCOPY, BONE SCAN, X-RAYS, CT SCAN, and ULTRASOUND. A CORE NEEDLE BIOPSY is sometimes used for a definitive diagnosis. However, a potential bleeding problem may rule that out and require, instead, exploratory surgery.

Following is the National Cancer Institute's (NCI) staging for adult liver cancer:

- Localized resectable—cancer appears to be confined to a portion of the liver; complete surgical removal of the tumor may be possible
- Localized unresectable—cancer appears to be confined to the liver, but it is not possible to remove the entire tumor
- Advanced—the tumor has spread through much of the liver and/or to other parts of the body
- Recurrent—cancer has returned to the original site or to another part of the body after treatment.

Treatment depends on the stage of the disease, the general state of health of the patient, and other factors. Treatment for liver cancer includes surgery (removal of the part of the liver where the cancer has been found), RADIATION THERAPY, CHEMOTHERAPY, CHEMOEMBOLIZATION, and LIVER TRANSPLANT. HYPOTHERMIA and BIOLOGICAL THERAPY are being investigated. For specific information on the latest state-of-the-art treatment, by stage, call NCI's Cancer Information Service at 1-800-4-CANCER (1-800-422-6237), or for a TTY: 1-800-332-8615.

liver cancer/childhood   a rare cancer that arises in the liver in both infants and children. There are two types: hepatoblastoma, which is most common in children under the age of three and rarely seen in children over the age of six, and hepatocellular carcinoma, which occurs most often in male children between the ages of 10 and 12. It is much more common in adults.

Following is the National Cancer Institute's (NCI) staging for childhood liver cancer:

- Group I—the tumor can be completely removed by surgery
- Group II—the tumor can be completely removed by surgery after RADIATION THERAPY and CHEMOTHERAPY
- Group IIB—any tumor left in the liver after surgery is confined to one lobe of the liver
- Group III—both lobes of the liver are involved
- Group IV—the cancer has spread to other areas of the body, regardless of the extent of liver involvement
- Recurrent—the cancer has returned to the original site or to another part of the body after treatment.

Treatment depends primarily on the stage of the disease. The treatments for liver cancer include surgery, radiation therapy, and chemotherapy. For specific information on the latest state-of-the-art treatment, by stage, call NCI's Cancer Information Service at 1-800-4-CANCER (1-800-422-6237), or for a TTY: 1-800-332-8615. Much of the information for adult liver cancer applies also to childhood liver cancer.

See also LIVER CANCER/ADULT.

liver metastases (mě-tas′tah-sēz)   a secondary cancer that has spread to the liver from some other sites most commonly the colon, stomach, breast, lung, or pancreas. The liver is a common site of metastatic disease. An enlarged or tender liver in a patient at HIGH RISK, in which cancer commonly metastasizes to the liver, is an indication that there may be metastases in the liver. Diagnostic procedures include a physical examination, LIVER SCAN, ULTRASOUND, CT SCAN, and ALKALINE PHOSPHATASE TEST.

Treatment and biopsy of liver metastases depends on a number of factors, including the number of metastases, their location in the liver, and the primary site of the cancer. The chances for long-term survival are greatest when the entire tumor can be surgically removed CHEMOTHERAPY is also used. For specific information on the latest state-of-the-art treatment by primary site, call the National Cancer Institute's Cancer Information Service at 1-800-4-CANCER (1-800-422-6237), or for a TTY: 1-800-332-8615.

See also LIVER CANCER.

liver scan an examination of the structure and function of the liver after the administration of a small amount of a RADIOACTIVE substance. The normal tissue absorbs the substance, and abnormalities are highlighted. An abnormal liver scan can be a result of cancer as well as other disorders, such as cirrhosis of the liver. A liver scan is commonly used in the diagnosis of LIVER CANCER and LIVER METASTASES.

See also NUCLEAR SCAN.

liver transplant replacing the diseased liver with a healthy liver donated by someone else. Very few patients with liver cancer are eligible for this treatment.

living will a signed document that describes under what conditions a person wants life-sustaining equipment to be used. It is a flexible document and can spell out exactly which types of treatment would not be acceptable, such as cardiopulmonary resuscitation, ventilation (use of a respirator), and intubation (inserting a tube for breathing). A living will can also designate another person as a proxy to make medical decisions for the patient in the event that the patient is unable to make his or her treatment wishes known.

Since 1977, most states have passed some kind of legislation making a living will a legally binding document. The living will has been upheld in court and is accepted by many doctors and hospitals. Although not all states require that aliving will be notarized, notarization is further proof of the person's seriousness of intent. See "Concern for the Dying" in Appendix I.

LLETZ See LEEP.

lobe a well-defined portion of a body organ, especially of the brain, breast, liver, and lung.

Cancer can develop in a lobe, such as lobular breast carcinoma.

lobectomy (lo-bek'to-me) surgical removal of a lobe of any organ or gland in the body. In cancer, a lobectomy may be performed in the treatment of such cancers as lung, thyroid, and liver.

lobular breast carcinoma in situ (LCIS) (lob'u-lar kar"sĭ-no'mah) [lobular neoplasia] a type of BREAST CANCER in which tiny cancers are confined to the lobules of the breast and have not invaded adjacent tissue. When diagnosed it can be found in one or both breasts. The cancer may never become invasive, and life threatening, but in some cases it may develop into, or be associated with, either infiltrating (invasive) lobular or ductal carcinoma. There is no way to determine which cancers will become invasive and which will remain noninfiltrating. Diagnosis of this type of breast cancer can be difficult; it can neither be felt nor identified by mammogram, and its treatment is controversial, with strategies evolving.

lobular neoplasia See LOBULAR BREAST CARCINOMA IN SITU.

local anesthesia (an-es-the'ze-ah) ANESTHESIA that is administered and confined to one part of the body. The anesthesia blocks the sensation of pain in a specific location on the body. A "local" is given for many minor surgical procedures, particularly those that can be done on an outpatient basis.

local recurrence the return of cancer to the original site in which it occurred after it has been treated. In a local recurrence, there are no signs of cancer in nearby LYMPH NODES or tissue. Cancer that has recurred locally generally has the best prognosis (outlook). Cancer can also undergo a REGIONAL RECURRENCE (in nearby lymph nodes or tissue) and METASTASIZE (appear in other parts of the body). A local recurrence of cancer may be treated by additional surgery or other treatments such as CHEMOTHERAPY (anticancer drugs), RADIATION THERAPY, and BIOLOGICAL THERAPY. The prognosis depends on a number of factors, including the type of cancer, the likelihood of successful surgery, etc. For the latest state-of-the-art treatment for recurrent cancer, call the National Cancer Institute's Cancer Information Service at 1-800-4-CANCER (1-800-422-6237), or for a TTY: 1-800-332-8615.

local wide excision surgical removal of the malignant (cancerous) tumor with a layer of the healthy tissue surrounding it. Although a LUMPEC-TOMY may be referred to as a local wide excision, this procedure may be performed in the treatment of a number of different cancers.

localized cancer cancer that is confined to the site where it originated with no sign that it has METASTASIZED.

localized radiation RADIATION THERAPY that is directed to one specific site.

lomustine   See CCNU.

LOOP diathermy   See LEEP.

LOOP electrosurgical excision procedure   See LEEP.

lower gastrointestinal series   See LOWER GI SERIES.

lower GI (gastrointestinal) series [barium enema] an examination of the colon (the lower part of the intestines) by X-RAY after administration of the CON-TRAST MEDIUM barium to the patient. Before the procedure is started, the bowel must be completely empty. Any substance remaining in the bowel, no matter how small, can distort the finding. The barium is inserted, via catheter, into the rectum and colon, and the X-rays are taken. Additional pictures are taken when the barium has been expelled by the patient. In some cases, air may be carefully injected into the colon in order to take an AIR-CONTRAST X-RAY as well, which can show POLYPS. The lower GI series can be done at a doctor's office or on an out-patient basis at the hospital. The procedure has a minimal risk but can be quite uncomfortable and tiring. It takes about an hour. A lower GI series may be performed in the diagnosis of COLON CANCER and many other disorders.

low-grade lymphoma   See NODULAR POORLY DIF-FERENTIATED LYMPHOMA.
See also NON-HODGKIN'S LYMPHOMA.

L.P. (lumbar puncture)   See SPINAL TAP.

L-PAM   See ALKERAN.

L-phenylalanine mustard   See ALKERAN.

L-Sarcolysin   See ALKERAN.

Lukes and Collins' lymphoma classification a method of describing NON-HODGKIN'S LYMPHOMA. It was proposed in 1974 and is based on the immunologic characteristics of lymphoid cells.

lumbar puncture (L.P.)   See SPINAL TAP.

lumpectomy (lum-pek'to-me) [excisional biopsy, breast conservation, wedge resection, local wide excision, partial mastectomy, quadrantectomy, quadrant excision, hemimastectomy, tylectomy] removal of a cancerous lump and the tissue surrounding it in the breast. The lumpectomy was first used in the treatment of breast cancer in Finland in the 1930s. The researcher showed that the survival rate for women undergoing RADICAL MASTECTOMY and women undergoing lumpectomy with radiation produced just about the same results if the tumor in the breast was two CENTIMETERS (cm) (about three-fourths of an inch) or less in diameter. In 1976 the National Cancer Institute undertook a 10-year study comparing lumpectomy with mastectomy in more than 1,800 women whose tumors were under 4 cm. The study found no significant differences in survival rates. And in 1990 a federal advisory panel concluded that a lumpectomy with radiation and a mastectomy achieves the same results in treating early-stage breast cancer.

Not all women are candidates for a lumpectomy. Among those who might benefit from other treatment, such as a mastectomy, are those women who have small breasts; or have a lump that adheres to the skin or underlying muscle, a lump that is very large, or more than one cancerous lump or area in the breast; or are too ill to have the radiation therapy following a lumpectomy. The absolute need for radiation following lumpectomy is being reevaluated.

See also MASTECTOMY.

lumpy breasts   See FIBROCYSTIC CHANGES.

lung   a cone-shaped organ in the chest composed of soft, pinkish gray, spongy tissue. The lungs are part of the respiratory system. They are located in the chest cavity on either side of the MEDIASTINUM containing the heart, windpipe, esophagus, thymus gland, and LYMPH NODES.

lung cancer   a disease in which a primary cancer develops in the tissues of the lungs; the lung tissue takes in oxygen and releases CO_2. Lung cancer was first described by doctors in the mid-1800s. At the turn of the century, it was still considered a rarity; that has changed dramatically. What has not changed is the difficulty in detecting lung cancer in its earliest stage when it has the greatest chance of being successfully treated. Lung cancer is the leading cause of death from cancer among both men and women; more people die of lung cancer than of colon, breast, and prostate cancers combined. Lung cancer is fairly rare in people under the age of 40.

The average age of people found to have lung cancer is 70.

The American Cancer Society estimated there would be about 172,570 new cases of lung cancer in the United States in 2005: 93,010 among men and 79,560 among women, with some 163,510 deaths from the disease: 90,490 men and 73,020 women in 2005.

People at the greatest risk of getting lung cancer are

- men over 60
- people who have smoked one or more packs of cigarettes a day for 20 years or longer
- people who began to smoke before age 20 and are still smoking
- workers in an industrial plant with a high-risk material (such as asbestos) who also smoke
- people who have a persistent or violent smokers cough

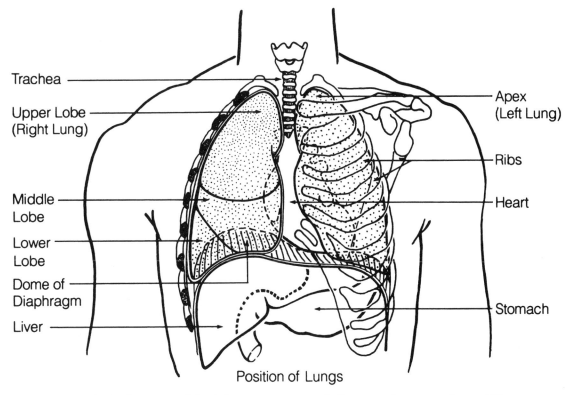

Lung cancer is the leading cause of death from cancer among both men and women.   Courtesy NCI.

- people who do not smoke, but are exposed to PASSIVE SMOKE.

Workers exposed to CARCINOGENS who smoke face an even greater chance of developing lung cancer.

Numerous studies all over the world have shown a link between cigarette SMOKING and lung cancer (as well as other cancers), with an increase in cigarette smoking followed by an increase in lung cancer. RADON, a naturally occurring radioactive gas, is also considered to be a cause of lung cancer. In 1991 the Environmental Protection Agency estimated that 16,000 Americans would die of lung cancer caused by radon. Again, people who smoke are at a much higher risk when exposed to radon than are nonsmokers. ASBESTOS, a group of naturally occurring mineral fibers used in many products, is also considered to be a cause of lung cancer. Workers

exposed to asbestos are at a greater risk of developing lung cancer. The risk is multiplied in smokers.

Other possible causes of lung cancer include exposure to the chemicals bischloromethyl ether (BCME) and chloromethyl methyl ether (CMME). Studies in the United States, Germany, and Japan have confirmed a high incidence of lung cancer among workers exposed to these chemicals. Studies of copper smelter workers exposed to arsenic, a known carcinogen, show an increased incidence of lung cancer. The role of genetic factors is not clear, but there are families that appear to have an inherited susceptibility to the carcinogenic effects of these exposures.

There are two basic kinds of lung cancer—SMALL CELL LUNG CANCER (also called undifferentiated small cell and oat cell), accounting for 20 to 25% of all lung cancers, and NON-SMALL CELL LUNG CANCER, accounting for 75 to 80% of lung cancers. The latter is broken down further into large cell carcinoma, SQUAMOUS CELL LUNG CANCER (also called epidermoid carcinoma), and ADENOCARCINOMA, including BRONCHIOLOALVEOLAR LUNG CANCER.

The most common symptom of lung cancer is a cough—caused by blockage of the air passage to the lung as the tumor grows. Other symptoms may include chest pain, shortness of breath, repeated pneumonia or bronchitis, coughing up blood, hoarseness, or swelling of the neck and face.

Procedures used in the diagnosis and evaluation of lung cancer may include a chest X-RAY followed by BRONCHOSCOPY, PERCUTANEOUS NEEDLE BIOPSY, MEDIASTINOSCOPY, THORACOTOMY, CT SCAN, MRI, ANGIOGRAPHY, and BRONCHOGRAPHY.

For STAGING and treatment see NON-SMALL CELL LUNG CANCER and SMALL CELL LUNG CANCER.

See also SMOKING, LUNG METASTASES.

lung function test   See PULMONARY FUNCTION TEST.

lung metastases   a secondary cancer that has spread (metastasized) to the lung from some other site. It is very common since the entire cardiac output (all the blood from the heart) flows through the lungs. Among the most common cancers to spread to the lungs are testicular, breast, and colon/rectal, melanoma, GERM CELL TUMORS, SOFT TISSUE SARCOMAS, OSTEOSARCOMAS, and other cancers. Treatment of metastatic cancer to the lung generally relies on

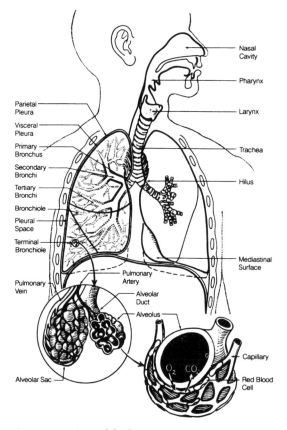

A cutaway view of the lung structure. Courtesy NCI.

systemic therapy for the primary cancer. A few tumors that metastasize almost exclusively to the lung can, on rare occasion, be cured by treatment of the primary site along with surgical removal of the metastases in the lungs. For specific information on the latest state-of-the-art treatment, by primary site, call the National Cancer Institute's Cancer Information Service at 1-800-4-CANCER (1-800-422-6237), or for a TTY: 1-800-332-8615.

lung scan examination of the lung after administration of a small amount of a virtually harmless RADIOACTIVE substance. The substance is administered by IV (injected into a vein). Depending on which scanner is used, this procedure can take anywhere from 10 minutes to an hour and a half. It can be performed in a doctor's office or on an outpatient basis at a hospital. A lung scan is generally used in the diagnosis of other disorders but may occasionally be used in the diagnosis of LUNG CANCER.

See also NUCLEAR SCAN.

Lupron [LEUP, leuprolide, LHRH agonist leuprolide, leuprolide acetate] a drug that blocks the production of male hormones by the testicles. When Lupron is combined with FLUTAMIDE or Casodex (an antiandrogen), it may be an alternative treatment (total androgen blockade) to surgical removal of the testicles in the treatment of PROSTATE CANCER. It is self-administered subcutaneously (injection under the skin) daily. Long-acting DEPOT preparations (pellets of the drug inserted under the skin) that can be given once a month are also being used to treat prostate cancer. Side effects may include impotence and hot flashes. Lupron is an important drug in the treatment of cancer.

luteinizing hormone-releasing hormone (LHRH) (lu"te-in"i'zing) [gonadotropin-releasing hormone] a HORMONE that controls the production of sex hormones in men and women. LHRH drugs are used in the treatment of PROSTATE CANCER and BREAST CANCER.

L-VAM a combination of the anticancer drugs LUPRON, VINBLASTINE, ADRIAMYCIN, and MUTAMYCIN sometimes used in the treatment of kidney, bladder, and prostate cancer. See individual drug listings for side effects.

See also COMBINATION CHEMOTHERAPY.

lymph (limf) a nearly colorless liquid that bathes the body tissues and contains cells that help the body fight infection. See LYMPH SYSTEM.

lymph glands See LYMPH NODES.

lymph node [lymph gland] one of many small, bean-shaped organs of the IMMUNE SYSTEM linked by LYMPHATIC VESSELS throughout the body. Lymph nodes make and store many different immune cells that fight infections. They filter germs and foreign bodies from the lymph and trap them, which is why swollen glands can be an indication of disease. Lymph nodes are found throughout the body—under the arms, behind the ears, in the neck, in the groin, in the abdominal cavity, behind the knee, and in many other areas.

lymph node biopsy removal and microscopic examination of one of the LYMPH NODES, the small, bean-shaped organs of the immune system, for cancer cells.

See also LYMPHADENECTOMY.

lymph node involvement cancer from another site that has spread to the LYMPH NODES. The term *lymph node involvement* is commonly used when discussing breast cancer as well as other cancers. Doctors check to see if a cancer has spread from its original (primary) site to lymph nodes by surgically removing some of them and performing a biopsy. This is important information needed for the staging of the cancer and its treatment.

lymph system the part of the body responsible for fighting infections. It is composed of a network of lmphatic vessels, thin tubes like blood vessels, that carry lymph, a watery, colorless fluid, throughout the body, and the tissue and organs that produce and store the white blood cells that fight infection. Those cells, LYMPHOCYTES, are contained in the lymph. Clusters of LYMPH NODES, which make and store white blood cells, are found at different points in the lymph system. The other organs of the lymph system, some of which also produce white blood cells, but in a much smaller amount, are the bone marrow, spleen, thymus, adenoids, appendix, and the tonsils. When cancer arises in the lymph system, it is known as LYMPHOMA.

lymphadenectomy (lim-fad″ĕ-nek′to-me) surgical removal and biopsy of LYMPH NODES to evaluate the extent of disease. A LYMPH NODE BIOPSY is performed in many cancers when they are being staged. When there is LYMPH NODE INVOLVEMENT, it means the cancer has spread from the primary site and is more likely to spread to other sites. A lymphadenectomy may also be performed when a recurrence of cancer is suspected. Lymphadenectomy is sometimes performed, as well, in the treatment of cancer (such as removal of the lymph nodes in the abdomen of men with stage A and B nonseminomatous testicular cancer).

lymphangiogram   See LYMPHANGIOGRAPHY.

lymphangiography (lim-fan″je-og′rah-fe) [lymphography]   an X-RAY examination of the abdomen, pelvis, or chest for enlarged lymph nodes. A blue dye is injected into the lymphatic passages of the legs through the toes. It can take an hour for enough dye to enter the lymphatic system, after which X-RAYS are taken. The patient returns the following day for additional X-rays. The X-ray, called a lymphangiogram, can show enlarged nodes and a distorted pattern of lympathic flow. This procedure may be used in the diagnosis and/or evaluation of HODGKIN'S DISEASE, LYMPHOMAS, GYNECOLOGIC CANCERS, and TESTICULAR CANCER.

lymphangiosarcoma (lim-fan″je-o-sar-ko′mah) a type of SOFT-TISSUE SARCOMA that originates in the LYMPHATIC VESSELS.

lymphatic organs (lim-fat′ik) the organs in the body that are concerned with the growth, development, and deployment of the white blood cells LYMPHOCYTES. These organs include BONE MARROW, the THYMUS, SPLEEN, and LYMPH NODES as well as the TONSILS, ADENOIDS, and APPENDIX.

lymphatic system (lim-fat′ik) the tissues and organs—including the bone marrow, spleen, thymus, and lymph nodes—that produce and store cells that fight infection, and the network of channels that carry LYMPH fluid.

lymphatic vessels (lim-fat′ik) the thin, tubelike structures that make up the LYMPH SYSTEM.

lymphedema (lim″fĕ-de′mah) an accumulation of fluid that may collect in the arms or legs when lymph vessels or LYMPH NODES are blocked or removed. Lymphedema is most often associated with breast cancer but can result from treatment of other cancers. Following are the cancers and risk factors from treatment of the cancers:

- breast cancer—removal of lymph nodes; radiation therapy
- melanoma of the arms or legs with radiation treatment—removal of lymph nodes under the arm or the groin
- prostate cancer—surgery; radiation therapy to the entire pelvic area
- advanced gynecologic cancer—surgery with lymph node removal or radiation therapy
- advanced ovarian, testicular, colorectal, pancreatic, or liver cancer that has spread

Lymphedema can occur any time after treatment, even years later. It is frequently painful and uncomfortable but can be painless. And it may be acute or chronic.

Following is a guide for the prevention and control of lymphedema:

- Keep the affected arm or leg elevated above the level of the heart when possible.
- Avoid rapid circular movements that cause pooling of fluids in the hands or feet.
- Clean and apply lotions to the skin of the arm or leg daily.
- Use an electric razor for shaving.
- Wear gardening and cooking gloves, use a thimble when sewing.
- Maintain good hand and foot nail care; do not cut cuticles.
- Wear foot coverings for ocean bathing.
- Keep hands and feet clean and dry; wear cotton socks.
- Use a sunscreen; tan gradually.
- Clean breaks in the skin with soap and water, then use an antibacterial ointment.
- Use gauze wrapping instead of tape.
- Consult physician about rashes.
- Avoid hypodermic needles and intravenous infusions in the affected arm or leg.
- Avoid extreme hot or cold to affected arm or leg.

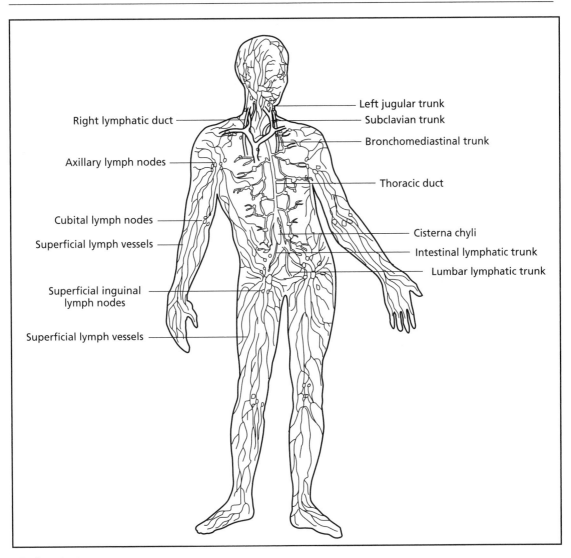

The lymphatic system. Infobase Publishing.

- Avoid prolonged and strenuous work with the affected arm or leg.
- Do not cross legs while sitting.
- Wear loose jewelry and clothes with no tight bands.
- Do not carry handbag on affected arm.
- Do not have blood pressure taken on affected arm.
- Do not use elastic bandages and stockings with constrictive bands.

- Do not sit in one position without moving for more than 30 minutes.
- At any signs of infection call your doctor.
- Keep regular follow-up appointments with your doctor.
- Practice drainage-promoting exercises regularly.
- Use affected hand to test temperatures, e.g., for bath water or cooking.
- Eat a well-balanced, protein-rich, low-salt diet.

Although lymphedema is rarely cured, it can be controlled by elevating the arm or leg; wearing special custom-fitted compression garments; keeping the skin clean to prevent infection; and weight control. Medication is available for pain and infections.

For additional information call the National Lymphedema Network at 800-541-3259.

lymphedema sleeve (lim″fĕ-de′mah) an elasticized apparatus used in the treatment of LYMPHEDEMA, fluid buildup in an arm. The device goes over the swollen arm like a sleeve. The pressure that is exerted on the arm helps to reduce the swelling by forcing the fluids back into the LYMPH SYSTEM. It can be used once or twice a day. It can help control the lymphedema but cannot cure it.

lymphoblastic non-Hodgkin's lymphoma (lim″fo-blas′tik) [formerly called lymphosarcoma] a type of NON-HODGKIN'S LYMPHOMA in children. It usually starts in the chest.

See also LYMPHOMA.

lymphocyte (lim′fo-sīt) a type of WHITE BLOOD CELL. Produced in the LYMPHOID ORGANS, lymphocytes are the most important cells in the immune system, responsible for regulating and carrying out most of its activities. There are about 1 trillion lymphocytes in the average body, constituting between 20 and 40% of all the white blood cells. The three main kinds of lymphocytes are T CELLS, B CELLS, and NATURAL KILLER CELLS. T cells attack and destroy virus infected cells, foreign tissue, and cancer cells. B cells produce antibodies—proteins that help destroy foreign substances. Natural killer cells destroy cancer cells and virus-infected cells through PHAGOCYTOSIS and produce substances that can kill cancer and virus-infected cells. A deficiency in lymphocytes may result in LYMPHOCYTOPENIA.

lymphocyte predominant See HODGKIN'S DISEASE.

lymphocyte depleted See HODGKIN'S DISEASE.

lymphocytic leukemia See ALL and CLL.

lymphocytic lymphoma (lim″fo-sit′ik lim-fo′mah) a type of NON-HODGKIN'S LYMPHOMA in which the cancer cells are small, resembling LYMPHOCYTES.

lymphocytopenia (lim″fo-si″to-pe′ne-ah) a condition in which there is a deficiency in the number of LYMPHOCYTES in the blood. Since the lymphocytes play a major role in the body's immune system, a person with lymphocytopenia is more susceptible to infections. In cancer, lymphocytopenia can be a result of various cancer treatments such as RADIATION THERAPY and CHEMOTHERAPY. A decrease in lymphocytes occurs in the progression of AIDS.

lymphogram See LYMPHANGIOGRAPHY.

lymphography See LYMPHANGIOGRAPHY.

lymphoid organs (lim′foid) organs of the IMMUNE SYSTEM where LYMPHOCYTES develop and congregate. Among the lymphoid organs are bone marrow, thymus, lymph nodes, spleen, and other various clusters of lymphoid tissue.

lymphokine-activated killer cells See LAK CELLS.

lymphokines (lim′fo-kīnz) powerful chemical substances secreted primarily by the T CELLS in minute quantities. There are about 50 different types of lymphokines. They play a major role in the body's IMMUNE SYSTEM—encouraging cell growth, promoting cell activation, directing cellular traffic, destroying target cells, and inciting macrophages. BIOLOGICAL TECHNOLOGY has made it possible to produce lymphokines in great quantities, making them far more available. In the past, large amounts of blood were needed to get a tiny sample.

Some of the more well known lymphokines are GAMMA INTERFERON and INTERLEUKIN-2. Lymphokines are being investigated in their role in the BIOLOGICAL THERAPY of cancer.

See also LAK CELLS.

lymphoma (lim-fo′mah) a general term for cancers that develop in the LYMPHATIC SYSTEM, affecting the body's IMMUNE SYSTEM. Most lymphomas develop in the lymph nodes, with the rest arising in lymphoid tissue elsewhere in the body. There are two basic kinds of lymphomas: HODGKIN'S DISEASE and NON-HODGKIN'S LYMPHOMA (which is composed of a number of different lymphomas). There are also other rarely occurring lymphomas. Hodgkin's disease has unique characteristics that distinguish it from the other lymphomas. It is identified by the presence of the REED-STERNBERG CELL and is more likely to follow a more predictable and limited pattern of spread than that of the other lymphomas, thereby giving it a better PROGNOSIS. Non-Hodgkin's lymphomas are more likely to develop outside the lymph nodes, in organ such as the bones and liver, than is Hodgkin's disease.

The Leukemia and Lymphoma Society estimated that about 63,740 Americans would be diagnosed with lymphoma in 2005 (7,350 cases of Hodgkin's disease and 56,390 cases of non-Hodgkin's lymphoma). The incidence of Hodgkin's lymphoma is consistently lower than that of non-Hodgkin's lymphoma.

Non-Hodgkin's lymphoma is the sixth most common cancer in males and the fifth most common cancer in females in the United States. The age-adjusted incidence of non-Hodgkin's lymphoma rose by 74% from 1975 to 2002—an annual average percentage increase of 2.7%.

See also BURKITT'S LYMPHOMA, MYCOSIS FUNGOIDES, ATLL, and LYMPHOBLASTIC NON-HODGKIN'S LYMPHOMA.

lymphoplasmacytic disorders   See CLL.

lymphoproliferative disorders   See CLL.

lymphosarcoma   See LYMPHOBLASTIC NON-HODGKIN'S LYMPHOMA.

Lynch syndrome   See HEREDITARY NONPOLYPOSIS COLORECTAL SARCOMA

Lysodren   See MITOTANE.

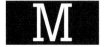

M-2 a combination of the anticancer drugs VIN-CRISTINE, BCNU, Cytoxan, melphalan (ALKERAN) and PREDNISONE sometimes used in the treatment of MYELOMA. See individual drug listings for side effects.

See also COMBINATION CHEMOTHERAPY.

MACC a combination of the anticancer drugs METHOTREXATE, ADRIAMYCIN, Cytoxan, and CCNU sometimes used in the treatment of NON-SMALL CELL LUNG CANCER. See individual drug listings for side effects.

See also COMBINATION CHEMOTHERAPY.

Macleron [dromostanolone propionate] See ANDROGENS.

macrobiotic diet a diet consisting mostly of cereal products, such as brown rice. Sugar, meat, or animal products are not allowed in a macrobiotic diet. Some supporters claim a macrobiotic diet is an effective primary treatment for cancer. Others claim that it can be effective when combined with other forms of treatment. The American Medical Association, the Food and Drug Administration, and nutrition experts say a macrobiotic diet can be harmful. The National Cancer Institute and the American Cancer Society believe that strict adherence to it poses a serious health hazard and is not effective in preventing or treating cancer, and that there is no scientific evidence supporting its use,

either alone or combined with standard cancer treatment.

See also UNCONVENTIONAL TREATMENT METHOD.

macrocalcifications (mak″ro-kal″sĭ-fĭ-ka′shuns) when used in regard to cancer, coarse calcium deposits in the breast that can be seen in a mammogram (X-RAY of the breast). Macrocalcifications usually are degenerative changes in the breast resulting from old injuries, inflammations, or aging of the breast arteries and are usually benign (noncancerous). They usually do not require a biopsy. Macrocalcifications occur in about half the women in the United States who are over 50, and in about 10% of the women under the age of 50.

See also MICROCALCIFICATIONS and BREAST CALCIFICATIONS.

macroglobulinemia See MYELOMA and WALDENSTROM'S MACROGLOBULINEMIA.

macrophage (mak′ro-fāj) a type of WHITE BLOOD CELL that plays many roles in the body, including an important role in the IMMUNE SYSTEM. Macrophages engulf and destroy foreign material such as bacteria in the body. They secrete a large array of powerful chemical substances including enzymes, proteins, and regulatory factors such as INTER-LEUKIN-1. Macrophages are also called "scavengers" because they rid the body of worn-out cells and other debris. Various forms of macrophages are found in tissue throughout the body. They are being investigated for their role in the BIOLOGICAL THERAPY of cancer.

magnetic resonance imaging   See MRI.

mainstream smoke   See PASSIVE SMOKE.

maintenance therapy [continuation therapy] additional chemotherapy (anticancer drugs) for people with acute myelogenous leukemia (AML) and acute lymphocytic leukemia (ANLL) after they have gone into remission. Its purpose is to destroy any cancer cells that may still be in the body. There are multiple schedules of maintenance therapy, which is generally given for a planned/fixed amount of time and then stopped.

male breast cancer   a rare occurrence of cancer in the male breast. The American Cancer Society estimated there would be some 1,690 new cases of invasive breast cancer diagnosed among men in the United States in 2005, with about 60 deaths. Breast cancer accounts for about 0.22% (two tenths of a percent) of cancer deaths among men. The number of breast cancer cases relative to the population has been increasing in the last 20 years for unknown reasons.

Risk factors may include radiation exposure, and familial tendencies. An increased incidence is seen in men who have a number of female relatives with breast cancer. An increased risk of male breast cancer has been reported in families in which the BRCA2 BREAST CANCER GENE appears. Middle-aged and older men are at the greatest risk of getting breast cancer. Almost all breast cancers in men are CARCINOMAS; there are also occurrences of INFLAMMATORY CARCINOMA OF THE BREAST and PAGET'S DISEASE. The symptoms for male breast cancer are similar to those for BREAST CANCER in women, including a painless lump (usually discovered by self-examination), nipple discharge, nipple retraction, and a lump under the arm. Diagnostic procedures are the same as those used for women. Therapeutic principles are also generally the same. Breast cancer is about 100 times more common among women.

male reproductive cancers   See TESTICULAR CANCER, PROSTATE CANCER, and PENILE CANCER.

malignant   poisonous, life threatening. When used in a medical setting, it means "cancerous" and commonly refers to a MALIGNANT TUMOR. The main characteristic of a malignant tumor (as opposed to a BENIGN TUMOR) is that it is likely to penetrate the tissues or organ in which it originated as well as move to other sites (METASTASIZE), eventually causing death, unless effectively treated.

malignant ascites   See ASCITES.

malignant effusions   See EFFUSIONS.

malignant fibrous histiocytoma (MFH) (mah-lig'nant fi'brus his''te-o-si-to'mah)   a malignant (cancerous) tumor in the bone generally found in the ends of long bones such as those in the legs or arms, especially around the knee. It is a SARCOMA that is most common in men in their 50s and 60s. Treatment generally is surgery and CHEMOTHERAPY. For the latest state-of-the-art treatment, call the National Cancer Institute's Cancer Information Service at 1-800-4-CANCER (1-800-422-6237), or for a TTY: 1-800-332-8615.

See also BONE CANCER.

malignant giant cell   a type of BONE CANCER affecting the leg or arm. It frequently starts in the knee. It is one of the few bone cancers to which women are more susceptible than men. Symptoms may include pain, local tenderness, and decreased motion in the adjacent joint. A benign (noncancerous) condition, GIANT CELL TUMOR OF THE BONE, may occasionally become cancerous. Another form of giant cell tumor begins as a sarcoma. Giant cell tumors can recur locally, but rarely metastasize (spread).

See also SOFT TISSUE SARCOMA.

malignant melanoma   See MELANOMA.

malignant mesothelioma   See MESOTHELIOMA.

malignant mixed mullerian tumor   See MULLERIAN TUMOR.

malignant pericardial effusion   See PERICARDIAL EFFUSION.

malignant pleural effusion   See PLEURAL EFFUSION.

malignant thymoma   See THYMOMA.

malignant tumor (mah-lig'nant) a cancerous growth with the following characteristics:

- its cells divide rapidly without stopping, above the needs of the tissue or organ; the cells have a higher rate of growth than the normal tissue where they originate
- the cells have a different appearance from the cell from which they originate
- the cells fail to maintain the normal boundaries of the organ
- the cells are undifferentiated (immature); they lack normal structure or function
- the cells are capable of breaking away and entering other areas of the body and destroying areas to which they have spread.

  See also BENIGN TUMOR and TUMOR.

malt (mucosa-associated lymph tissue) lymphoma a form of non-Hodgkin's lymphoma. Malt lymphoma of the stomach is closely associated with chronic gastritis 2°-*H. Pylori* infection. Regression of some MALTs have followed treatment of the infection. CHEMOTHERAPY is also used. See NON-HODGKIN'S LYMPHOMA.

mammaplasty (mam'ah-plas"te) plastic surgery of the breast to enlarge it, reduce it, or reconstruct it. See BREAST RECONSTRUCTION.

mammary dysplasia   See FIBROCYSTIC CHANGES.

mammogram   See MAMMOGRAPHY.

mammography (mam-og'rah-fe) an X-RAY procedure used in the screening and diagnosis of BREAST CANCER. A mammogram can reveal a tumor in the breast long before it can be felt during a BREAST SELF-EXAMINATION or by a doctor. That is very significant because the earlier breast cancer is detected, the better the chance for a cure. In addition to breast masses it can show MACROCALCIFICATIONS (coarse deposits of calcium) and MICROCALCIFICATIONS (minute deposit of calcium) as well as abnormal tissue that may indicate a cancer in the breast.

Mammography is not a new technique. A German pathologist used it as early as 1913. From

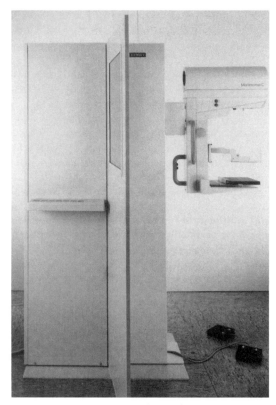

Siemen's "Mammomat C" for performing mammography screenings. Courtesy Siemen's Medical Systems, Inc.

that time on, it was used to a limited extent in the United States and abroad. The value of annual breast examinations (breast self-exams and mammograms) in detecting early breast cancer was conclusively shown in the National Cancer Institute (NCI)/American Cancer Society (ACS) Breast Cancer Detection Demonstration Project. The project found a 30% reduction in breast cancer deaths among women over the age of 50 who had annual physician and mammographic screenings and a 24% reduction in deaths among women aged 40 to 50. The American Cancer Society and the National Cancer Institute recommend that women age 40 and older have a mammogram every year and should continue to do so for as long as they are in good health; they also recommend that women in their 20s and 30s have a clinical breast exam (CBE) as part of a periodic (regular) health exam by a health professional preferably every three years. Starting at age 40, women should have a breast exam by a health professional every year.

The procedure takes just a few minutes. The breast is put in a device in the X-ray machine that squeezes it and spreads it out so that the pictures of the breast will be as precise as possible. Generally two pictures of each breast are taken, from above and from the side. There may be some minor discomfort when the mammogram is done, but it is generally a painless procedure.

There have been many technological advances that have made mammography a very safe procedure. The amount of radiation exposure a woman receives when getting a mammogram has been lowered by new and better machines. It is important for a woman to go to a facility that has high-quality mammography machines and well-trained technicians. Following are guidelines for choosing a facility:

- the machine used for the mammogram should be "dedicated" (used only for mammography)
- the person administering the exam should be a trained, registered technologist; he or she should be certified by the American College of Radiological Technologists or be licensed by the state
- the radiologist who reads the mammogram should be board certified and should have taken special courses in mammography
- the American College of Radiology recommends the facility should perform at least ten mammograms per week
- the mammography machine should be calibrated at least once a year (there should be a sticker on the machine verifying this), and as of October 1994, all mammography facilities were required to have certification by the Food and Drug Administration (FDA).

See also SCREENING.

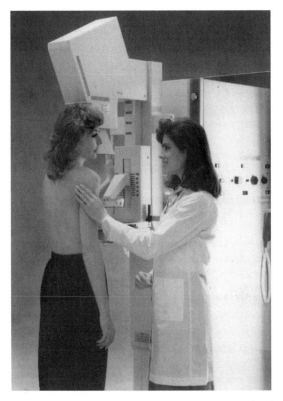

A woman getting a mammogram on a GE Medical Systems dedicated mammography system. Courtesy GE Medical Systems.

m-AMSA [amsacrine]   a drug being investigated for its use in acute nonlymphocytic leukemia (ANLL), LYMPHOMA, MELANOMA, and colon and breast cancer. It is administered by IV (injected into a vein). Common side effects may include nausea, vomiting, BONE MARROW DEPRESSION, and burning pain at the needle site if some of the drug leaks out during IV. Occasional or rare side effects may include liver problems, mouth sores, seizures, and heart problems.

mantle cell lymphoma   a form of NON-HODGKIN'S LYMPHOMA identified as a distinct entity in 1992, as one of the round cell lymphomas. It represents 6% of all NHL. The median age of onset is 60. The disease has an aggressive course and is not curable. CHEMOTHERAPY is standard treatment, R-CHOP being most widely used. Newer agents being explored include Velcade, Thalidomide, Flavopiradol, Pixantrone, M-tor inhibitors, et al.

mantle field   the part of the body comprising the neck, chest, and axilla (lymph nodes under the arm). RADIATION THERAPY to the mantle field may be used in the treatment of HODGKIN'S DISEASE and NON-HODGKIN'S LYMPHOMA.

MAP a combination of the anticancer drugs MUTAMYCIN, ADRIAMYCIN, and Platinol (CISPLATIN) sometimes used in the treatment of HEAD AND NECK CANCERS. See individual drug listings for side effects.

See also COMBINATION CHEMOTHERAPY.

marginal zone lymphoma a form of non-Hodgkin's lymphoma. See NON-HODGKIN'S LYMPHOMA.

margins in cancer, the area of normal tissue remaining after a malignant (cancerous) tumor has been removed. When a doctor says "the margins are clean," it means no cancer cells are present and all the cancer has been removed from the site. In the earliest stages of some cancer, this may be considered a cure. However, even with clean margins, ADJUVANT THERAPY (additional treatment) may be indicated.

marijuana (mar''ĭ-h wah'nah) [Marinol, Dronabinol] a member of the cannabis plant family, which can relax the mind and body, heighten perception, and cause mood swings when smoked or ingested. Marijuana's use as an ANTIEMETIC (antinausea drug) and ANALGESIC (pain reliever) has been investigated. One component of marijuana, delta-9-tetrahydrocannabino (THC/Dronabinol), is now available in a synthetic form for the treatment of nausea and vomiting in patients taking CHEMOTHERAPY (anticancer drugs). It is being sold under the brand names Marinol and Dronabinol and is taken orally. Some researchers believe that THC is as effective as other antiemetics in relieving or controlling nausea and vomiting. It can be of benefit for some patients whose treatment with other antiemetics has been unsuccessful. In some patients, THC can produce a sensation of unreality or loss of control that some people find unpleasant. This, along with the availability of numerous other antiemetics has tended to limit its use. In addition, the pain-relieving effects of marijuana have not proved to be consistent. The medical use of plant marijuana remains (in 2005) a contentious legal issue. Currently, 30 states and the District of Columbia have laws on the books that recognize marijuana's medical value. Eleven states have only "Therapeutic Research Program"

laws that do not give patients legal access to medical marijuana. Nine states and the District of Columbia have laws that "recognize" marijuana's medical value but do not protect patients from arrest.

Since 1996, nine states have enacted laws that allow patients to use medical marijuana despite federal laws to the contrary. A 10th state, Maryland, has established an "affirmative defense" law that protect medical marijuana users from jail, but not from arrest.

However, the states of Alaska, California, Colorado, Maine, Nevada, Oregon, and Washington, enacted laws via ballot initiatives that protect patients from jail and arrest for the medical use of marijuana. In Hawaii, a law was passed by the legislature and signed by the governor in June 2000. In Vermont, a law protecting patients was passed by the legislature and allowed to become the law of the state without the governor's signature in May 2004.

Marinol See MARIJUANA.

mast cell a large cell in body tissue that releases chemicals such as SEROTININ and HISTAMINE during inflammation and allergic reactions.

mastectomy (mas-tek'to-me) surgical removal of the breast, usually as treatment for BREAST CANCER. The first mastectomies were performed around the turn of the century. Before that, virtually no women survived breast cancer.

In the late 19th century, Dr. William Halsted, a surgeon from Baltimore, Maryland, devised the radical mastectomy, or "Halsted mastectomy," which bears his name. The procedure involved the removal of the breast and skin, the underlying muscle of the chest wall, the axillary LYMPH NODES, and fat tissue. From about 1895 to the mid-1970s about 90% of the women being treated for breast cancer in the United States underwent the radical, or Halsted, mastectomy.

A modified radical mastectomy was developed by an English surgeon in the 1930s. It required removal of the breast and axillary lymph nodes and was less disfiguring and debilitating than the radical. It gradually gained worldwide acceptance when

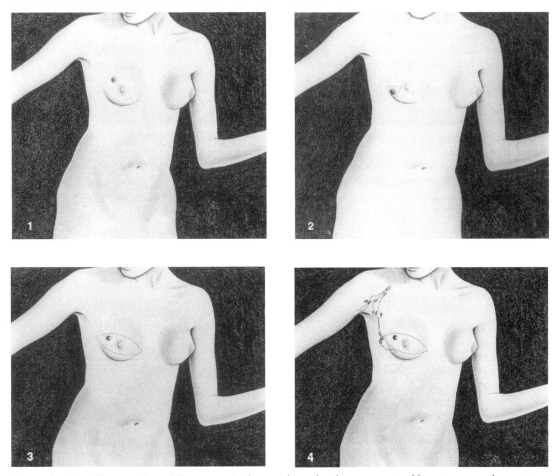

These drawings illustrate four different surgical procedures for the treatment of breast cancer: lumpectomy, partial or segmental mastectomy, total mastectomy, and modified radical mastectomy. From *The Breast Cancer Digest*, National Cancer Institute (1984).

studies showed it was as effective as the radical. By 1977 the modified radical mastectomy accounted for almost 70% of the surgeries performed on breast cancer patients in the United States.

In 1985, the results of a 10-year study conducted by the National Surgical Adjuvant Breast Project which followed more than 1,600 women, showed that a simple mastectomy, with removal of only the breast and a few axillary lymph nodes, had the same survival rate as the radical or modified mastectomy when used in the treatment of early breast cancers. In 1990 a federal advisory panel stated that a LUMPECTOMY, the removal only of the cancerous tumor with RADIATION THERAPY is just as effective in treating breast cancer in its early stages as a mastectomy.

It is important to note that each case is different and that the individual patient's condition may dictate one surgical procedure over another. Following are the different types of breast cancer surgical procedures being performed in the United States:

- RADICAL MASTECTOMY (also called Halsted mastectomy)—surgical removal of the breast, the underlying muscle, the lymph nodes in the armpit, and fat tissue; this is rarely performed
- MODIFIED RADICAL MASTECTOMY (total mastectomy with axillary dissection)—surgical removal of the breast and the lymph nodes in the armpit
- SIMPLE MASTECTOMY (total mastectomy, complete mastectomy)—surgical removal of the breast
- lumpectomy (quadrantectomy, partial mastectomy, segmental mastectomy, wedge resection, tylectomy, excisional biopsy, breast conservation)—surgical removal of a cancerous lump from the breast and the tissue surrounding it
- SUBCUTANEOUS MASTECTOMY—removal of the inner breast tissue through an incision under the skin

BREAST RECONSTRUCTION can be performed on many patients after the surgery. For many patients who want reconstruction it can be done at the same time that the surgery removing the breast is performed.

Masteril   [dromostanolone   propionate]   See ANDROGEN.

Matulane   See PROCARBAZINE.

maxillofacial prosthetic (mak-sil"o-fa'shal prosthet'ik)   an artificial body part made of plastic and/or silicone to replace a structure removed from the head during an operation, which may occur as a result of cancer. For example, in head and neck surgery, a patient may need a new jaw, cheekbone, or eye socket.

maxillofacial prosthodontist (mak-sil"o-fa'shal pros"tho-don'tist)   a dentist who is a specialist in evaluating and restoring the facial and oral tract after surgery—both cosmetically and functionally. He or she can restructure the face and head area using remaining tissue. A special MAXILLOFACIAL PROSTHETIC, used for speaking, eating, or swallowing, is inserted by the maxillofacial prosthodontist. A doctor who specializes in this field is a member of the American Academy of Maxillofacial Prosthetics.

m-BACOD   a combination of the anticancer drugs BLEOMYCIN, ADRIAMYCIN, CYTOXAN, ONCO-VIN (VINCRISTINE), DECADRON, and METHOTREXATE WITH LEUCOVORIN RESCUE sometimes used in the treatment of NON-HODGKIN'S LYMPHOMA. See individual drug listings for side effects.

See also COMBINATION CHEMOTHERAPY.

m-BACOS   a combination of the anticancer drugs BLEOMYCIN, ADRIAMYCIN, CYTOXAN, ONCOVIN (VINCRISTINE), and METHOTREXATE WITH LEUCOVORIN RESCUE sometimes used in the treatment of NON-HODGKIN'S LYMPHOMA. See individual drug listings for side effects.

See also COMBINATION CHEMOTHERAPY.

MBC   a combination of the anticancer drugs METHOTREXATE, BLEOMYCIN, and CISPLATIN sometimes used in the treatment of head and neck cancers. See individual drug listings for side effects.

See also COMBINATION CHEMOTHERAPY.

MC   a combination of the anticancer drugs MITOXANTRONE and cytarabine (ARA-C) sometimes used in the treatment of acute nonlymphocytic leukemia (ANLL). See individual drug listings for side effects.

See also COMBINATION CHEMOTHERAPY.

MDR   See MULTIDRUG RESISTANCE.

MDS   See MYELODYSPLASTIC SYNDROME.

mechlorethamine   See MUSTARGEN.

mediastinoscope   See MEDIASTINOSCOPY.

mediastinoscopy (me"de-as"tĭ-nos'ko-pe)   an examination of the MEDIASTINUM (the space in the chest between the lungs, breastbone, and spine). An instrument called a mediastinoscope (a thin, lighted tubular instrument and optical system) is inserted through a small incision in the neck just above the collarbone. It is passed behind the breastbone (sternum) so that it is right in front of the trachea (windpipe). The doctor can view the LYMPH NODES and other structures in the mediastinum and remove lymph nodes for BIOPSY. A mediastinoscopy is performed under general anesthesia in the hospital. It takes about an hour. It rarely has complications, and the patient can usually go home the same day. It may be used in the diagnosis of LUNG CANCER and/or to check on whether lung cancer has spread to the lymph nodes in the mediastinum.

See also MEDIASTINOTOMY.

mediastinotomy (me″de-as″tĭ-not′o-me) an examination of the area under the aorta (the main artery leaving the heart). A small incision is made to the right or left of the breastbone, and some rib cartilage is removed. The doctor can then view the LYMPH NODES and remove some for BIOPSY. A mediastinotomy is performed under general anesthesia in the hospital. It is performed to determine if tumors in the upper left lobe of the lung have spread to the lymph nodes under the aorta. Mediastinotomy is similar to a MEDIASTINOSCOPY, the only real difference being the incision and examination site.

mediastinum (me″de-as-ti′num) the space in the chest between the lungs, breastbone, and spine. Located in the mediastinum are the heart, great blood vessels, the thymus gland, part of the esophagus (tube connecting the throat to the stomach) and trachea (windpipe), and LYMPH NODES.

medical oncologist (on-kol′o-jist) a medical doctor who specializes in the treatment of cancer using medical treatment (drugs and hormones). This is a relatively new specialty, with certification by the American Board of Internal Medicine in 1972. After completing basic training in internal medicine, a doctor spends two to three additional years to meet the credential criteria of the American Board of Internal Medicine.

A medical oncologist is frequently the doctor who manages the cancer patient's course of treatment—consulting with other physicians when appropriate and referring the patient to other physicians for different tests and procedures when necessary. The medical oncologist is also the physician who most often "follows" the patient who is in remission or has been cured. A medical oncologist is sometimes referred to as a chemotherapist.

medical physicist See RADIATION THERAPIST.

Mediport See INFUSE-A-PORT.

Medrol [methylprednisolone] a corticosteroid hormonal drug sometimes used in the treatment of LYMPHOMA, HODGKIN'S DISEASE, acute leukemias, breast cancer, and MYELOMA. It is taken by mouth. Side effects may include an increased appetite, weight gain, fluid retention, mood changes, acne, increased blood pressure, elevated blood sugar, intestinal ulcers, lowered resistance to infection, and gastrointestinal upset.

See also ADRENOCORTICOIDS.

medroxyprogesterone [Provera, Depo-Provera] See PROGESTERONE.

medullary cancer (med′u-lār″e) a descriptive term for a cancer in the innermost portion of an organ or structure, such as MEDULLARY CARCINOMA OF THE BREAST and MEDULLARY CARCINOMA OF THE THYROID.

medullary carcinoma of the breast (med′u-lār″e kar″sĭ-no′mah) an uncommon type of BREAST CANCER accounting for some 3% of breast cancer cases. It grows within the ducts in the breast. It appears encapsulated and is frequently riddled with small white blood cells. Although it can grow quite large, it is not likely to spread beyond the breast. Primary treatment is surgical.

medullary carcinoma of the thyroid (med′u-lār″e kar″sĭ-no′mah) [C-cell carcinoma of the thyroid] an extremely rare THYROID CANCER arising from cells that migrate from the nervous system in the embryo. The cells produce the hormone calcitonin, which acts on calcium and bone metabolism. It accounts for about 5% of all thyroid cancers. They are slightly more common in women and in people in their 50s and 60s but can occur at any age. It may be familial (inherited; occurring in every generation) or sporadic (nonfamilial). In familial medullary carcinoma the cancer is usually in both lobes. In sporadic (nonfamilial) medullary carcinoma the tumor is usually in one lobe.

medulloblastoma (MDL) (mĕ-dul″-blas-to′mah) a type of BRAIN CANCER that originates in the lower part of the brain, occurring commonly in children. It is an invasive tumor. Symptoms include headaches, apathy, and unexplained vomiting followed by (not too much later) neurological signs such as difficulty in walking. Because the tumor grows quickly, symptoms are seen early.

See also GLIOMA.

MEG   See MEGACE.

Megace [MEG, megestrol, Pallace]   a hormonal anticancer drug. A type of progesterone, it may be used in the treatment of cancers of the breast, kidney, or uterus as well as other, noncancerous disorders. It is taken by mouth. The most common side effect that may occur is a change in vaginal bleeding (spotting, prolonged, or complete stoppage of bleeding). Other possible side effects include changes in appetite and weight, swelling of ankles and feet, and unusual tiredness or weakness. Because it can stimulate the appetite in some people, it is being used with many malnourished patients with cancer or AIDS. Megace is an important anticancer drug.

megavoltage (MeV) linear accelerator   See LINEAR ACCELERATOR.

megestrol   See MEGACE.

melanin (mel′ah-nin)   the pigment in the skin. The amount of melanin in the skin determines the color of the skin. The more melanin, the darker the skin color. The amount of melanin in the skin is a significant factor in the development of SKIN CANCER. Dark-skinned people have a much lower rate of skin cancer.

melanoma (mel″ah-no′mah) [cutaneous melanoma, malignant melanoma]   the most serious type of SKIN CANCER, which originates in the cells that produce MELANIN (the dark, protective pigment of the skin). Although most melanomas arise in the skin, they also may arise at other sites. The incidence of new cases of melanoma has been increasing steadily since the mid-1940s. More than half of all new cancers are skin cancers.

The American Cancer Society estimated there would be some 105,750 new cases of melanoma in 2005—46,170 IN SITU (NONINVASIVE) and 59,580 INVASIVE (33,580 men and 26,000 women). This is a 10% increase in invasive melanoma from 2004.

As of 2005, it was estimated that at current rates one in 34 Americans have a lifetime risk of developing melanoma and one in 62 Americans have a lifetime risk of developing invasive melanoma.

Melanoma occurs most frequently in white women and men over the age of 40 who have a lot of moles, light complexions, red or blond hair, and skin that freckles and burns easily. Women most often get melanoma on the arms and legs; men most often get it on the trunk (the part of the body between the shoulders and hips) or on the head or neck. There is a greater incidence of melanoma among people with DYSPLASTIC NEVI (one type of mole that can be inherited) as well as people with XERODERMA PIGMENTOSUM (a rare hereditary disease in which the skin and eyes are extremely sensitive to light). Few blacks, Asians, and others with dark skin are affected.

The four main types of melanoma are superficial spreading melanoma, nodular melanoma, acral-lentiginous melanoma, and lentigo maligna melanoma. INTRAOCULAR MELANOMA is a type of melanoma affecting the eye.

Warning signs of melanoma include a change in the size, shape, or color of a mole; oozing or bleeding from a mole; or a mole that feels itchy, hard, lumpy, swollen, or tender to the touch. Diagnosis of melanoma is by BIOPSY of the suspicious mole or area of the skin.

Melanoma can be staged in several different ways. Following is the NATIONAL CANCER INSTITUTE's (NCI) staging for melanoma with CLARK'S CLASSIFICATION SYSTEM of STAGING in parenthesis:

• Stage I—cancer is in the outer layer of the skin (epidermis) and/or the upper part of the inner layer of the skin (dermis); the cancer has not spread to nearby LYMPH NODES or distant sites; the tumor is less than 1.5 millimeters (mm) thick
(Clark's Level I—cancer involving only the epidermis; characterized by the abnormal growth of cells; sometimes called "in situ" and regarded, at times, as nonmalignant [noncancerous])
• Stage II—the tumor is 1.5 mm to 4 mm thick; it has spread to the lower part of the inner layer of the skin, but not into the tissue below the skin or into nearby lymph nodes
(Clark's Level II—cancer reaches into the papillary dermis [upper portion of the dermis])

- Stage III—(any of the following):
1. the tumor is more than 4 mm thick
2. the tumor has spread to the body tissue below the skin
3. there are additional tumor growths within one inch of the original tumor
4. the tumor has spread to nearby lymph nodes, or there are additional tumor growths between the original tumor and the lymph nodes in the area
(Clark's Level III—cancer extends to the bottom of the papillary dermis)
- Stage IV—the tumor has spread to other organs or to lymph nodes far away from the original tumor
(Clark's Level IV—cancer invades the lower part of the dermis)
(Clark's Level V—cancer penetrates through the layers of the skin into the underlying tissue)
- Recurrent—the cancer has returned after it has been treated; it may return in the original site or occur in another part of the body

Another way of staging melanoma is called MICROSTAGING. The thickness of the tumor and its depth in the skin are measured.

Treatment depends on the stage of the disease and other factors, but both BASAL CELL CARCINOMA and SQUAMOUS CELL CARCINOMA have a better than 95% cure rate if detected and treated early.

The four kinds of treatment being used are surgery (the most common treatment), CHEMOTHERAPY, RADIATION THERAPY, and BIOLOGICAL THERAPY. Following are the surgical procedures which may be used: conservative re-excision, the removal of any cancer remaining after the biopsy, and wide surgical excision, the removal of the cancer and some of the skin around it. Skin may have to be taken from another part of the body and put on the place where the cancer has been removed in a procedure called skin grafting. If the melanoma is on an arm or leg, chemotherapy may be administered by a technique called ISOLATION PERFUSION. Otherwise it is given in the conventional way. For specific information on the latest state-of-the-art treatment, by stage, call NCI's Cancer Information Service at 1-800-4-CANCER (1-800-422-6237), or for a TTY: 1-800-332-8615. (1-800-422-6237).

melphalan   See ALKERAN and CARCINOGENS.

MEN   See MULTIPLE ENDOCRINE NEOPLASIA.

meningeal carcinomatosis (mě-nin′je-al kar″sĭ-no-mah-to′sis)   METASTATIC CANCER that has spread over the surface of the brain and its lining. It can cause confusion and a variety of neurological symptoms. Diagnosis consists of performing a SPINAL TAP and BIOPSY to find abnormal cells in the spinal fluid. It is not unusual to have to perform several spinal taps before a diagnosis can be made. Treatment is usually with CHEMOTHERAPY instilled (administered drop by drop) into the spinal fluid or RADIATION THERAPY. Meningeal carcinomatosis has a very poor PROGNOSIS. See LEPTOMENINGEAL CARCINOMA.

meningioma (měe-nin″je-o′mah)   a brain tumor that arises from the meninges, the fibrous tissues that cover the brain's surface and spinal cord. Meningiomas seldom invade brain tissue. They account for about 15% of all BRAIN TUMORS and are usually benign (noncancerous), encapsulated, and slow growing. They are more common in women, and their incidence increases with age, beginning in middle adulthood. Meningiomas can cause many different symptoms including seizures.

meperidine   See DEMEROL.

mercaptopurine   See 6-MP.

Merkel cell carcinoma   a very rare small cell carcinoma of the skin appearing as painless red-purple skin NODULES, mostly in elderly patients. The two-year survival rate for this cancer stands at 50%. Primary treatment is surgical removal. The cancer may recur and may also METASTASIZE (spread). It is an aggressive cancer.

mesenchymoma (mes″en-ki-mo′mah)   a SOFT-TISSUE SARCOMA arising in the mixed tissue of the arms, legs, hands, and feet. These tumors are not always malignant (cancerous).

mesna [mesnex]   a chemical compound used with the drug IFOSFAMIDE in order to mitigate the toxic effects of this anticancer drug on the urinary bladder. It is a uro-protective. This is sometimes referred to as a "mesna rescue." Mesna appears to have low TOXICITY with both short- and long-term use. Side effects are rare, but may include skin rash or itching, diarrhea, nausea or vomiting, and an unpleasant taste.

mesna rescue   See MESNA.

mesna   uroprotection   See   IFOSFAMIDE   WITH MESNA.

Mesnex   See MESNA.

mesothelioma   (mes"o-the"le-o'mah)   [malignant mesothelioma]   a rare CANCEROUS TUMOR of the MESOTHELIUM, the lining of the chest (the pleura), the heart (the pericardium), and ABDOMINAL cavity (the PERITONEUM). There are between 1,000 and 1,500 cases diagnosed each year in the United States. It occurs nearly four times more often in men than in women—especially white men over the age of 50.

The major risk factor for acquiring mesothelioma is exposure to ASBESTOS, a group of minerals that occur naturally as masses of fibers. Inhalation of the fibers, which are too small to be seen by the naked eye, can lead not only to mesothelioma, but also to LUNG CANCER and a noncancerous, chronic disease of the lungs called ASBESTOSIS. Asbestos exposure was suspected as a risk factor for mesothelioma as far back as 1943. In 1960, a study of asbestos workers in South Africa established the link. Millions of American workers were exposed to asbestos during World War II while building asbestos-insulated ships.

Mesothelioma can develop some 30 to 40 years after exposure. Symptoms of mesothelioma in the lung may include shortness of breath and vague chest pain that may radiate to the shoulders or upper abdomen. Other symptoms may include loss of appetite, fatigue, hoarseness, weakness, and weight loss. Symptoms of mesothelioma in the abdominal cavity may include nausea, vomiting, bowel and urinary obstruction, and swelling of the legs and feet, and fever.

Procedures that may be used in the diagnosis of mesothelioma include chest X-RAYS (for pleural mesotheliotma) and CT SCANS (for both pleural and peritoneal). To get tissue samples for a BIOPSY (microscopic examination of cells for cancer), a THORACOSCOPY of the lung or a LAPAROSCOPY of the abdominal cavity may be done. If it is necessary to get a tissue sample through surgery, a THORACO-TOMY for pleural mesothelioma or a LAPAROTOMY for peritoneal mesothelioma may be performed. Diagnosis of mesothelioma can be difficult because its cancer cells are similar to a number of other cancer cells.

Mesothelioma is staged as follows:

- Localized (or limited)—the tumor appears only in the lining of the chest or the abdomen where it originated
- Advanced (or diffuse)—the tumor has spread beyond the lining of the chest or abdomen to other parts of the chest or abdomen
- Recurrent—the tumor has returned after it has been treated; it may return in the lining of the chest or abdomen or in another part of the body.

Treatment depends on the stage of the disease, the general state of health of the patient, and other factors. SURGERY is the most common treatment. RADIATION THERAPY and CHEMOTHERAPY may also be used. PEMETREXED (ALIMTA) was FDA-approved for malignant mesothelioma. For specific information on the latest state-of-the-art treatment, by stage, call the National Cancer Institute's Cancer Information Service at 1-800-4-CANCER (1-800-422-6237), or for a TTY: 1-800-332-8615.

mesothelium   a membrane that covers and protects internal organs of the body.

meta-analysis   a technique used in the reporting of data in which a large volume of information from previously reported series is pooled and the aggregate results summarized. It is a quantitative summary of research previously reported in a given area. Its place in helping to clarify issues in cancer management is controversial since it lumps together a large body of previously reported data, some of which may be incompatible. However, it may be a powerful tool in assessing the benefits of cancer treatment among a large population of cancer patients where previous studies have yielded conflicting information.

metastases   (mĕ-tas'tah-sēz)   the   plural   of METASTASIS.

metastasis (mĕ-tas′tah-sis) [mets] the transfer of disease from one part of the body to another. In cancer it is the spread of malignant (cancerous) cells from the primary (original) site to another part of the body. The term *metastasis* can also be used for the cancer that has spread. For example, a doctor might say a patient has a "breast metastasis in the lung." Metastasis is frequently referred to as a "secondary tumor." Newer research focuses on defining this as a sequential process that allows cancer cells to move from the primary tumor and grow elsewhere. This requires the establishment of a communications network between tumor cells and the nontransformed cells in the person. Recent clinical trials have examined the role of matrix metalloproteinase inhibitors as treatment.

See also METASTATIC CANCER.

metastasize (muh-tas′-tuh-size) to establish a second cancer site or multiple cancer sites away from the primary (original) site of cancer.

See METASTATIC CANCER.

metastatic brain tumor See BRAIN METASTASIS.

metastatic cancer (met″ah-stat′ik) cancer that has spread from its original or primary site. This happens when cancer cells in the primary tumor break away and travel through the LYMPH SYSTEM or bloodstream to another part of the body where they begin to multiply again, forming metastases. The lungs, bones, liver, and brain are frequent sites to which cancer metastasizes. The cancer cells that have spread from one part of the body to another are the same type as the cancer cells in the original cancer. For example, breast cancer that has spread to the lung is called "metastatic breast cancer." Metastatic cancer may also be called secondary cancer.

Metastatic cancer may occasionally be discovered before the primary cancer is found. This is more common in cancers, such as prostate cancer, that generally are not symptomatic in their early stages. A man whose prostate cancer has spread to the bones in the pelvis may have lower back pain before experiencing any symptoms from the prostate tumor itself. The cancer discovered in the pelvis is a secondary tumor that has spread from the original site, the prostate. On very rare occa-sions, the original site of a secondary cancer is never found despite extensive testing. That is referred to as an unknown primary or occult primary. Cancer that has metastasized is more difficult to treat and does not have as good a prognosis as cancer that has remained in the primary site.

Metastatic cancer may be treated with surgery, RADIATION THERAPY, CHEMOTHERAPY, HORMONE THERAPY, BIOLOGICAL THERAPY, or any combination of those treatments.

See also LIVER METASTASES, LUNG METASTASES, BONE METASTASIS, BRAIN METASTASIS, LEPTOMENIN-GEAL CARCINOMA, PLEURAL EFFUSION, PERICARDIAL EFFUSION, and ASCITES.

metastatic liver cancer See LIVER METASTASES.

metastatic workup (met″ah-stat′ik) a series of tests to determine if cancer has spread from its primary (original) site. This is usually done when cancer is first diagnosed. Depending on the site, some of the tests most commonly used are X-RAYS, scans (BRAIN SCAN, LIVER SCAN, BONE SCAN), ULTRASOUND, CT SCAN, BIOPSY, and BONE MARROW BIOPSY. These tests may also be done during or after treatment when there are suspicious symptoms or as follow-up after treatment.

methadone [Dolophine] a NARCOTIC drug used in the relief or control of pain. It is given by IM (injected into a muscle) or taken by mouth. It is available by prescription only.

Methosarb [Calusterone] See ANDROGEN.

methotrexate (meth″o-trek′sāt) [MTX, Mexate, amethopterin, Folex] an ANTIMETABOLITE anti-cancer drug sometimes used in the treatment of cancers of the breast, cervix, head and neck, colon, lung, and testes and acute LEUKEMIA SAR-COMA, LYMPHOMA, and MYCOSIS FUNGOIDES. It is given by IV (injection into a vein) or taken by mouth. Common side effects may include nausea, vomiting, diarrhea, mouth sores, and BONE MAR-ROW DEPRESSION. Occasional or rare side effects may include gastrointestinal problems, liver dam-age, kidney problems, cough, fever, hair thinning, headache, mental impairment, anemia, flank pain, and eye problems. Methotrexate is a widely used anticancer drug important in the treatment of cancer.

methotrexate with leucovorin rescue   See LEU-COVORIN RESCUE.

methoxsalen (mĕ-thok'sah-len) [8-MOP, 8-methoxypsoralen, Psoralen]   a drug used with ultraviolet light in two treatments—PUVA THERAPY and PHOTOPHERESIS—in the treatment of MYCOSIS FUNGOIDES and other diseases. When methoxsalen is given with ultraviolet light in these treatments, there is a ninefold increased risk of SQUAMOUS CELL SKIN CANCER.

methoxsalen with ultraviolet light   See PUVA THERAPY and PHOTOPHERESIS.

methyl-G   See METHYL-GAG.

methyl-GAG (meth'il gag) [MGBG, methylglyoxal-bis-guanylhydrazone, mitoguazone, methyl-G]   an anticancer drug being investigated for its role in the treatment of MELANOMA, LEUKEMIA, LYMPHOMA, MYELOMA, and cancers of the esophagus, lung, head, and neck. It is given by IV (injected into a vein) or intramuscularly (injected into a muscle). Common side effects may include flushing, numbness (usually in the facial areas but could involve the entire body), nausea, and mouth sores. Occasional or rare side effects may include BONE MARROW DEPRESSION, vomiting, bloody diarrhea, fatigue, and skin rash.

methylglyoxal-bis-guanylhydrazone   See METHYL-GAG.

methylprednisolone   See ADRENOCORTICOIDS.

methylprednisone   See ADRENOCORTICOIDS.

meticorten   See PREDNISONE.

metoclopramide [Reglan]   an ANTIEMETIC drug that may be given to a patient on CHEMOTHERAPY (anticancer drugs) before treatment to prevent nausea and vomiting. It is given by IV (injection into a vein) or taken by mouth. Side effects may include drowsiness and restlessness.

metrography   See HYSTEROGRAPHY.

metronomic chemotherapy   based on experimental studies, a concept proposed (2000) for the scheduling of cytotoxic drugs given regularly at subtoxic doses and having the activated endothelium as the principal target. This is a form of antiangiogenic therapy. Clinical trials are in progress to validate this.

mets   See METASTASIS.

Mexate   See METHOTREXATE.

MF   a combination of the anticancer drugs METHOTREXATE, 5-FU, and calcium LEUCOVORIN RESCUE sometimes used in the treatment of HEAD AND NECK CANCERS. See individual drug listings for side effects.
       See also COMBINATION CHEMOTHERAPY.

MFH   See MALIGNANT FIBROUS HISTIOCYTOMA.

MGBG   See METHYL-GAG.

MGUS (monoclonal gammapathy of unknown significance)   This entity is being found more frequently with the aging population. A person with MGUS has an abnormal lab test with no signs or symptoms of disease. For the most part the treatment is periodic observation. A few patients with MGUS may eventually develop myeloma; this risk is estimated at 1% per year. Premature treatment of MGUS is not recommended.

microcalcifications (mi"kro-kal"sĭ-fĭ-ka'shuns)   tiny specks of calcium in the breast that can be seen by MAMMOGRAPHY (X-ray of the breast). The residue left by rapidly dividing cells can appear as microcalcifications. Therefore, microcalcifications may indicate an area of the breast where cells are dividing rapidly. When many are seen in a cluster, they may indicate a small cancer. About half the cancers detected appear as these clusters. When microcalcifications are found by mammography, they may be biopsied (removed for microscopic examination for cancer cells) or simply followed, with another mammogram three to six months later.

See also BREAST CALCIFICATIONS and MACROCAL-CIFICATIONS.

micrographic surgery (mi"kro-graf'ik) a new surgical procedure in which the smallest amount of tissue possible is removed. The doctor removes the cancer and then microscopically examines the area to make sure no cancer cells remain. This is being investigated in the treatment of early-stage lip, oral, and skin cancer.

micrometastases (mi"kro-mĕ-tas'tah-sēz) very small numbers of cancer cells that have spread from the original cancer site, usually too small to be picked up in screening or diagnostic tests.

microstaging one way of classifying MELANOMA by measuring the thickness of the tumor and the depth of its invasion into the skin. The thicker the tumor and the greater its depth, the poorer the PROGNOSIS and the more likely it is that the cancer has metastasized (spread).

microwave oven an appliance that heats and cooks food using ELECTROMAGNETIC RADIATION. There is no data to suggest that the radiation from a microwave oven can cause cancer. All microwave ovens made after October 1971 are covered by a radiation safety standard enforced by the Federal Food and Drug Administration. The standard sets a limit on the amount of radiation that can leak from the oven over its lifetime. Any exposure to the radiation drops dramatically the farther away from the oven one moves. Someone 20 inches from the oven would receive about one-hundreth of the radiation as a person two inches away.

Mifepristone See RU486.

MINE a combination of the anticancer drugs IFOSFAMIDE WITH MESNA, MITOXANTRONE, and ETOPOSIDE sometimes used in the treatment of NON-HODGKIN'S LYMPHOMA. See individual drug listings for side effects.
See also COMBINATION CHEMOTHERAPY.

Miraluma test [scintimammography, sestamibi breast imaging] the first nuclear breast imaging test, approved by the Food and Drug Administration (FDA) in 1997, the Miraluma test is used as an adjunct to an abnormal mammography. It is not used in place of a mammogram or for screening but to provide further evaluation of a tumor in the breast. It is particularly useful in women who have breast implants or whose breasts are dense, which can limit the amount of information obtained from a mammogram.

In the Miraluma test, the woman is injected with a small amount of Miraluma—a radiopharmaceutical (imaging agent). She then lies face down on a table with her breasts protruding below. A gamma camera then provides images of the breasts. The whole procedure usually takes about an hour or less. See NUCLEAR SCAN and SCINTIGRAPHY.

MITH See MITHRACIN.

Mithracin (mith'rah-sin) [MITH, Mithramycin, plicamycin] an ANTIBIOTIC anticancer drug sometimes used in the treatment of testicular cancer and PAGET'S DISEASE of the bone. It is also used for its calcium-lowering property in the condition of HYPERCALCEMIA, which may be associated with a variety of cancers. It is given by IV (injection into a vein). Common side effects may include severe nausea, vomiting, and diarrhea. Occasional or rare side effects may include bleeding, BONE MARROW DEPRESSION, liver and/or kidney damage, mouth sores, fever, headaches, depression, drowsiness, and facial flushing.

mithramycin See MITHRACIN.

MITO See MUTAMYCIN.

mitoguazone See METHYL-GAG.

mitolactol See DIBROMODULCITOL.

mitomycin See MUTAMYCIN.

mitomycin-C See MUTAMYCIN.

mitosis (mi-to'-sis) the process by which cells in the body divide or reproduce. In cancer, mitosis is abnormal with too many cells being produced.
See also CELL CYCLE.

mitotane (mi'to-tān) [Lysodren, O,P'-DDD lyso-dren]   an anticancer drug sometimes used in the treatment of ADRENOCORTICAL CANCER. It is taken by mouth. Common side effects may include nausea and vomiting. Occasional and rare side effects may include diarrhea, mental depression, tremors, visual disturbances, skin rash, lethargy, drowsiness, headache, hypertension, fever, and general aching.

mitotic inhibitor (mi-tot'ik) a substance that prevents a cell from dividing by interrupting the cell cycle. Some CHEMOTHERAPY (anticancer drugs) function as mitotic inhibitors.

mitoxantrone (mi-toks'an-trōn") [Novantrone, DHAD]   an anticancer drug being used in the treatment of LEUKEMIA, LYMPHOMA, and BREAST CANCER. It is being used palliatively with corticosteroids to treat patients with advanced hormone-refractory prostate cancer. It was the first CHEMOTHERAPY approved for the treatment of hormone refractory prostate cancer. It is given by IV (injection into a vein). It was developed as a possible alternative to ADRIAMYCIN. Although mitoxantrone has many of the same side effects as Adriamycin, they are generally not as harsh. Common side effects may include BONE MARROW DEPRESSION, mild nausea, vomiting, mouth sores, and green urine. Occasional and rare side effects may include hair loss, heart problems, blue streaking in or around the vein, and liver problems. Mitoxantrone is an important anticancer drug in the treatment of cancer.

mixed cellularity   See HODGKIN'S DISEASE/ADULT.

mixed tumor   a TUMOR made up of two or more cell types or tissue types. PROGNOSIS and treatment may be effected.

MM   a combination of the anticancer drugs 6-MP and METHOTREXATE sometimes used in the treatment of acute lymphocytic leukemia (ALL). See individual drug listings for side effects.
See also COMBINATION CHEMOTHERAPY.

MoAb   See MONOCLONAL ANTIBODY.

modified radical mastectomy (mas-tek'to-me) [total mastectomy with axillary dissection] removal of the breast and axillary (armpit) lymph nodes. It was developed by a British surgeon in the 1930s. The modified radical mastectomy gradually replaced, in most instances, the much more disfiguring RADICAL MASTECTOMY when studies showed no difference in survival rates of women who had a radical mastectomy and those who had a modified mastectomy. It is the most common treatment for early-stage BREAST CANCER, although studies now show that a LUMPECTOMY is just as effective in women for whom it is appropriate.
See also MASTECTOMY.

Mohs' micrographic surgery (mōz mi"kro-graf'ik)   a treatment for SKIN CANCER in which layers of tissue are removed one by one, until a layer is found that has no cancer cells. As each layer of tissue is removed, it is sent immediately to a pathologist for examination for cancer cells. Because the removal of one layer of tissue can take anywhere from 15 minutes to an hour, the procedure can take several hours. This technique was first described by Dr. Frederick Mohs in the late 1930s. Since then it has been refined and simplified. Mohs' surgery has the highest cure rate of all the treatments available for nonmelanoma skin cancers.

molar pregnancy   See HYDATIDIFORM MOLE.

mole [nevus, pigmented nevus (plural is nevi)] a common skin growth that is usually colored and may have hair growing from it. Most people have between 15 and 50 on their body. About 20 to 30% of MELANOMAS begin in moles. Generally moles are only a problem when they change in size or color, bleed, or ulcerate. When that occurs, they should be shown to a doctor. Some researchers advise removal of all moles that are:

• present at birth no matter what the size
• one CENTIMETER in diameter or larger
• in hard-to-see places such as the scalp, mouth, vagina, or anus where they cannot be easily monitored.

Any mole that appears after the age of 30, itches, or is tender should also be shown to a doctor.

molecular (cell) biology (mo-lek'u-lar) a general term for the study of the role of DNA and genes in causing human illness. The field of study that weds biochemistry to the function of cells, the drive of this is the explosion in knowledge of the role of DNA and genes as the central components of life. Recent advances in the understanding of how cell components communicate inside the cell has led to the development of many new pharmaceutical compounds. Molecular biology also encompasses investigation of activity at the CELL surface and its interaction with materials in the milleu. The technological advances of the past 30 years has created a vast amount of information. The terminology of this new biology and its application to drug development is quite technical and does require some educational background in science. The AMERICAN SOCIETY OF CLINICAL ONCOLOGY (ASCO) has aided this educational effort by developing a glossary, available either in print or online at www.jco.org.

See BIOLOGICAL THERAPY.

monoclonal antibody (MoAb) (mon″o-klōn′al an′tĭ-bod″e) a laboratory produced substance that reacts with a specific protein antigen. MoAbs are specific for a particular antigen, and researchers are investigating ways to create MoAbBs specific to antigens found on cancer cells. MoAbs are made by injecting human cancer cells into mice, whose immune systems make antibodies against those cancer cells. The mouse cells that are producing these antibodies are removed and fused with a laboratory-grown immortal cell to create a "hybrid" cell called a hybridoma. Hybridomas are like factories that can indefinitely produce large quantities of these pure antibodies or MoAbs.

MoAbs may be used in cancer treatment in a number of ways:

- react with specific types of cancer to enhance a patient's to enhance the immune response to the cancer
- link to anticancer drugs, radioactive substances (radioisotopes), BRMs, or other toxins. When the antibodies latch onto cancer cells, they deliver these poisons directly to the tumor, helping to destroy it
- may also prove useful in diagnosing certain cancers (radioscope-linked MoAbs)
- may help destroy any cancer cells in a patient's bone marrow before an autologous bone marrow

transplant, in which bone marrow is removed from a patient, stored, and later given back to the patient after high-dose chemotherapy and/or radiation therapy.

MoAbs are currently being tested in clinical trials in patients with lymphomas, colorectal cancer, lung cancer, leukemia, and a rare childhood cancer called neuroblastoma.

Because the MoAbs originally produced from hybridomas were foreign (mouse) proteins, patients often developed an immune response to them, producing human antimouse antibodies (HAMA). Newer MoAbs have been engineered to minimize this problem. Rituximab, approved by the FDA in late 1997, is the first approved MoAb in the United States for treating cancer.

See also BIOLOGICAL THERAPY.

monocyte (mon′o-sīt) a WHITE BLOOD CELL that can envelop and destroy foreign material in the body. Monocytes circulate through the blood before entering tissue in the body, where they develop into MACROPHAGES.

monocytic leukemia (mon″o-sit′ik) a rare form of acute nonlymphocytic leukemia.

See ANLL.

monokine (mon′o-kīn) a powerful chemical substance in the body produced by MONOCYTES and MACROPHAGES. Monokines help direct and regulate immune responses. INTERLEUKIN-1 is a monokine.

MOPP a combination of the anticancer drugs MUSTARGEN, ONCOVIN (VINCRISTINE), PROCARBAZINE, and PREDNISONE used in the treatment of HODGKIN'S DISEASE. See individual drug listings for side effects.

See also COMBINATION CHEMOTHERAPY.

morbidity the condition of being ill or diseased. The term can also be used when referring to the adverse side effects of a treatment.

morbidity rate the number of people with a disease compared with the number of people without the disease in a given population during a specific period of time.

morphine (mor'fēn) a strong NARCOTIC drug commonly used to relieve or control pain in the management of cancer. It can be administered by IV (INTRAVENOUSLY), IM (INTRAMUSCULAR, into a muscle) or taken orally. It is available in slow-release tablets, which means its effects can last longer. It is available by prescription only.

See also MS CONTIN and ANALGESIC.

mortality rate   the number of deaths per standard unit of population during a year. In cancer, the mortality rate can be calculated for a specific type of cancer, age, race, or sex. For example, the mortality rate may be five deaths from STOMACH CANCER per 100,000 people.

Motrin   See NONSTEROIDAL ANTI-INFLAMMATORY DRUG.

mouth cancer   the presence of cancer cells in the mouth (oral cavity), including the lip, gums, cheeks, tongue, tonsils, and floor of the mouth. According to the Oral Cancer Foundation, some 30,000 Americans would be diagnosed with oral or pharyngeal cancer in 2005, with more than 8,000 deaths from these cancers. More men than women are affected.

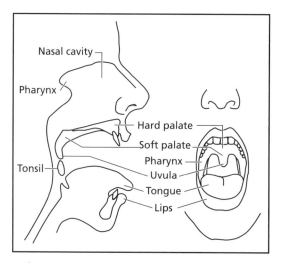

Side cutaway view and front view of the mouth. Courtesy NCI.

The primary cause of mouth cancer is tobacco use—SMOKING, chewing, and dipping (keeping powdered or finely ground tobacco tucked between the lip and gum, the cheek, and gum, or beneath the tongue). Smokers are four to 15 times more likely to develop cancer of the mouth. Another cause of this cancer is chronic or excessive alcohol consumption. Epidemiological research has indicated that the risk of cancer is higher among people who drink, even if they don't smoke. If they do smoke, the risk is multiplied. The risk of oral cancers is elevated more than 35-fold in heavy smokers and drinkers over abstainers.

Other risk factors include certain nutritional deficiencies. A lack of B vitamins and vitamin A, as well as the PLUMMER-VINSON SYNDROME, has been linked to the development of mouth cancer. Oral cancer can also develop in people with precancerous conditions such as LEUKOPLAKIA and ERYTHROPLAKIA. Leukoplakia is a whitish patch that may appear anywhere in the mouth. Erythroplakia is a reddened velvety patch that may appear in the mouth.

Another possible cause is poorly fitting dentures and bridges. Some studies have also shown that sharp or broken teeth that produce chronic irritation and/or infection may increase the risk of oral cancer. Too much sun can cause some cases of cancer of the lower lip, most often among white men over 40.

People who have had one oral cancer are at an increased risk of developing a new oral cancer, especially if they continue to smoke or drink.

Early cancers of the mouth may appear as red, slightly raised areas with ill-defined borders. Leukoplakia may also be present. Another symptom may be a lump that can be felt with the tip of the tongue or a sore that does not heal. Eating or drinking may be difficult and cause some soreness.

A symptom of lip cancer may be an enlarging growth that repeatedly forms a dry crust that bleeds when removed. It may not be painful unless it becomes an open sore or gets infected.

Cancer of the gum may appear as a toothache, loose teeth, or a sore that does not heal. Bleeding and mild pain may occur if the area is injured. Leukoplakia is frequently present.

A persistent sore is the most common symptom of cancer of the hard palate. The earliest symptom of cancer of the soft palate may be a sore throat that is made worse by eating or drinking.

The most common symptom of tongue cancer is a mild irritation. Pain may only occur during eating or drinking. Extensive involvement of the muscles of the tongue can affect speech and swallowing. Advanced tumors may produce a foul smell.

Cancer in the tonsils often does not produce any symptoms until it is somewhat advanced, at which point there may be a sore throat that is aggravated by eating and drinking, and an earache.

All of the symptoms described above may be symptoms of many other disorders besides cancer. A doctor should be consulted when symptoms persist and/or worsen.

Diagnostic procedures may include a manual exam by the doctor (or dentist), X-RAYS, and BIOPSY (microscopic examination of cells for cancer).

Following is the National Cancer Institute's (NCI) staging for cancer of the mouth:

- Stage I—cancer is no more than two CENTIMETERS (cm) (about one inch) and has not spread to LYMPH NODES in the area
- Stage II—the cancer is more than 2 cm but less than 4, and has not spread to lymph nodes
- Stage III
  — the cancer is more than 4 cm or
  — the cancer is any size but has spread to only one lymph node on the same side of the neck as the cancer; that lymph node is no larger than 3 cm
- Stage IV
  — the cancer has spread to tissues around the lip and oral cavity; the lymph nodes may or may not contain cancer or
  — the cancer is any size and has spread to more than one lymph node on the same side of the neck as the cancer, to lymph nodes on one or both sides of the neck, or to any lymph nodes that measures more than 6 cm or
  — the cancer has spread to other parts of the body
- Recurrent—the cancer has returned to the original site or to another part of the body after treatment

Treatment depends on the stage of the disease, its location, the general state of health of the patient, and other factors. The two standard treatments for mouth cancer are surgery, the most common treatment, and RADIATION THERAPY. For spe-cific information on the latest state-of-the-art treatment, by stage, call NCI's Cancer Information Service at 1-800-4-CANCER (1-800-422-6237), or for a TTY: 1-800-332-8615.

See also HEAD AND NECK CANCER.

mouth sores   See STOMATITIS.

mouthwash   a possible carcinogen. Studies suggest that people who use mouthwash with an alcohol content of 25% or greater are at a slightly increased risk of developing lip, tongue, mouth, or pharynx cancer. Men are at a greater risk than women.

MP [Leukerin]   See 6-MP.

MP   a combination of the anticancer drugs ALKERAN and PREDNISONE that may be used in the treatment of MYELOMA. See individual drug listings for side effects.

See also COMBINATION CHEMOTHERAPY.

M-Protein   an abnormal monoclonal protein (immunoglobulin) produced in measurable quantities by certain plasma cell disorders (see MYELOMA and MGUS). The measure of this protein in the plasma or urine may be diagnostic and act as a TUMOR MARKER to be followed with treatment over time. For myeloma, the level of the M-Protein reflects the quantity of plasma cell tumor bulk (see PLASMACYTOMA).

MRI (magnetic resonance imaging) [formerly known as "nuclear magnetic resonance"]   a highly sophisticated technique to examine the body. MRI produces internal pictures of the body using powerful electromagnets, radiofrequency waves, and a computer. It can produce images of blood vessels, blood flow, cerebro spinal fluid, cartilage, bone marrow, muscles, ligaments, and the spinal cord. It is used, along with other procedures, in the diagnosis and evaluation (the extent) of disease and to monitor for the recurrence of cancer as well as other disorders.

In 1946 two American scientists demonstrated the basic principles of MRI. They used it to analyze small chemical samples by exposing them to magnetic fields. Since then, it has been used by industry in the development of drugs, plastics, and other

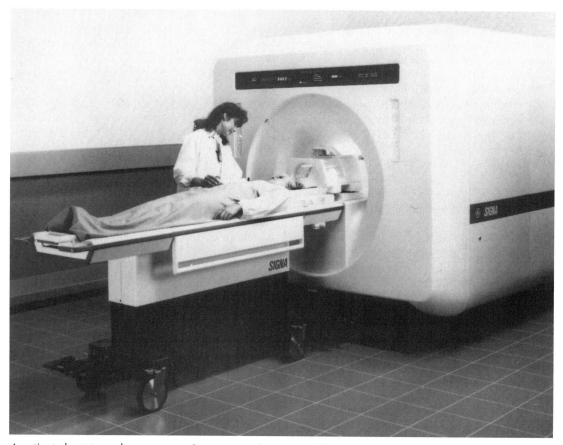

A patient about to undergo a magnetic resonance imaging (MRI) scan. Courtesy GE Medical Systems.

materials. In the mid-1970s a British company produced the first MRI of a human head. In 1989 there were some 1,200 MRI scanners operating in the United States.

MRI produces pictures similar to those taken by the CT SCAN but with greater definition. MRI is considered a safer procedure because RADIATION is not used, and dyes are rarely used. People with heart pacemakers, joint pins, surgical metal clips, artificial heart valves, an IUD, shrapnel, or any other electronic or metal implant may not be candidates for MRI. MRI may be done in conjunction with a CT SCAN and/or ULTRASOUND.

The scan takes approximately 30 minutes to an hour. The patient lies still, on a table, and the pic-

tures are taken. The patient's position does not have to be changed during the procedure. Parents can stay with a child while the scan is done.

MRI appears to be the most effective procedure for diagnosis of HEAD AND NECK CANCERS. Investigation of the neurological system (brain and spinal cord) is best accomplished by MRI.

MS Contin the NARCOTIC drug MORPHINE in a continuously acting pill. Its effects last longer so it can be taken less frequently. It is available by prescription only.

MSI (microsatellite instability) Microsatellites sequences are short sequences repeated up to hundreds of times that occur normally in DNA. However, where DNA repair systems are abnormal, such as when there are mutations in mismatch repair genes, abnormally long or short microsatellite sequences tend to accumulate. High levels of MSI are suggestive of the presence of HNPCC-related mutations, which may suggest an increased risk of colon cancer.

MTP-PE [muramyl tripeptide phosphatidyl-ethanolamine]   a synthetic drug that can activate the WHITE BLOOD CELLS called MONOCYTES and MACROPHAGES in the IMMUNE SYSTEM (primarily in the lungs and liver). Its role in the treatment of cancer is under investigation.

MTX   See METHOTREXATE.

mucinous breast carcinoma (mu'sĭ-nus kar"sĭ-no'mah)   a type of BREAST CANCER. It accounts for about 2% of all breast cancers. It appears in the ducts and produces mucus. It is usually slow growing and does not tend to spread outside the breast.

mucositis   See STOMATITIS.

mucous membrane (mu'kus)   the delicate tissues lining the inside of the nose, mouth, throat, vagina, and other tissues.

mullerian tumor (mil-e're-an)   a rare cancer of the uterus, ovary, or fallopian tubes (tubes that connect the ovaries with the womb) that arises from remnants of embryonic tissue (tissue left in the body from the first seven or eight weeks of the developing fetus). It occurs most often in women aged 55 to 60. One symptom may be vaginal bleeding, although this is also a symptom for other disorders. Diagnosis is usually made by performing a D & C. The primary treatment is surgical removal of the uterus, fallopian tubes, and ovaries. For the latest state-of-the-art treatment, call the National Cancer Institute's Cancer Information Service at 1-800-4-CANCER (1-800-422-6237), or for a TTY: 1-800-332-8615.

multicentric disease [polycentric disease]   the development of disease in different sites in the same part of the body—for example, the presence of more than one cancerous tumor in a breast or the bladder. This is *not* METASTATIC CANCER (cancer that has spread).

multicolony-stimulating factor   See INTERLEUKIN-3.

multi-CSF   See INTERLEUKIN-3.

multidrug chemotherapy   See COMBINATION CHEMO-THERAPY.

multidrug resistance (MDR)   a condition in a person in which certain cancer cells exhibit broad resistance to multiple CHEMOTHERAPY (anticancer drugs). This has been associated with a measurable protein, P-glycoprotein. MDR is associated with a genetic mutation of the P-glycoprotein gene. See PSC-833.

multifocal osteosarcoma (os"te-o-sar-ko'mah)   cancer that occurs in several bones spontaneously or that arises in just one bone and metastasizes (spreads) to other bones without affecting the lungs. It does not have a good prognosis. See OSTEOSARCOMA.

multi-modality treatment   See COMBINATION TREATMENT.

multiple basal cell carcinoma syndrome   a rare hereditary condition resulting in skin that is very sensitive to ULTRAVIOLET RADIATION, one type of radiation from the sun. People with this syndrome are at a greater risk of developing SKIN CANCER. They can develop skin cancers on many areas of the body, including those of the palms of the hands and soles of the feet, where skin cancer usually does not occur.

multiple endocrine neoplasia [MEN] (en'do-krin ne"o-pla'ze-ah)   a small group of genetically transmitted syndromes involving different ENDO-CRINE components (THYROID, ADRENAL GLAND, etc). This was initially described in 1954 and occurs in children. These rare tumors should be seen by endocrinologists. They may be benign or malignant. Additional components of MEN may be ISLET CELL CARCINOMA of the pancreas and PARATHYROID GLAND CANCER.

See also ENDOCRINE CANCERS.

multiple myeloma   See MYELOMA.

muramyl tripeptide phosphatidylethanolamine
See MTP-PE.

mustard gas   an odorless, colorless, oily liquid that was used in chemical warfare during World War I. Several studies have shown an increased mortality from respiratory tract cancer among individuals exposed to mustard gas. See CARCINOGENS.

Mustargen (mus'tar-jen) [mechlorethamine, HN2, nitrogen mustard]   an ALKYLATING anticancer drug sometimes used in the treatment of HODGKIN'S DISEASE, NON-HODGKIN'S LYMPHOMA, LUNG CANCER, and MYCOSIS FUNGOIDES. NITROGEN MUSTARD was the first anticancer drug to be investigated in a clinical trial and found to produce responses in patients with cancer of the lymph glands, LYMPHOMA. It was used in gas warfare during World War II, and when American seamen were accidentally exposed to it, their lymph glands were affected. It was then given to patients with lymphoma and evaluated. It is given by IV (injection into a vein). Side effects may include severe nausea, vomiting, irritation of veins, and burning pain where the needle was inserted if the drug leaks out during the IV. Occasional and rare side effects may include BONE MARROW DEPRESSION, hair loss, skin rash, menstrual irregularities, and fever.

Mutamycin (mu''tah-mi'sin) [MITO, mitomycin-C, mitomycin]   an ANTIBIOTIC anticancer drug sometimes used in the treatment of cancers of the breast, stomach, pancreas, cervix, colon, and bladder. It is given by IV (injection into a vein). Common side effects may include nausea and vomiting. Occasional or rare side effects may include BONE MARROW DEPRESSION, kidney problems, hair loss, fatigue, lung problems, diarrhea, fever, mouth sores, and blurred vision. A unique side effect is the development of HEMOLYSIS, which may be fatal.

MV   a combination of the anticancer drugs MITOXANTRONE and VePesid (ETOPOSIDE) sometimes used in the treatment of ANLL. See individual drug listings for side effects.
See also COMBINATION CHEMOTHERAPY.

MVAC   See M-VAC.

M-VAC [MVAC]   a combination of the anticancer drugs METHOTREXATE, VINBLASTINE, ADRIAMYCIN, and CISPLATIN sometimes used in the treatment of cancers of the kidney, pancreas, and bladder. See individual drug listings for side effects.
See also COMBINATION CHEMOTHERAPY.

MVPP   a combination of the anticancer drugs MUSTARGEN, VINBLASTINE, PROCARBAZINE, and PREDNISONE sometimes used in the treatment of HODGKIN'S DISEASE. See individual drug listings for side effects.
See also COMBINATION CHEMOTHERAPY.

myasthenia gravis (mi''as-the'ne-ah)   a condition characterized by profound muscle weakness, fatigue, mouth dryness, dysarthria (stammering; difficulty in pronouncing words), dysphasia (difficulty swallowing), blurred vision, and muscle pain. It may occur as a primary disorder or as a result of cancer. It has been associated with THYMOMA.

myasthenic syndrome (mi''as-then'-ik) [Eaton-Lambert syndrome]   a rare condition that has been associated with SMALL CELL LUNG CANCER. As many as 6% of the people diagnosed with it are affected. The symptoms are the same as those that occur with MYASTHENIA GRAVIS. Treatment of combination chemotherapy for the cancer will frequently relieve a patient of these symptoms as well.

mycosis fungoides (mi-ko'sis fun-goi-'dēs) [cutaneous T-cell lymphoma, T-cell lymphoma]   a rare cancer of the LYMPHOCYTES (WHITE BLOOD CELLS) affecting the skin. It is related to NON-HODGKIN'S LYMPHOMA and LEUKEMIA. It was first described by J. L. Alibert in Paris in 1806. He named it mycosis fungoides because of the mushroom-like appearance of the tumors in an advanced stage of the disease. (The disease is not related to fungus.)
Mycosis fungoides is believed to be caused by the uncontrolled growth of helper T cells (a type of white blood cell that regulates the antibody production of B cells). It is commonly preceded by a long history of skin disorders such as chronic eczema (an itching disease of the skin) and psoria-

sis (a chronic skin disease characterized by red scaly patches on the skin).

The first symptoms are usually a generalized itching and areas of raised, reddened skin. It can appear just about anywhere on the body—the face, scalp, arms, legs, etc. Mycosis fungoides frequently progresses very slowly, and it can appear as raised patches of skin for many years. The patches of skin (tumors) may eventually ulcerate as the disease progresses, and the LYMPH NODES may become enlarged and appear as lymphomas.

Following is the NATIONAL CANCER INSTITUTE'S (NCI) STAGING for mycosis fungoides:

- Stage I—localized redness and/or some raised surfaces of the skin that may involve either a minimal amount or the majority of the skin; skin tumors are not present and lymph nodes are not enlarged
- Stage II—skin tumors or ulcers, or clinically enlarged lymph nodes that on biopsy are benign (noncancerous)
- Stage III—a general redness of the entire skin; cancer cells are nearly always circulating in the blood; there may be enlarged lymph nodes that are benign
- Stage IV—cancer has spread to the lymph nodes or internal organs, most often the liver or lung; cancer cells are often circulating in the blood
- Recurrent—cancer has returned to the same site or to another location in the body after treatment.

Treatment depends on the stage of the disease and other factors. The most common form of treatment is RADIATION THERAPY. Other treatments may include PHOTODYNAMIC THERAPY, PHOTOPHERESIS, PUVA THERAPY, BIOLOGICAL THERAPY, and CHEMO-THERAPY. For specific information on the latest state-of-the-art treatment, by stage, call NCI's Cancer Information Service at 1-800-4-CANCER (1-800-422-6237), or for a TTY: 1-800-332-8615. See SEZARY SYNDROME.

myeloblastoma See CHLOROMA.

myelocyte See GRANULOCYTE.

myelodysplastic syndrome (mi″ĕ-lo-dis-plas′tik) **(MDS)** [preleukemia and smoldering leukemia]

hematologically (relating to issues of the blood) diverse group of STEM CELL MALIGNANCIES that have a varied course, a complex nomnclature and until 2004, no specific therapy. The end result of MDS is ineffective hematopoesis (blood cell production), involving one or more cell lines (red blood cells, white blood cells, PLATELETS). MDS progresses to ACUTE MYELOGENOUS LEUKEMIA (AML) in 35% of patients. An older name for some in this grouping was preleukemia or SMOLDERING LEUKEMIA.

MDS can occur as a primary disorder or secondary to prior exposure to certain CHEMOTHERA-PEUTICS or RADIATION. Genetic abnormalities provide a useful guide to prognosis (see 50 MINUS SYNDROME). Put another way, MDS is a clonal disorder of multilineage blood CELL precursors. In the BONE MARROW there is ineffective blood cell production with resulting peripheral cytopenias (low cell counts). As the marrow fails, patients may succumb to infections or to AML. Symptoms relate to which blood cell line is depressed (causing ANEMIA, INFECTION, or bleeding). There are approximately 25,000 new cases in the United States each year; the median age of onset is over 60 years of age.

Mortality from MDS is about 50% over three to four years. The standard treatment has been "supportive care" for most (such as antibiotics, growth factors, and transfusions). CHEMOTHERAPY has been ineffective. ALLOGENEIC STEM CELL TRANSPLANTA-TION is potentially curative but only available to a minority of patients because of the advanced age of most people when they get MDS.

In 2004, the chemotherapeutic drug AZACYTA-DINE (AZC OR Vidaza) was the first drug approved by the FDA specifically to treat MDS. DECYTADEN, a more potent AZC is currently being evaluated. These drugs are thought to restore healthy differentiation to the AML cells. THALIDOMIDE is also useful in some patients and clinical studies are ongoing. For specific information on the latest state-of-the-art treatment, call the NCI information service at 1-800-4-CANCER (1-800-422-6237) or for a TTY: 1-800-332-8615.

myelofibrosis (mi″ĕ-lo-fi-bro′sis) a disease in which the BONE MARROW is replaced by fibrous tissue. This may occur as a primary pathologic process or may be part of another underlying illness, such as chronic myelogenous leukemia. See CML and MYELOPROLIFERATIVE DISORDERS.

myelogram   See MYELOGRAPHY.

myelography (mi″ĕ-log′rah-fe) an examination of the spinal cord. An X-RAY of the spinal cord is taken after injection of a CONTRAST MEDIUM into the fluid surrounding the cord. The dye makes the outline of the spinal cord and adjacent structures visible on the X-ray film (the myelogram).

myeloma (mi″ĕ-lo′mah) cancer arising in the plasma cells in the BONE MARROW. It is the primary cancer of the several conditions that fall under the general term of "plasma cell neoplasms" or "plasma cell dyscrasias." The two other plasma cell neoplasms are macroglobulinemia and PLASMACYTOMA (plasma cell tumor). (When there are multiple plasmacytomas, it is called multiple myeloma.) Heavy chain disease is a rare form of multiple myeloma.

The American Cancer Society estimated there would be some 15,980 new cases of multiple myeloma (8,600 in men and 7,380 in women) in 2005, with about 11,300 (5,660 men and 5,640 women) deaths from the disease in 2005. It occurs about equally in men and women. It can develop in any age range, starting at young adulthood, but occurs most commonly in people in their 50s.

Although the cause of myeloma is not known, there is some evidence to suggest that genetic factors may predispose some people to developing myeloma. The number of myeloma cases seems to be increased in first-degree relatives. Other factors that may play a role in the development of myeloma are exposure to petroleum products in the workplace and exposure to high levels of radiation.

The first symptom of myeloma is bone pain (which is a symptom of many other disorders as well). The bone pain is caused by the infiltration of the plasma cells into the bone marrow, resulting in gradual destruction of the bone. The pain may start out as a mild annoyance, or it may be quite severe, often resulting from a spontaneous bone fracture. Eventually there can be deformities in the skeleton, particularly of the ribs and sternum (breastbone), and a shortening of the spine. Other symptoms may include abnormal bleeding, painful swelling on the ribs, and susceptibility to infections. Almost all patients suffer from ANEMIA either at the time of diagnosis or as the disease progresses. There is also an increased susceptibility to shingles (a viral infection of the nerve path). Hypercalcemia may be a problem.

Procedures used in the diagnosis and evaluation of myeloma may include X-RAYS, BONE MARROW ASPIRATION, blood and urine tests, and the ERYTHROCYTE SEDIMENTATION RATE. The presence of the BENCE JONES PROTEIN in the urine may be an indication of myeloma.

Following is the National Cancer Institute's (NCI) staging for myeloma and other plasma cell neoplasms:

- Stage I—multiple myeloma—relatively few malignant (cancerous) cells have spread throughout the body; bone X-rays are normal or show only one localized growth (plasmacytoma) in the bone; the level of M-protein in the blood or urine is low; the red blood cell count is normal
- Stage II—multiple myeloma—a moderate number of malignant cells have spread throughout the body
- Stage III—a relatively large number of cancer cells have spread throughout the body, more than three bone lesions are present, or there are high levels of M-protein in the blood or urine
- isolated plasmacytoma of the bone—a single plasma cell tumor is in the bone, generally without further evidence of disease
- extramedullary plasmacytoma—isolated plasma cell tumors of soft tissues occurring most commonly in the bones or areas around the nose; no signs of tumors in the bones
- macroglobulinemia—an increase in the plasma blood cells producing a specific M-protein; enlarged lymph nodes and spleen; usually no tumors in the bones
- monoclonal gammopathy of undetermined significance—elevation of low levels of the M-protein in the blood; there are no other symptoms, signs, or evidence of disease. (see MGUS)

Treatment depends on the stage of the disease, the general state of health of the patient, and other factors. In a very early stage it may not be immediately treated. Generally treatment consists of CHEMOTHERAPY (anticancer drugs), RADIATION THERAPY, and occasionally surgery. For specific information on the latest state-of-the-art treatment, by stage, call NCI's Cancer Information Service at 1-800-4-CANCER (1-800-422-6237), or for a TTY: 1-800-332-8615.

myeloproliferative disorders (mi″ĕ-lo-pro-lif′er-a″tiv)   a term used to describe three different blood disorders, only one of which, chronic myelogenous leukemia (CML), is cancerous. The others are:

- polycythemia vera—a disorder characterized primarily by uncontrolled production of RED BLOOD CELLS. There may also be an increase in the WHITE BLOOD CELLS and PLATELETS. With treatment, many patients can live with this condition for years. One possible complication is the development of chronic myelogenous leukemia.
- agnogenic myeloid metaplasia—a disorder in which red and white blood cells and platelets, which may not have matured, are produced outside the BONE MARROW, primarily in the liver and/or spleen, resulting in an enlarged liver or spleen.
- essential thrombocythemia—a disorder in which the platelet count may be much higher than normal without an increase in red blood cells.

There is no formal STAGING for these disorders. Treatment depends on the particular disorder and other factors. Myeloproliferative disorders are treated by hematologists. A substantial number of cases will transform into acute myelogenous leukemia. For specific information on the latest state-of-the-art treatment, call the National Cancer Institute's Cancer Information Service at 1-800-4-CANCER (1-800-422-6237), or for a TTY: 1-800-332-8615. or visit the NCI Web site at http://www.cancer.gov.

myeloproliferative disorders, chronic   These are POLYCYTHEMIA VERA (or P. Vera), ESSENTIAL THROMOCYTHEMIA (ET), AND idiopathic (of unknown origin) MYELOFIBROSIS. They arise from a multipotent progenitor cell.

myelosuppression (mi″ĕlo-sŭ-pre′shun)   a condition in which the BONE MARROW has a decreased production of the elements it normally, primarily blood cells. This can be a side effect of CHEMOTHERAPY (anticancer) or RADIATION THERAPY. In certain instances myelosuppression is intentionally induced.

See MYELOSUPPRESSION CHEMOTHERAPY.

myelosuppression chemotherapy (mi″ĕ-lo-sŭ-pres′shun ke″mo-ther′ah-pe)   using anticancer drugs to intentionally decrease the bone marrow's production of blood cells. Myelosuppression may be used in the treatment of primary disease of the bone marrow such as LEUKEMIA, polycythemia vera (an increase in the red blood cells), essential thrombocythemia (a high platelet count with no increase in red blood cells), and other disorders. Myelosuppression can also be an unwanted side effect of CHEMOTHERAPY and RADIATION THERAPY.

myleran   See BUSULFAN.

MYX   See METHOTREXATE.

myxoma (milk-so′mah)   an uncommon, benign (noncancerous) soft-tissue tumor.

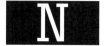

nandrolone decanoate [Deca-Durabolin] See ANDROGEN.

nandrolone phenpropionate [Durabolin] See ANDROGEN.

narcotic the most potent of the ANALGESIC drugs. Narcotics are known as "controlled substances" because they are regulated by both federal and state authorities. They are opiate derivatives and are available only with a doctor's prescription. Narcotics are the strongest painkillers available. They are regularly used after surgery for short-term control of pain for a few days. For chronic pain associated with cancer, they are usually given at regular intervals, the goal being to keep the patient pain free. Sometimes they are given in combination with antidepressants and/or mild sedatives. Over time, some patients may need higher doses of the narcotic as they build up tolerance for the drug, or are given a different narcotic.

Among the more commonly prescribed narcotics are CODEINE, PERCODAN, oxycodone in Percodan, MORPHINE, MS CONTIN, DILAUDID (hydromorphone), METHADONE (Dolophine), DEMEROL (meperidine), LEVODROMORAN (levorphanol), and NUMORPHAN (oxymorphone). HEROIN is also a narcotic that has been used in England as a pain medication. Several studies conducted in the United States have concluded that heroin does not appear to be any better than morphine in controlling pain.

Narcotics work by targeting and attaching to specific receptors in the brain that register pain. When the receptors are blocked, the pain is lessened. Side effects of narcotics may include sedation, nausea, vomiting, constipation, and depressed respiration. A "bowel regimen" is recommended to prevent constipation.

nasal cavity cancer See PARANASAL SINUS/NASAL CAVITY CANCER.

nasogastric tube (na"zo-gas'trik) a CATHETER that is inserted through the nose and throat and into the stomach. A nasogastric tube may be used in a patient with CANCER who is not getting sufficient nutrients. Supplemental nutrients can be administered through the tube.

nasopharyngeal cancer (na"zo-fah-rin'je-al) cancer of the lining of the area of the pharynx above the palate that connects the mouth and nose with the esophagus (the tube connecting the stomach and throat). This is a fairly uncommon cancer in the United States, occurring about three times as often in men as in women. About 20% of the people developing this cancer are younger than 30.

Symptoms may include pain and pressure in the cheek, a toothache, persistent draining of the sinus after tooth extraction, a nasal quality to the voice, a lump in the cheek, or bloodstained discharge from the nose.

Diagnostic procedures may include X-RAYS of the facial bones, examination by a head light and mirror, NASOPHARYNGOSCOPY, and BIOPSY.

Following is the National Cancer Institute's (NCI) staging for nasopharyngeal cancer:

- Stage I—the tumor, if visible, is confined to one area of the nasopharynx and there is no evidence of spread to the LYMPH NODES or to other parts of the body
- Stage II—the tumor involves more than one area of the nasopharynx and there is no evidence of spread to lymph nodes or to other parts of the body
- Stage III
  — the tumor extends into the nasal cavity or oropharynx but has not spread to lymph nodes or other parts of the body or
  — the primary tumor is confined to the nasopharynx but has spread to only single lymph node on the same side of the neck and is three CENTIMETERS (cm) or less in its greatest dimension
- Stage IV
  — the primary tumor has invaded the skull and/or involves cranial nerves; there is no spread to distant parts of the body and there is no more than one lymph node involved by tumor on the same side of the neck as the primary tumor and is no more than 3 cm in greatest dimension or
  — there is one abnormal lymph node larger than 3 cm in its greatest dimension, there are multiple abnormal nodes of any size on the same side of the neck as the primary tumor, there are abnormal nodes of any size on both sides of the neck or there is one or more abnormal nodes on the opposite side of the neck from the primary or
  — there is evidence of spread to distant parts of the body
- Recurrent—the cancer has returned after treatment to the original location or another part of the body

Treatment depends on the stage of the disease, the general state of health of the patient, and other factors. The most common treatment is RADIATION THERAPY. EXTERNAL RADIATION THERAPY or INTERNAL RADIATION may be used. Surgery may be performed if the cancer does not respond to radiation therapy. CHEMOTHERAPY (anticancer drugs) may also be used. For specific information on the latest state-of-the-art treatment, by stage, call NCI's Cancer Information Service at 1-800-4-CANCER (1-800-422-6237), or for a TTY: 1-800-332-8615.

See also HEAD AND NECK CANCER.

nasopharyngoscope See NASOPHARYNGOSCOPY.

nasopharyngoscopy (na"zo-fah"rin-gos'ko-pe) an examination of the upper airway. A nasopharyngoscope, a flexible instrument for viewing the upper airway, is used for this diagnostic procedure. During the examination the nasopharyngoscope may be used to obtain tissue for a BIOPSY. It may be used in the diagnosis of NASOPHARYNGEAL CANCER.

nasopharynx (na"zo-far'inks) the part of the pharynx that lies above the palate. Air from the nasal cavities passes through the nasopharynx.

National Cancer Act legislation passed in the United States in 1937. The National Cancer Act guaranteed, for the first time, the use of federal funds for research into cancer. The act also established the NATIONAL CANCER INSTITUTE (NCI). The NCI has been the mainstay of cancer research in the United States and has served worldwide as a model for cancer research.

National Cancer Institute (NCI) an agency of the United States government charged with conducting cancer research for treatment, detection, diagnosis, prevention, control, and rehabilitation of the disease. The National Cancer Institute is the largest of the 12 National Institutes of Health in Bethesda, Maryland.

NCI was founded in 1937 when the NATIONAL CANCER ACT was passed. Its programs were intensified in 1971 after passage of a second National Cancer Act.

NCI supports the CLINICAL CANCER CENTERS that have been established in many medical centers and designates as COMPREHENSIVE CANCER CENTERS those institutions that offer the most extensive range of cancer treatment in the United States. NCI also encourages and supports CLINICAL TRIALS at institutions all over the country.

NCI's immediate goal is to eliminate the suffering and death due to cancer: a challenge to cancer by 2015. To achieve this goal, the institute will focus on the concept of preemption with four objectives: by striving to prevent cancer before it starts, identify cancers that do develop at the earliest stage, eliminate cancers through innovative treatment interventions, and biologically control those cancers that we cannot eliminate so they become manageable, chronic diseases. NCI STAGING guidelines are used for most cancers. NCI's Web site is a comprehensive tool for learning about all facets of cancer in general as well as specific cancers; the address is: http://www.cancer.gov/ and includes a live, online interactive service during specified business hours. NCI also maintains a Cancer Information Service that may be reached at 1-800-4-CANCER (1-800-422-6237), or for a TTY: 1-800-332-8615.

National Center for Complementary and Alternative Medicine (NCCAM) The National Center for Complementary and Alternative Medicine is one of the 27 institutes and centers that make up the National Institutes of Health (NIH). The NIH is one of eight agencies under the Public Health Service (PHS) in the Department of Health and Human Services (DHHS). Founded in 1992 by congressional mandate as the Office of Alternative Medicine, it was upgraded to a center in October 1998. Its purpose is to facilitate the evaluation of complementary and alternative medical (CAM) treatments. Its budget went from $2 million in 1992 to $122,692,000 appropriated by Congress for fiscal year 2006. NCCAM has 75 full-time employees. As of 2005, there were 29 NCCAM funded research centers in the United States to study alternative and complementary treatments for specific health conditions. Two of the 29 centers are devoted to the study of CAM treatments and modalities for cancer. These are: The Johns Hopkins Center for Cancer Complementary Medicine (see www.hopkinsmedicine.org/CAM/about/organization.html). The center is devoted to the study of antioxidant effects of herbs in cancer cells; the antioxidant and anti-inflammatory properties of soy and tart cherry on aspects of cancer pain in four animal models; and the safety and efficacy of fish oil supplements for weight mainte-

nance in pancreatic cancer patients. The other center is the Specialized Center of Research in Hyperbaric Oxygen Therapy University of Pennsylvania, where researchers are conducting four projects to examine the mechanisms of action, safety, and clinical efficacy of hyperbaric oxygen therapy for head and neck tumors. The center will develop and validate a model to predict who benefits from hyperbaric oxygen treatment after laryngectomy; examine the effects of hyperbaric oxygen on growth of blood vessels and tumors; characterize the effects of hyperbaric oxygen on cell adhesion and growth of metastatic tumor cells in the lung; and test the effects of elevated oxygen pressures on cellular levels of nitric oxide.

Other CAM treatments for cancer that are being studied include massage therapy, acupuncture, electrochemical DC current, music therapy, imagery and relaxation, macrobiotic diet, hypnosis, garlic, green tea, and other teas, antioxidant vitamins, and yoga. The NCCAM Web site offers comprehensive, searchable information: http://nccam.nih.gov/

National Surgical Adjuvant Breast and Bowel Project (NSABP) a program organized in 1957 by the NATIONAL CANCER INSTITUTE to conduct studies on the treatment of BREAST CANCER. The program expanded to study issues surrounding COLORECTAL CANCER. Some of the studies have resulted in new standards of treatment. The NSABP also provides a way for physicians throughout the United States and abroad to share information from various CLINICAL TRIALS being conducted. The Office of the Chairman and the NSABP Operations Center are located on the campus of Allegheny General Hospital, and the group's Biostatistical Center is at the University of Pittsburgh.

In 1958, the NSABP undertook a study to evaluate the effectiveness of adjuvant CHEMOTHERAPY following breast cancer surgery. Patients were treated with low doses of anticancer drugs for two days after surgery. Premenopausal women with four or more positive lymph nodes who received the chemotherapy had an improved five- and 10-year survival rate.

In 1971, the NSABP undertook a 10-year study to evaluate the various types of MASTECTOMY used as treatment for breast cancer. More than 1,600 women in the United States and Canada who had undergone simply mastectomy (removal of only the breast; a few axillary lymph nodes may be removed), radical mastectomy, and modified mastectomy were followed. The results of the study, published in 1985, concluded that the simple mastectomy had the same survival rate as the radical or modified mastectomy when used in the treatment of early breast cancers.

In 1976, the NSABP undertook another study to compare LUMPECTOMY, with and without radiation, with simple mastectomy. More than 1,800 women in the United States and abroad who were all either stage I or stage II with tumors no larger than four CENTIMETERS took part in the study. The study found that lumpectomy with radiation therapy was as effective as a simple mastectomy in terms of five-year survival. In addition, it was the NSABP's breast cancer studies that led to the establishment of lumpectomy plus RADIATION over RADICAL MASTECTOMY as the standard surgical treatment for breast cancer. The NSABP was the first to demonstrate that adjuvant therapy could alter the natural history of breast cancer, increasing survival rates, and the first to demonstrate on a large scale the preventive effects of the drug TAMOXIFEN in breast cancer.

The NSABP continues to conduct studies into the most effective treatments for breast cancer. (See the NSABP Web site: http://www.nsabp.pitt.edu)

natural killer cell [NK cell]   a type of large lymphocyte (WHITE BLOOD CELL) that contains potent chemicals and attacks tumor cells and infected body cells. Natural killer cells kill on contact by binding to the "target" cell and then releasing a lethal burst of chemicals. Normal cells are not affected by natural killer cells. Natural killer cells are thought to play a major role in cancer prevention by destroying abnormal cells before they have a chance to pose a real threat.

nausea and vomiting   one of the most common side effects of CHEMOTHERAPY (anticancer drugs). It can also be a side effect of RADIATION THERAPY to the gastrointestinal tract, liver, or brain or be a result of the cancer itself. It is one of the most dreaded side effects and can have a physical as well as psychological impact on a patient. Nausea and vomiting can lead to nutrition depletion and a general deteriora-

tion of the patient's physical condition. It can also lead to the patient's quitting a treatment that could be potentially curative or useful as well as to a decrease in self-care and functional ability.

Acute nausea and vomiting can occur from within minutes to several hours of the administration of the chemotherapy and subside within 24 hours. Delayed nausea and vomiting may occur after several hours and last several days. Drugs associated with delayed nausea and vomiting are CISPLATIN, Cytoxan, Adriamycin, and IFOSFAMIDE. In some patients nausea and vomiting occurs before the chemotherapy is administered. This is known as ANTICIPATORY NAUSEA AND VOMITING and is a conditioned response.

Not all patients experience nausea and vomiting, although a common misconception is that anyone on chemotherapy does. Among patients who do experience it, its severity can vary depending on many factors, including the particular drug, the dose, its schedule of administration, and the patient. In general, children are not as affected as adults. Not experiencing nausea and vomiting does not mean the chemotherapy is not working.

Progress has been made in understanding the mechanisms that cause nausea and vomiting as well as its management. Antiemetic (antinausea) drugs are the greatest defense against nausea and vomiting. They may be given before administration of the chemotherapy, during its administration, and/or after its administration. Combination antiemetics may also be given. Other methods of controlling nausea and vomiting may include HYPNOSIS, ACUPUNCTURE, distraction, RELAXATION TECHNIQUES, and IMAGERY.

Investigation into new and more effective ways of managing nausea and vomiting continues.

Navelbine [vinorelbine, NVP]   an anticancer drug used alone or in combination with CISPLATIN for the treatment of patients with unresectable, advanced NON-SMALL CELL LUNG CANCER, BREAST CANCER, and OVARIAN CANCER. Possible side effects may include anemia, nausea and vomiting, hair loss, chest pain, difficulty breathing, fatigue, constipation, pain in jaw, or tumor. It is taken orally or by IV (injected into a vein).

NCI   See NATIONAL CANCER INSTITUTE.

neck dissection   the surgical removal of lymph glands and some surrounding structures within the neck.

needle aspiration biopsy (as"pĭ-ra'shun bi'op-se) [aspiration biopsy, fine needle biopsy, fine needle aspiration (FNA), and suction biopsy]   removal of a small piece of tissue or fluid (in the case of a cyst) from a suspicious mass in the body by hypodermic needle and syringe. The tissue is then microscopically examined for cancer cells.

Needle aspiration biopsy is performed frequently. It is less costly, causes less discomfort, and has a lower risk of infection than a SURGICAL BIOPSY. It can be done in the doctor's office and has a high level of accuracy.

A needle aspiration biopsy is frequently used in the diagnosis of breast cancer. It may also be used in the biopsy of cancers of the eye, lung, liver, gallbladder, thyroid, prostate, bile ducts, and pancreas and myeloma among others. A CORE NEEDLE BIOPSY is similar to the needle aspiration but uses a wider needle in order to get a bigger tissue sample.

needle biopsy   See CORE NEEDLE BIOPSY.

needle implant   See INTERSTITIAL RADIATION.

needle localization   a technique to locate a small, suspicious area on the breast identified during MAMMOGRAPHY so that a BIOPSY can be performed. The radiologist uses the mammogram to find the area and marks the skin directly above it with a pen. A thin, hollow needle with a wire, about the size of a strand of hair, is then inserted into the breast at that spot. Another mammogram is done to make sure that the needle is in the right place. When it is confirmed that it is, the needle is removed and the wire is left in the breast. The wire enables the surgeon performing the biopsy to find the area, which cannot be seen with the naked eye. The surgeon removes the suspicious area as well as the wire.

neoadjuvant therapy (ne"o-ad'ju-vant) therapy given before the primary treatment (surgery) in order to shrink the cancerous tumor. This may be done because the tumor is too large to be removed. Shrinking it may make its removal possible.

Shrinking the tumor also makes the surgery less extensive. In Italy researchers are using neoadjuvant chemotherapy (anticancer drugs) to shrink large breast cancer tumors so that the mastectomy can be replaced with breast conservation surgery. Researchers think in some cases of very early cancer, neoadjuvant therapy might eliminate the need for surgery, with the administration of radiation therapy after the chemotherapy (anticancer drugs) to eliminate any remaining cancer cells. Neoadjuvant therapy is being used in France, where researchers are using chemotherapy to treat breast cancer in women with early-stage disease.

neocarzinostatin   See ZINOSTATIN.

neo-hombreol [testosterone   propionate] See ANDROGENS.

neoplasm (ne'o-plazm) an abnormal growth or tumor. Although it may be benign (noncancerous) or malignant (cancerous), the term usually refers to a malignancy.

neoplastic   referring to NEOPLASM.

Neosar   See CYTOXAN.

nephrectomy (nĕ-frek'to-me) [simple   nephrectomy] surgical removal of a kidney, a common treatment for KIDNEY CANCER as well as other disorders.

nephroblastoma   See WILMS' TUMOR.

nephrotomogram   See NEPHROTOMOGRAPHY.

nephrotomography (nef"ro-to-mog'rah-fe) a test to examine the kidneys. This procedure uses X-RAYS to obtain a three-dimensional picture of the kidneys after administration of a CONTRAST MEDIUM. It may be used in the diagnosis of KIDNEY CANCER as well as other disorders.

nephroureterectomy (nef"ro-u"re-ter-ek'to-me) surgical removal of the kidney, ureter, and top part of the bladder. It may be performed in the treatment of TRANSITIONAL CELL CANCER OF THE RENAL PELVIS AND URETER.

nerve block a technique using anesthesia to temporarily or permanently relieve pain in a specific area. A local anesthetic, which may be combined with CORTISONE, is injected into or around a nerve to numb or deaden the nerve fibers to give temporary relief of pain. For pain relief of longer duration, phenol (a strong antiseptic) or alcohol may be injected into the site. A side effect may be the loss of all feeling in the area, which makes a patient more vulnerable to injury. A nerve block is usually not performed until other, more conventional methods of pain relief have proved to be inadequate.

nerve root clipping a technique to relieve pain. Nerve roots high in the neck are cut to interrupt pain passages in the upper part of the body. This treatment is done generally after other, more conventional methods of pain relief have been unsuccessful.

nerve-sparing prostatectomy a surgical procedure used in the treatment of prostate cancer in which nerves are kept intact when the prostate is removed. Impotence and incontinence can result when the nerves are severed. The nerve-sparing procedure was developed in 1982 by a doctor at Johns Hopkins University and is used by most surgeons familiar with it. However, sparing the nerves is not always possible, and the procedure is not performed if treatment would be compromised in any way.

nervous system See CENTRAL NERVOUS SYSTEM.

Neulasta (pegfilgrastim) a long-lasting COLONY STIMULATING FACTOR indicated to decrease the incidence of infection, as manifested by FEBRILE NEUTROPENIA in patients with non-myeloid malignancies receiving MYELOSUPPRESSIVE anticancer drugs associated with a clinically significant incidence of FEBRILE NEUTROPENIA. The drug is given by subcutaneous injection.

Neumega See INTERLEUKIN-11.

Neupogen (nu'po-jen) See G-CSF.

neurinoma See NEUROMA.

neuroblastoma (nu"ro-blas-to'mah) a tumor that can arise anywhere in the sympathetic nervous system (the system that regulates tissues such as the glands, muscles, and the heart) but most commonly occurs in the abdomen. It is the fourth most common childhood cancer, occurring two-thirds of the time in children under the age of five. Alcohol, hair dye, and certain medicines taken during pregnancy may be a prenatal risk factor.

Symptoms may include signs of chronic illness such as slow growth rate, weight loss, lack of interest, irritability, intermittent diarrhea, fever, and abdominal pain. Diagnostic procedures may include an IVP, ULTRASOUND, X-RAYS of the chest and entire skeleton, a BONE MARROW TEST, and urinalysis for chemicals that are made by some tumor cells.

There are three different staging systems currently in use in the United States. Following is the National Cancer Institute's (NCI) staging for neuroblastoma:

- Localized resectable—the cancer is found only within the tissue where it first began and can be completely removed by surgery
- Localized unresectable—the cancer is only in one area where it began and cannot be completely removed during surgery
- Regional—the cancer has spread beyond the tissue where it first began, to adjacent tissues or to LYMPH NODES on both sides of the body
- Disseminated—the cancer has spread to other structures in the body such as the bones, organs, or distant lymph nodes
- Stage IVS (special)—usually occurs in infants; the primary tumor is relatively small but there is evidence of spread to the liver, skin, or bone marrow (but not the bones)
- Recurrent—cancer has returned to the same site or to another part of the body after treatment.

Treatment depends on the stage of the disease, the general state of health of the patient, and other factors including age. The most common treatment is SURGERY. CHEMOTHERAPY (anticancer drugs) and RADIATION THERAPY may also be used. For specific information on the latest state-of-the-art treatment, by stage, call NCI's Cancer Information Service at 1-800-4-CANCER (1-800-422-6237), or for a TTY: 1-800-332-8615.

See also EMBRYONAL CANCER.

neurofibroma   See NEUROMA.

neurofibromatosis (nu"ro-fi'bro-mah-to'sis) [Von Recklinghausen's disease, "elephant man" disease] an inherited disorder characterized by developmental changes in the nerves, muscles, bones, and skin. It may result in lumps all over the body. Although it is rarely fatal, as many as 25% of the people with this disorder develop cancer of the brain, spinal cord, ear, and eye. People with neurofibromatosis are also at an increased risk of developing kidney and pancreatic cancer. Fifty percent of the children and brothers and sisters of someone with this disease will develop it.

neurological cancer   See BRAIN CANCER.

neurological workup [neurological exam] a series of diagnostic tests for the presence of a tumor in the brain. A neurologist can frequently spot a problem by performing a series of simple, noninvasive procedures with the patient, using pins, tuning forks, reflex hammers, colored charts, and memory and other mental tests. Other diagnostic procedures that may be part of the workup include X-RAYS, CT SCANS, MRI, EEG, vision tests, spinal tap, and BRAIN SCANS.

neurologist (nu-rol"o-jist)   a medical doctor who specializes in disorders of the brain and central nervous system.

neuroma (nu-ro'mah) [neurofibroma, neurinoma] a noncancerous tumor composed of nerve cells and nerve fibers in the brain. It occurs most frequently in adults over 40. The most common neuroma is acoustic schwannoma neuroma occurring in the nerve of the ear. Neuromas are usually slow growing.
See also BRAIN CANCER.

neuron-specific enolase (NSE)   an enzyme detected in patients with neuroblastoma, small cell lung cancer, Wilms' tumor, melanoma, and cancers of the thyroid, kidney, testicle, and pancreas. Studies of NSE as a TUMOR MARKER have concentrated primarily on patients with neuroblastoma and small cell lung cancer. Levels in patients with those two diseases can provide information about the extent of the disease and the patient's prognosis, as well as about the patient's response to treatment, mostly in an investigational setting.

neuropathy [peripheral or sensory neuropathy] A problem in peripheral nerve function (any part of the nervous system except the brain and spinal cord) that causes pain, numbness, tingling, swelling, and muscle weakness in various parts of the body.

neuro-oncologist   an oncologist specializing in cancers of the brain or spinal canal (the neurologic system).

neuroradiologist (nu"ro-ra"de-ol'o-jist)   a medical doctor who specializes in making images of the brain using X-RAYS, CT SCANS, MRI, EEG, and BRAIN SCANS.

neurosurgeon (nu"ro-sur'jun)   a medical doctor who specializes in surgery of the brain, spinal cord, and nerves. Qualification as a neurosurgeon requires certification as a surgeon, plus four years in neurological surgery.

neurotoxic chemotherapy   a group of chemotherapeutics whose toxicity profile features significant peripheral NEUROPATHY. This group includes taxanes, platinum compounds, and vinca alkyloids.

neutron therapy   See PARTICLE BEAM THERAPY.

neutropenia (nu"tro-pe'ne-ah) [granulocytopenia, agranulocytosis]   a blood condition characterized by the virtual absence of NEUTROPHILS, one type of WHITE BLOOD CELL that is crucial to the body's defense against infection. Neutrophils account for about 60% of all the white blood cells. A person with neutropenia is more susceptible to infections and ulcerations of the mucous membrane.
    In a cancer patient neutropenia may be a result of CHEMOTHERAPY (anticancer drugs), which can enter the BONE MARROW and cause a decrease in granulocytic production, or of radiation therapy, which can cause BONE MARROW DEPRESSION. Neutropenia can also be caused by cancer or leukemia cells that infiltrate the bone marrow, or by a BONE MARROW TRANSPLANTATION.

If neutropenia is caused by chemotherapy, stopping the administration of the drugs usually reverses the condition in about one week and there is a good PROGNOSIS.

Neutropenia may be induced intentionally in some patients with LEUKEMIA during bone marrow transplantation. When bone marrow transplantations are performed in other cancers, neutropenia would be an undesired side effect. After a prolonged period of neutropenia, the body's IMMUNE SYSTEM is dangerously compromised and is defenseless against infection.

neutrophil (nu′tro-fil) a type of WHITE BLOOD CELL that plays a major role in the body's defense against bacteria, viruses, and fungi. It is an important PHAGOCYTE (the most prevalent of the three kinds of GRANULOCYTES). Approximately 60% of the white blood cells circulating in the body are neutrophils. They can pass through capillary walls to engulf and destroy invading bacteria. A deficiency of neutrophils in the blood, NEUTROPENIA, increases the risk of infections and ulcerations of the mucous membrane.

nevus (ne′vus) the medical term for MOLE, a skin growth that is usually colored and may sprout hair.

NHL See NON-HODGKIN'S LYMPHOMA.

nicotine patch [transdermal nicotine patch] a patch worn on the body which gradually releases nicotine through the skin into the body. It can reduce some of the side effects of withdrawal when someone quits smoking. There are a number of patches available, including Habitrol and Nicoderm. It is worn on the shoulder, back, or upper chest.

Nilandrone See NILUTAMIDE.

nilutamide [Nilandrone] an antiandrogen used in combination with surgical removal of the testes for metastatic prostate cancer. Possible side effects may include shortness of breath; abdominal pain; dark urine; nausea/vomiting; yellow eyes or skin; chest pain; cough; fever; frequent, painful, or difficult urination. It is taken orally.

Nipent See DEOXYCOFORMYCIN.

nipple banking saving the nipple of a diseased breast that is removed in a MASTECTOMY by temporarily grafting the nipple to another part of the body. This is done in the treatment of BREAST CANCER for use during BREAST RECONSTRUCTION. During reconstruction the nipple is removed from the part of the body where it was stored and grafted onto the new breast.

nipple discharge fluid leaving the nipple of the breast. It may be a symptom of breast cancer, especially if it is bloody or milky, or green or brown in color.

nipple retraction when the nipple on the breast is pulled inward. This may be caused by an underlying tumor or inflammation and can be a sign of BREAST CANCER. A woman with a retracted nipple should see a physician. A retracted nipple is different from an inverted nipple, which is considered normal. Nipple retraction is a developed condition that was not always present, and it is usually found on just one breast.

nitrate (ni′trāt) a chemical that is added to some cured meats and cheeses as a preservative. Nitrates are spontaneously turned into nitrites at room temperature and when it is combined with normal bacteria in the mouth. When nitrites combine with other compounds containing nitrogen, nitrosamines can be formed. There is increasing evidence to suggest that nitrosamines (known CARCINOGENS) are associated with the development of STOMACH CANCER. In the United States the amount of nitrate in prepared foods has been set by the Food and Drug Administration at the minimum level needed to prevent food contamination.

nitrite See NITRATE.

nitrogen mustard See MUSTARGEN.

nitrosamines See NITRATE.

Nizoral See KETOCONAZOLE.

NK cell See NATURAL KILLER CELL.

nodal involvement (no′dal)   the spread of cancer from the original (primary) site to the nearby LYMPH NODES. When cancer is diagnosed, the lymph nodes are frequently checked as part of the STAGING process. In many cancers, the lymph nodes are the first place to which the cancer spreads. With nodal involvement the PROGNOSIS is not as good as with primary cancers that have not spread. Nodal involvement may also be the first indication that the cancer has recurred (come back after treatment).

node   a small protuberance or swelling. See LYMPH NODES.

nodular melanoma (nod′u-lar   mel″ah-no′mah) one type of MELAMONA that arises from a preexisting mole or as a new growth.

nodular poorly differentiated lymphoma (NPDL) (nod′u-lar   lim-fo′mah) [low-grade   lymphoma] one type of NON-HODGKIN′S LYMPHOMA. It accounts for about 70% of the low grade lymphomas.

nodular sclerosis   See HODGKIN′S DISEASE.

nodule (nod′ūl)   small node; small group of cells.

Nolvadex   See TAMOXIFEN.

non-Hodgkin′s lymphoma/adult   a term for a group of different cancers that develop in the LYMPH SYSTEM. Although non-Hodgkin′s lymphoma has some of the characteristics of HODGKIN′S DISEASE, they are different disorders and are treated differently. Non-Hodgkin′s lymphoma is also far more unpredictable than Hodgkin′s disease and has a poorer PROGNOSIS.

Most non-Hodgkin′s lymphomas arise in the LYMPH NODES although it is not unusual for them to start in other parts of the body such as the liver or bones.

The American Cancer Society estimated there would be some 53,370 cases of NHL (28,850 men and 25,520 women) diagnosed in the United States in 2005, with about 19,410 deaths from the disease. It is the fifth most common cancer in the United States. Slightly more men than women are affected, and there is a greater incidence in the white population than the black population. It is rare for someone under 40 years of age to develop non-Hodgkin′s lymphoma; people most affected are over 44. Recently, an increased incidence has been seen in young men who are HIV POSITIVE.

The cause of non-Hodgkin′s lymphoma is not firmly established. In Japan, there were a greater number of cases among survivors of the atomic bomb at Hiroshima than would be expected in the normal population. People with damaged IMMUNE SYSTEMS, caused by immune disorders or immuno-suppressive drugs, are more likely to develop non-Hodgkin′s lymphoma. Kidney transplant patients, whose immune systems are medically suppressed to avoid organ rejection, are 40 to 100 times more likely to develop non-Hodgkin′s lymphoma, often within a year. Scientists think that in some way a viral infection may play a role in the development of many non-Hodgkin′s lymphomas.

Non-Hodgkin′s lymphoma is broken down into two basic types: aggressive and indolent. Aggressive non-Hodgkin′s lymphomas include:

• nodular histiocytic lymphoma
• diffuse histiocytic lymphoma
• diffuse mixed lymphocytic histiocytic lymphoma
• diffuse undifferentiated lymphoma and
• diffuse lymphoblastic lymphoma

About half of all non-Hodgkin′s lymphomas are the aggressive type. They are the most common form affecting children.

Indolent lymphoma types include:

• nodular or diffuse poorly differentiated lymphocytic nodular
• mixed lymphoma
• diffuse well-differentiated lymphocytic lymphoma
• diffuse intermediate differentiated lymphocytic lymphoma

Indolent non-Hodgkin′s lymphoma affects primarily adults over the age of 40 and is slow growing. Other forms of non-Hodgkin′s lymphoma are MYCOSIS FUNGOIDES and BURKITT′S LYMPHOMA.

Symptoms may include painless swelling of the lymph nodes in the neck, groin, or underarm, fevers, night sweats, tiredness, weight loss, itching, and reddened patches on the skin. Sometimes there is nausea, vomiting, or abdominal pain.

Diagnosis and evaluation of non-Hodgkin's lymphoma may include a thorough physical exam, X-RAYS, TOMOGRAPHY, CT SCAN, blood test, urinalysis, BONE MARROW TEST, LYMPHANGIOGRAPHY, and a BIOPSY of tissue from an enlarged lymph node.

Following is the National Cancer Institute's (NCI) staging for non-Hodgkin's lymphoma:

- Stage I—involvement of one group of lymph nodes in an area of the body or a single extranodal organ site without lymph node involvement
- Stage II—involvement of more than one group of lymph nodes that are either all above or all below the diaphragm, or involvement of one extranodal organ and an adjacent group of lymph nodes on the same side of the diaphragm
- Stage III—involvement of lymph nodes both above and below the diaphragm with or without involvement of the spleen (considered part of the lymph system) and with or without localized (limited) extralymphatic involvement
- Stage IV—widespread involvement of one or more extranodal organ sites (often the BONE MARROW and/or liver) with or without widespread involvement of the lymph nodes
- Recurrent—cancer has returned after treatment

The pathological description of the NHLs has undergone multiple systems of classification over the past 50 years by people such as Rappaport, Lukes-Collins, and Kiel. An organization, The Working Formulation, offered a system of classification, and now the World Health Organization [WHO]) offers its own. This has led to a confusing terminology and a bewildering array of categories that transcends the scope of this book. It does, however, help in recognizing that the NHLs are a group of illnesses.

Treatment depends on the stage of the disease, the general state of health of the patient, and other factors. Generally treatment is RADIATION THERAPY or CHEMOTHERAPY (anticancer drugs). BONE MARROW TRANSPLANTATION is a fairly new option. For specific information on the latest state-of-the-art treatment, by stage, call NCI's Cancer Information Service at 1-800-4-CANCER (1-800-422-6237), or for a TTY: 1-800-332-8615.

See also LYMPHOMA and NON-HODGKIN'S LYMPHOMA/CHILDHOOD.

non-Hodgkin's lymphoma/childhood   cancer that originates in the lymph cells but usually causes masses or tumors outside the LYMPH SYSTEM. The most common sites are the abdomen, bone marrow, or chest. Combined with HODGKIN'S DISEASE, it is the third most common cancer affecting children and young adults under the age of 21. Boys are three times as likely to get it as girls.

The two major kinds of childhood non-Hodgkin's lymphoma are lymphoblastic lymphoma and non-lymphoblastic lymphoma, which includes

- undifferentiated lymphoma,
- BURKITT'S LYMPHOMA,
- non-Burkitt's lymphoma, and
- large-cell lymphoma.

Symptoms may include coughing and difficulty in breathing when the thymus gland is enlarged; swelling and pain if there is an abdominal mass; or vomiting when there is obstruction in the bowel. Procedure for diagnosing and evaluating childhood non-Hodgkin's lymphoma may include a complete blood test, X-RAYS, BONE MARROW ASPIRATION, CT SCAN, and ULTRASOUND.

Following is the National Cancer Institute's (NCI) staging for childhood non-Hodgkin's lymphoma:

- Stage I—a single tumor or nodal area outside the abdomen and MEDIASTINUM (chest cavity)
- Stage II
  - a single tumor with regional LYMPH NODE involvement or
  - two or more tumors or nodal areas on one side of the diaphragm or
  - a primary gastrointestinal tract tumor with or without regional lymph node involvement
- Stage III—tumor of lymph node areas on both sides of the diaphragm and affecting the chest, abdomen, spine, or brain
- Stage IV—disease in the BONE MARROW or CENTRAL NERVOUS SYSTEM regardless of other sites
- Recurrent—the cancer has returned to the same site or another part of the body after treatment

The treatment of childhood non-Hodgkin's lymphoma depends on the cell type, the stage of the disease, where it has spread, and other factors. Treatment is usually COMBINATION CHEMOTHERAPY. RADIATION THERAPY is used less often. For specific information on the latest state-of-the-art treatment, by stage, call the NCI's Cancer Information Service at 1-800-4-CANCER (1-800-422-6237), or for a TTY: 1-800-332-8615.

noninfiltrating ductal papillary carcinoma   See DUCTAL BREAST CARCINOMA IN SITU.

noninvasive   when used to describe cancer, meaning the cancer has not invaded, entered, or harmed tissue bordering the tumor. It is the earliest stage of many cancers and has the best PROGNOSIS. About half the patients diagnosed with noninvasive cancer will be cured with PRIMARY TREATMENT. Noninvasive cancer may also be referred to as in situ.

nonopioids   Non-narcotic drugs used to treat mild or moderate pain. Acetaminophens and nonsteroidal anti-inflammatory drugs (NSAIDS) are examples of nonopioids, which can usually be bought over the counter.

nonseminoma   (non-se″mĭ-no′mah)   a   general term for TESTICULAR CANCER that arises in specialized sex cells called germ cells. There are four types of nonseminomas: embryonal cell carcinoma, teratoma, teratocarcinoma (yolk sac tumor), and CHORIOCARCINOMA. Nonseminomas account for approximately 46 to 63% of all testicular tumors. The other major form of testicular cancer is SEMINOMA.

non-small cell lung cancer (NSCLC)   a disease in which cancer cells are found in the tissue of the lungs. Overall, this grouping makes up approximately 75 to 80% of all LUNG CANCER cases. (SMALL CELL LUNG CANCER is considered separately because of its different behavior and treatment strategy.)

NSCLC is a general term for three types of lung cancer: adenocarcinoma (includes bronchiolalveolar), squamous cell (or epidermoid) carcinoma, and large cell carcinoma.

In adenocarcinoma of the lung, the cells grow in patterns resembling glands, cube- or column-shaped cells. They often develop along the outer edges of the lungs and under the membranes lining the bronchi (tubes in the lungs). It is the most common type of lung cancer in the United States and the most commonly diagnosed lung cancer in women.

Squamous cell lung cancer is characterized by cells that are flat and scale-like. It often begins in the large bronchi and tends to remain localized in the chest for longer periods than other types of lung cancer. It is the only type of lung cancer that goes through phases. The precancerous phase can last for years. Squamous cell cancers are generally the most responsive to treatment.

Large cell carcinoma is a catch-all term for lung cancers that do not fit into other categories. It accounts for between 10 and 20% of all lung cancer cases, frequently arising in the smaller bronchi.

The major risk factor in developing NSCLC is smoking. Other possible risk factors include exposure to certain industrial substances such as arsenic, certain organic chemicals, and ASBESTOS, particularly for people who smoke, and exposure to radiation from occupational, medical, and environmental sources. Radon in the home may increase the risk, especially in smokers. Passive smoke increases the risk for nonsmokers.

NSCLC frequently has no symptoms until it is fairly advanced. Symptoms that may be associated with it include a chronic cough, blood in the sputum, wheezing unrelated to asthma, repeated episodes of pneumonia, fever, weakness, weight loss, and chest pain. Other symptoms that may accompany more advanced disease include hoarseness, shortness of breath, enlargement of lymph glands in the neck, shoulder and arm pain, difficulty in swallowing, and drooping of the upper eyelids. There can also be symptoms in other parts of the body caused by lung cancer that has metastasized (spread).

Procedures used in the diagnosis and evaluation of NSCLC may include chest X-RAYS, CT SCAN, BRONCHOSCOPY, MEDIASTINOSCOPY, MEDIASTINOTOMY, THORACOTOMY, PERCUTANEOUS NEEDLE BIOPSY, and/or NEEDLE ASPIRATION BIOPSY.

NSCLC can be characterized by the appearance of the tumor cells. Cells that are poorly differentiated are immature and very different from normal cells. Poorly differentiated cancer cells tend to grow more rapidly than well-differentiated cancer cells, which resemble normal cells.

Following is the National Cancer Institute's (NCI) STAGING for NSCLC:

• Occult stage—cancer cells are found in the sputum but no tumor is found in the lung

- Stage 0 or in situ—cancer is found only in a local area and only in a few layers of cells; it has not grown through the top lining of the lung
- Stage I—the cancer is only in the lung, with normal tissue around it
- Stage II—the cancer has spread to nearby LYMPH NODES
- Stage III—the cancer has spread to the chest wall or diaphragm near the lung; or the cancer has spread to the lymph nodes in the area that separates the two lungs (mediastinum), or to the lymph nodes on the other side of the chest or in the neck
- Stage III
  — IIIA (surgery can be performed)
  — IIIB (surgery cannot be performed)
- Stage IV—the cancer has spread to other parts of the body
- Recurrent—the cancer has returned after previous treatment.

Treatment depends on the stage of the disease, the general state of health of the patient, and other factors. Treatment of choice is surgery, when possible. RADIATION THERAPY is also used. For specific information on the latest state-of-the-art treatment, by stage, call NCI's Cancer Information Service at 1-800-4-CANCER (1-800-422-6237), or for a TTY: 1-800-332-8615.

See also ADENOCARCINOMA OF THE LUNG and SQUAMOUS CELL LUNG CANCER.

nonsteroidal anti-inflammatory drugs (NSAIDS) (non-ster-oi'dal) drugs used primarily in the treatment of arthritis. NSAIDs are similar to aspirin and are effective for reducing inflammation and pain, especially in the joints. When NSAIDs were first introduced in the early 1970s, they were available only by a doctor's prescription. Today many can be bought over the counter. Three of the brands currently available are Nuprin, Motrin, and Advil. Stronger doses, such as Rufen, are still available only by prescription. (There is also a large group of NSAIDs available by prescription primarily for patients with arthritis.) In cancer patients, NSAIDs may be useful in controlling mild pain and inflammation either alone or in combination with other drugs. Possible side effects may include stomach irritation and water retention.

See also ANALGESIC and NONOPIOIDS.

nose cancer cancers that occur in the nasal fossa (nasal cavity), paranasal sinuses (sinus), and nasopharynx (tube that connects the mouth and nose with the esophagus). Symptoms of nose cancer may include a reddish, easily bleeding mass in the nose, pain and pressure in the check, a toothache, lump in the check, or a bloody discharge from the nose.

See also NASOPHARYNGEAL CANCER.

Novantrone See MITOXANTRONE.

NOVP a combination of the anticancer drugs Novantrone (MITOXANTRONE), Oncovin (VINCRISTINE), VINBLASTINE, and PREDNISONE sometimes used in the treatment of HODGKIN'S DISEASE. See individual drug listings for side effects.

See also COMBINATION CHEMOTHERAPY.

NPC (Nutritional Prevention of Cancer) study a NUTRITIONAL INTERVENTION STUDY focused on the effect of selenium supplements on the rate of BASAL CELL and SQUAMOUS CELL SKIN CANCER. Overall, selenium had no significant effect on these or other cancers.

NPDL See NODULAR POORLY DIFFERENTIATED LYMPHOMA.

NSAIDs See NONSTEROIDAL ANTI-INFLAMMATORY DRUGS.

NSCLC See NON-SMALL CELL LUNG CANCER.

NSE See NEURON-SPECIFIC ENOLASE.

nuclear medicine the use of RADIOACTIVE chemicals to diagnose and treat disease. After a radioactive substance is swallowed or injected into the body, its distribution in the body can be watched via a special machine. The doctor can study the structure and function of an organ and identify conditions of disease. Nuclear medicine includes many commonly used NUCLEAR SCANS in the diagnosis and evaluation of cancer. Radioactive iodine is a major treatment for thyroid cancer.

nuclear power plant a facility that produces energy using radioactive substances. Exposure to excessive amount of radiation can cause cancer. There is still a great deal of controversy over the need for and safety of nuclear power plants. Opponents point to the accident at the plant in Chernobyl in 1986 in the Soviet Union and the deaths and cancers it has caused. Proponents of nuclear power say the possibility of a nuclear accident is minuscule and that the benefits far outweigh any risks. Although there have been reports of so-called clusters of cancer cases around nuclear plant facilities, studies have not shown that any clusters appear more often at nuclear facility sites than in the general population.

nuclear scan [radioactive scan, radioisotope scan, isotope scan]   a diagnostic procedure using a RADIOACTIVE substance to examine different organs in the body. Among the substances used are RADIOACTIVE ISOTOPES, including GALLIUM and TECHNESIUM.

In the procedure, a virtually harmless amount of radioactive substance is injected into a vein in the body or orally ingested by the patient. Certain radioactive substances concentrate in areas of the body where cells are dividing rapidly. In some scans, a "locking" agent may be given first, to keep the radioactive substance from going to other parts of the body. Once the radioactive substance has reached the target organ, the person receiving the scan lies in a prone position under a very sensitive radiation-measuring device, which takes a scintiscan, a two-dimensional picture of the organ. The image shows whether an organ is functioning normally or if it has an abnormal area or mass. Increased or decreased amounts of radioactivity on the scintiscan may be an indication of cancer as well as other disorders.

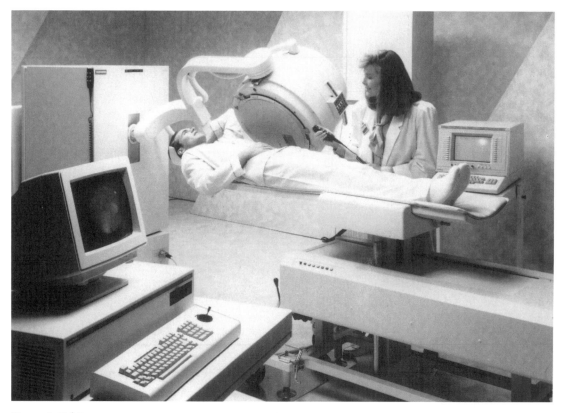

Siemen's Orbiter gamma camera. Courtesy Siemen's Medical Systems, Inc.

Two different machines are used to perform scans. The gamma camera is the newest. One kind of gamma camera stays in one place while doing the scan. The rotating gamma camera can move while the data for the image is being obtained. The older rectilinear scanner as a narrower field of vision and takes longer.

Scans can be done on virtually any part of the body. The most common include LUNG SCAN, BRAIN SCAN, LIVER SCAN, BONE SCAN, KIDNEY SCAN, THYROID SCAN, and PANCREAS SCAN, among others.

null-cell acute lymphocytic leukemia (lim-fo-sit′ik) [undifferentiated ALL]   accounts for about 8% of acute lymphocytic leukemia (ALL) cases. It occurs primarily in older children and adults. Null-cell ALL affects grossly immature stem cells that exhibit no DIFFERENTIATION.

See ALL.

Numorphan [oxymorphone]   a NARCOTIC drug used in the relief or control of pain. It is given by injection into a muscle or rectal suppository. It is available by prescription only.

Nuprin   See NONSTEROIDAL ANTI-INFLAMMATORY DRUGS.

NutraSweet   See ARTIFICIAL SWEETENERS.

nutritional intervention study   a study in which researchers are trying to isolate a particular dietary component as preventive against cancer. These are methodologically difficult to control and interpret and usually require large numbers of patients and years to complete. Other examples of such studies include the ATBC STUDY, CARET, NPC, PHS, and WHS.

NVP   See NAVELBINE.

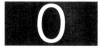

O,p′-DDD See MITOTANE.

oat cell carcinoma See SMALL CELL LUNG CANCER.

oat cell lung cancer See SMALL CELL LUNG CANCER.

obesity the state of being extremely overweight. Obesity has been identified as a possible risk factor in the development of endometrial cancer.

Oblimersen sodium an antisense compound being investigated for treatment of LEUKEMIA.

obserable survival rate See SURVIVAL RATE.

obstruction a blockage, as of the bowel, a duct, or another place on the body.

OC See ORAL CONTRACEPTIVES.

occult blood stool test (ŏ-kult′) [guaiac test, blood stool test, stool blood test, stool guaiac test] examination of stool for traces of blood not visible to the naked eye. This is an easy and inexpensive test obtained from a doctor and usually done at home; it is capable of identifying a large number of people who should be given further tests for possible COLON/RECTAL CANCER. Because bleeding can be intermittent, the samples of stool are usually taken from three consecutive bowel movements. For as accurate a result as possible, a meat-free and high-fiber diet should be followed for two days prior to doing the test. Upon completion, the test is returned to the doctor or sent directly to a laboratory for analysis. Blood in the stool is a possible sign of cancer as well as many other disorders.

See also SCREENING.

occult primary malignancy See UNKNOWN PRIMARY.

occupational therapist See PHYSICAL THERAPIST.

Octreotide [Sandostatin] a therapeutic drug which is an analog of SOMATOSTATIN, used in therapy of carcinoid tumor and syndrome or other vasoactive intestinal peptide-secreting tumors. It is a potent inhibitor of serotonin. It is given by subcutaneous injection.

See SANDOSTATIN.

Octreotide scan a nuclear medicine scan used in the diagnostic evaluation of carcinoid tumors and other neuroendocrine tumors.

ocular referring to the eyes.

ocular melanoma See INTRAOCULAR MELANOMA.

Office of Alternative Medicine See NATIONAL CENTER FOR COMPLEMENTARY AND ALTERNATIVE MEDICINE.

off-label usage applies to the use of a drug, usually based on published scientific data, in a condition that has not been given formal approval by the Food and Drug Administration (FDA). Physicians may decide to use drug in this way if they believe (based on data) that it will benefit the patient with an acceptable risk/benefit ratio. However, it is important to note that insurance companies may not cover/reimburse for a drug prescribed for "off-label" usage. Patients should check with their pharmacists or insurance plans to see if a drug prescribed in this way will be considered a covered benefit under their specific plan.

Oldfield's syndrome a rare hereditary condition in which there are multiple POLYPS in the colon. People with this condition are at a greater risk of developing COLON CANCER.

oligodendrocytoma (ol″ĭ-go-den″dro-si-to′mah) a soft, slow-growing tumor in the brain. Over time it can transform into a more malignant (cancerous) grade of cell type. It occurs most often in people of middle age. An oligodendrocytoma tumor can be present for many years before it causes symptoms and is diagnosed. It is one type of GLIOMA brain cancer.
    See also BRAIN CANCER.

oligodendroglia (ol″ĭ-go-den-drog′le-ah) a type of brain tumor beginning in brain cells called oligodendrocytes that provide support and nourishment for the cells that transmit nerve impulses.
    See BRAIN CANCER.

oligodendroglioma (ol″ĭ-go-den″dro-gli-o′mah) a rare tumor of the brain that grows very slowly and is frequently benign (noncancerous), although malignant (cancerous) forms are possible. They can be present for many years before they are detected and diagnosed. Survival for many years after is not uncommon.
    See BRAIN CANCER.

Ommaya reservoir (o-mi′ah) a special device used to deliver CHEMOTHERAPY (anticancer drugs) to the fluid surrounding the brain. The small device, a soft plastic dome and thin tubing, is placed in the head by a neurosurgeon. The tube goes into a small pouch of the brain where CEREBROSPINAL FLUID is formed. The Ommaya reservoir enables chemotherapy to be administered without pain by eliminating the need for painful, multiple spinal taps. The Ommaya reservoir may be used in the treatment of LEPTO-MENINGEAL METASTASES, and MENINGEAL LEUKEMIA.

Cerebrospinal fluid may also be removed from the reservoir to detect any abnormal cells during an Ommaya reservoir tap. An Ommaya tap usually takes about 15 or 20 minutes and is performed in an operating room under general anesthesia. The reservoir may be removed if it is no longer needed.

Ommaya reservoir tap See OMMAYA RESERVOIR.

Oncaspar See PEGASPARGASE.

oncofetal antigen See CEA.

oncogene (ong′ko-jēn) [cancer gene] one of a family of genes that when mutated foster malignant accelerated growth. Researchers believe that *every* person carries one or more oncogenes in every body cell and that the oncogene remains harmless until it is triggered by something. When that happens, the oncogene can transform some normal cells into malignant (cancerous) cells.

The existence of oncogenes was discovered in 1910 by Peyton Rous, who found that liquid from a sarcoma in a chicken, from which all the cancerous cells had been removed, caused sarcomas in other birds. The liquid contained an oncogene that transformed cells infected with a virus into tumor cells. Without the viral infection, the oncogenes would be harmless.

There appear to be at least three types of oncogenes that act in different ways to promote or cause the development of cancer. How they work is still being actively investigated. The major areas of oncogene investigation are:

- how oncogenes become activated to transform normal cells into cancer cells
- how the activation of oncogenes can be prevented
- once activated, how to reverse the process and prevent it from perpetuating through future generations in the course of cell division.

Researchers see great potential in the continuing investigation into oncogenes, which they think will eventually result in ways to use oncogenes in cancer prevention, diagnosis, and treatment. Oncogenes have been found in association with a number of cancers. Identified oncogenes include RAS, associated with bladder cancer; P53, a mutated version on chromosome 17 involved in a variety of cancers, including breast, ovary, and lung; HER-2/neu, associated with breast and ovarian cancer. Development in this field continues at a rapid pace.

oncogenic (ong"ko-je'ik)   cancer causing.

oncologic surgeon (ong"ko-loj'ik) [surgical oncologist]   a doctor who specializes in cancer surgery.

oncologist (ong-kol'o-jist)   a doctor who specializes in the diagnosis and treatment of cancer. Medical oncologists treat the patient with CHEMO-THERAPY and HORMONE THERAPY and frequently serve as the main caretaker; radiation oncologists specialize in treating cancer patients with RADIA-TION THERAPY; surgical oncologists specialize in cancer surgery and may also serve as the main caretaker; and pediatric oncologists treat children with cancer.

oncology (ong-kol'o-je)   the study of cancerous tumors.

oncology nurse (ong-kol'o-je)   a nurse trained in caring for cancer patients. The oncology nurse can provide a number of important services for the patient, including:

- the administration of CHEMOTHERAPY (anticancer drugs)
- conducting educational programs for the patient before, during, and after treatment, such as preparing a patient for chemotherapy by explaining what it is, how it is performed, the side effects, etc.
- providing special care for patients undergoing operations that change their body function or lifestyle, such as removal of a breast or an OSTOMY for colon or bladder cancer
- helping plan at-home care and rehabilitation
- helping the patient and the patient's family with psychosocial issues.

National certification for nurses trained in oncology has been available since 1984 by the Oncology Nursing Certification Corporation (ONCC; see http://www.oncc.org). There are more than 21,000 oncology certified nurses, including 19,191 oncology-certified nurses (OCN's), 978 certified pediatric ongology nurses (CPON's), and 1,495 advanced oncology certified nurses (AOCN's), 48 advanced oncology certified nurse practitioners (AOCNPs), and 18 advanced oncology certified clinical nurse specialists (AOCNS).

ONCC is accredited by the American Board of Nursing Specialties and the National Commission for Certifying Agencies.

oncor test   the first gene-based test approved by the Federal Drug Administration for predicting whether a cancer will recur. The test measures the number of copies of the HER-2/neu gene in a patient with breast cancer. Five to 10 copies per cell increases the risk of recurrence. Most people have two copies per cell.

OncotypeDX   an ancillary diagnostic test done by a pathologist to predict breast cancer recurrence using a multigene panel as an assessment tool. This test is done on breast cancer tissue and attempts to assign a level of risk of recurrence. It is costly and not universally covered by insurance.

Oncovin   See VINCRISTINE.

Ondansetron   See ZOFRAN.

ONTAK [denikeukin diffitoxin]   an intravenous (IV) CHEMOTHERAPEUTIC indicated for treatment of persistent or recurrent cutaneous T CELL LYMPHOMA whose MALIGNANT cells express the CD25 component of the IL2 receptor. Side effects include VASCU-LAR LEAK SYUNDROME and an acute hypersensitivity reaction.

oophorectomy (o"of-o-rek'to-me) [ovariectomy] surgical removal of one or both OVARIES. Removal of one ovary is called a unilateral oophorectomy; removal of both is a bilateral oophorectomy. Oophorectomy was first performed for menstrual irregularities and psychological disorders in the early 1870s by an American gynecologist who continued its use until 1910 despite a high MORTALITY RATE. In 1896, a British surgeon reported that removing the ovaries of patients who had BREAST CANCER delayed a recurrence of the cancer. Oophorectomy was then performed in the treatment of breast cancer in premenopausal women routinely for some 50 years. The rationale was that elimination of the ovaries, the major producer of ESTROGEN, would slow the growth of the TUMOR, which was stimulated by estrogen. However, several large clinical trials in the 1960s found that oophorectomies did not improve survival rates and the surgery is now rarely done for that purpose. HORMONE THERAPY, using new medical agents that can block estrogen, have eliminated the need for surgery in most cases. The development of the ESTROGEN RECEPTOR TEST and PROGESTERONE RECEPTOR TEST has also played a role in eliminating oophorectomies by identifying women who are most likely to benefit from HORMONE THERAPY. With the discovery of the BREAST CANCER GENE, which increases a woman's risk of breast and ovarian cancer, oophorectomy may be the choice of some women who test positive for the gene as a prophylactic measure against OVARIAN CANCER. For appropriate patients, it can be a simple one-day procedure done by laparoscopy.

OPEN a combination of the anticancer drugs Oncovin (VINCRISTINE), PREDNISONE, ETOPOSIDE, and MITOXANTRONE sometimes used in the treatment of NON-HODGKIN'S LYMPHOMA. See individual drug listings for side effects.

See also COMBINATION CHEMOTHERAPY.

ophthalmologist (of"thal-mol'ŏ-jist) a medical doctor who diagnoses and treats diseases of the eye and the surrounding structure. An ophthalmologist can perform surgery. To become certified by the American Board of Ophthalmology, the ophthalmologist must be a licensed doctor of medicine, have had three years of residency in ophthalmology, one year of independent practice or research, and passed the written and oral exams given by the board.

ophthalmoscope See OPHTHALMOSCOPY.

ophthalmoscopy (of-thal-mos'ko-pe) an examination of the eye. An instrument called an ophthal-moscope is used by an eye doctor to view the retina and other posterior portions of the globe of the eye. This can be done in the doctor's office. An ophthalmoscopy is one of the examinations that may be performed in the diagnosis of EYE CANCER.

opioids a class of drugs used to treat moderate to severe pain. Morphine and codeine are two examples. A doctor's prescription is needed for these drugs.

See NARCOTIC.

OPM (occult primary malignancy) See UNKNOWN PRIMARY.

opportunistic infection an INFECTION that would not usually occur in someone whose IMMUNE SYSTEM was functioning normally.

Opreleukin See INTERLEUKIN.

oral cancer See MOUTH CANCER.

oral cavity cancer See MOUTH CANCER.

oral contraceptives (OC) hormones that a woman takes, usually in pill form, to prevent conception.

Currently, two types of OCs are available in the United States. The most commonly prescribed OC contains two man-made versions of natural female hormones (ESTROGEN and PROGESTERONE) that are similar to the hormones the ovaries normally produce. Estrogen stimulates the growth and development of the uterus at puberty, causes the endometrium (the inner lining of the uterus) to thicken during the first half of the menstrual cycle, and influences breast tissue throughout life, but particularly from puberty to menopause.

The second type of OC available in the United States is called the minipill. It contains only a progestogen. The minipill is less effective in preventing pregnancy than the combination pill, so it is prescribed less often.

Because medical research suggests that cancers of the female reproductive organs depend on naturally occurring sex hormones for their development and growth, scientists have been investigating a possible link between OC use and cancer risk. Researchers have focused a great deal of attention on OC users over the past 40 years. This scrutiny has produced a wealth of data on OC use and the development of certain cancers, although results of these studies have not always been consistent.

In June 1995, the NATIONAL CANCER INSTITUTE (NCI) reported an increased risk of BREAST CANCER among women under age 35 who had used birth control pills for at least six months, compared with those who had never used them, and a slightly lower but still elevated risk among women aged 35 to 44. A higher risk level was also seen among long-term users, especially those who had started to take the pill before age 18. A later study found that the risk of developing breast cancer returned to a normal level 10 years or more after discontinuation of use.

There is some evidence that long-term use of OCs may increase the risk of CERVICAL CANCER. However, the exact nature of the association between OC use and risk of cervical cancer remains unclear. Most studies have found that the pill reduces the risk of OVARIAN CANCER. Reduced risk is seen in women who have used OCs for as as little as three to six months. The longer a woman uses the pill, the lower her risk. In addition, this lowered risk persists long after the pill is no longer being taken. Researchers estimate that OC use averts more than 1,700 cases of ovarian cancer in the United States each year. The labels on oral contraceptive products now warn of the possible risk of cervical cancer and advise users to have a yearly PAP SMEAR to monitor for any changes.

Here are some key points that the NCI offers regarding OCs and cancer risk:

- There is evidence of an increased risk of breast cancer for women under age 35 who are recent users of OCs.
- Studies have consistently shown that using OCs reduces the risk of ovarian cancer.
- There is evidence that long-term use of OCs may increase the risk of CANCER OF THE CERVIX.
- There is some evidence that OCs may increase the risk of certain CANCEROUS LIVER TUMORS.
- For additional information, see the NCI's Web site, which includes a page on oral contraceptives and cancer risk (http://www.cancer.gov/cancertopics/factsheet/Risk/oral-contraceptives).

oral gallbladder test   See CHOLECYSTOGRAPHY.

Orasone   See PREDNISONE.

Ora-Testryl [fluoxymesterone, Halotestin]   See ANDROGEN.

orchiectomy (or″ke-ek′to-me)   surgical removal of a testicle, the source of male sex hormones. Removal of both testicles is called bilateral or radical orchiectomy. Removal of both testicles usually results in INFERTILITY, however, it generally does not interfere with the ability to have an erection. An orchiectomy may be used as the primary treatment for TESTICULAR CANCER. Orchiectomy may also be used in the treatment of prostate cancer by removing the male hormones, which stimulate its growth. With the availability of drugs, orchiectomy is less commonly performed.

orderly carcinoma   See TUBULAR DUCTAL BREAST CANCER.

Oreton   See ANDROGEN.

oropharyngeal cancer (o″ro-fah-rin′je-al)   cancer of the oropharynx, the middle part of the throat (also called the pharynx). The pharynx is a hollow tube about five inches long that starts behind the nose and goes down to the neck to become part of the tube that goes to the stomach (the esophagus). Air and food pass through the pharynx on the way to the esophagus. The oropharynx includes the soft palate (the back of the mouth), the base of the tongue, and the tonsils.

The American Cancer Society estimated there would be some 29,370 new cases (19,100 in men and 10,270 in women) of oral cavity and oropharyngeal cancer in the United States in 2005, with an estimated 7,320 deaths from the disease in the same year (4,910 men and 2,410 women).

Oral cavity and oropharyngeal cancer occurs more often in blacks than in whites. The number of new cases of this disease has been dropping during the past 20 years. In 2003 and 2004, the number of new cases dropped by 5% a year. Along with this, the death rate for oral cavity and oropharyngeal cancer has been decreasing since the late 1970s.

Symptoms may include a mild but persistent sore throat, a lump in the back of the tongue, difficulty swallowing, a voice change, a pain in the ear, and emergence of velvety red patches, some of which are open sores. Occasionally there is difficulty in breathing and lumps in the neck. Diagnostic procedures may include a LARYNGOSCOPY and a BIOPSY.

Following is the NATIONAL CANCER INSTITUTE's (NCI) STAGING for oropharyngeal cancer:

- Stage I—the tumor is two CENTIMETERS (cm) or less and there is no evidence of spread of the tumor to LYMPH NODES or other parts of the body
- Stage II—the tumor is not more than 4 cm and there is no evidence of spread of the tumor to lymph nodes or to other parts of the body
- Stage III
  - the tumor is bigger than 4 cm but there is no evidence of spread to the lymph nodes
  - the tumor is any size (except massive, as in stage IV) and there is spread to a single lymph node less than 3 cm on the same side of the neck as the primary tumor
- Stage IV
  - the primary tumor is more than 4 cm and invades deeply to involve adjacent structures, even if there is no spread to distant parts of the body; there is no more than one lymph node involved by tumor that is both on the same side of the neck as the primary tumor and no more than 3 cm
  - regardless of the size of the primary tumor, there is one abnormal lymph node larger than 3 cm; there are multiple abnormal nodes of any size on both sides of the neck; or there is one or more abnormal nodes on the opposite side of the neck from the primary tumor
  - there is evidence of spread to distant parts of the body
- Recurrent—the cancer has returned to the same site or to another part of the body after treatment

Treatment depends on the stage of the disease, the general state of health of the patient, and other factors. The treatment for oropharyngeal cancer may be SURGERY, RADIATION THERAPY, and CHEMOTHERAPY. For specific information on the latest state-of-the-art treatment, by stage, call NCI's Cancer Information Service at 1-800-4-cancer (1-800-422-6237), or for a TTY: 1-800-332-8615.

See also HEAD AND NECK CANCER.

oropharynx (o"ro-far'inks) The area in the body from the base of the tongue to the back of the throat. It lies below the nasopharynx, through which air passes from the nasal cavities. Below the oropharynx is the hypopharynx, through which food passes before it enters the esophagus.

orphan drug a drug used to treat rare diseases affecting 200,000 people or less. Because pharmaceutical companies do not consider it commercially viable to manufacture these drugs. The Food and Drug Administration's (FDA) Orphan Drug Act of 1983 was passed to ensure development of drugs even if they would have a limited market. Orphan drug status is granted before FDA approval. Among the incentives offered to drug companies to develop orphan drugs is seven years of marketing exclusivity after FDA approval.

orthopedic surgeon (or"tho-pe'dik) A surgeon who is a specialist in the diagnosis and treatment of disorders, including cancers, of the bones, joints, tendons, and muscles. Requirements for certification by the American Board of Orthopedic Surgery include being a licensed doctor for four years, four years of general surgery, two years of orthopedic surgery, and passing oral and written exams given by the board.

orthovoltage treatment RADIATION THERAPY using relatively low energy rays, usually less than one megavolt.

osteogenic sarcoma See OSTEOSARCOMA.

osteosarcoma (os"te-o-sar-ko'mah) [osteogenic sarcoma] the most common form of BONE CANCER in teenagers. It usually arises in areas of rapid bone growth, in the leg bones, upper arm, or hip, which occurs during puberty. According to The American Cancer Society, there are about 900 new cases of osteosarcoma diagnosed in the United States each year. About 400 of these cases occur in children and adolescents younger than 20 years old. Osteosarcoma is about 50% more common in males than in females. Most osteosarcomas occur between the ages of 10 and 30. Teenagers are the most commonly affected age group, but it can occur at any age. About 10% of all osteosarcomas develop in people over the age of 60.

Five-year survival rates have significantly improved over the last few years, and in 2005 were around 65% to 70% for children. Although adults have not been as well studied, doctors think they will do as well if they can take the same type of treatments as children do. Until the 1970s, the PROGNOSIS for someone with osteosarcoma was very bleak, with a cure rate of 10 to 20%. However, the discovery of effective CHEMOTHERAPY (anticancer drugs) has radically altered the prognosis.

Osteosarcoma may also occur in a bone that was previously exposed to RADIATION. The normal bone is destroyed and replaced by cancer cells. As a result, the bone is softer and can break easily, seemingly for no apparent reason (pathologic fracture).

There are three types of osteosarcoma: PAROSTEAL OSTEOSARCOMA, MULTIFOCAL OSTEOSARCOMA, and SOFT-TISSUE SARCOMA. Symptoms may include swelling or pain in the lower leg or forearm. Procedures used in the diagnosis and evaluation of osteosarcoma may include X-RAYS, CT SCAN, FLUOROSCOPY, BONE SCAN, and BIOPSY.

Osteosarcoma is staged by the NATIONAL CANCER INSTITUTE (NCI) as local, confined within the bone of the area immediately around the bone where the cancer arose;metastatic, the tumor having spread beyond the bone where it arose to other parts of the body. The most common site of metastatic disease from bone cancer is the lungs. The last stage is described as recurrent, the cancer has come back (recurred) after it has been treated. It may come back in the tissues where it first started or it may come back in another part of the body.

Treatment depends on the stage of the disease, its type, location, the general state of health of the patient, and other factors. Surgery is the primary treatment whenever possible. Other treatment options include RADIATION THERAPY, preoperative CHEMOTHERAPY, chemotherapy after the surgery, and LOCALIZED RADIATION. For specific information on the latest state-of-the-art treatment, by stage, call NCI's Cancer Information Service at 1-800-4-CANCER (1-800-422-6237), or for a TTY: 1-800-332-8615.

ostomy (os'to-me) [urostomy]   surgical creation of an artificial opening (stoma) through the abdominal wall for elimination of body waste that may be used in the treatment of cancer as well as other disorders. Variations of this procedure include COLOSTOMY, and ILEOSTOMY. The disease and its location are two of the factors that dictate which procedure is performed. See Appendix I for support organizations for those who have undergone this procedure.

otolaryngologist (o"to-lar"in-gol'o-jist) [sometimes referred to as an ENT (ear, nose, throat) specialist]   a medical doctor who specializes in the examination and treatment of the ear, nose, throat, larynx, and air tubes to the lungs. An otolaryngologist can perform surgery and is often referred to as a head and neck surgeon. To become certified by the American Board of Otolaryngology, an otolaryngologist must be a licensed medical doctor, have had at least one year of residency in surgery, three years of residency in otolaryngology, and have passed written and oral exams given by the board. Some otolaryngologists specialize in cancer.

otoscopy   An examination of the ear using an otoscope, an instrument with a light and lens which can be inserted in the ear.

ovarian cancer [ovarian epithelial cancer]   cancer of the female reproductive organs in which the ova, or eggs, are formed. There are two ovaries, one on either side of the uterus. The ovaries also produce ESTROGEN.

The American Cancer Society estimated there would be some 22,220 new cases of ovarian cancer

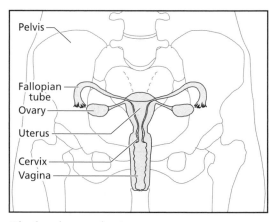

The female reproductive organs. Courtesy NCI.

in the United States and about 16,210 deaths from the disease. It is the fourth most frequent cause of death from cancer in women. A woman's chances of getting ovarian cancer in her lifetime are about 1.7 percent, or one in 58. A woman's lifetime chance of dying from the disease is about 1.0 percent or one in 98. Ovarian cancer is most common in women aged 50 to 59. It is unusual for a woman under the age of 35 to be diagnosed with ovarian cancer. Women at a greater risk of getting ovarian cancer are those with family members who have had it. Three distinct hereditary patterns have been identified: ovarian cancer alone, ovarian and breast cancers, or ovarian and colon cancers. The most important risk factor for ovarian cancer is a family history of a first-degree relative (mother, daughter, or sister) with the disease. The highest risk appears in women with two or more first-degree relatives with ovarian cancer. The risk is somewhat less for women with one first-degree and one second-degree (grandmother, aunt) relative with ovarian cancer. Other risk factors include women who have had few or no children; women with a history of menstrual problems; and women who have had cancer of the breast, intestine, or rectum.

The cause of ovarian cancer is not known, although a number of factors have been associated with its occurrence. It appears that HORMONES play a role in the development of ovarian cancer. This is based on data showing that women who have been pregnant are half as likely to develop this cancer as those who have not been pregnant. The use of birth control pills also seems to lower the risk, quite possibly because they create a hormone balance similar to that found during pregnancy. Women who have had breast cancer are twice as likely to develop ovarian cancer.

Exposure to high levels of radiation may also cause ovarian cancer. Studies of Japanese women following the atomic bomb explosion in Hiroshima found almost twice the expected number of ovarian cancer cases. One study showed that women working in places where they were exposed to high levels of ASBESTOS were also at a greater risk of developing ovarian cancer.

The most common type of ovarian cancer, accounting for about 90% of all ovarian cancers, are epithelial carcinomas that arise in the ovary's outer layer. They are classified as:

- serous cystadenocarcinoma
- mucinous cystadenocarcinoma
- endometroid adenocarcinoma
- hclear cell cystadenocarcinoma

OVARIAN GERM CELL TUMOR AND STROMAL TUMOR account for less than 10% of ovarian cancers.

Frequently there are no symptoms in the early stages of ovarian cancer, making it difficult to obtain an early diagnosis, when there is the greatest chance for effective treatment. An ovarian tumor can grow for some time before pressure or pain can be felt or other problems are noticed. When symptoms do occur, they may include abdominal swelling or bloating, discomfort in the lower part of the abdomen, feeling full after a light meal, nausea, vomiting, not feeling hungry, gas, indigestion, losing weight, constant need to urinate, diarrhea or constipation, or nonmenstrual bleeding. (These symptoms may be an indication of many other disorders, and a doctor should be consulted if any persist.)

Procedures used in the diagnosis and evaluation of ovarian cancer may include an internal (pelvic) exam of the uterus, vagina, ovaries, fallopian tubes, bladder, and rectum (in which the doctor feels for lumps or changes or enlarged ovaries), A PAP SMEAR, ULTRASOUND, blood and urine tests, and X-RAYS. Additional procedures that may be done are CT SCAN, LYMPHANGIOGRAPHY, IVP, LOWER GI SERIES, an exploratory LAPAROTOMY, and BIOPSY, which is the only definitive way to reach a diagnosis.

A number of TUMOR MARKERS are being investigated for their role in the diagnosis of ovarian cancer and the follow-up evaluation of its treatment. For example, high levels of CA 125, a MONOCLONAL ANTIBODY, may indicate that cancer cells are still present following initial treatment. However, it is not unusual for levels to be in the normal range even though cancer remains in the body. An increased level of CEA may also be found in some patients with advanced ovarian cancer.

Following is the NATIONAL CANCER INSTITUTE'S (NCI) STAGING for ovarian cancer:

- Stage I—cancer is in one or both ovaries
- Stage II—cancer is in one or both ovaries and has spread to the uterus and/or the fallopian tubes (the pathway used by the egg to get from the ovary to the uterus) and/or other body parts within the pelvis

• Stage III—cancer is in one or both ovaries and has spread to LYMPH NODES or to other body parts inside the abdomen, such as the surface of the liver or intestine

• Stage IV—cancer is in one or both ovaries and has spread outside the abdomen or has spread to the inside of the liver

• Recurrent—the cancer has returned after treatment, or did not respond to the initial therapy. It may recur in the ovary that is left after surgical removal of a diseased ovary, or in another place.

Treatment depends on the stage of the disease, the general state of health of the patient, and other factors. Treatment for ovarian cancer may be SURGERY alone in early stages, RADIATION THERAPY and CHEMOTHERAPY, INTRA-PERITONEAL THERAPY, and other treatments being investigated in CLINICAL TRIALS. In January 2006, a study from Johns Hopkins indicated that there was a substantial benefit in survival in patients given both intravenous and intraperitoneal therapies after debulking surgery. This, along with existing, previous data, prompted the National Cancer Institute to issue a major clinical announcement in January 2006, suggesting that these therapies should be the new standard of care in a select group of patients. The procedure had been under active study for some 20 years. Surgical options include a TOTAL ABDOMINAL HYSTERECTOMY, UNILATERAL SALPINGO-OOPHOREC-TOMY, BILATERAL SALPINGO-OOPHORECTOMY, and TUMOR DEBULKING (taking out as much of the cancer as possible). (See INTRAPERITONEAL THERAPY.) For specific information on the latest state-of-the-art treatment, by stage, call NCI's Cancer Information Service at 1-800-4-CANCER (1-800-422-6237), or for a TTY: 1-800-332-8615. See also GILDA RADNER FAMILIAL REGISTER.

ovarian germ cell tumor and stromal tumor [sex cord tumor]   two rare ovarian cancers that make up less than 10% of the ovarian cancers diagnosed. Germ cell tumors affect the special cells that give rise to the ovaries during fetal development.

The most frequently seen stromal tumors are granulosa cell tumors and Sertoli-Leydig tumors. The most common germ cell tumors, found primarily in teenage girls and young women, are dysgermi-noma, endodermal sinus tumor, embryonal carcinoma, malignant teratoma, and CHORIOCARCINOMA.

Symptoms, which usually do not occur until late stages of the disease, may include a swelling in the abdomen without a weight gain in other places or vaginal bleeding after menopause. Procedures in the diagnosis and evaluation of ovarian germ cell tumor and stromal tumor may include an internal (pelvic) exam, blood test and urinalysis, ULTRA-SOUND, and CT SCAN.

Following is the National Cancer Institute's (NCI) staging for ovarian germ cell tumor and stromal tumors:

• Stage I—cancer is in one or both ovaries

• Stage II—cancer is in one or both ovaries and/or has spread to the uterus and/or the fallopian tubes (the pathway used by egg cells to get from the ovary to the uterus) and/or other body parts within the pelvis

• Stage III—cancer is in one or both of the ovaries and has spread to LYMPH NODES or to other parts of the body in the abdomen, such as the surface of the liver, or intestine

• Stage IV—cancer is in one or both ovaries and has spread outside the abdomen or to the inside of the liver

• Recurrent—the cancer has returned to the original site or appears in another place in the body after it has been treated

Treatment depends on the stage of the disease, the general state of health of the patient, and other factors. The three types of treatment that may be used in ovarian germ cell tumor and stromal tumor are SURGERY, RADIATION THERAPY, and CHEMOTHERAPY. For specific information on the latest state-of-the-art treatment, by stage, call NCI's Cancer Information Service at 1-800-4-CANCER (1-800-422-6237), or for a TTY: 1-800-332-8615.

ovariectomy   See OOPHORECTOMY.

ovaries   two small, round organs on each side of the uterus that produce eggs and female HORMONES. See OVARIAN CANCER.

oxycodone   See PERCODAN.

oxymorphone   See NUMORPHAN.

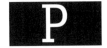

p27 a newly discovered ONCOGENE in the body that may be able to predict how aggressive a cancer is, thereby identifying those patients at greatest risk of not surviving the cancer. Lower levels of p27 in BREAST, PROSTATE, LUNG, COLON, and ESOPHAGEAL cancers could indicate a need for the most aggressive treatment possible. It is a prognostic indicator that is not readily available and has not been validated.

P53 gene a tumor-suppressing ONCOGENE that controls other growth-related genes. A mutation of this tumor-suppressing gene has been found in a wide variety and large number of cancers and is the most common alteration in human cancer. When P53 is inactivated, a block of cell proliferation is removed, enabling unregulated cell growth that can lead to cancer.

PABA (para-aminobenzoic acid) a chemical used in sunscreen and sunblock products to help protect the skin from the harmful ULTRAVIOLET RADIATION from the sun. PABA can be listed in different ways, including para-aminobenzoic acid, glycerol PABA, octyldimethyl PABA, padimate O, and padimate A. Some people have an allergic reaction to PABA and should seek a product without PABA.

PAC a combination of the anticancer drugs Platinol (CISPLATIN), ADRIAMYCIN, and CYTOXAN sometimes used in the treatment of ovarian cancer. See individual drug listings for side effects.
See also COMBINATION CHEMOTHERAPY.

paclitaxel See TAXOL.

Paget's disease (paj'ets) In BREAST CANCER Paget's disease tumor cells grow through ducts in the breast onto the surface of the nipple. The disease accounts for 3% of all breast cancers and is usually noninvasive. Symptoms may include itching and burning of an eczema-like eruption around the nipple, sometimes accompanied by an oozing or bleeding.
Paget's disease is also a noncancerous disease of the bone resulting in bone degeneration or the formation of bone spurs. The bones affected can become large and misshapen. It may also occur in bones that have been exposed to RADIATION THERAPY. Men are more commonly affected than women. It is sometimes associated with OSTEOSARCOMA.
See also BONE CANCER.

pain a sensation that hurts, that causes discomfort. Pain can range from mild to very severe. It can occur in just one place, or in several areas of the body. Pain can be described in various ways, as sharp or dull, throbbing or steady. Acute pain is usually severe and lasts a relatively short time. Chronic pain may be mild or severe and last for long periods of time.
Besides discomfort, pain can have other effects on the body and psyche. It can cause physical symptoms such as nausea, headache, dizziness, drowsiness, constipation, and diarrhea. Pain can also cause psychological or emotional symptoms

such as fear, anger, DEPRESSION, crying, irritability, and suicidal feelings. It can affect sleep as well as appetite. Pain can affect basic lifestyle, preventing a person from working, taking part in habitual recreational activities, and interfering with personal relationships.

Among cancer patients, the degree of pain depends on the type of cancer, the stage of disease, and the patient's pain tolerance. Pain associated with cancer may be a result of:

- pressure on a nerve by a tumor
- infection or inflammation
- poor blood circulation because of blocked blood vessels
- blockage of an organ or tube in the body
- bone fractures caused by cancer cells that have spread to the bone
- after effects of surgery, stiffness from inactivity, or side effects from medications, as constipation or mouth sores
- after affects of RADIATION THERAPY or CHEMO-THERAPY
- nonphysical responses to illness such as tension, depression, or anxiety.

Much research is being conducted in the understanding of the causes of pain and its treatment.

See also PAIN MANAGEMENT.

pain management eliminating/controlling pain in the cancer patient. This is a major component in the comprehensive treatment of cancer. The treatment of pain has undergone dramatic changes since the mid-1970s, when researchers discovered how opiates relieve pain and isolated natural substances in the body called endorphins and enkephalins that fight pain. New and far more effective ways of administering pain medication, surgical procedures, and nonmedical techniques have been developed.

Many hospitals have pain specialists, physicians who specialize in the treatment and management of pain. These specialists do an initial assessment and evaluation of the individual cancer patient's pain—to determine its source and the patient's perception of it and the best way to treat it. They regularly reassess the patient's response to the pain therapy and make modifications when needed. Referral to a pain management center or an organized pain con-

trol team is a viable option for any cancer patient suffering uncontrolled pain.

The most common method of pain control is the use of medication known as ANALGESICS. Analgesics do not affect the cause of the pain; they relieve pain temporarily by suppressing it. Analgesics come in different degrees of strength. Those that are used for mild to moderate pain are called nonopioids and generally can be purchased over the counter (eg., aspirin, Tylenol, ibuprofen) without a prescription. Nonsteroidal anti-inflammatory drugs (NSAID), some of which can be bought over the counter, are also part of the group known as NONOPIOIDS.

OPIOIDS are used to treat moderate to severe pain. These are the strongest analgesics, which always require a doctor's prescription.

Over-the-counter analgesics are generally the first drugs to be used. Some of the over-the-counter analgesics include aspirin and acetaminophen. If they are not sufficiently effective they may be used in combination with other analgesics, or the next level of analgesics may be used. In patients with more severe pain, over-the-counter drugs may be used to potentiate the effects of narcotics.

Narcotics are used when other drugs have not been effective in controlling pain. Some patients can develop a tolerance of the drug and require larger and larger doses for it to be effective. While some patients may become physically dependent on the narcotic, it is important to note that physical dependence is different from addiction, which has a strong psychological factor. The misguided fear of addiction unnecessarily prevents many patients from receiving adequate treatment to relieve or control their pain. Following are some of the common narcotics used in the treatment of pain:

- morphine
- codeine
- *Percocet (Oxycodone Hcl)*
- Percodan (oxycodone)
- Levo-Dromoran (levorphanol)
- Dilaudid hydromorphone
- Demerol (meperidine)
- methadone (Dolophine)
- Numorphan (oxymorphone)
- Fentanyl citrate (duragesis)
- *Vicodin (hydroxycodone and APAP)*

Analgesics are generally taken by mouth or given by injection into a muscle, but they can be administered in a number of ways including:

- orally—by tablet, capsule, or liquid
- IV—injected into a vein
- IM—injected into a muscle
- subcutaneous injection—injected just under the skin using a small needle
- epidural or intrathecal injections—placed directly into the back using a small tube
- transdermal patch—a patch that is placed on the skin
- indwelling reservoir—a thin tube that extends outside of the body and is anchored into a large vein in the body
- analgesic pump—amount of narcotic entering body is regulated by patient
- rectal suppository—the medicine placed in the rectum and absorbed by the body

One of the newer methods of pain medication administration, the analgesic pump, is commonly referred to as patient controlled analgesia (PCA). The patient can turn the pump on and off and control the rate of drug delivery. Epidural administration is another recent development. Tiny doses of morphine are placed into the space just outside of the spinal cord by the physician. A method approved late in 1998 is a lollyipop called ACTIQ (contains fentanyl citrate), which starts relieving pain as the patient disolves the lozenge in the mouth.

Other techniques that may be used in controlling pain are nerve blocks (medication is injected directly around a nerve or into the spine to block the pain), tranquilizers, alcohol (drinking small amounts may relieve pain and increase appetite), antidepressants, and anticonvulsants (which can relieve tingling and burning pain and which when working with other pain medications can achieve greater pain control), and steroids (which can help relieve bone pain, pain caused by spinal cord and brain tumors and pain caused by inflammation). These may be called co-analgesics.

Surgical methods of pain relief include pain NERVE ROOT CLIPPING (cutting nerves high in the neck), CORDOTOMY (cutting nerves in the spinal column), EPIDURAL DORSAL COLUMN STIMULATOR (implantation of electrodes), RHIZOTOMY (cutting

nerves close to the spinal cord), surgery (removal of all or part of tumor that is causing pain by putting pressure on nerves or other body parts).

Radiation therapy can reduce pain by shrinking a tumor.

Other methods of pain control include transcutaneous electric nerve stimulation and percutaneous cordotomy.

Nonmedical treatment methods of pain include BIOFEEDBACK, ACUPUNCTURE, ACUPRESSURE, HYPNOSIS, IMAGERY, and various RELAXATION TECHNIQUES.

Investigations into new and more effective methods of pain control are ongoing.

palate (pal'at)   the roof of the mouth.

Pallace   See MEGACE.

Palladone   the extended-release version of Dilaudid; HYDROMORPHONE extended-release capsule. A narcotic ANALGESIC given orally every 24 hours for relief of persistent severe pain.

See also DILAUDID.

palliative treatment (pal'e-a"tive)   the use of medical remedies to relieve pain, symptoms, and/or prevent further complications rather than to cure. The term *palliative care* is often used when palliative treatment alone is given for the comfort of the patient when a cure is not possible—to improve the patient's quality of life. Palliation can be achieved with drugs (palliative chemotherapy), radiation (palliative radiation), or surgery (palliative surgery). For example, radiation to a METASTASIS in a bone will not cure the cancer but can relieve the pain. In advanced BLADDER CANCER, surgery may be performed to make a way for urine to flow out of the body so that it does not go into the bladder, in order to relieve or reduce symptoms. The use of optimum pain medications, to keep a person as pain-free as possible, is also palliative.

palpable mass (pal'pah-bl')   a growth or lump in the body that can be felt by pressing the hands on the surface of the skin.

palpate (pal'pāt)   to examine or explore the body by touch using the hands. Palpation is a basic technique in a medical examination and can be done by an individual as well as a doctor. For example, in a BREAST SELF-EXAMINATION a woman palpates the entire surface of each breast to check for lumps.

pamidronate disodium   See AREDIA.

Pancoast tumor [superior sulcus tumor] a cancerous tumor found in the apex or groove along the top edge of the lung. It is one form of NON-SMALL CELL LUNG CANCER. It grows slowly and can cause pain by affecting adjacent nerves. It is named for the Philadelphia radiologist Henry Khanrath Pancoast.

pancreas (pan′kre-as) a gland located behind and below the stomach. It is pear shaped and about six inches long. It has two basic functions: producing juices for food digestion, which is done by the part of the gland known as the EXOCRINE PANCREAS; and producing hormones, such as insulin, that regulate how the body stores and uses food, which is a function of the ENDOCRINE PANCREAS.

See also PANCREATIC CANCER.

pancreas scan an examination of the pancreas after administration by IV (injected into a vein) of a

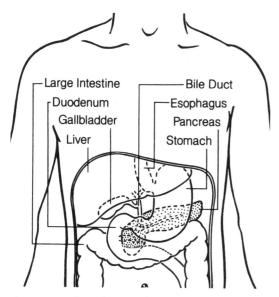

A cutaway view showing the relative size and position of the pancreas in the digestive system. Courtesy NCI.

small, virtually harmless amount of a radioactive substance to a patient. A picture produced by a scanning machine can show areas of concentration of the radioactive substance, where cells are dividing rapidly, which could be a result of cancer. The scan can take between one and two hours. A LIVER SCAN can be done at the same time. Although a pancreas scan can be done on an outpatient basis, many doctors prefer that the patient be hospitalized.

See also NUCLEAR SCAN.

pancreatic cancer (pan″kre-at′ik) [exocrine cancer] cancer of the large, elongated gland behind the stomach that secretes the hormone insulin and juice containing digestive enzymes. Although pancreatic cancer itself is not common, nine cases per 100,000 in the United States, it is the fifth most common cause of death from cancer. The American Cancer Society estimated there would be some 32,180 (16,100 men and 16,080 women) new cases of cancer of the pancreas during 2005. Over the past 15 to 25 years, rates of cancer of the pancreas have slowly dropped in men and women.

An estimated 31,800 Americans (15,820 men and 15,980 women) will die of pancreatic cancer in 2005, making this type of cancer the fourth leading cause of cancer death overall.

Only about 23% of patients with cancer of the exocrine pancreas will be alive one year after their diagnosis; only about 4% will live five years after diagnosis. Even for those people diagnosed with local disease (has not spread to other organs), the five-year RELATIVE SURVIVAL RATE is only 15%. It is more common among men than women, and more common in blacks than whites. It usually develops in people over the age of 60.

There are two types of pancreatic cancer: exocrine and endocrine. Exocrine pancreatic cancer accounts for about 95% of cases of pancreatic cancer and originates primarily in the head of the organ and less commonly in the body or tail. Some are diffused throughout the pancreas. The most common type is called ductal adenocarcinoma. It arises in the duct cell membrane of the pancreas. Other, rare exocrine tumors include giant cell carcinoma and acinar cell carcinoma. Cancer of the endocrine pancreas, or ISLET CELL CARCINOMA, is very rare, accounting for several hundred cases a year in the United States. Islet cell carcinomas are slow growing and generally have a better PROGNOSIS than exocrine pancreatic cancer.

The most common risk factor for pancreatic cancer is smoking. Studies have indicated that people who smoke may increase their risk as much as sixfold. People who stop smoking eventually reduce their risk of getting pancreatic cancer to the risk nonsmokers face. Coffee drinking, which was at one time considered a risk factor in the development of pancreatic cancer, is no longer considered to be any kind of risk in this disease.

Some studies have indicated that diets high in fat and meat may be related to the disease, and that fruits and vegetables may be preventive. Although alcohol has been mentioned as a possible risk, its role has not been established.

The role that exposure to known carcinogens in the workplace plays in the development of pancreatic cancer has not been established. What has been found, however, is that the percentage of pancreatic cancer patients who have worked in occupations where they were exposed to solvents and petroleum compounds is greater than the percentage of patients with other types of cancer who have had similar exposure.

There is some data indicating a hereditary factor in the development of pancreatic cancer, although it has been seen in some hereditary disorders including hereditary pancreatitis (inflammation of the pancreas), FAMILIAL MULTIPLE POLYPOSIS OF THE COLON, and neurofibromatosis, sometimes called "elephant man" disease.

Early symptoms, such as abdominal pain and discomfort, nausea, diarrhea, belching, a feeling of fullness, intolerance for fatty foods, weight loss, loss of appetite, and loss of strength and energy, resemble those of other digestive disorders. Thus, pancreatic cancer may be difficult to detect and is usually not diagnosed in an early stage when there is the greatest possibility of effective treatment. Later symptoms may include jaundice (which may be a very subtle yellow discoloration of the skin due to blockage of the biliary duct system), severe back pain, and itchy skin (due to backing up of bile pigment).

Among the procedures that may be used in diagnosing pancreatic cancer are ULTRASOUND, CT SCANS, MRI, percutaneous transhepatic cholangiog-

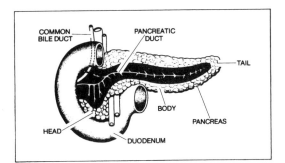

The pancreas. Courtesy NCI.

raphy, X-RAYS, ENDOSCOPIC RETROGRADE CHOLANGIOPANCREATOGRAPHY, CA 19-9 and CEA. For a definitive diagnosis a LAPAROTOMY with a biopsy is generally required. However a PERCUTANEOUS NEEDLE BIOPSY may also be sufficient to achieve a diagnosis, thereby eliminating the need for surgery.

Following is the NATIONAL CANCER INSTITUTE'S (NCI) STAGING for pancreatic cancer:

- Stage I—the cancer is entirely confined to the pancreas or has started to spread to nearby tissue such as the small intestine, bile duct, stomach, or tissues around the pancreas
- Stage II—the cancer has spread further to involve adjacent organs such as the stomach, spleen, or colon but has not entered the LYMPH NODES
- Stage III—the cancer has spread to the lymph nodes near the pancreas; it may or may not have spread to nearby organs
- Stage IV—the cancer has spread to distant sites, most commonly the liver or lungs
- Recurrent—the cancer has returned in the pancreas or in another part of the body.

Treatment depends on the stage of the disease, the general state of health of the patient, and other factors. Treatment for pancreatic cancer includes surgery, CHEMOTHERAPY, and RADIATION THERAPY. Surgical options may include a PANCREATODUODENECTOMY (the WHIPPLE PROCEDURE), a TOTAL PANCREATECTOMY, or a DISTAL PANCREATECTOMY. For specific information on the latest state-of-the-art treatment, by stage, call NCI's Cancer Information Service at 1-800-4-CANCER (1-800-422-6237), or for a TTY: 1-800-332-8615.

pancreatic oncofetal antigen See POA and CA-19-9.

pancreatoduodenectomy (pan″kre-ah-to-du″o-dĕ-nek′to-me) surgical removal of most of the pancreas gland and the adjacent duodenum (first eight to 10 inches of the small intestine). This operation, known as a WHIPPLE PROCEDURE, is a common surgical treatment for PANCREATIC CANCER in which the head of the pancreas is removed.

pancytopenia (pan″si-to-pe′ne-ah) a decrease in all three major BLOOD CELL LINES—white, red, and PLATELETS. There are different causes for this—for example, failure of the bone marrow to produce cells, or an increase in the destruction of blood cells (e.g., by an enlarged spleen or by immunological destruction). Many primary BONE MARROW diseases may cause pancytopenia. HAIRY CELL LEUKEMIA is commonly associated with pancytopenia. Many drugs/chemicals and RADIATION may cause pancytopenia.

Pap smear [Pap test] the microscopic examination of cells from the vagina or the cervix (of the uterus). It is a quick and painless screening test for the detection of precancerous stages of CERVICAL CANCER. The Pap smear is named for Dr. George Papanicolaou, who developed it more than 50 years ago. It can show the presence of infection, inflammation, abnormal cells, or cancer.

The Pap smear is usually done in a doctor's office. The woman lies on the examination table. A speculum is inserted into the vagina to widen the opening. A cotton swab, a cervical brush, or a wooden spatula is then used to remove a sample of cells from the surface of the vagina and cervix. The cells are smeared on a glass slide, which is sent to a lab for microscopic examination. A positive Pap smear—or a Pap smear that is not negative—is not proof of cancer but may indicate the need for further diagnostic tests.

The NATIONAL CANCER INSTITUTE (NCI) recommends that all women 18 or older or who have had sexual intercourse have an annual Pap smear done. After a woman has had three normal Pap smears, the exam may be done less frequently, as her doctor advises. Women who are at an increased risk of developing cervical cancer may need more frequent Pap smears.

There has been some controversy over how Pap smear results are reported. Following are the class numbers frequently used and a brief explanation of what each means:

- Class 1—the Pap smear is completely normal; there are no abnormal cells present.
- Class 2—some cells are abnormal, but none suggests cancer. The abnormal cells may be due to an inflammation and/or infection. The Pap smear should be repeated in three to six months.
- Class 3—DYSPLASIA is present. A follow-up Pap smear and a BIOPSY may be needed.
- Class 4—carcinoma in situ is found; a follow-up Pap smear and biopsy are needed.
- Class 5—the Pap smear reveals invasive cancer of the cervix. A biopsy is needed.

In 1988, an NCI-sponsored workshop proposed a new reporting system called the "Bethesda system." It is less ambiguous than the class system and allows for clearer communication between the lab examining the cells and the physician who is treating the patient.

The Bethesda system uses very specific, descriptive diagnoses rather than class numbers. It also evaluates the adequacy of the smear sample, thereby reducing the likelihood of a false-negative result due to an insufficient sample of cells. For example, under the Bethesda system, the lab will report whether the specimen examined was satisfactory for interpretation, less than optimal, or unsatisfactory. If the sample was not satisfactory, it will explain why. There are eight possibilities listed, including poor fixation or preservation, obscuring blood, presence of a foreign material such as a lubricant, etc. The Bethesda system is much more sophisticated and comprehensive than the class numbers system and provides the physician with much more information. It has been endorsed by many professional organizations. Its use is widespread and it is the standard of reporting. Screening by computer is also available in general as a quality assurance tool.

See also SCREENING.

Pap test See PAP SMEAR.

PAP test See PROSTATIC ACID PHOSPHATASE TEST.

papillary cancer of the bladder (pap'ĭ-ler"e) one type of BLADDER CANCER that starts on the wall of the bladder and grows into the bladder cavity, while staying attached to the wall. The tumor cells appear to be almost normal. It is sometimes referred to as superficial bladder cancer and is staged 0 (in situ).

papilloma virus See HUMAN PAPILLOMAVIRUS.

para-aminobenzoic acid See PABA.

paracentesis (par"ah-sen-te'sis) [peritoneocentesis] insertion of a thin needle or tube into the peritoneal cavity (space between the membrane lining the abdomen and the membrane covering the abdominal organs) to remove fluid. This can be performed to relieve symptoms or for diagnosis, in which case some of the fluid that is extracted is microscopically examined for cancer cells or other abnormalities.

paramethasone See ADRENOCORTICOIDS.

paranasal sinus/nasal cavity cancer cancer of the paranasal sinuses, small hallow spaces around the nose. The sinuses are lined with cells that make mucus, which keeps the nose from drying out; the sinuses are also a space through which the voice can echo to make sounds when one talks or sings. The nasal cavity is the passageway just behind the nose through which air passes on the way to the throat when breathing. It is a very rare cancer occurring in about one in 100,000 people each year in the United States. These cancers appear about twice as often in men and usually occur after the age of 40. People at the greatest risk of developing this cancer appear to be those who work in occupations that are associated with wood dust and in other occupations where there is a lot of dust, such as baking and the flour-making industry.

Symptoms may include blocked sinuses that don't clear, sinus infection, nose bleeding, a lump or sore in the nose that doesn't heal, frequent headaches or pain in the sinus region, swelling or other trouble with the eyes, pain in the upper teeth, or problems with dentures.

Following is the NATIONAL CANCER INSTITUTE'S (NCI) STAGING for paranasal sinus/nasal cavity cancer:

- Stage I—cancer is confined with no bone erosion (wearing away) or destruction; there is no evidence of spread to LYMPH NODES or to other parts of the body
- Stage II—there is erosion or destruction of the bone; there is no evidence of spread to lymph nodes or to other parts of the body
- Stage III—there is no evidence of spread to other parts of the body and
  — the cancer is more extensive and invades the skin of the cheek and/or other nearby areas or
  — the cancer has spread to a single lymph node three CENTIMETERS (cm) or less on the same side of the neck as the primary cancer
- Stage IV
  — the cancer is massive and has invaded nearby parts of the body including the base of the skull; there may be no spread to distant parts of the body and there is no more than one lymph node involved no more than 3 cm and on the same side as the primary tumor or
  — there is one abnormal lymph node larger than 3 cm; or there are multiple abnormal nodes of any size on the same side of the neck; or there is one abnormal lymph node (or more) on the opposite side of the neck from the primary tumor or
  — the cancer has spread to distant parts of the body
- Recurrent—the cancer has returned to the same site or to another part of the body after treatment

Treatment depends on the stage of the disease, the general state of health of the patient, and other factors. Treatment is generally SURGERY CHEMO-THERAPY or RADIATION THERAPY. For specific information on the latest state-of-the-art treatment, by stage, call NCI's Cancer Information Service at 1-800-4-CANCER (1-800-422-6237), or for a TTY: 1-800-332-8615.

See also HEAD AND NECK CANCER.

paraneoplastic syndrome (par"ah-ne"o-plas'tik) symptoms caused by a tumor that appears elsewhere in the body and would not normally be associated with the presence of that cancer. For example, in lung cancer, hormones are produced by some lung cancer cells. One of those is argine vasopressin, which acts on the kidneys, causing a drastic reduction of the level of sodium in the body. That can result in confusion and even a coma, which is not a typical symptom of lung cancer. Another paraneoplastic symptom is an increase in body fat and hair growth caused by the increased production of the hormone adrenocorticotropic (ACTH) or parathormone (PTH).

Paraneoplastic syndromes can play a role in the diagnosis and treatment of cancer, and it is important that they be recognized for the following reasons:

- their appearance can be the first sign of cancer and can enable the cancer to be detected early, when it is most treatable
- they may erroneously be diagnosed as METASTATIC cancer, thereby preventing the patient from receiving appropriate or even curative treatment
- conversely, treatable metastatic complications may be perceived as a paraneoplastic syndrome, leading to inappropriate treatment
- a paraneoplastic syndrome may serve as a TUMOR MARKER in previously treated patients to detect recurrence, or in patients undergoing ADJUVANT THERAPY to guide further treatment
- treatment of the paraneoplastic syndrome in a patient with metastatic disease may be an effective PALLIATIVE TREATMENT

Paraplatin   See CARBOPLATIN.

parathyroid gland cancer (par"ah-thi'roid)   a rare cancer of the four small glands behind the thyroid gland in the lower mid-neck that regulate the balance of calcium and phosphorus in the body. Symptoms of parathyroid gland cancer may include bone pain, formation of kidney stones, irregular heartbeat rhythm, and symptoms of hypercalcemia (too much calcium in the blood) such as fatigue, muscle weakness, depression, anorexia, nausea, and constipation.

Parathyroid gland cancer is staged by the NATIONAL CANCER INSTITUTE (NCI) as localized, metastatic, or recurrent. Localized means that the tumor may have invaded adjacent tissues but not the regional lymph nodes. Metastatic means that the tumor has spread to the regional lymph nodes or distant sites. *Recurrent* means that the cancer has come back (recurred) after it has been treated. It may come back in the original place or in another part of the body.

Treatment depends on the stage of the disease, the general state of health of the patient, and other factors. The usual treatment is surgery or radiation therapy. For specific information on the latest state-of-the-art treatment, by stage, call NCI's Cancer Information Service at 1-800-4-CANCER (1-800-422-6237), or for a TTY: 1-800-332-8615.

parenteral nutrition (pah-ren'ter-al) [total parenteral nutrition (TPN)]   providing a malnourished patient with nutrients by injection into the bloodstream or tissues. Parenteral nutrition may be used to reverse a condition of malnutrition in the patient with cancer, either before treatment (to build up the patient's health) or after treatment. Hospitalized cancer patients have the highest rate of malnutrition of any group of hospital patients, lessening the effectiveness of therapy. The malnutrition may be a result of:

- an extreme loss of weight because of a lack of appetite, caused either by the cancer itself or by the treatment of the cancer (surgery, anticancer drugs, and/or radiation therapy)
- an inability to eat because of the cancer or its treatment
- an inability of the body to metabolize nutrients.

Parenteral fluids contain a mixture of amino acids, fat, sugar, vitamins—all the known essential nutrients. Although many patients have standard nutritional requirements and can receive a "standard" solution, others have specific needs that require a specially designed parenteral fluid.

Parenteral nutrition may also be used with a patient who no longer has to be hospitalized. It can be administered by IV (injected into a vein) at the patient's home.

There is some controversy regarding parenteral nutrition—whether it works and who will benefit from it. Some question whether parenteral nutrition actually alters the patients metabolism and improves the patient's tolerance of and response to treatment, and whether the parenteral nutrition supports, or even promotes or accelerates, the growth of the tumor (feeds the tumor).

See also HYPERALIMENTATION and CACHEXIA.

parosteal osteosarcoma (par-os'te-al os"te-o-sar-ko'mah) [parosteal sarcoma, juxtacortical osteosarcoma]   a type of OSTEOSARCOMA that generally affects young people between the ages of 10 and 25. The cancer usually involves the midshaft of the long bones rather than the ends. This is a slow-growing cancer.

See also BONE CANCER.

parosteal sarcoma   See PAROSTEAL OSTEOSARCOMA.

parotid gland cancer (pah-rot'id)   a rare cancer arising in the large salivary gland, which is near the ear. Most tumors found in the parotid gland are benign (noncancerous). Symptoms of parotid gland cancer may include the presence of a slowly growing lump in the cheek next to the ear. Occasionally there is a dull pain that gets worse and facial nerve paralysis. Diagnostic procedures may include a CT SCAN or MRI and BIOPSY.

Treatment depends on the extent of the disease and other factors. The primary treatment is surgery, which may be followed by RADIATION THERAPY. In some cases CHEMOTHERAPY may be used. Clinical trials are evaluating new treatment. For specific information on the latest state-of-the-art treatment, call the National Cancer Institutes's Cancer Information Service at 1-800-4-CANCER (1-800-422-6237), or for a TTY: 1-800-332-8615.

partial laryngectomy (lar"in-jek'to-me) [hemilaryngectomy]   surgical removal of part of the larynx (voice box). During the procedure a hole (tracheostomy) for breathing is made in the windpipe. The tracheostomy is temporary, and normal breathing is usually restored within a few days. This is a treatment that may be used for LARYNGEAL CANCER.

partial mastectomy   See LUMPECTOMY.

partial nephrectomy (nĕ-frek'to-me)   surgical removal of only the cancerous tumor in the kidney. The normal kidney tissue and function of the kidney are preserved. This is a treatment that may be used in very early KIDNEY CANCER or in patients who have only one kidney.

partial penectomy (pe-nek'to-me)   surgical removal of the part of the penis that contains the urethra (the tube that carries urine from the bladder to outside the body). This may be performed in the treatment of URETHRAL CANCER.

partial remission (PM)   See REMISSION.

particle beam therapy [neutron beam therapy, proton beam therapy, high linear energy transfer (LET) radiation]   a type of RADIATION THERAPY using fast-moving subatomic particles, such as protons and neutrons traveling close to the speed of light. It can deliver high energy radiation to tumor cells while avoiding damage to surrounding normal tissue. It requires the use of a very expensive and sophisticated radiation machine. Particle beam therapy may be used alone or with CHEMOTHERAPY (anticancer drugs) in the treatment of many cancers, including cancers of the lung, brain, uterus, head and neck, gastrointestinal tract, pancreas, and urinary tract.

passive smoke [environmental tobacco smoke (ETS), secondhand smoke]   tobacco smoke in the environment made up of sidestream smoke (emitted by the burning end of a cigarette) and mainstream smoke (emitted by the smoker) in an enclosed space. See SECONDHAND SMOKING.

passive smoking   See SECONDHAND SMOKING.

pathologist (pah-thol'o-jist)   a doctor who specializes in the examination of normal and diseased tissue. A pathologist microscopically examines tissue for the presence of cancer cells, the type of cell, their origin, their rate of reproduction, their grade (degree of DIFFERENTIATION), and other factors that may affect treatment and prognosis.

pathology (pah-thol'o-je)   the study of disease and its effect on body tissue. See PATHOLOGIST.

PCA (patient-controlled analgesia)   See ANALGESIC PUMP and PAIN MANAGEMENT.

PCB   See PROCARBAZINE.

PCR   See POLYMERASE CHAIN REACTION.

PDGF (platelet-derived growth factor)   a family of proteins involved in the proliferation pathway.

PDGFR   the receptor for PDGF.

PDQ (Physician Data Query)   a computer data base for retrieval of cancer treatment information supported by the NATIONAL CANCER INSTITUTE (NCI). The database has three major files:

- a file that summarizes the latest cancer treatment for both patients, written in layperson's language, and physicians
- a file of ongoing CLINICAL TRIALS that are accepting patients
- a directory of doctors who provide cancer treatment and health care organizations that have programs of cancer care.

The treatment information is developed and refined with the assistance of more than 400 cancer specialists in the United States and is updated monthly. It is considered state-of-the-art treatment information because it includes the latest and best available treatments for a specific type of cancer, by STAGE.

PDQ is available on the Internet at http://www.cancer.gov/cancertopics/pdq/cancerdatabase. Cancer patients and the general public can get PDQ information by calling the NCI's Cancer Information Service at 1-800-4-CANCER (1-800-422-6237), or for a TTY: 1-800-332-8615.

PDR   *Physician's Desk Reference.*

PDT   See PHOTODYNAMIC THERAPY.

pediatric cancers   See CHILDHOOD CANCERS.

pediatric oncologist (ong-kol'o-jist)   a doctor who specializes in childhood cancers.
See also MEDICAL ONCOLOGIST.

PEG   See PERCUTANEOUS ENDOSCOPIC GASTROSTOMY.

pegaspargase [Oncaspar, PEG-L-asparaginase] an anticancer drug used in the treatment of patients with acute lymphoblastic leukemia who have developed a hypersensitivity to the native forms of L-asparaginase. It is given by IV (into a vein) or IM (into a muscle).
See also L-ASPARAGINASE.

Pegfilgrastim   See NEULASTA.

PEG-L-asparaginase   See PEGASPARGASE.

Pel-Epstein fever (pel-eb'stīn)   a persistent but remittent, unexplained fever or intermittent cyclic episodes of fever; it may be a symptom of HODGKIN'S DISEASE as well as other disorders.

pelvic exam   the part of a gynecological (referring to a woman's sexual organs) exam that focuses on the VAGINA, VULVA, CERVIX, FALLOPIAN TUBES, OVARIES, and UTERUS. A pelvic exam is done routinely when a woman goes to her doctor, generally a gynecologist, for a check-up and for diagnostic purposes. After disrobing from the waist down, the woman lies on her back on an examination table. Her knees are bent and her feet are elevated and in stirrups. A pelvic exam has several different parts. The doctor inserts one or two gloved and lubricated fingers into the vagina while placing the other hand on the lower abdomen to feel the size, shape and position of the ovaries and uterus. Then a SPECULUM is inserted into the vagina which enables the doctor to view the inside of the vagina and the cervix and to remove some tissue for a PAP SMEAR. The last part is the rectal examination in which the doctor inserts one gloved, lubricated finger into the rectum and another into the vagina to feel for any abnormalities. The entire pelvic exam takes under half an hour. It is relatively painless (there may be a moment or two of some discomfort).
See also SCREENING.

pelvic exenteration (eks-en"ter-a'shun)   surgical removal of the uterus, fallopian tubes, ovaries, regional lymph nodes, part of the vagina, the bladder, and rectum. This very extreme surgery may be performed for very advanced CERVICAL CANCER or VULVAR CANCER.

pelvic lymph node dissection   surgical removal of the LYMPH NODES in the abdomen. This may be performed in the diagnosis and evaluation of PROSTATE CANCER and TESTICULAR CANCER.

pelvis   the bony part of the body between the thighs and abdomen.

pemetrexed   See ALIMTA.

penectomy (pe-nek'-to-me) surgical removal of the penis. This may be done in the treatment of PENILE CANCER or URETHRAL CANCER. When a penectomy is performed, plastic surgery may be done to construct a new penis.

penile cancer (pe'nīl) cancer of the penis, which is very rare in the United States, accounting for 0.2% of all cancers and 0.1% of deaths in males. It is more common in elderly men and blacks. The rate of incidence increases steadily after age 55. The American Cancer Society estimated that in the United States about 1,470 new cases of penile cancer would be diagnosed, and an estimated 270 men would die of penile cancer in 2005. While penile cancer is very rare in North America and Europe, it is much more common in some parts of Africa and South America, where it accounts for up to 10% of cancers in men.

Epidemiological studies have shown a higher rate of penile cancer among men in cultures where circumcision (removal of all or part of the foreskin on the penis shortly after birth) is not practiced. Phimosis, a condition caused by a lack of cleanliness, has been associated with penile cancer. It is possible, as well, that dietary factors may play a role in penile cancer.

Symptoms of penile cancer may include a painless, small nodule, warty growth, or ulcer on the penis. Other symptoms that may appear later include pain, bleeding during erection or intercourse, a foul-smelling discharge, or a lump in the groin. Diagnosis of penile cancer is fairly routine because of the organ's accessibility. A NEEDLE ASPIRATION BIOPSY of LYMPH NODES or surgical removal of a node may be done to evaluate lymph node involvement. Lymphography may also be performed to diagnose METASTASES.

Following is the NATIONAL CANCER INSTITUTE'S (NCI) STAGING for penile cancer:

- Stage I—a tumor that is limited to the glans (end part of the penis) and the foreskin but does not involve the shaft of the penis
- Stage II—a tumor that has invaded the shaft of the penis but has not spread to lymph nodes
- Stage III—a tumor that has spread to the regional lymph nodes in the groin
- Stage IV—extensive and inoperable involvement of lymph nodes in the groin and/or has spread to other parts of the body

- Recurrent—cancer has returned to the same site or to another part of the body after treatment.

Treatment depends on the stage of the disease and other factors. Surgery is the most common treatment. RADIATION THERAPY, CHEMOTHERAPY, or BIOLOGICAL THERAPY may also be used. For specific information on the latest state-of-the-art treatment, by stage, call NCI's Cancer Information Service at 1-800-4-CANCER (1-800-422-6237), or for a TTY: 1-800-332-8615.

penile implant (pe'nīl) a prosthesis (an artificial substitute for a missing part) surgically implanted into the penis to make sexual intercourse possible. The devices are either semi-rigid or inflatable. The treatment of some cancers, such as prostate cancer, may result in IMPOTENCY (the inability to get an erection).

penis cancer See PENILE CANCER.

pentamadine isethionate [Lomidine] an ANTIBIOTIC that is effective against the protozoan *P. carinii,* which can cause fatal pneumonia in some patients with cancer and AIDS. In treating pneumonia, it is given intravenously. It is also available as an aerosol as a preventative and is widely used by many HIV POSITIVE patients.

pentostatin [deoxycoformycin, VP/Vidaribine, DCF, Nipent] an anticancer drug being used in the treatment of HAIRY CELL LEUKEMIA (HCL) with active disease as defined by clinically significant anemia, neutropenia, thrombocytopenia, or disease-related symptoms. Side effects may include skin rashes, nausea, vomiting, lack of energy and nervous disorders. It is given by IV (injected into a vein).

Percocet a NARCOTIC drug containing oxycodone and ACETAMINOPHEN, used for the relief or control of pain. It is taken orally and is available by prescription only.

See also ANALGESIC and PAIN MANAGEMENT.

Percodan a NARCOTIC drug containing oxycodone used for the relief or control of pain. It is taken orally and is available by prescription only.

See also ANALGESIC.

percutaneous (PTC) (per″ku-ta′ne-us) a term used to describe procedures performed through the skin. Many medical procedures are done percutaneously. For example, in a PERCUTANEOUS NEEDLE BIOPSY, a needle is inserted through the skin to remove tissue for biopsy. A radioactive substance may also be delivered percutaneously.

percutaneous cordotomy (per″ku-ta′ne-us kor-dot′o-me) a technique for relieving or controlling pain. Using an X-RAY for guidance, the doctor inserts a needle through the skin into the pain nerve bundle in the spinal cord. An electric current then passes through the needle into the nerve bundle, destroying it, and the transmission of the sensation of pain to the patient's brain and conscious level is interrupted. It is most commonly used in the treatment of pain arising in the abdomen, chest, arms, and legs.

See also CORDOTOMY.

percutaneous endoscopic gastrostomy (PEG) (per″ku-ta′ne-us en″do-skop′ik gas-tros′to-me) a procedure in which a tube is placed into the stomach through the abdominal wall to allow feeding and medication in a patient with a disorder or dysfunction of the mouth or esophagus. It is done under direct inspection of the stomach via the gastroscope, a thin, lighted tube.

percutaneous needle biopsy (per″ku-ta′ne-us bi′op-se) a commonly performed procedure in which a thin needle is inserted through the skin to obtain a sample of tissue from a part of the body (lung, pancreas, breast, internal lymph nodes) to microscopically examine for the presence of cancer cells.

See also NEEDLE ASPIRATION BIOPSY.

percutaneous nephrostomy (per″ku-ta′ne-us nef-ros′to-me) a procedure in which the kidney is punctured to provide drainage of urine when the ureter leading from the kidney to the bladder is blocked.

percutaneous transhepatic cholangiography (PTC) (per″ku-ta′ne-us trans″he-pă′tik ko″lan-je-og′rah-fe) a procedure used to examine the pancreas and bile duct system. Dye is injected through the skin into the liver. When the dye travels through the gallbladder and bile duct systems, any blockage at the head of the pancreas can be seen. This method has a high degree of accuracy as a diagnostic tool and may be used in the diagnosis of PANCREATIC CANCER. Possible complications may include hemorrhage or infection.

performance status (PS) a statement as to the degree of impact the presence of CANCER has on a patient. PS measures ambulatory capacity, symptoms, and need for assistance. Two systems in current clinical use are the Karnofsky scale and the Eastern Co-operative Oncology Group (ECOG) scale. These are rough but useful guides to PROGNOSIS and response to TREATMENT. A fit person with minimal symptoms may be expected to have a better outcome than one debilitated, severely symptomatic, and bed-bound. Many CLINICAL TRIALS exclude people with the poorest PS.

The ECOG scale is as follows:

ECOG PS	Detail
0	normal activity
1	symptoms but ambutlatory and able to carry out normal activity
2	out of bed more than 50% of day; may need minimal assistance
3	in bed more than 50% of time; requires skilled care
4	100% bed-bound

perfusion administration of CHEMOTHERAPY (anti-cancer drugs) by adding it directly to the blood that is going to an affected limb or body part. In this way, a larger dose reaches the tumor. This technique may be used in the treatment of MELANOMA, when it occurs on an arm or leg. Perfusion chemotherapy, which started out as a treatment for melanoma, is now being more widely explored in the treatment of LIVER CANCER and cancers at other sites.

pericardial effusion collection of fluid in the sac that surrounds the heart, a possible sign of cancer as well as many other conditions. When it is caused by cancer, it can be result of either direct spread of cancer from adjacent organs like the lung, or by metastatic spread from other parts of the body.

See also PERICARDIOCENTESIS.

pericardiocentesis (per″ĭ-kar″de-o-sen-te′sis) a procedure in which a needle is used to remove fluid from the pericardial sac around the heart. The fluid that has been extracted is microscopically examined for cancer cells or other abnormalities.

See also PERICARDIAL EFFUSION.

pericardium (per″ĭ-kar′de-um) a thin lining of tissue surrounding the heart.

perineal prostatectomy (per″ĭ-ne′al pros″tah-tek′to-me) one way of performing a RADIAL PROSTATECTOMY (removal of the prostate and surrounding tissue). The doctor cuts into the space between the scrotum and the anus (the perineum). This may be performed in the treatment of PROSTATE CANCER.

peripheral neuroepithelioma (nu″ro-ep″ĭ-the″le-o′mah) a rare non–central nervous system tumor. It is found most commonly in children and young adults. It arises most often in the chest wall, pelvis, or extremity, either in bone or soft tissue. Evaluation and treatment is the same as for EWING'S SARCOMA.

peripheral stem cell transplantation the removal, storage, and reinfusion of very early cells (stem cells) that produce blood cells. Stem cells are restored in order to reconstitute blood-producing bone marrow in patient's whose bone marrow has been destroyed by high-dose chemotherapy. Blood cells are removed by a technique called pheresis in which the stem cells can be separated from the rest of the blood. The removed stem cells are frozen and stored until the patient is ready to receive them. The recovery time involved in peripheral stem cell support is shorter than for bone marrow transplantation and costs less. Peripheral blood stem cell transplantation has a shorter recovery time than bone marrow transplantation; the stem cells are easier to harvest than bone marrow (it is like drawing blood); and the procedure is less costly. In most instances peripheral stem cell transplantation has replaced bone marrow transplantation as the rescue system used after the administration of high-dose chemotherapy.

See also BONE MARROW TRANSPLANTATION.

peritoneal cavity the lower part of the ABDOMEN that contains the intestines (last part of the digestive tract), the stomach, and the liver.

peritoneal cavity cancer See MESOTHELIOMA.

peritoneocentesis See PARACENTESIS.

peritoneography (per″ĭ-to-ne-og′rah-fe) an X-RAY examination of the peritoneum, the membrane that lines the abdomen.

peritoneoscope See LAPAROSCOPY.

peritoneoscopy See LAPAROSCOPY.

peritoneovenous shunting a small surgical procedure to reduce fluid in the peritoneal cavity (ASCITES) by draining it into the venous system. It may be performed to alleviate persistent ascites due to malignancy where other methods have failed.

peritoneum (per″ĭ-to-ne′um) the membrane that encases the abdominal cavity.

permanent section biopsy examination of tissue for cancer cells. The tissue taken for the BIOPSY is put through a series of solutions that eliminate water and fatty substances. It is then saturated with warm liquid paraffin (wax). When it gets hard, it is cut into thin slices. The slices are placed on slides and stained to bring out cell formations and their nuclei. While a FROZEN SECTION BIOPSY can take minutes, a permanent section biopsy can take a few days. However, a permanent section is more accurate, and a permanent section is always performed, regardless of whether a frozen section was done. The biopsy slides used for the permanent section may be kept indefinitely as a permanent record of the procedure for patient care as well as for medical research and legal reasons.

Permastril [dromostanolone propionate] See ANDROGEN.

pernicious anemia (per-nish'us ah-ne'me-ah) a condition in which a decrease in the RED BLOOD CELLS affects the gastrointestinal and neurological systems. It is caused by the lack of a substance that is essential to the absorption of vitamin B_{12} and the maturation of red blood cells and other cells. Symptoms of pernicious anemia are the same as for ANEMIA and may include paleness, shortness of breath, fatigue, palpitations or heart fluttering, soreness in the tongue and mouth, and a yellowing of the skin. If the nervous system is affected, there may be difficulty walking, tingling in the hands and feet, memory loss, confusion, and depression. Ten percent of the people with pernicious anemia develop STOMACH CANCER.

petechiae (pe-te'ke-ah) small red and/or brown spots on the skin, which are tiny hemorrhages. They can appear as a rash on the skin. Petechiae are

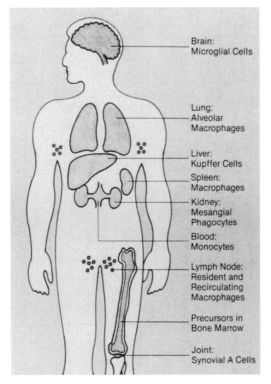

Phagocytes play an important role in the immune system, destroying foreign particles. Courtesy NCI.

caused by a low blood count and decreased clotting function and may be a result of CHEMOTHERAPY, LEUKEMIA, and other disorders.

PET-CT scan the union of a PET NUCLEAR SCAN to traditional CT SCAN technology, currently used as a diagnostic test and one to follow the course of treatment.

PET (positron emission tomography) scan a diagnostic NUCLEAR SCAN introduced to widespread use in imaging in 2002. It is based on the concept that neoplastic tissue is more avid for the tracer radioactive material compared to background tissue. The PET scan does not use X-RAYS but measures emissions from a RADIOACTIVE ISOTOPE injected into the blood. The nuclear equipment used for the scan produces pictures of the organs in slices or planes. For example, in the brain it can show where oxygen is not being metabolized.

Peyer's patches lymphoid tissue in the small intestine. Peyer's patches play a role in the IMMUNE SYSTEM.

PFT See PULMONARY FUNCTION TEST.

phagocytes (fag'o-sīts) any large WHITE BLOOD CELL that can engulf and eat microorganisms and foreign particles. They play an important role in the IMMUNE SYSTEM. Some important phagocytes are MONOCYTES, MACROPHAGES, and NEUTROPHILS.

phagocytosis (fag"o-si-to'sis) the engulfing of microorganisms and other cells and foreign particles by PHAGOCYTES.

phantom pain pain experienced in an arm, leg, or breast that has been removed by surgery. The sensation can also be one of numbness, pins and needles "tingling," and even an itch. Although it is not known why a patient experiences phantom pain, doctors say it is experienced as a real sensation in the brain. It can last for weeks, months, or an indefinite period of time. Various methods of pain therapy have been tried, including spinal surgery, additional surgery at the original site, RELAXATION TECHNIQUES, and HYPNOSIS, which work for some patients.

pharyngeal cancer See OROPHARYNGEAL CANCER.

pharyngeal speech (fah-rin'je-al) a method of speaking after the voice box has been removed. Air that goes into the mouth and nose is blocked by the tongue, causing the air to vibrate against the roof of the mouth. With practice, speech formed this way can sound very close to normal.

pharynx (far'inks) the upper part of the throat, just behind the mouth.

pharynx cancer See OROPHARYNGEAL CANCER.

phenacetin See CARCINOGENS.

phenobarbital (fe"no-bar'bĭ-tal) a drug that may be used as an anticonvulsant to prevent seizures in patients with BRAIN CANCER. It is a central nervous system depressant that slows down the nervous system. Phenobarbital is available by prescription only and is taken by mouth.

phenytoin See DILANTIN.

pheochromocytoma (fe-o-kro"mo-si-to'mah) a rare form of ADRENAL CANCER believed to be inherited. People with pheochromocytoma frequently have hypertension as a result of the release of large amounts of the hormone catecholamine. Symptoms may include headaches, sweating, palpitations, anxiety, and constipation. Diagnostic procedures may include blood tests, urinalysis, CT SCAN, and MRI.

The following stages are used for pheochromocytoma:

  localized benign pheochromocytoma—tumor is found in only one area and has not spread to other tissues
  regional pheochromocytoma—cancer has spread to lymph nodes in the area or to other tissues around the original cancer
  metastatic pheochromocytoma—cancer has spread to other parts of the body
  recurrent pheochromocytoma—the cancer has come back (recurred) after it has been treated. It may come back in the area where it started or in another part of the body

Treatment is generally SURGERY. RADIATION THERAPY and CHEMOTHERAPY may be used. For the latest state-of-the-art treatment, call the National Cancer Institute's Cancer Information Service at 1-800-4-CANCER (1-800-422-6237), or for a TTY: 1-800-332-8615.

Philadelphia chromosome (Ph) an abnormal-appearing CHROMOSOME discovered in 1960 associated with CHRONIC MYELOGENOUS LEUKEMIA (CML). This is a chromosome rearrangement that causes the production of an aberrant protein, a TYROSINE KINASE which causes the disease. This translocation produces an abnormal fusion gene, the BCR-ABL gene, which produces the abnormal protein. The therapeutic drug GLEEVIC was designed to block the activity of this tyrosine kinase, causing APOPTOSIS of the BCR-ABL positive cells.

photochemotherapy See PHOTODYNAMIC THERAPY.

photocoagulation (fo"to-ko-ag"u-la'shun) the use of heat to incapacitate the blood vessels that deliver needed nutrients to cancer cells. Blood vessels entering the tumor are heated by a light beam and destroyed. This treatment is being investigated in the treatment of small ocular melanoma tumors of the eye. It may be used in combination with RADIATION THERAPY.

photodynamic therapy (PDT) [phototherapy; previously known as photochemotherapy and photoradiation therapy (PRT)] a treatment for cancer in which light and a photosensitizer, a substance that makes cells more sensitive to light, interact to destroy tumor tissue.

The photodynamic process was first reported in 1900 by a German scientist who discovered that microorganisms could be inactivated by certain dyes in the presence of light. By the 1920s, researchers had discovered a group of compounds that were selectively retained in cancer cells. Cancer patients were first treated with PDT in the 1960s. The photosensitizer used was hematoporphyrin (HPD).

In photodynamic therapy, patients are injected with a light-activated photosensitizer, PHOTOFRIN, that makes their body sensitive to light. Cancer cells retain the drug. Fiber-optic probes are then used to expose the cancer to laser light and activate the photosensitizer. When it is activated, the photosensitizer produces a toxic reaction, destroying the tumor. Relatively little harm is done to the normal tissue.

Photodynamic therapy has several positive features. Cancer cells can be selectively destroyed while most normal cells are spared; the damaging effects of HPD occur only when it is exposed to light; and the side effects are relatively few. One limiting factor is that the laser light being used in the process can not pass through more than a centimeter of tissue (little more than a third of an inch). Because of the limited range of this technique, its value remains limited to early, superficial lesions or obstructions that are best approached by an endoscope, such as in the lung, esophagus, bladder, and female pelvis.

Side effects may include skin sensitivity for four or more weeks. Exposure to sunlight can produce a severe sunburn. Other side effects may include some pain in the treatment area, a skin reaction similar to a mild sunburn, nausea, vomiting, metallic taste, eye sensitivity to light, and mild liver toxicity. The side effects are reversible.

No longer investigational, the use of photodynamic therapy is still undergoing evaluation and expansion as a new technology. Endoscopists are interested in its possible use in treating of early cancers as well as of obstructing lesions in the esophagus and bronchus. It is not a treatment for metastatic cancers.

Photofrin [porfimer]   a photosensitizing agent for use with PALLIATIVE PHOTODYNAMIC THERAPY of patients with completely or partially obstructing ESOPHAGEAL CANCER who cannot be satisfactorily treated with laser therapy. It is also used in the treatment of microinvasive endobronchial NON-SMALL CELL LUNG CANCER (NSCLC) in patients for whom SURGERY and RADIOTHERAPY are not indicated. Photofrin is given by IV (injected into a vein).

photons (fo′tons)   one type of energy used in RADIATION THERAPY. Photons can take the form of X-RAYS and GAMMA RAYS.

photopheresis (fo″to-fĕ-re′sis)   a treatment procedure using ULTRAVIOLET RADIATION to activate a drug. The patient takes the drug methoxsalen (8-MOP) by mouth. Blood is then taken from the patient, exposed to the ultraviolet light, and then returned to the patient. Photopheresis was approved for the treatment of MYCOSIS FUNGOIDES by the Food and Drug Administration in 1987. It is also used in cutaneous T-cell lymphoma and chronic GRAFT VERSUS HOST DISEASE.

photoradiation   therapy   See   PHOTODYNAMIC THERAPY.

photosensitivity   sensitivity to sun and light. This can be a side effect of CHEMOTHERAPY and result in a severe sunburn with relatively little exposure to sunlight. People receiving chemotherapy should avoid exposure as much as possible, wear protective clothing (a wide-brimmed hat, long-sleeved shirt, etc.), and use a sunblock with a sun protection factor (SPF) of 15 or more.

phototherapy   See PHOTODYNAMIC THERAPY.

PHS (Physicians′ Health Study)   a NUTRITIONAL INTERVENTION STUDY, launched in the United States to study the effect of ASPIRIN and beta carotene on cardiovascular disease and cancer. A total of 22,071 male physicians age 40–84 years old were entered into the study. Reported in 1996, neither agent affected cancer rates positively or negatively.

phymotoxin (fi″mo-toks′in)   an extract of the mandrake plant. ETOPOSIDE, a derivative of phymotoxin, is a very active anticancer drug.

physiatrist (fiz″e-at′rist)   a doctor who specializes in helping patients who are bedridden or have been immobilized for a long period of time exercise and stimulate their muscles to regain strength and independence. The physiatrist also helps people acclimate to artificial limbs and relearn some of the activities of normal everyday life. This therapist can help define for the patient the expected disabilities and outline rehabilitation goals, institute an appropriate rehabilitation program, and supervise treatment and follow-up.

physical therapist   a specialist, trained by a PHYSIATRIST, who can teach patients exercises and other techniques to overcome disabilities as well as help patients become facile in the use of artificial limbs or braces.

physical therapy   teaching a person to perform skills that were done prior to an illness or accident, or how to use an artificial limb. This is usually done by a physical therapist. The physical therapy program for the particular patient may be designed by a PHYSIATRIST.

Physician Data Query   See PDQ.

pigmented nevi   See MOLES.

pineal gland tumors (pin′e-al)   a very rare tumor in the pineal gland, a small structure, about the size of a pea, located near the center of the brain. There are four different kinds of benign (noncancerous) pineal tumors. They occur most frequently in children and young adults. Symptoms may include problems in movement, mental deterioration, and a difficulty in looking up because the pineal gland is near the nerve center that controls upward movement of the eyes. Although surgery is difficult because of the location of the gland, it is being used successfully more and more frequently. RADIATION THERAPY to reduce the tumors is also a treatment being used.

See also BRAIN CANCER.

pituitary adenoma   See PITUITARY TUMOR.

pituitary   tumor (pĭ-tu′ĭ-tar″-e) [pituitary adenoma]   a growth in the pituitary gland, a small organ, about the size of a pea, in the center of the brain just above the back of the nose. Most pituitary tumors are benign (noncancerous), though they frequently produce too many HORMONES, which can cause problems in other parts of the body. Symptoms may include headaches, difficulty seeing, nausea, or vomiting or any of a fairly wide range of symptoms, which depend on the type of pituitary tumor. The symptoms for the particular tumor are included in the staging. Diagnostic procedures may include lab tests for hormone levels, a CT SCAN, and MRI.

Following is the NATIONAL CANCER INSTITUTE'S (NCI) STAGING by type of tumor:

- ACTH-producing tumors—a tumor that makes the hormone adrenocorticotropic hormone

(ACTH), this can result in CUSHING'S DISEASE. Cushing's disease causes a fat buildup in the face, back, and chest while the arms and legs become very thin. Other symptoms may include too much sugar in the blood, weak muscles and bones, a flushed face, and high blood pressure
- prolactin-producing tumor—a tumor that makes prolactin, a hormone that stimulates a woman's breasts to produce milk during and after pregnancy. It can also cause the breasts to make milk and menstrual periods to stop when a woman is not pregnant. In men, it can cause impotence
- growth hormone-producing tumor—a tumor that makes the growth hormone that can cause acromegaly or giantism (larger than normal hands, feet, and face; or the whole body may be larger than normal)
- nonfunctioning pituitary tumor—a tumor that does not make hormones
- recurrent pituitary tumor—a tumor that has returned to the pituitary or another part of the body after treatment

Treatment depends on the type of tumor, how far it has spread into the brain, the age of the patient, and general state of health of the patient. SURGERY is a common treatment. A TRANSPHENOIDAL HYPOPHYSECTOMY or CRANIOTOMY may be performed. RADIATION THERAPY may be used, as well as certain drugs that block the pituitary from making too many hormones. For specific information on the latest state-of-the-art treatment, by stage, call NCI's Cancer Information Service at 1-800-4-CANCER (1-800-422-6237), or for a TTY: 1-800-332-8615.

See also BRAIN CANCER.

placebo (plah-se′bo)   a harmless, inactive substance given to some patients while other patients are given a medication in CLINICAL TRIALS. It can be in tablet or capsule form or given by injection and looks like the medication that is being evaluated. The patient does not know if the substance he or she is receiving is the medication or the placebo. A placebo is used to eliminate any psychological effects that may occur if the patient knows he or she is on the medication. For example, if a pain medication is being tested for how effective it is in relieving pain, just knowing that he or she is getting the medication may make the patient feel better. When the patients do not know which group they are in, the group getting the medication or the group getting the placebo, it is called a "single-blind" study. When the doctor also does not know which patients are getting what, it is called a "double-blind" study. A placebo would only be used in a clinical trial with a new drug when there is no evidence that any current drug or treatment is effective.

placebo effect (plah-se'bo)   a beneficial effect that cannot be attributed to the medical technology used. It is often considered to be psychologically engendered, a belief on the part of the patient that the treatment or technology is beneficial.

placenta cancer   See CHORIOCARCINOMA.

plant alkaloid   See ALKALOIDS.

PLAP   See PLACENTAL ALKALINE PHOSPHATASE.

plasma (plaz'mah)   the colorless fluid part of the blood containing mostly water (more than 90%) in which the blood cells are suspended. Plasma contains ANTIBODIES, HORMONES, salts, electrolytes, nutrients, wastes, and blood-clotting factors.

plasma cell (plaz'mah) [plasmacyte]   large, antibody-producing WHITE BLOOD CELLS that are produced by B lymphocytes. Each plasma cell can produce millions of identical ANTIBODIES, which are released into the bloodstream.

plasma cell dyscrasias   See MYELOMA.

plasma cell leukemia   See LEUKEMIA.

plasma cell neoplasm   See MYELOMA.

plasma cell tumor   See PLASMACYTOMA.

plasma exchange (plaz'mah)   a treatment for conditions thought to be caused by abnormal material circulating in the PLASMA. Its role as a standard treatment for any condition has not been proved. Essentially, the patient's plasma is removed and replaced by material of similar nature that is devoid of the offending agent.

plasma platelet pheresis   See PLATELETPHERESIS.

plasmacyte   See PLASMA CELL.

plasmacytoma (plaz"mah-si-to'mah) [plasma cell tumor]   a MALIGNANT (cancerous) tumor of PLASMA CELLS. When there are multiple plasmacytomas in the body, it is called (multiple) MYELOMA. A single malignant plasma cell can be used in the production of HYBRIDOMAS, which are used to make MONOCLONAL ANTIBODIES.

plasmapheresis (plaz"mah-fĕ-re'sis)   the removal of PLASMA from withdrawn blood. The blood goes through a pheresis machine, which extracts the plasma and separates it from the red and white blood cells and platelets. The blood cells are then returned to the donor. This procedure may be performed in patients with WALDENSTROM'S MACRO-GLOBULINEMIA to reduce the thickness of the blood, which can cause HYPERVISCOSITY SYNDROME. After the blood is separated, the plasma is removed and replaced with a substitute, which is returned to the patient along with the blood cells. Plasmapheresis is also a method of harvesting plasma from healthy people for therapeutic use in a diseased patient.
See PLATELETPHERESIS.

platelet (plāt'let) [thrombocyte]   blood cells that help the blood to clot. They help prevent abnormal or excessive bleeding and hemorrhaging by traveling to the site in the body that is cut or injured. Platelets are produced in the BONE MARROW.

plateletpheresis (plāt"let-fĕ-re'sis) [thrombocytopheresis]   the removal of PLATELETS from withdrawn blood. The blood is passed through a pheresis machine, which extracts the platelets and separates it from the red and white blood cells. The remaining blood cells are then returned to the donor. This procedure may be used for the transfusion of platelets to patients with LEUKEMIA, preventing or limiting hemorrhaging.

Platinol   See CISPLATIN.

platinum   See CISPLATIN.

pleocytosis (ple"o-si-to'sis)   an increase in the number of cells in the spinal fluid. This may be an indication of BRAIN CANCER.

pleomorphic lymphoma (ple"o-mor'fik lim-fo'mah) a type of NON-HODGKIN'S LYMPHOMA occurring in children. It can occur in the chest, abdomen, pelvis, or neck.

pleura the membrane surrounding the lungs.

pleural cavity (ploor'al) a space enclosed by the thin pleura tissue covering the lungs and lining the interior walls of the chest cavity.

pleural effusion (ploor'al) an accumulation of fluid in the pleural cavity, the space between the lungs and the interior walls of the chest. If the cause of this is cancer, this is called malignant pleural effusion.

About 12% of LUNG CANCER patients have this at the time of diagnosis. It may also be the result of cancers of the breast, gastrointestinal tract, pancreas, or ovary, or metastases that have spread to the lung or the pleural cavity, as well as many other, noncancerous disorders.

See also EFFUSION.

pleural tap See THORACENTESIS.

pleurectomy (ploor-ek'to-me) surgical removal of a portion of the pleura, the tissue covering the lungs and the pleural cavity. This may be performed in the treatment of MESOTHELIOMA.

pleuropneumonectomy (ploor"o-nu"-mo-nek'to-me) [extrapleural pneumonectomy] removal of the lung and the surrounding pleura along with the adjacent portions of the diaphragm and pericardium (sac surrounding the heart). This may be performed in the treatment of MESOTHELIOMA.

pleuroscopy (ploor-os'ko-pe) examination of fluid in the PLEURAL CAVITY. An ENDOSCOPE is inserted into the pleural space through a small incision in the chest wall. The area can be examined visually, and fluid and biopsy samples can be obtained. This procedure, infrequently used, can cause moderate chest wall discomfort, but other complications are rare.

plicamycin See MITHRACIN.

ploidy (ploi'de) characterizing a cancer cell by how "cancerous" it is. This is determined by comparing it with a normal cell using FLOW CYTOMETRY. DIPLOID cells are normal; ANEUPLOID cells are abnormal. The more abnormal the cell is, the more aggressive the cancer is. This information can be useful in treatment planning.

Plummer-Vinson syndrome a wasting away of the mucous membranes of the mouth, pharynx, and esophagus caused by dietary deficiencies of vitamins and iron. It is not a cancerous condition but may precede MOUTH CANCER.

pneumoalveolography (nu"mo-al"ve-o-log'rah-fe) an X-RAY examination of the alveoli (air sacs) of the lung.

pneumoangiography (nu"mo-an"je-og'rah-fe) an X-RAY examination of the blood vessels of the lung after the administration of a CONTRAST MEDIUM. The substance is injected directly into the blood vessels surrounding the lungs.

pneumography (nu-mog'rah-fe) an X-RAY examination of a specific part of the body after the injection of a gas such as oxygen. This procedure may be used to view the bladder, stomach, brain, spinal column, and MEDIASTINUM.

See also AIR-CONTRAST X-RAYS.

pneumomassage See LYMPHEDEMA.

pneumonectomy (nu"mo-nek'to-me) surgical removal of the right or left lung. A pneumonectomy may be performed in the treatment of NON-SMALL CELL LUNG CANCER.

pneumothorax (nu"mo-tho'raks) air leakage into the pleural cavity, causing the lung to collapse. This happens in 5 to 20% of patients receiving a NEEDLE ASPIRATION BIOPSY in the lung. It can occur as a result of many other conditions as well.

POA (pancreatic oncofetal antigen) a TUMOR MARKER under investigation for its role in detecting PANCREATIC CANCER.

See CA-19-9.

polycentric disease See MULTICENTRIC DISEASE.

polychemotherapy the use of a number of different anticancer drugs used in combination with hormones for the treatment of cancer. It is COMBINATION CHEMOTHERAPY with a hormonal component added.

polycythemia vera See MYELOPROLIFERATIVE DISORDERS.

polymerase chain reaction (PCR) a biochemical technique used in molecular biology to amplify minute quantities of nucleic acid material. This is done to enhance detection and sensitivity. For example, a lymph node looked at by standard microscopy may not show evidence of cancer but by using the PCR technique cancerous DNA may be identified. This is also known as RT-PCR (reverse transcriptase).

polymorphonuclear cell See GRANULOCYTE.

polypectomy the surgical removal of a small, bulging piece of tissue (polyp). A polypectomy may be performed in the treatment of colon cancer when a cancerous polyp is found on the colon.

polyps (pol'ips) small, noncancerous growths in the mucous membrane, most commonly found in the colon (the lower part of the intestines). They may also occur in the nose, uterus, and bladder. Polyps may eventually become cancerous and generally should be removed.

porfimer See PHOTOFRIN.

portogram See PORTOGRAPHY.

portography (por-tog'rah-fe) an examination by X-RAY of the portal vein (the large vein that carries blood to the liver from the veins of the stomach, intestine, spleen, and pancreas). For greater visibility of the portal vein, a substance that shows up in X-ray pictures is injected into the vein or spleen.

positron emission tomography See PET SCAN.

power lines See ELECTROMAGNETIC FIELDS.

PR (partial remission) See REMISSION.

precancerous a term used to describe a condition that may become cancerous.

precursor a sign or symptom that precedes another; in cancer, one condition that is known to occur before the onset of another condition.

prednisolone See ADRENOCORTICOIDS.

prednisone (pred'nĭ-sōn) [Deltasone, Meticorten, Orasone] an ADRENOCORTICOID drug used frequently in combination with other drugs in the treatment of many cancers, including BREAST CANCER, LEUKEMIA, HODGKIN'S DISEASE, NON-HODGKIN'S LYMPHOMA, and MYELOMA. It is taken by mouth. Common side effects may include gastrointestinal upset, weight gain, and fluid retention. Occasional or rare side effects may include ulcers, increased susceptibility to infection, increased appetite, sleeplessness, agitation, skin rash, increased blood sugar and blood pressure, and increased bruising.

preleukemia See MYELODYSPLASTIC SYNDROME.

Premarin [conjugated equine estrogen] See ESTROGEN.

preventive mastectomy (mas-tek'to-me) the removal of one or two breasts to ensure that BREAST CANCER does not occur. A woman may decide to have a second breast removed after cancer is detected in the first breast, especially if it is the type of breast cancer with a high probability of occurring in the second breast. Or she may decide to have both breasts removed because she is at a high risk of developing breast cancer. This is a controversial procedure and is considered by many physicians to be, in most cases, too extreme. A woman who is at a greater risk than the average woman is usually advised to be followed regularly by a physician with an exam several times a year.

See also PROPHYLACTIC SUBCUTANEOUS MASTECTOMY and MASTECTOMY.

preventive surgery surgical removal of a growth that is considered precancerous, such as POLYPS in the colon and MOLES on the skin. Surgery may also be performed on a person at high risk of developing a particular cancer. For example, a woman who has a family history of breast cancer and is considered to be at a greater risk of getting breast cancer than women in the general population might choose to have her breasts removed in order to prevent getting breast cancer.

See also CHEMOPROPHYLAXIS.

primary cancer [primary site, primary tumor]   the original site where cancer occurs. Generally, determining the primary site is fairly routine. However, in rare cases of an UNKNOWN PRIMARY, the primary site is never discovered. When the primary site of the cancer is not known, it is more difficult to determine the appropriate treatment. Occasionally the primary site is discovered after the cancer has already METASTASIZED (spread to other parts of the body). Discovery of the cancer through its metastases, rather than at the primary site, is most likely to happen when the primary cancer is a type that does not show symptoms in its earliest stages. For example, prostate cancer may be diagnosed after it has metastasized to the bones, causing pain and other symptoms in the bones.

See also SECONDARY CANCER.

primary site   See PRIMARY CANCER.

primary treatment   the standard or first procedure used to treat cancer. SURGERY is generally, but not always, the primary treatment for cancer. RADIATION THERAPY, CHEMOTHERAPY, and BIOLOGICAL THERAPY may, at times, be the primary treatment.

See also ADJUVANT THERAPY.

procarbazine (pro-kar′bah-zēn) [PCB, Matulane] an anticancer drug sometimes used in the treatment of lung and brain cancer, HODGKIN'S DISEASE, and NON-HODGKIN'S LYMPHOMA. It is taken by mouth. Common side effects include nausea, vomiting, mental depression, and confusion. Procarbazine is a commonly used anticancer drug important in the treatment of cancer.

Procrit   See EPOGEN.

procto exam   an examination of the lower part of the colon and rectum by a PROCTOSCOPY or SIGMOIDOSCOPY.

proctologist (prok-tol′o-jist)   a physician who specializes in the examination and treatment of dis-orders of the colon and rectum. A proctologist can perform surgery. To be certified by the American Board of Colon and Rectal Surgery, the proctologist must be a licensed medical doctor, have four years of training in general surgery and one year of training in colon and rectal surgery, and pass written and oral exams by the board.

proctoscope   See PROCTOSCOPY.

proctoscopy (prok-tos′ko-pe)   an examination of the anus and rectum using a thin, lighted instrument about six inches long called a proctoscope. The patient either lies face down with the knees drawn up, or on his or her side with the knees drawn up to the chest. The proctoscope is inserted in the rectum. A small sample of tissue may be removed for BIOPSY (microscopic examination for cancer cells). This is a simple procedure that is done without anesthesia in the doctor's office and takes only a few minutes. While there may be minor discomfort, it is generally not painful. This may be used as a screening device for RECTAL CANCER. The proctoscopy is very similar to the SIGMOIDOSCOPY. Sometimes the terms are used interchangeably. However, they are not the same. The proctoscopy examines a smaller area than the sigmoidoscopy.

proctosigmoidoscopy   See SIGMOIDOSCOPY.

progesterone (pro-jes′tĕ-ron)   a female sex HORMONE that causes the buildup of the uterine lining and the other body changes before conception. It is also released by the adrenal glands in tiny amounts in both men and women. Progesterone has been linked with BREAST CANCER and CERVICAL CANCER. Progesterone has been used along with ESTROGEN in ESTROGEN REPLACEMENT THERAPY to help prevent endometrial buildup, which may eventually lead to cancer.

Progesterone has been used in the treatment of some cancers such as BREAST, KIDNEY, and ENDOMETRIAL. Some of the more commonly used forms are MEGACE, MEDROXYPROGESTERONE, DEPO-PROVERA, and PROVERA.

progesterone receptor level   See PROGESTERONE RECEPTOR TEST.

progesterone receptor test (pro-jes'tĕ-ron) a test done during the BIOPSY of cancerous breast tissue to determine whether progesterone receptors are present. The presence of progesterone receptors indicates that the tumor is dependent on the hormone PROGESTERONE. Women with a positive progesterone receptor level may benefit from HORMONE THERAPY. Women who have both estrogen and progesterone receptors have a better prognosis—they have an 80% chance of responding to hormone therapy. Some studies suggest that the progesterone receptor status may be a better indicator of prognosis than the ESTROGEN RECEPTOR TEST.

prognosis a prediction of the course and outcome of a disease. In cancer, the prognosis is based on many factors, including the type of cancer, its stage at the time of diagnosis, the available treatments, and the general state of health of the patient. Generally, the earlier the cancer is detected and treated, the better the prognosis, or prospect of recovery.

Prokine See GM-CSF.

Proleukin See INTERLEUKIN-2.

prolymphocytic leukemia (PLL) (pro-lim"fo-sit' ik) an extremely rare form of LEUKEMIA primarily affecting men over the age of 60. It usually involves B CELLS, although T-CELL involvement has been found. See LEUKEMIA.

ProMACE a combination of the anticancer drugs PREDNISONE, METHOTREXATE WITH LEUCOVORIN RESCUE, ADRIAMYCIN, CYTOXAN, and ETOPOSIDE sometimes used in the treatment of NON-HODGKIN'S LYMPHOMA. See individual drug listings for side effects.
See also COMBINATION CHEMOTHERAPY.

promyelocyte (pro-mi'ĕ-lo-sīt) a primitive GRANULOCYTE (WHITE BLOOD CELL) that fights INFECTIONS.

promyelocytic leukemia See ANLL.

prophylactic cranial irradiation (pro"fĭ-lak'tik kra'ne-al ĭ-ra"de-a'shun) radiation of the brain after treatment of LUNG CANCER in order to kill any

cancer cells that may have metastasized (spread) to the brain. This is done more commonly in patients with SMALL CELL LUNG CANCER. This is a somewhat controversial procedure because of data on survival benefits and possible side effects associated with radiation to the brain.

prophylactic oopherectomy elective surgical removal of both ovaries to prevent development of OVARIAN CANCER, especially in women who carry the BRCA mutation.

prophylactic subcutaneous mastectomy (pro"fĭ-lak'tik sub"ku-ta'ne-us mas-tek'to-me) removal of 85 to 90% of the breast tissue through an incision under the breast when there is no disease present. The skin, nipple, and areola are saved. An implant is then inserted. This is sometimes done when a woman is at greater risk of BREAST CANCER than the rest of the population. This is a controversial procedure and not generally recommended. Cancer may develop after this procedure, and it may give a false sense of security. In addition, some hidden cancer cells in the breast may grow behind or alongside the implant and be difficult to detect. Some doctors instead advise women who are at a higher risk to do a monthly BREAST SELF-EXAMINATION, be checked by a physician several times a year, and get a MAMMOGRAPHY starting at age 35 or 40.
See also PREVENTIVE MASTECTOMY and MASTECTOMY.

prophylactic treatment (pro"fĭ-lak'tik) the use of medical procedures or remedies to prevent or defend against a disease. Prophylactic measures are used in some cancers. For example, in patients with SMALL CELL LUNG CANCER, PROPHYLACTIC CRANIAL (BRAIN) IRRADIATION may be used because of the likelihood of METASTASIS to the brain. To prevent breast cancer, some women at high risk opt for a preventive mastectomy, removal of a breast or both breasts before there is any evidence of disease.
See also PREVENTIVE SURGERY, PROPHYLACTIC CRANIAL IRRADIATION, and CHEMOPROPHYLAXIS.

Proscar [finasteride] a drug in tablet form used to treat BENIGN PROSTATIC HYPERPLASIA (BPH), a noncancerous condition. It is being investigated for possible use in the prevention of PROSTATE CANCER.

prostate   one of the male sex glands located just below the bladder and in front of the rectum. It is about the size of a walnut and is wrapped around part of the urethra. It produces fluid that becomes part of the semen (the fluid that contains sperm). The gland may develop PROSTATE CANCER.

prostate cancer   cancer in the prostate, the male sex glands just below the bladder and in front of the urethra. It is the second most common cancer in men, after skin cancer. The American Cancer Society estimated that during 2005 about 232,090 new cases of prostate cancer would be diagnosed in the United States. About one man in six will be diagnosed with prostate cancer during his lifetime, but only one man in 34 will die of this disease. A little more than 1.8 million men in the United States are survivors of prostate cancer. Prostate cancer occurs most frequently in older men—the average age of diagnosis is 73. Only 2% of the cases of prostate cancer occur in men under 50. Black Americans have the highest incidence rate in the world. Prostate cancer is more common in northwestern Europe and North America. Among men diagnosed with prostate cancer, about 99% survive at least five years, 92% survive at least 10 years, and 61% survive at least 15 years. These figures include all stages and grades of prostate cancer. The results are better for men whose cancer is discovered at an early stage. A recent review of death rates in men with localized prostate cancer found that they had nearly the same five- and 10-year survival as men without prostate cancer.

The role of the prostate in causing bladder obstruction was first noted in 1530. The first reference to cancer of the prostate was made in 1794. In the mid-1930s it was shown that regression of a prostate carcinoma could be induced by endocrine (hormonal) manipulation.

Not much is known about the causes of prostate cancer. It is believed to develop very slowly over a period of many years. Some studies have suggested a genetic link. An increased risk has been associated with the presence of the BRCA1 or BRCA2 gene. HORMONES appear to be a factor in the development of prostate cancer. It has been found that men whose testicles, a major source of male hormones, were removed before puberty have little

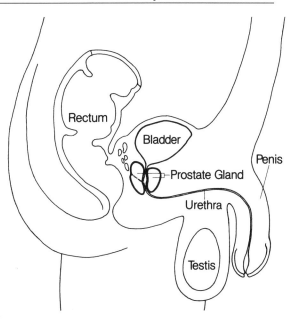

A cutaway view of the prostate glands. Courtesy NCI.

risk of getting this cancer. However, the precise role that hormones play has yet to be determined.

Some studies have shown that workplace exposure to cadmium, a metallic element used in welding, electroplating, and the production of alkaline batteries may increase the risk of prostate cancer. There is also some evidence that workers in the rubber industry may be at an increased risk. Diet may also play a role in the development of prostate cancer. Epidemiological studies suggest a link between the consumption of large amounts of animal fat and prostate cancer.

Symptoms of prostate cancer may include weak or interrupted urine flow; inability to urinate, or difficulty starting or stopping the urine flow; the need to urinate frequently, especially at night; blood in the urine; pain or burning on urination; and pain in the lower back, pelvis, or upper thighs. These symptoms can result from many other disorders, but a doctor should be seen if any persist.

The American Cancer Society and the NATIONAL CANCER INSTITUTE recommend that all men over age 40 have a DIGITAL RECTAL EXAM every year. Recently, use of a PROSTATE-SPECIFIC ANTIGEN (PSA) blood test in conjunction with an ULTRASOUND has been found to be highly sensitive in detecting early cancer and is becoming widely used for that purpose. Other diagnostic procedures may include URINALYSIS, blood tests, IVP, PELVIC LYMPH NODE DISSECTION, X-RAYS, CT SCAN, FLOW CYTOMETRY, MRI, and BIOPSY.

Following is the National Cancer Institute's (NCI) STAGING of prostate cancer:

- Stage I(a)—the cancer cannot be felt and causes no symptoms; it is only in the prostate and is usually found accidentally when surgery is performed for other reasons such as BENIGN PROSTATIC HYPERPLASIA
  A1—cancer cells are found in only one area of the prostate
  A2—cancer cells are found in many areas of the prostate
- Stage II(b)—the tumor can be felt during a rectal exam but the cancer cells are found only in the prostate
- State III(c)—cancer cells have spread outside the covering of the prostate to tissues around the prostate; the glands that produce semen may have cancer in them
- Stage IV(d)—cancer cells have metastasized (spread) to LYMPH NODES or to organs and tissues far away from the prostate
  D1—cancer cells have spread to lymph nodes near the prostate
  D2—cancer cells have spread to lymph nodes far from the prostate or to other parts of the body such as the bone, liver, or lungs
- Recurrent—the cancer has returned to the same location or another part of the body after treatment.

Treatment depends on the stage of the disease, the general state of health of the patient, and other factors. The three forms of treatment commonly used are surgery, RADIATION THERAPY, and HORMONE THERAPY. Surgical procedures include a RADICAL PROSTATECTOMY, nerve-sparing prostatectomy, cryosurgery, and a TRANSURETHRAL RESECTION. CHEMOTHERAPY is also used occasionally. BIOLOGICAL THERAPY is being investigated in CLINICAL TRIALS. For specific information on the latest state-of-the-art treatment, by stage, call NCI's Cancer Information Service at -800-4-CANCER (1-800-422-6237), or for a TTY: 1-800-332-8615.

Prostate Cancer Prevention Trial (PCPT) a study being done to see if finasteride can prevent prostate cancer. Of the 18,000 men in the trial, half are taking finasteride and the rest are taking a PLACEBO. Finasteride is known to lower PSA levels in men taking the drug, and the trial will enable researchers to more precisely measure the effect of finasteride on PSA levels.

See PROSCAR.

prostatectomy   See RADICAL PROSTATECTOMY.

prostate-specific antigen (PSA)   a protein in the blood produced by prostate tissue that serves as a TUMOR MARKER.

See PROSTATE-SPECIFIC ANTIGEN TEST.

prostate specific antigen test (PSA)   an analysis of blood for levels of a protein that is produced by PROSTATE. An elevated level may be an indication of PROSTATE CANCER. Because elevated blood levels may also be present in patients with other prostate problems such as BENIGN PROSTATIC HYPERPLASIA (BPH) it is not an ideal screening device, although it is gaining more and more acceptance in a screening role. In screening, it is generally used in combination with a DIGITAL RECTAL EXAM and ULTRASOUND. If the PSA level is high, the doctor may perform a BIOPSY, which is the only way to make a definitive diagnosis of cancer. Researchers are trying to find ways to increase the accuracy of PSA tests to help doctors distinguish BPH from PROSTATE CANCER, and thereby avoid unnecessary followup procedures, including BIOPSIES. The use of PSA as a screening measure is controversial. It is not known whether using PSA to screen for prostate cancer actually saves lives. The test is FDA-approved.

PSA is very useful in monitoring patients after a RADICAL PROSTATECTOMY. PSA is more sensitive than a BONE SCAN and may lead to an early detection of recurrence.

See SCREENING.

prostatic acid phosphatase (PAP) (pros-tat′ik fos″fah-tās) an enzyme in the blood that may serve as a TUMOR MARKER in PROSTATE CANCER. See ACID PHOSPHATASE TEST.

prostatic hyperplasia See BENIGN PROSTATIC HYPERPLASIA.

prostatic hypertrophy See BENIGN PROSTATIC HYPERPLASIA.

prosthesis (pros-the′sis) an artificial replacement for a missing body part, such as a breast or a leg. It may be functional, such as a leg; cosmetic, such as a breast; or both. Prostheses can be made of many different materials and may be permanent or removable. See Appendix I for organizations for specific cancers as well as general organizations such as the American Cancer Society that can help patients choose a prosthesis and adjust to its use.

protein an organic compound made up of amino acids. Proteins are one of the major constituents of plant and animal cells.

protocol in medicine, protocol usually refers to the outline or plan for use of an experimental procedure or experimental treatment. It states the clinical treatment rationale, its goal, and hypothesis. If drugs are involved, it describes which ones, method of administration, dose, and duration. If radiation is involved, it describes the type of radiation, method of administration, dose, and duration. The protocol also lists the criteria for participants. Protocol may also be used to describe a particular, standardized treatment program.

proton beam therapy See PARTICLE BEAM THERAPY.

Provera See PROGESTERONE.

pruritus (pru-ri′tus) a condition in which there is intense itching of the skin. It can occur in one location on the body or be widespread and is frequently related to dry skin.

In a patient with cancer, pruritus can be a side effect of CHEMOTHERAPY (anticancer drugs), RADIATION THERAPY, BIOLOGICAL THERAPY, or the cancer itself. It occurs frequently in patients with AIDS and less frequently in patients with HODGKIN'S DISEASE, NON-HODGKIN'S LYMPHOMA, and LEUKEMIA as well as other cancers. Pruritus can also be a symptom of a cancer not yet detected or an infection in the body. Pruritus may occur in the early stages of Hodgkin's

disease and other lymphomas. The itching sensation can be set off by a number of things, including heat, inflammation, a lack of humidity, dehydration, chemical irritants, and restrictive clothing.

There are a number of remedies for alleviation (or control) of pruritus. A doctor may prescribe antihistamines for general itching, corticosteroid creams for small localized areas, or antibiotics if the pruritus is the result of an infection.

Other steps patients can take to ease the itching include

- skin lubrication with a water-based moisturizer
- drinking at least eight glasses of fluid a day
- protection of the skin from wind and extreme temperatures
- avoidance of the sun on very hot days
- use of lukewarm or cool water for baths or showers
- the use of cornstarch on irradiated skin after bathing
- maintenance of a humid environment (e.g., using a humidifier)
- application of cool wet packs to affected areas
- use of a cotton flannel blanket if needed
- use of loose-fitting, lightweight cotton clothes
- use of DISTRACTION, RELAXATION TECHNIQUES, and IMAGERY.

Aggravating factors that should be avoided include:

- scratching, which only makes the itching worse
- wool, corduroy, or other scratchy fabrics
- tight, restrictive clothing
- sheets and clothing laundered with detergents
- bathing in hot water
- use of soaps that contain detergents
- frequent or extended bathing
- underarm deodorants or antiperspirants
- genital deodorants or bubble bath
- use of ointments such as petroleum or mineral oil
- dry environment
- stress.

Pruritus generally diminishes as the disease is treated but may reappear when there is a recurrence of the disease.

PSA test See PROSTATE-SPECIFIC ANTIGEN TEST.

Psoralen See METHOXSALEN.

PSC-833 an agent undergoing investigation for its possible role in reversing MULTIDRUG RESISTANCE (MDR).

psychotherapy a way of treating psychological problems. Cancer evokes many emotions in patients, as well as in their families, including depression, anger, hostility, hopelessness, guilt and fear, which can affect quality of life. There is ongoing research into the role emotions may play in the development of cancer, its recurrence and the patient's response to treatment. Some studies suggest that a cancer patient with a "positive" attitude and support from family members and/or friends fares better. This is still fairly controversial. However, it can be said with some certainty that a cancer patient with a positive outlook will have a better quality of life, whatever its length.

psychotropic drug (si″ko-trop′pik) drugs used in the treatment of sleep and psychological disorders. They appear to be useful, as well, in the treatment of nausea and vomiting caused by CHEMOTHERAPY (anticancer drugs).

PTC See PERCUTANEOUS and PERCUTANEOUS TRANSHEPATIC CHOLANGIOGRAPHY.

PTK-787 an investigational antiangiogenesis agent. In 2005, in clinical trials sponsored by NCI, PTK-787 showed promise as therapy of NSCLC.

pulmonary (pul′mo-ner″e) relating to the lungs.

pulmonary cytology (pul′mo-ner″e si-tol′o-je) the microscopic examination of samples of sputum-containing cells from the bronchial passages (tubes from the mouth or nose to the windpipe) or the pleural fluid in the lungs for cancer cells.
    See SPUTUM CYTOLOGY EXAM.

pulmonary fibrosis (pul′mo-ner″e fi-bro′sis) a condition in which delicate tissue in the lung is scarred. This may occur in a variety of conditions and may be caused by RADIATION THERAPY or CHEMOTHERAPY.
    See also RADIATION FIBROSIS.

pulmonary function test (PFT) (pul′mo-ner″e) [lung function test] a procedure to measure breathing and the patient's ability to get oxygen into the blood. The test measures the amount of air moving into and out of the lungs. It can also indicate an obstruction in the air passages.
    The pulmonary function test consists of various breathing exercises and blood tests. While this test is not painful, it can take as long as two hours to complete. Radioactive materials and a camera or a computer may be used. This test may be used in the diagnosis of LUNG CANCER. It may also be used to see if a patient can tolerate serious surgery.

punch biopsy See EXCISIONAL BIOPSY.

purging (pur′jing) the removal of cancer cells from BONE MARROW or STEM CELLS that have been removed from a patient undergoing an AUTOLOGOUS BONE MARROW TRANSPLANT or PERIPHERAL BLOOD STEM CELL TRANSPLANT. The purging is done with anticancer drugs and other methods. The marrow or stem cells are then frozen and stored until it is needed for reinfusion into the patient.

Purinethol See 6-MP.

PUVA therapy [topical photochemotherapy] a treatment in which the patient takes METHOXSALEN (8-MOP) by mouth and is then exposed to ULTRAVIOLET RADIATION. The light activates the drug, which then binds to DNA and causes cell death. Because the ultraviolet light does not penetrate beyond the skin, the effects are confined to the skin. This procedure may be used in the treatment of MYCOSIS FUNGOIDES as well as other skin disorders such as vitiligo (the skin loses color) and psoriasis (the skin develops red, scaly patches). One possible side effect of PUVA treatment, for mycosis fungoides, is the development of secondary skin cancers.
    See also PHOTOPHERESIS.

pyelography See IVP.

pyriform sinus cancer See HYPOPHARYNGEAL CANCER and OROPHARYNGEAL CANCER.

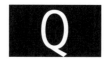

Q-TWiST [quality-adjusted time without symptoms and toxicity] a method devised to factor quality of life into decisions about treatment. This represents a philosophical shift for some medical professionals. The goal of cancer treatment, or any disease, had been to prolong life as long as possible. Now many patients are questioning whether it is worth undergoing a rigorous treatment with devastating side effects that offers no hope of cure but will give them another few weeks or months to live. Q-TWiST uses standardized questions to help a patient weigh the benefits of aggressive treatment against its likely impact on the quality and length of life.

quack in medicine, a slang expression for a person who falsely represents him- or herself as having medical skill or curative powers. The term *quack* or quackery implies a knowing intent to misrepresent. In 1983 the Senate Committee on Aging noted that quackery was the most frequent and lucrative fraud affecting the elderly. Also in 1983, an FBI probe uncovered 39 diploma mills, some of which specialized in phony medical credentials. An example of quackery in cancer treatment was the promotion of LAETRILE, a widely touted cancer "cure" in the 1970s and 1980s even though a study had shown that it was never proven to be an effective treatment for cancer.

See also UNCONVENTIONAL TREATMENT METHOD.

Quadramet (samarium Sm-153 lexidronam injection) a radioisotope used in the treatment of pain associated with metastatic bone cancer most commonly occurring in advanced prostate, breast, and lung cancers.

quadrant excision See LUMPECTOMY.

quadrantectomy See LUMPECTOMY.

quality of life (QOL) the assessment of the impact of cancer treatment on the patient in terms of psychosocial adjustment, daily activity, economic impact, mobility, pain, sense of wellness, sexual function, et al. Assessment of QOL is becoming more commonplace in clinical studies where no major changes in survival are expected. See Q-TWiST.

R

RAD (radiation absorbed dose) the measurement that was used for the amount of RADIATION that is absorbed by the body. It was the traditional method of describing doses of radiation by radiation therapists. The term *RAD* has recently been replaced by the term *Gray* (Gy). One gray equals 100 RADs.

radiation energy in the form of waves or particles. Types of radiation include (from short to long wave length), GAMMA RAYS, X-RAY, ULTRAVIOLET, RADIATION, visible light, and infrared rays (radiant heat) and particles. Radiation can be used in the diagnosis, treatment, and follow-up treatment of cancer.

See also RADIATION THERAPY.

radiation enteritis (en″ter-i′tis) inflammation of the intestinal tract as a result of RADIATION THERAPY to the abdomen, pelvis, or rectum. This is a fairly common side effect of radiation therapy. Some of its symptoms include nausea, vomiting, abdominal cramping, watery diarrhea, rectal pain, and rectal bleeding. A doctor can prescribe or recommend over-the-counter medications for alleviation or reduction of some of the problems.

Patients with radiation enteritis are advised to eat fish, poultry, and meat that is broiled, or roasted; bananas, peeled apples and applesauce, white bread, pasta, potatoes, mild cooked vegetables and mild processed cheese, eggs, smooth peanut butter, buttermilk, and yogurt. Foods that should be avoided include milk and milk products (with the exceptions noted above), whole bran bread and cereals, nuts, seeds, fried foods, fresh and dried fruits, raw vegetables, popcorn, potato chips, chocolate, coffee, tea, alcohol, and tobacco.

Radiation enteritis can occur after the first treatment. The symptoms usually disappear within two to three weeks after the last treatment. In about 5 to 15% of patients radiation enteritis can continue long after treatment, for months or even years.

radiation fibrosis (fi-bro′sis) scarring of tissue as a result of RADIATION THERAPY to the esophagus or lungs. Symptoms may include a dry or sore throat and a sense of difficulty in swallowing or breathing. It can be a temporary side effect of radiation therapy for lung or esophageal cancer occurring early in the treatments, or it may develop months or years after the radiation treatment has concluded.

radiation implants See INTERSTITIAL RADIATION.

radiation oncologist (on-kol′o-jist) a doctor who specializes in using radiation to treat disease. The radiation oncologist decides what type of RADIATION THERAPY is best, plans the treatment, and monitors the patient. To receive certification from the American Board of Radiologists, the radiation oncologist must be a medical doctor, spend three to four years of residency training in radiation oncology, and pass oral and written exams.

radiation physicist [medical physicist]   a person trained to oversee the RADIATION THERAPY a patient receives and ensure that the radiation machine is working correctly and delivers the right amount of radiation to the treatment site. Radiation physicists design and select radiation equipment and conduct safety measurements on a regular basis. Radiation physicists have a doctorate or master's degree. They typically have one to two years of clinical physics training and are certified by either the American Board of Radiology or the American Board of Medical Physics.

radiation pneumonitis (nu"mo-ni′tis)   inflammation of the lung tissue. This can be a side effect of RADIATION THERAPY to the lung and is more apt to occur in someone who has a preexisting lung problem such as bronchitis. It occurs several months after radiation therapy and may cause reduced lung function and be painful. It usually subsides in time, although in very weak patients it may not. There may be permanent scarring.

See also RADIATION FIBROSIS.

radiation recall   a side effect of RADIATION THERAPY that may occur when CHEMOTHERAPY is given after the radiation. It can take place weeks or months after the radiation therapy. Radiation recall usually takes the form of patches of redness and shedding or peeling of the skin that was irradiated. Less common are blisters and wet, oozing areas of skin that peel. There are several steps a patient with radiation recall can take. The skin should be gently cleansed using a mild soap and tepid water. The area should be patted dry with a soft towel. Creams with vitamins A, D, and E can be applied to alleviate dry skin. For itchiness, the doctor may prescribe a cortisone cream or spray.

radiation simulation   a procedure performed before the start of RADIATION THERAPY. X-RAYS are taken to locate the precise area of the body that will be treated, called the treatment port; the area is marked on the skin with tiny dots of semipermanent ink. If they start fading, they are redrawn to ensure that the radiation is always delivered to the

exact location. The amount of radiation, how it will be delivered, and how many treatments will be given are based on information obtained in the simulation and from other tests, as well as the patient's medical history. There can be more than one treatment port, and this process may take several days.

radiation therapist [radiotherapist, therapeutic radiologist]   a person specially trained to operate radiation equipment. Radiation therapists treat each patient according to a doctor's instructions and keep daily records and regularly check the treatment machines to make sure they are working properly.

radiation therapy [radiation treatment, radiotherapy, X-ray therapy or treatment, irradiation, electron beam therapy, cobalt treatment]   the use of high-energy penetrating rays or subatomic particles to treat or control disease. Radiation therapy dates from the 1890s when the French physicist Henri Becquerel discovered uranium and Marie and Pierre Curie discovered radium, a substance even more radioactive than uranium. Experiments were done using radiation to treat skin cancer. Radiation was also found to be effective in the treatment of some cervical cancers. The development in the early 1950s of radioactive cobalt, an artificial isotope that can deliver radiation deep in the body with less skin irritation, made radiation a much more viable therapy for many cancers.

In the 1960s, more technological advances produced higher energy machines that could deliver radiation even more deeply into the body with even less skin damage. Most radiation therapy units are now equipped with several types of machines that can treat different parts of the body. Half of all cancer patients are treated with some kind of radiation treatment, either alone or in combination with other treatments.

Radiation works by killing and eliminating cancer cells and tumors; shrinking a tumor; or preventing cancer cells from growing and dividing. The radiation is targeted to the DNA in the malignant (cancerous) cell. The DNA of a malignant cell is more susceptible to radiation damage than a normal cell. The destruction of the cancer cell can take hours or even days. Most normal cells generally recover more fully than cancer cells from the effects of radiation.

Computers and diagnostic tests are frequently used to determine the correct dose of the radiation and the exact location in the body where it should be directed. After the total dose is calculated, it is broken down into treatments to cause the most damage to the cancer cells and the least damage to the normal cells and nearby organs. Radiation is generally administered over a period of several weeks. The radiation may be directed to the same area in the body from different directions in order to minimize skin damage.

Radiation can be given in two ways, externally by a special machine, or internally, by placing radioactive substances in the body. External radiation is more commonly used. Sometimes both methods are used, one after the other.

In EXTERNAL RADIATION THERAPY, a machine delivers radiation to the cancer inside the body. Different radiation machines are used depending on the location of the cancer. Some are most effective in treating cancers near the surface of the skin. Others are better for cancers deeper in the body.

In the type of INTERNAL RADIATION THERAPY called INTERSTITIAL RADIATION, a radioactive substance is sealed in a small container such as a wire, seed, capsule, needle, or tube called an implant. The implant is placed directly into the tumor or into a body cavity. It generally stays in the body for one to seven days. For some cancer sites, it may be permanently implanted. Unsealed radiation in liquid form may also be used. It may be injected or swallowed. In a technique called afterloading, the containers (e.g., needles, tubes) for the radioactive substance are placed in the body and the radioactive substance is then inserted into the containers. The other types of internal radiation are INTRACAUTIONARY RADIATION and BRACHYTHERAPY.

Radiation therapy can treat cancer in most locations in the body. Its success in eliminating the cancer depends on several factors, including the location of the cancer and the dose that can be administered. Due to physical condition or age, some patients are not able to tolerate the dose of radiation that would wipe out the cancer. Radiation may also be used before surgery to shrink a tumor to provide the best chance of successful removal. It may be used after surgery to eliminate any remaining cancer cells. Radiation therapy is frequently used as palliative treatment to shrink tumors and reduce pressure, bleeding, pain, or other symptoms of a cancer that cannot be cured.

Radiation has various side effects, depending on the part of the body being treated and the person receiving the radiation. The side effects usually start about two weeks after the beginning of treatment. Some patients experience more serious problems while others have no side effects or mild ones. The most common side effects are fatigue, skin changes, and loss of appetite. Fatigue can result from the effects of the radiation on normal cells, stress related to the cancer, and the daily trips for treatment. Skin changes in the treatment area include redness, irritation, sunburn, tan, dryness, itching, discomfort, or soreness. Loss of appetite can be stress related, a result in changes in normal cells, or a loss or change in the taste sensation. Most side effects stop after a time.

Following are some of the side effects associated with radiation to different parts of the body:

- *head and neck area*
  — redness and irritation in the mouth, dry mouth
  — difficulty in swallowing
  — changes in taste, or a loss of taste
  — earaches (caused by hardening of ear wax)
  — swelling or drooping of skin under the chin
  — change in skin texture
  — hair loss (when radiation is directed to the head)
- *breast, chest, and lung*
  — difficulty or pain when swallowing
  — coughing
  — decrease in blood counts
  — breast soreness and swelling (in women with breast cancer)
  — PNEUMONITIS
  — PULMONARY FIBROSIS
- *stomach and abdomen*
  — an upset stomach, nausea, or diarrhea
- *pelvis*
  — bladder irritation resulting in discomfort and/or frequent urination
  — upset stomach, nausea, or diarrhea
  — in women, vaginal dryness, itching, and burning, cessation of menstruation
  — in men, reduction in the sperm count and fertility

Some symptoms that should be reported to a doctor if they persist include: a pain that does not go away; lumps, bumps, or swelling; nausea, vomiting, diarrhea, or loss of appetite; unexplained weight loss; a fever or cough that does not go away; unusual rashes; and bruises or bleeding. Radiation therapy can also have long-term side effects of second cancers such as sarcomas many years after the initial treatment.

See also HYPERFRACTIONATED RADIATION THERAPY, SUPERFRACTIONATED RADIATION THERAPY, and RADIOIMMUNOTHERAPY.

radical cystectomy (sis-tek′to-me) surgical removal of the bladder and the tissue around it. In women, the uterus, ovaries, fallopian tubes, part of the vagina, and urethra are also removed. In men, the prostate and the glands that produce fluid that is part of the semen are also removed, and the urethra may be removed as well. The LYMPH NODES in the pelvis may also be removed. A radical cystectomy may be performed in the treatment of BLADDER CANCER.

radical hysterectomy (his″ter-ek′to-me) [Wertheim's operation] surgical removal of the cervix, uterus, and part of the vagina. LYMPH NODES may also be removed. A radical hysterectomy may be performed in the treatment of CERVICAL CANCER or ENDOMETRIAL CANCER.

See also HYSTERECTOMY.

radical inguinal orchiectomy (ing′gwĭ-nal or-ke-ek′to-me) [radical orchiectomy] surgical removal of one or both testicles and all adjoining tissue through an incision in the groin. Some of the lymph nodes in the abdomen may also be removed. A radical inguinal orchiectomy may be performed in the treatment of TESTICULAR CANCER.

radical mastectomy (mas-tek′to-me) [Halsted mastectomy] surgical removal of the breast, the underlying muscle of the chest wall (both major and minor), the LYMPH NODES in the adjacent armpit, and fat tissue as a treatment for BREAST CANCER. This was first performed by Dr. William Halsted, a surgeon in Baltimore in the early 1880s. He published information on the procedure in 1894, and the radical or Halsted mastectomy became the treatment for breast cancer through the

early 1970s. The Halsted mastectomy is now seldom performed, having been replaced by the modified mastectomy or LUMPECTOMY, which have proven to be just as effective as the radical with far fewer side effects and much less disfigurement and debilitation.

See MASTECTOMY.

radical neck dissection surgical removal of a block of tissue from the collarbone to the jaw and from the front of the neck to the back. The muscle on the side of the neck used for rotating, flexing, or extending the neck is also removed along with the major vein on the side of the neck. This may be performed in the treatment of a tumor in the neck when a cure is thought to be possible.

radical nephrectomy (nĕ-frek′to-me) surgical removal of the kidney with the tissue around it. Some lymph nodes in the area may also be removed. This may be performed in the treatment of KIDNEY CANCER.

The radical nephrectomy was first performed in the 1950s and in most instances has now replaced the NEPHRECTOMY as the surgical treatment of choice.

radical orchiectomy See RADICAL INGUINAL ORCHIECTOMY.

radical prostatectomy (pros″tah-tek′to-me) surgical removal of the prostate and the tissue surrounding it. This may be performed by cutting into the space between the scrotum and the anus (the perineum) in an operation called a perineal prostatectomy or by cutting into the lower abdomen in an operation called a retropubic prostatectomy. A radical prostatectomy may be performed in the treatment of PROSTATE CANCER. If the cancer has spread to the LYMPH NODES, a radical prostatectomy may not be performed, and other treatment such as RADIATION THERAPY, HORMONE THERAPY, or CHEMOTHERAPY may be used instead.

A common side effect of a radical prostatectomy has been impotence. A new, nerve-sparing procedure, developed by a doctor at the Johns Hopkins University in Baltimore, Maryland, is reducing the occurrence of impotency. However, the new procedure is generally appropriate only for smaller tumors confined to the prostate, and most doctors agree that attempts to preserve potency are less important than complete removal of the tumor. Other less common side effects may be urinary incontinence and stricture (narrowing of the urethra).

radical vulvectomy (vul-vek′to-me) surgical removal of the vulva, clitoris, and LYMPH NODES in the groin and thigh. A radical vulvectomy may be performed in the treatment of VULVAR CANCER.

radioactive emitting energy in the form of waves or particles. Any living thing or object may become radioactive, and give off radiation, after receiving a high dose of radiation. This can be accidental or a side effect of RADIATION THERAPY. For example, in 1986, after the nuclear accident at Chernobyl in the Soviet Union in which high levels of radiation were released, there was worldwide concern over the possibility of widespread radiation contamination of food products. Radiation therapy to treat cancer using RADIATION IMPLANTS can cause a person to become temporarily radioactive. When a patient is radioactive, visits to the patients are limited to 10 to 30 minutes and visitors are told to stay at least six feet from the patient. Children under 18 and pregnant women are usually not allowed to visit while the patient is radioactive. This condition is temporary.

radioactive implant See INTERSTITIAL RADIATION.

radioactive iodine one type of RADIOACTIVE ISOTOPE that may be used in a THYROID SCAN. Radioactive iodine may also be used as a treatment for THYROID CANCER.
See also NUCLEAR SCAN.

radioactive isotope (i′so-tōp) [radioisotope, radionuclide] an isotope that emits RADIATION (X-RAYS or charged particles). It can be used in scans to diagnose cancer. It can also be used in the treatment of cancer. It can be administered by IV (injected into the vein) or taken by mouth.

radioactive scan See NUCLEAR SCAN.

radioactive seeds seeds about the size of grains of rice containing iodine-125. The seeds can be injected into the prostate using ultrasound in the treatment of prostate cancer. Implanting the seeds,

a form of brachytherapy, requires less recovery time and may eliminate the need for surgical removal of the prostate and its side effects, which can be impotence and/or incontinence.

radiocurability refers to a condition in which a curative dose of radiation will not cause excessive damage to normal tissue. Examples of some radiocurable tumors are cancer of the breast, cervix, larynx, and prostate and HODGKIN′S DISEASE.

radio-frequency ablation a surgical technique using a small instrument to destroy a discrete tumor by using high energy. Most often applied to liver metastasis and often approached via laparoscopy.

radioimmunoglobulin therapy See RADIOIMMUNOTHERAPY.

radioimmunotherapy (ra″de-o-im″u-no-ther′ape) [radioimmunoglobulin therapy] treatment that delivers radiation directly to the cancer by way of the bloodstream. In the laboratory radioactive isotopes are attached to antibodies against components of the cancer cells. When injected back into the body, the antibodies, carrying the radioactive isotopes, travel through the bloodstream to the tumor, where the isotopes attach to the tumor and attack and kill cells. This is one use of MoAbs (see MONOCLONAL ANTIBODY).

radioisotope See RADIOACTIVE ISOTOPE.

radioisotope scan See NUCLEAR SCAN.

radiologist (ra″de-ol′o-jist) a doctor who specializes in using radiation to diagnose or treat disease.
See also RADIATION THERAPIST and DIAGNOSTIC RADIOLOGIST.

radiology the use of X-RAYS and other forms of RADIATION THERAPY to diagnose and treat disease.

radionuclide scan See NUCLEAR SCAN.

radiopharmaceutical a drug combining an agent with a radioactive isotope designed to target a specific cell or receptor. Examples are BEXXARR and ZEVALIN.

radioprotector a substance that protects the normal cells from the effects of radiation. This enables a larger dose of radiation to be given.

radioresistant a cancer whose cells are not sufficiently sensitive or susceptible to a radiation dose that would not cause excessive damage to normal tissue.

radioresponsiveness the amount of regression of a tumor after RADIATION THERAPY. This can be affected by the tumor's radiosensitivity as well as other factors. Some cancers are more radioresponsive than others.

radiosensitivity the degree to which a cell is affected by radiation. The more radiosensitive a cell is, the more susceptible it is to being destroyed by radiation.

radiosensitizer a substance or procedure that makes a cancer cell more susceptible to the effects of RADIATION THERAPY, thereby boosting the effect of the radiation dose. One example is HYPERTHERMIA THERAPY, which uses heat to increase the cancer cell's sensitivity to radiation. Investigations into radiosensitizers are ongoing.

radiotherapist See RADIATION THERAPIST.

radiotherapy See RADIATION THERAPY.

radium (ra′de-um) a highly radioactive metallic element that may be used as a source of radiation in radiation therapy.

radium implant See INTERNAL RADIATION.

radon (ra′don) a naturally occurring radioactive gas that comes from uranium and rock. You cannot smell, feel, or see radon. Radon is a known CARCINOGEN. In 1998 a National Research Council committee estimated that 19,000 lung cancer deaths would be caused by inhalation of radon. Radon is not a problem outdoors. It becomes a problem when it gets into a confined area, such as a home or office, where the radon breaks down and attaches to dust particles that are inhaled. The higher the level of radon, the bigger the risk.

Smokers are at a higher risk of developing lung cancer as a result of inhaling radon than are nonsmokers.

raloxifene (Evista) the first in a class of new drugs known as selective estrogen receptor modulators (SERMs). Raloxifene, like TAMOXIFEN, is a synthetic drug that blocks the action of estrogen, which is known to encourage the growth of breast tumors.

In 1997, raloxifene was approved by the Food and Drug Administration as a treatment to reduce the risk of osteoporosis in postmenopausal women. Although it does not offer the same protection that estrogen does, it can be used by women who cannot take estrogen.

randomized clinical trial a study in which patients with similar characteristics, such as type and extent of disease, are selected randomly (by chance) for placement into groups that are comparing different treatments to determine which treatment is better. Because irrelevant factors or preferences do not influence the distribution of patients, the treatment groups can be considered comparable and results of the different treatments used in different groups can be compared. Neither the patient nor the doctor can choose which treatment the patient will receive.

See CLINICAL TRIALS.

Rappaport classification of non-Hodgkin's lymphoma one of several ways of describing NON-HODGKIN'S LYMPHOMA. Developed in 1966, the Rappaport system is based on the relationship between cell histology (microscopic cell structure) and PROGNOSIS.

R-CHOP the chemotherapy combination of RITUXAN (rituximab) with CHOP (CYTOXAN, hydroxydoxorubicin (ADRIAMYCIN), ONCOVIN, AND PREDNISONE) widely used in treatment of lymphomas. See individual drug listings for side effects.

See also COMBINATION CHEMOTHERAPY.

Reach to Recovery the first support group for women with BREAST CANCER. The program was started in 1956 by Terese Lasser, a women in New York who had undergone a MASTECTOMY. Based on her own experience, she felt that women with breast cancer had very little emotional support. The program is now run by the American Cancer Society. At the request of a patient's doctor, Reach to Recovery volunteers who have had breast cancer visit women in the hospital to share their experience and offer practical information about acquiring a PROSTHESIS (they bring the patient a temporary prosthesis), clothing, BREAST RECONSTRUCTION, and exercises for the arm and shoulder. In some areas of the country patients who have been discharged from the hospital can call their local ACS office and request a visit from a Reach to Recovery volunteer. See American Cancer Society and other support groups listed in Appendix I.

von Recklinghausen's neurofibromatosis   See NEUROFIBROMATOSIS.

recombinant DNA   DNA that has been altered by inserting into its chain a sequence not originally present; a laboratory technique.

recombinant DNA technology   (re-kom'bĭ-nant) a highly sophisticated way of altering cells and making identical copies of a substance. DNA from the genes of different species is divided and spliced together in a laboratory to produce new kinds of cells, which can be reproduced in great quantities. This relatively new technology is seen as having great potential in BIOLOGICAL THERAPY.

reconstructive mammoplasty   See BREAST RECONSTRUCTION.

reconstructive surgeon   a medical doctor with special training to perform operations to reconstruct or restore parts of the body. He or she can perform grafts of the skin, bone, and cartilage and can transfer tissue from one part of the body to another. The reconstructive surgeon also plays a key role in planning, initiating, and coordinating the overall rehabilitation of the patient. She or he helps patients who have had debilitating surgery that has limited their ability to speak, hear, or see to lead as normal a life as possible.

rectal cancer   cancer of the lowest four to six inches of the intestinal tract adjoining the anus.

According to the American Cancer Society, approximately 40,340 people would be diagnosed with rectal cancer in 2005, with 56,290 deaths from the combined diseases of colon and rectal cancer in the same year.

Cancer of the rectum occurs more frequently in men than in women. People at the greatest risk of getting rectal cancer are over 40; have a family history of cancer of the colon, rectum, or the female organs; hereditary conditions, such as familial POLYPOSIS, familial NONPOLYPOSIS syndromes, a cancer family syndrome (autosomal dominant); and/or have a history of ulcerative colitis (ulcers in the lining of the large intestines). However, these high-risk groups account for only 23% of all COLORECTAL CANCERS.

Symptoms may include rectal bleeding, blood in the stool, jet-black stool, a change in bowel habits, alternating between constipation and diarrhea, crampy abdominal pain, weakness, loss of weight, and loss of appetite. (These symptoms may also be caused by other, NONCANCEROUS conditions.)

Diagnostic and evaluation procedures may include DIGITAL RECTAL exam, PROCTOSCOPY, COLONOSCOPY, SIGMOIDOSCOPY, endorectal ultrasound, LOWER GI SERIES, CEA, and BIOPSY.

Following is the NATIONAL CANCER INSTITUTE's (NCI) STAGING for rectal cancer along with DUKES' STAGING SYSTEM:

- Stage 0 or carcinoma in situ—cancer is found only in the top lining of the rectum
- Stage I or Dukes A—cancer has spread beyond the top lining of the rectum to the second and third layers and involves the inside wall of the rectum, but has not spread to the outer wall of the rectum or outside the rectum
- Stage II or Dukes B—cancer has spread outside the rectum to nearby tissue, but it has not gone into the LYMPH NODES
- Stage III or Dukes C—cancer has spread to nearby lymph nodes but has not spread to other parts of the body
- Stage IV or Dukes D—cancer has spread to other parts of the body
- Recurrent—the cancer has returned after treatment, either to the original site or to another part of the body. Recurrent rectal cancer is often found in the liver and/or lungs

Treatment depends on the stage of the disease, the general state of health of the patient, and other factors. Surgery is the most common treatment. Depending on the stage, FULGURATION, COLONOSCOPY, WEDGE RESECTION, or BOWEL RESECTION may be performed as well as other surgical procedures. Other possible treatments include RADIATION THERAPY and CHEMOTHERAPY, BIOLOGICAL THERAPY is being investigated in the treatment of rectal cancer. For specific information on the latest state-of-the-art treament, by stage, call NCI's Cancer Information Service at 1-800-4-CANCER (1-800-422-6237), or for a TTY: 1-800-332-8615.

See also COLON/RECTAL CANCER.

rectal exam See DIGITAL RECTAL EXAM.

rectilinear scanner See NUCLEAR SCAN.

rectus abdominous reconstruction See BREAST RECONSTRUCTION.

recurrence [relapse] the reappearance of an illness and its symptoms after treatment. In cancer the recurrence can be local (in the same site), regional (in tissue near the original site), or metastatic (in another part of the body).

red blood cell [erythrocytes] the blood cells that carry oxygen from the lungs throughout the body. Most blood cells are red. Red blood cells contain the pigment hemoglobin, an iron-rich protein that can take up oxygen as the blood passes through the lungs and release it to the tissues. Having too few blood cells results in ANEMIA, which may spur feelings of weakness, shortness of breath, fatigue, dizziness, headaches, and irritability.

See also WHITE BLOOD CELLS and PLATELETS.

Reed-Sternberg cell a giant, abnormal cell with several nuclei that appears in patients with HODGKIN'S DISEASE. The Reed-Sternberg cell is one of the characteristics of Hodgkin's disease that distinguishes it from NON-HODGKIN'S LYMPHOMA. The diagnosis of Hodgkin's disease is rarely made without the presence of Reed-Sternberg cells. However, the presence of these cells alone cannot provide a definitive diagnosis of Hodgkin's disease since similar cells may also be found in patients with mononucleosis and other diseases. Research is ongoing in an attempt to define the exact cell of origin of the Reed-Sternberg cell.

refractory a term commonly used to describe a cancer that does not respond to therapy, or a cancer that was responding to the treatment being used until losing its sensitivity. In order to achieve a response when the original treatment is no longer effective, a patient may have to undergo alternative treatment.

regional anesthesia (an″es-the′ze-ah) the blockage of sensation from one part of the body by interrupting the transmission of sensory nerve conduction. It is more extensive, affecting a larger part of the body, than LOCAL ANESTHESIA.

regional chemotherapy a general term used to describe the administration of CHEMOTHERAPY (anticancer drugs) to a particular body part or organ. This is done to increase the effect of the drug at the cancer site while at the same time decreasing the toxic effects of the drug on other parts of the body.

See also CHEMOEMBOLIZATION and REGIONAL PERFUSION.

regional enteritis See CROHN'S DISEASE.

regional ileitis See CROHN'S DISEASE.

regional involvement refers to the spread of cancer to adjacent tissue and/or nearby LYMPH NODES. Regional involvement of the cancer is one criterion for the STAGING of most cancers.

regional pancreatectomy (pan″kre-ah-tek′to-me) surgical removal of the pancreas, the duodenum, bile duct, gallbladder, spleen, most of the adjacent lymph nodes, and part of the arterial and venous systems. Doctors who favor this very extensive surgery believe it offers a better chance of a cure for PANCREATIC CANCER. However, there is little evidence that it achieves any longer survival.

regional perfusion a method of administering CHEMOTHERAPY (anticancer drugs) mainly to the cancerous tumor. It works best with tumors in body extremities such as arms or legs. The chemotherapy is injected into the cancerous area through an artery. A tourniquet is used to prevent the drug from reaching and affecting the rest of the body. After the drug has "traveled" through the cancerous area, it is removed through a vein using special tubes. It is recirculated—into the artery, out the vein—repeatedly by means of a pump oxygenator. Regional perfusion enables a greater dose of the toxic chemotherapy to be administered while decreasing the toxic effects of the drug on other parts of the body.

See also CHEMOEMBOLIZATION.

regional recurrence   in cancer, return of the disease in the LYMPH NODES or tissue near the original site after treatment. In a regional recurrence there is no evidence that the cancer has spread (metastasized) to a distant location.

See also LOCAL RECURRENCE METASTASIS.

Reglan   See METOCLOPRAMIDE.

regression   in cancer, refers to a tumor growing smaller or, eventually, disappearing.

relapse   a term originating from early experience with successful chemotherapy treatment of leukemia in which the cancer was thought to be in remission. When over time it was found to be active again it was called a relapse.

See RECURRENCE.

relative survival rate   a way to measure survival. In cancer, the rate is calculated by adjusting the observed SURVIVAL RATE to remove the effects of all causes of death except cancer. This rate is commonly expressed in terms of five-year survival.

relaxation techniques   techniques to produce a relaxed state in the body, used to minimize sensations of discomfort or pain in cancer patients. Relaxation techniques can be used to induce sleep and to reduce stress. They can be energizing and helpful in dealing with pain and unpleasant side effects of cancer treatment.

There are many different ways to practice relaxation. Frequently people modify a technique to make it as effective as possible for themselves.

Following are brief descriptions of a few techniques:

- tension relaxation—this is usually done in a prone position. People using this technique breathe in slowly and deeply. As they breathe in, they tense a muscle or group of muscles—one example is stiffening the legs. While holding their breath, they keep the muscles tense for a few seconds. Then, they exhale and let the legs go limp while the tension drains out of the legs and the body. This can be done with every part of the body. Audio tapes with relaxation exercises are available. Some people make their own.
- rhythm technique—deep breaths are taken in a slow and steady rhythm. The person may think, or say, "In, one, two; out, one, two." Each time the person breathes out, the body relaxes and goes limp. Rhythmic breathing can be done anywhere, anytime for a few seconds or several minutes. To end rhythmic breathing, count silently from one to three.
- distraction—doing any activity that takes the mind off the problems that are present. It sounds perfectly simple and obvious—and it is. Watching television or reading an engrossing book, working on needlework, doing some carpentry, painting pictures (or the walls) are all activities that can be involving. Each individual has her or his own "distractions." Involvement in an activity can help one keep from thinking about or noticing pain and other problems.

See also HYPNOSIS, IMAGERY, SIMONTON TECHNIQUE, and BIOFEEDBACK.

REM (Roentgen equivalent man)   a way to measure RADIATION; the quantity of any ionizing radiation that has the same biological effectiveness as one RAD of X-RAYS.

remission   the decrease or disappearance of disease. Remission may also refer to the disease-free period. Although remission is a word that can be used in relation to any cancer, it is most associated with LEUKEMIA and HODGKIN'S DISEASE and the other lymphomas. In complete remission (CR) there is no evidence of cancer present in the body. In a partial remission (PR) the tumor is reduced by at least 50% but the cancer is still present.

renal pertaining to the kidneys.

renal adenocarcinoma See KIDNEY CANCER.

renal arteriogram See SELECTIVE RENAL ARTERI-
OGRAPHY.

renal arteriography See SELECTIVE RENAL ARTERI-
OGRAPHY.

renal cell cancer See KIDNEY CANCER.

renal cell carcinoma See KIDNEY CANCER.

renal pelvis the innermost part of the kidney,
called the medulla. It is hollow.

renal pelvis tumors See TRANSITIONAL CELL CAN-
CER OF THE RENAL PELVIS AND URETER.

renal scan See KIDNEY SCAN.

reproduction See INFERTILITY and SEXUAL ACTIVITY.

rescue process a term used in BONE MARROW
TRANSPLANTATION to describe the infusion of the
donated marrow or the patient's own marrow to the
patient. This is usually done shortly after administration of the chemotherapy (anticancer drugs)
and/or radiation treatment.

resection a surgical procedure in which part of
the body tissue is cut out, such as the removal of a
segment of an organ. A resection is performed most
frequently when cancer is in an early stage and the
entire tumor can be removed, with clean MARGINS,
no signs of cancer cells in the tissue around the
cancer, without removing the entire organ. One
example of a common resection is a LUMPECTOMY
in breast cancer. The cancerous lump is removed,
leaving the rest of the breast intact.

response a term used in the treatment of cancer
to describe a positive result of treatment. A "complete response" (CR) means the disappearance of
all measurable evidence of the cancer. A CR is not
intended to imply a cure, as recurrence may
develop over time. A response is the purpose of
treatment.

retching [dry heaves] the urge and attempt to
vomit without bringing anything up. This can be a
side effect of chemotherapy and other treatments.
See NAUSEA AND VOMITING.

reticulocyte (rĕ-tik'u-lo-sīt) a young red blood
cell. An increase in reticulocytes may be seen as a
healthy response to abrupt blood loss. A reticulocyte count may be done along with a COMPLETE
BLOOD COUNT in the evaluation of ANEMIA.

reticulum cell sarcoma [histiocytic lymphoma]
See BONE CANCER.

retinoblastoma (ret″ĭno-blas-to′mah) a rare and
sometimes hereditary cancer of the eye occurring
primarily in infants and young children. About
40% of the cases are hereditary (see HEREDITARY
RETINOBLASTOMA). When retinoblastoma is inherited, it is not unusual for it to occur in both eyes.
Patients with the hereditary form are at risk of
developing a secondary malignancy (cancer), particularly OSTEOSARCOMA. The annual incidence of
retinoblastoma in the United States ranges from
one in 15,000 to one in 34,000.

Retinoblastoma arises from the retina. It is
highly curable, and if detected and treated early
enough, eyesight may be preserved. Symptoms may
include the development of a squint or the appearance of a white area in the center of the pupil.
Because young children who are not likely to com-
plain about visual problems are primarily affected,
early detection can be difficult. At the time of diagnosis most patients have extensive disease.

Diagnostic procedures may include examination
by OPHTHALMOSCOPY, FLUORESCEIN ANGIOGRAPHY,
CT SCAN, ULTRASOUND, and CORE NEEDLE BIOPSY.

There is no standard STAGING for retinoblastoma. It is broken down into two classifications:

- intraocular—cancer is localized to the eye; confined to the retina or extending to involve the
globe; does not extend outside the eye into tissues around the eye or other parts of the body
- extraocular—cancer is extended outside the eye;
confined to the tissue around the eye or spreading to other parts of the body

Treatment depends on the extent of the disease
and other factors. Treatments that may be used in

retinoblastoma include RADIATION THERAPY, CRYO-SURGERY, CHEMOTHERAPY, and PHOTOCOAGULATION. For specific information on the latest state-of-the art treatment, call the National Cancer Institute's Cancer Information Service at 1-800-4-CANCER (1-800-422-6237), or for a TTY: 1-800-332-8615.

See also EYE CANCER.

retinoic acid   See ACCUTANE.

retinoids (ret′ĭ-noids)   vitamin A and synthetic compounds similar to vitamin A. Synthetic retinoids are being investigated in their possible role blocking the action of cancer-causing agents. Vitamin A itself cannot be used because the amount that would be needed to be effective causes harmful side effects.

retracted nipple   See NIPPLE RETRACTION.

retrograde   the direction that is opposite to the way a fluid usually flows.

retrograde ejaculation [dry orgasm]   a condition in which semen shoots backward into the bladder at the time of orgasm instead of out through the penis. Retrograde ejaculation can be a side effect of some cancer treatments such as abdominoperineal resection (removal of the rectum and lower colon), RADICAL PROSTATECTOMY, CYSTECTOMY TRANSURETHRAL RESECTION, or retroperitoneal lymph node dissection (removal of the LYMPH NODES in the ABDOMEN).

retrograde pancreaticoduodenography   See ENDOSCOPIC RETROGRADE CHOLANGIOPANCREATOGRAPHY.

retrograde pyelography (pi″ĕ-log′rah-fe) [retrograde urography]   an examination of the urinary system (kidneys, ureters, and bladder) by X-RAY. This is very similar to an IVP, but instead of the CONTRAST MEDIUM being injected into a vein, it is inserted directly into the ureter. A fluoroscope is used to check the progress of the filling of the internal structures of the kidneys. The X-ray films that are taken can show conditions that impede or block passage of urine from the kidneys to the bladder. A retrograde pyelography may be performed in the diagnosis of kidney cancer—in addi-

tion to an IVP, or in place of it if the patient is allergic to the IVP medium or if the patient has a kidney condition that prevents the contrast medium from being filtered out from the blood.

retrograde urography   See RETROGRADE PYELOGRAPHY.

retroperitoneal lymph node dissection (RPLND) (re″tro-per″ĭ-to-ne′al limf nōd)   a major surgical procedure performed deep in the abdomen removing the LYMPH NODES that filter lymph from the testes. This may be performed in the STAGING of TESTICULAR CANCER to determine the extent of disease. It may also help control spread of NONSEMINOMA testicular cancer, since nonseminoma spreads first to the retroperitoneal lymph nodes. A common side effect of RPLND may be infertility because the procedure disrupts nerve pathways that control ejaculation. However, it seldom affects the ability to have an erection and orgasm. Doctors are now using new nerve-sparing surgical techniques that preserve normal ejaculation. Researchers are trying to find ways to stage testicular cancer without having to use surgical techniques and to develop better CHEMOTHERAPY (anticancer drugs) so that RPLND may not be necessary for some patients.

retroperitoneum (re″tro-per″ĭ-to-ne′um)   an area behind the smooth, transparent membrane that lines the abdominal cavity and part of the pelvic region.

retropubic prostatectomy (ret″ro-pu′bik pros″tah-tek′to-me)   surgical removal of the PROSTATE GLAND and surrounding tissue. An incision is made from the navel to the pubic bone to permit removal of the prostate and pelvic LYMPH NODES. This is one way in which a RADICAL PROSTATECTOMY is performed.

Retrovir   See AZT.

retrovirus   a large group of viruses characterized by their ability to reproduce "backward," instead of the way genes normally reproduce. Since the early 1900s retroviruses have been known to cause cancer in animals. In 1980, researchers at the National

Cancer Institute found an association between some leukemia and lymphoma patients and a retrovirus. The first identified human retrovirus was HTLV-1. The HTLV-III (HIV) retrovirus is considered to be the cause of AIDS. Retroviruses in humans can be devastating, as can be seen in the case of AIDS. Researchers are investigating the role retroviruses may play in the treatment of cancer. They appear to be able to serve as vehicles for transplanting genes from one species to another. Retroviruses are a major component in GENE THERAPY.

Revici, Emanual   a doctor in the United States who developed "biologically guided chemotherapy," a treatment that he claimed could be used for cancer as well as a wide range of other disorders including AIDS, Alzheimer's, arthritis, chronic pain, and schizophrenia. Revici wrote that his treatment "when correctly applied, can, . . . in many cases, bring under control even far-advanced malignancies." The only published clinical study of biologically guided chemotherapy appeared in the *Journal of the American Medical Association* in 1965. It concluded that "the Revici method of treatment of cancer is without value." There has not been a controlled CLINICAL TRIAL to evaluate the safety and efficacy of Revici's treatment.

See also UNCONVENTIONAL TREATMENT METHOD.

Revlimed   See LENALIDOMIDE.

rhabdomyosarcoma (rab"do-mi"o-sar-ko'mah) a fairly rare, soft tissue cancer originating in the skeletal muscles (muscles attached to the bone). This is the most common SOFT TISSUE SARCOMA among children, most often affecting young children aged two to six and children in their teens. It accounts for 8 to 13% of the malignant (cancerous) solid tumors of childhood. The most common site of occurrence is the head and neck, the eyes, and the genitourinary system, especially in young children. In teens it more commonly occurs in the arms and legs. Although rhabdomyosarcoma is not as common in adults, it does occur in adults, generally in men and women in their 40s and 50s. It is most commonly found, in adults, in the thigh, shoulder, or upper arm.

Symptoms of rhabdomyosarcoma vary because the disease can occur in so many different parts of the body. In general, swelling, bleeding, or an unusual mass found in the head, neck, eyes, genitourinary system, extremities, chest, and abdomen are possible symptoms for rhabdomyosarcoma, as well as many other disorders. A symptom of rhabdomyosarcoma in the eye may be a marked protrusion or bulging of the eye. Procedures used in the diagnosis and evaluation of rhabdomyosarcoma, depending on the location of the symptoms, may include X-RAY, CT SCAN, ULTRASOUND, and BIOPSY as well as other exams when necessary.

Following is the NATIONAL CANCER INSTITUTE's (NCI) STAGING for childhood rhabdomyosarcoma:

Stage 1—cancer is found in the eye, head, and/or neck, or near the sex organs and bladder
Stage 2—cancer is located in only one area (but in none of the areas in Stage 1), is smaller than two inches (5 cm) across in size, and has not spread to the lymph nodes
Stage 3—cancer is located in one area (but not one of the areas in Stage 1), is greater than two inches (5 cm) across in size, and may have spread to the lymph nodes found nearby the cancer
Stage 4—cancer has spread and is found in more than one place at the time of diagnosis
Recurrent—the cancer has come back (recurred) after it has been treated. It may come back in the area where it started or in another part of the body

Treatment depends on the stage of the disease, its location, the general state of health of the patient, and other factors. Treatment procedures include surgery, CHEMOTHERAPY, RADIATION THERAPY, and CLINICAL TRIALS. BONE MARROW TRANSPLANTATION is being studied for its role in the supportive treatment of rhabdomyosarcoma. For specific information on the latest state-of-the-art treatment, by stage, call NCI's Cancer Information Service at 1-800-4-CANCER (1-800-422-6237), or for a TTY: 1-800-332-8615.

See also EMBRYONAL CELL CANCER, SOFT-TISSUE SARCOMA, and EYE CANCER.

rhizotomy (ri-zot'o-me)   a method of blocking or controlling pain through the use of surgery. A neurosurgeon cuts a nerve close to the spinal column to prevent the transmission of sensation. This not only stops the sensation of pain, but the sensation of pressure and temperature as well. Without the protective reflexes evoked by those sensations, there is greater potential for injury in the area affected.

See also PAIN MANAGEMENT.

rhythm technique   See RELAXATION TECHNIQUES.

ribonucleic acid   See RNA.

r-IFN-beta   See INTERFERON BETA.

RIL-2   See INTERLEUKIN-2.

risk factor   in cancer, a substance or condition that increases the chance of developing a particular cancer. A risk factor can be natural or synthetic or a combination of both. The degree of risk each factor poses depends on a number of different things and can vary from person to person. Risk factors can complement one another resulting in a twofold, threefold or more increase in risk than the person would face if exposed to just one of the factors.

Cigarette SMOKING is a risk factor created by people. People who smoke are at a much greater risk of developing lung cancer, as well as other cancers; the risk is reduced by stopping smoking. People who are exposed to passive smoke can reduce their risk by avoiding people and places where there is passive smoke. Much new legislation protects nonsmokers as cities throughout the United States have enacted laws requiring smoke-free areas in restaurants and other public places.

A naturally occurring risk factor that has been enhanced by humans is ULTRAVIOLET RADIATION from the Sun. Destruction of the ozone layer, a natural "sun blocker," has increased the risk of exposure to the sun. Generally, the fairer complected the person, the greater risk of developing skin cancer. The risk can be mitigated by using sunscreen or sunblock, wearing protective clothing, and avoiding the sun during the time of the day when it is strongest.

Many risk factors can be controlled or avoided. For example, people can minimize their exposure to RADON, a naturally occurring substance known to be a risk factor in lung cancer, by testing their home and taking corrective measures if dangerous levels are present. Of course, many risks present in the environment cannot be controlled; nor can hereditary factors, which can increase the risk of developing cancer, be changed.

See also DIET and CARCINOGENS.

risk/benefit ratio   the relationship between the risks and benefits of a new or experimental treatment or procedure. Before setting up a CLINICAL TRIAL, an Institutional Review Board (IRB) where the study is to take place determines whether the risk involved in the trial is reasonable compared with the potential benefits. Ultimately, it is up to the patient to decide if the potential benefits outweigh the potential risks, before deciding whether to take part in the trial. The risk/benefit ratio may also be used by a patient in deciding which, if any, standard treatment to take.

Rituxan [rituximab]   a chimeric mouse/human antibody that binds to cancer cells after they track them down, stimulating the body's IMMUNE SYSTEM to destroy the cancer cells. It is used in the treatment of NON-HODGKIN'S LYMPHOMAS that express CD-20. When it was approved by the Food and Drug Administration in late 1997, it became the first monoclonal antibody available in the United States for treating cancer. Side effects may include rigors, rashes, hypotension, wheezing, and infections. It is administered by IV (injected into a vein).

rituximab   See RITUXAN.

RNA (ribonucleic acid)   one of the two nucleic acids found in all cells. The other is DNA (deoxyribonucleic acid). RNA transfers genetic information from DNA to proteins produced by the cell.

Roentgen equivalent man   See REM.

Roentgen knife   See STEREOTACTIC RADIOSURGERY.

Roentgen ray   See X-RAY.

Roferon-A   See ALPHA INTERFERON and INTERFERON.

RPLND   See RETROPERITONEAL LYMPH NODE DISSECTION.

RT-PCR   See POLYMERASE CHAIN REACTION.

RU486 [mifepristone] a drug developed in France that is used to induce abortions. It works by interfering with certain hormones, including progesterone, which is vital to healthy pregnancies. It acts as an antiprogesterone and also has antiangiogenesis properties. This drug is under investigation for treatment of certain cancers, including metastatic BREAST CANCER, OVARIAN CANCER, endometriosis, PROSTATE CANCER, as well as meningliomas (BRAIN TUMORS).

RU 486 has been surrounded by controversy in the United States because of its use in abortions in France.

Rubidomycin   See DAUNOMYCIN.

saccharin See ARTIFICIAL SWEETENERS.

saddle block a form of spinal anesthesia. The anesthesia is injected into the lower part of the spinal cord. It is used during surgery in the rectum or genital areas

SAHA (subeoyleanilide hydroxamic acid) an oral histone deacetylase inhibitor being investigated for treatment of cutaneous T-CELL LYMPHOMA.

saline implant (sa'lēn) an implant filled with a salt-water solution that may be used in BREAST RECONSTRUCTION or breast augmentation (plastic surgery to increase the size of the breasts).

salivary gland a gland in the mouth that secretes saliva. There are major salivary glands (parotid, submandibular, and sublingual) and minor glands (oral mucosa, palate, uvula, floor of the mouth, posterior tongue, retromolar area, and peritonsillar area).

See also SALIVARY GLAND CANCER.

salivary gland cancer cancer of the salivary glands, which secrete saliva. Most tumors that occur in the salivary glands are benign (noncancerous). Tumors can affect different glands. Approximately 20 to 25% of parotid tumors, 35 to 40% of submandibular tumors, 50% of palate tumors, and 95 to 100% of sublingual gland tumors are malignant (cancerous). People at the greatest risk are those who have had radiation to the head and neck area and those who smoke. Symptoms of cancer in the salivary glands may be the presence of a slowly growing lump in the cheek next to the ear. There may be a dull and indefinite but progressive pain and facial-nerve paralysis. Diagnostic procedures may include an MRI, CT SCAN with contrast, and BIOPSY.

Following is the NATIONAL CANCER INSTITUTE'S (NCI) STAGING for salivary glands cancer:

- Stage I—the tumor is less than four CENTIMETERS (cm) in size and is confined to the salivary glands
- Stage II
  — the tumor is less than 4 cm in size and extends to local tissues
  — the tumor is 4 to 6 cm in size and does not extend to local tissue
- Stage III
  — the tumor is any size (except greater than 6 cm with extension into local tissue) with spread to a single layer of LYMPH NODES on the same side of the neck but not distant sites or
  — the tumor is 4 to 6 cm in size with invasion of local tissue but without spread to lymph nodes or distant sites or
  — the tumor is greater than 6 cm and is confined to the salivary glands
- Stage IV
  — the tumor is greater than 6 cm in size and extends to local tissues

— the tumor is any size with extensive spread to lymph nodes

— the tumor is any size and has spread to distant sites

• Recurrent—the tumor has returned to the original site or to a distant location after treatment.

Treatment depends on the stage of the disease, the general state of health of the patient, and other factors. Treatment may be SURGERY, RADIATION THERAPY, CHEMOTHERAPY, or CLINICAL TRIALS. For specific information on the latest state-of-the-art treatment, by stage, call NCI's Cancer Information Service at 1-800-4-CANCER (1-800-422-6237), or for a TTY: 1-800-332-8615.

salpingectomy (sal"pin-jek'to-me) surgical removal of one or both fallopian tubes. This may be performed in the treatment of different cancers of the female reproductive organs as well as other disorders.

salvage therapy medical jargon for the administration of an alternative treatment when the PRIMARY TREATMENT failed or is no longer effective.

samarium Sm-153 lexidronam injection See QUADRAMET.

Sandostatin [SSTN, octreotide] See OCTREOTIDE.

sarcoma (sar-ko'mah) a malignant (cancerous) tumor arising in the bone, cartilage, fibrous tissue, or muscle. Sarcomas are broadly divided into two groups—those that arise from the bone (BONE CANCER); and those that arise from the soft tissue (SOFT-TISSUE SARCOMA).

sargramostim See GM-CSF.

SCA (self-controlled analgesia) See PAIN MANAGEMENT and PCA PUMP.

scan a view or image of the interior of the body that can show abnormalities in structure and function. The many different scans include nuclear, CT, PET, MRI, and ultrasound. Different scans are used for different parts of the body and to obtain different information. Scans play a major role in the diagnosis and STAGING of many different cancers.

They are also used in follow-up to evaluate the effectiveness of treatment and to monitor for recurrence after treatment. Scans are also used in the diagnosis of many other disorders besides cancer.

One scan widely used is the NUCLEAR SCAN. A small, relatively harmless amount of a radioactive substance is inserted in the body, either by IV (injected into a vein) or orally. A two-dimensional picture of the radiation rays given off by the substance can show functional and structural abnormalities.

The CT scan uses an X-RAY and computer to produce cross-sectional pictures. Abnormalities in different parts of the body can be seen. It does not require the use of a radioactive substance.

ULTRASOUND uses sound waves to detect a mass or tumor in the body. It is noninvasive and does not use a radioactive substance in the body.

The PET SCAN, can pinpoint changes in metabolic activity that may indicate abnormalities.

The MRI uses powerful electric magnets, radio frequency waves, and a computer to take internal pictures of the body.

See also BONE SCAN, BRAIN SCAN, KIDNEY SCAN, LIVER SCAN, LUNG SCAN, PANCREAS SCAN, and THYROID SCAN.

scavenger cells See MACROPHAGE.

Schiller test an examination of cells in the vagina and cervix. The exam can be performed in a doctor's office. An iodine solution is swabbed on the walls of the cervix and vagina. Normal cells are stained brown. Abnormal cells do not absorb the solution and may appear to be pink or white. A Schiller test may be used in the diagnosis of VAGINAL CANCER or CERVICAL CANCER.

schwannoma See NEUROMA.

scintigram See SCINTIGRAPHY.

scintigraphy [scintiscan] a two-dimensional picture of the radioactive rays emitted by a radioactive substance that has been injected into the body. A special camera scans the body for radioactivity and takes a photograph (scintigram), which will show areas of rapidly dividing cells. Concentrations of the substance can indicate abnormalities. A scintiscan may be performed in the diagnosis of cancer in many different organs such as the bones, brain, kidney, or thyroid. It may also be used to detect metastatic cancer. The word *scan* is frequently interchangeable with scintiscan, although not all scans are scintiscans.

scintimammography See SCINTIGRAPHY and MIRALUMA TEST.

scintiscan See SCINTIGRAPHY.

scirrhous (skir'us) a term used to describe a cancer that has become hard because of the formation of dense connective tissue in the stroma (the supporting tissue or framework) of an organ.

SCLC See SMALL CELL LUNG CANCER.

screening a mass examination of a population, without symptoms, for the existence of a particular disease. For example, in cancer, there may be a mass screening for skin cancer, with many people being examined for possible signs of skin cancer.

Screening may also be done on an individual basis. An individual can be screened for different cancers, screened regularly for just one cancer, or screened regularly for a cancer that he or she may be at a greater risk of developing than the general population. Screening is done to detect cancer as early as possible when it is most treatable. A screening procedure can indicate an abnormal condition that may be cancerous. Follow-up with diagnostic procedures, including a BIOPSY, are then needed. Some screening procedures, such as the BREAST SELF-EXAMINATION and TESTICULAR SELF-EXAMINATION, can be performed by an individual.

Screening for cancer appears to, and does in fact, have many advantages, including:

- saving the life of someone who would have died had the cancer not been detected by screening
- requiring less radical treatment for some cancers that are detected early
- lower treatment cost if a less radical treatment is needed
- reassuring those patients who receive negative results.

However, cancer screening also carries with it some disadvantages, including:

- for patients whose PROGNOSIS would be the same—no matter when the cancer was detected—a longer period of "being ill"
- overtreatment of borderline abnormalities, many of which might never have been detected without the screening, with its associated costs
- false reassurance for those with false negative results who may then ignore warning signs
- false positive results, which result in expenditure for additional tests and tremendous anxiety.

The effectiveness of screening for different cancers is being investigated in the United States and abroad. For example, one study on breast cancer screening found a reduced mortality rate in women who received a physical exam and mammography throughout 18 years of follow-up. Several studies in the United States have been conducted on the effectiveness of screening for lung cancer, using X-rays and sputum tests, in over 30,000 men. The findings indicated that while the screening successfully located early-stage lung cancer that could be surgically treated, *long-term survival was not significantly affected.* It was therefore concluded that large-scale screening for lung cancer is not justified.

Following are the cancers for which there are screening guidelines and the source of the guidelines:

- Breast
  — women 20 to 40—monthly breast self-exam for any lumps or changes; physical exam of breasts by doctor every three years; baseline mammography between the ages of 35 and 40
  — women 40 and older—monthly self-exam; yearly exam of breasts by doctor; yearly mammography
  — women with personal or family histories of breast cancer—check with doctor about the need for more frequent examinations (American Cancer Society)
- Cervix
  — women who are sexually active or 18 and older—PAP SMEAR and pelvic exam; after three normal Pap smears in three consecutive years, the doctor may recommend it be done less frequently
  — women exposed to DES before birth—a pelvic exam and pap smear starting at (whichever comes first) age 14 or when menstruation begins

— women who have had a hysterectomy—a regular pelvic exam and pap smear (National Cancer Institute)

• Colon/Rectal
  Adults 50 and older—one of the examination schedules listed should be followed:
  — occult blood stool test yearly and a flexible sigmoidoscopy every five years
  — colonoscopy—every 10 years
  — double-contrast barium enema every five to 10 years
  — a digital rectal exam should be done at the same time as a sigmoidoscopy, coloscopy, or double-contrast barium enema. People at an increased risk of colon/rectal cancer should discuss the appropriate screening schedule with their doctor (American Cancer Society)

• Prostate
  — men 50 and older—a yearly rectal exam (Prostate Cancer Education Council and National Cancer Institute)
  — men 50 and older—a yearly PSA (American Cancer Society). The U.S. Preventive Services Task Force does not recommend routine PSA and digital rectal examination. The American Urological Association recommends annual PSA and digital rectal exams for men who have at least a 10-year life expectancy beginning at age 50 or to younger men at higher risk

• Skin
  — individuals should examine their skin thoroughly on a regular basis
  — physicians should examine skin during periodic health exam
  — anyone who has had skin cancer should be checked regularly (National Cancer Institute)

• Testicular—monthly testicular self-exam for any lumps or changes (National Cancer Institute)

scrotum (skro′tum)   a sac of loose skin that contains the testicles and which lies directly below the penis.

scrotum cancer (skro′tum)   a rare condition, significant for its contribution in the understanding of the role environmental/occupational factors play in cancer. In the late 1700s, in England, an association was noted between chimney sweeps and scrotum cancer. It was found that it could be eliminated

if they washed after work. Since then, many environmental occupational risks have been identified.

sebaceous hyperplasia (sĕba′shus hi″per-pla′ze-ah)   a benign (noncancerous) skin condition characterized by shiny, yellow, waxy-oily tumors. They rarely become cancerous.

seborrheic keratoses (seb″o-re′ik ker″ah-to′sis)   a benign (noncancerous) skin condition with raised and warty-looking bumps. They appear to be stuck on the skin but can be scraped off with a fingernail. It rarely becomes cancerous.

second-line therapy   medical jargon for a treatment after the best primary treatment is no longer effective

second-look laparotomy (lap-ah-rot′-o-me) [second-look surgery]   a surgical procedure in the abdomen that is performed in people with OVARIAN CANCER and, on rare occasion, in other cancers and disorders. It may be done for diagnostic purposes, to evaluate treatment's effectiveness, and to determine if it needs to be continued, or to determine if a tumor, which had been inoperable, has been sufficiently reduced by the treatment so that it can be removed. It may also be performed, following completion of chemotherapy or radiation therapy, to evaluate whether treatment was effective or to see if there has been a recurrence. Second look surgery is also an opportunity to remove remaining cancer cells that are found.

second-look surgery   a term usually used in the management of ovarian cancer after a period of treatment to assess results and plan possible future treatment. See SECOND-LOOK LAPAROTOMY.

second opinion   a consultation with a doctor who specializes in the treatment of the cancer with which the patient has been diagnosed. This is very commonly done when there is a diagnosis of cancer, as well as with many other disorders. Generally, a second opinion is sought right after diagnosis and before treatment starts. A second opinion may also be sought when the treatment is not producing the hoped-for result. However, a patient can seek a second opinion anytime.

A second opinion by a specialist may be requested by the patient's doctor because of the importance of correctly identifying the specific subcategory of the cancer so that the best treatment for that specific cancer can be given. The opinion of the second doctor does not always agree with the opinion of the original doctor. The patient then has several options. He or she can ask the two doctors to discuss the treatment or the patient can seek a third opinion. A patient may also seek a second opinion on the PATHOLOGIST'S report, generally when a BIOPSY is positive. There is a possibility that the pathologist has made an error, or it may be important, psychologically, for a patient who is having a problem accepting the diagnosis.

Most physicians will support a patient's decision to get a second opinion; some will encourage a patient to do so. Patients can find a cancer specialist for a second opinion by asking their doctor for a referral. They can call their local Medical Society Office listed in the telephone book, and ask for a doctor specializing in their type of cancer. Another source for a second opinion is a COMPREHENSIVE CANCER CENTER, a CLINICAL CANCER CENTER, a teaching hospital or medical school, or a hospital with a cancer program approved by the American College of Surgeons. Another possible way to find a doctor for a second opinion is to call the local American Cancer Society or the National Cancer Institute's Cancer Information Service at 1-800-4-CANCER (1-800-422-6237), or for a TTY: 1-800-332-8615.

second primary cancer [secondary cancer] cancer that originates in a site different from the PRIMARY CANCER site where the cancer was originally diagnosed. This is different from cancer that has metastasized (spread) from the original site to another location in the body. A second primary cancer is a new cancer in a different location in the body. People who have had cancer are at an increased risk of developing another type of cancer. In most cases a new cancer is not related in any way to the original cancer. In very rare instances, a second primary cancer may be a result of the CHEMOTHERAPY or RADIATION THERAPY administered for the treatment of the first (original) cancer.

secondary liver cancer   See LIVER METASTASES.

secondary tumor   See METASTATIC CANCER.

secondhand smoke   See PASSIVE SMOKE.

secondhand smoking [environmental tobacco smoke (ETS), involuntary smoking, passive smoking]   inhalation of tobacco smoke by nonsmokers. Secondhand smoke includes sidestream smoke from the burning end of a cigarette or smoke exhaled by a smoker. Data from epidemiological studies indicate that nonsmokers exposed to cigarette smoke are at an increased risk of lung cancer and other diseases. In 1993, the Environmental Protection Agency called secondhand smoke a carcinogen responsible for some 3,000 lung cancer deaths a year among nonsmokers.

Health hazards associated with involuntary smoking may be specially significant for specific groups of people. Children of smoking parents have more repiratory infections and symptoms than children of nonsmoking parents. There may be differences of lung function in children, as well as adults, exposed to passive smoke over a long period of time. Unborn children (involuntary smokers) of mothers who smoke weigh on average seven ounces less at birth than children of nonsmoking mothers. They are also at greater risk for spontaneous abortion, fetal death, and death shortly after birth (including sudden infant death syndrome).

See also SMOKING.

SEER (Surveillance, Epidemiology, and End Results) a program of the NATIONAL CANCER INSTITUTE'S (NCI) Division of Cancer Prevention or Control. It is NCI's main tool for tracking, assembling, and reporting data on cancer in the United States and ascertaining national trends. SEER has been monitoring the annual occurrence of cancer and patient survival since 1973. Those figures are compiled in a report called the Cancer Statistics Review (CSR). The purpose of the CSR is to summarize the key measures of cancer's impact on the population—number of new cases, number of deaths, number of survivors living for a specific period of time after diagnosis. It may also include measures of other factors such as long-term behavior trends (e.g., smoking), cancer knowledge (e.g., awareness of risk factors), and use of early detecting methods (e.g., mammography).

segmental cystectomy (sis-tek'to-me) surgical removal of part of the bladder. This operation is used only in those cases of bladder cancer in which the cancer is in only one area.

segmental mastectomy See LUMPECTOMY.

segmental resection surgical removal of a cancerous tumor, leaving the rest of the organ. This can only be done if an adequate MARGIN of clean (cancer-free) tissue can be removed from around the tumor. Segmental resection may be performed in many different cancers, especially when the cancer is in an early stage.

selective renal arteriography (ar"te-re-og'rah-fe) an examination of the kidney's blood vessels by X-RAY. A substance that enables the doctor to see the veins and arteries that serve the kidney is injected into the bloodstream. This test helps show the extent of a mass of tissue and is 95 to 98% accurate in diagnosing kidney cancer. This is virtually the last step in diagnosing kidney cancer, although a NEEDLE ASPIRATION BIOPSY may also be performed to confirm the diagnosis.

selenium an essential mineral that acts as an ANTIOXIDANT and can substitute for vitamin E in some of that vitamin's antioxidant activities. A 10-year cancer prevention trial, ended three years early in 1996, suggested that dietary supplements of selenium may significantly lower the incidence of prostate, colorectal, and lung cancers in people with a history of skin cancer. There were no adverse effects in the people who were given selenium. A 1998 study at Harvard University found a reduced risk of advanced prostate cancer with higher selenium levels. There is some indication that a selenium deficiency may increase the risk of cancer, though the link is being investigated and there is no hard data. Too much selenium can cause loss of hair and nails, nervous system and skin lesions, and possibly damage to the teeth.

self-controlled analgesia (SCA) See PAIN MANAGEMENT and ANALGESIC PUMP.

self-examination of the breast See BREAST SELF-EXAM.

self-examination of the testicles See TESTICULAR SELF-EXAM.

seminoma (se"mǐ-no'mah) one of two main types of TESTICULAR CANCER. Seminomas occur primarily in men aged 25 to 45 and account for between 30 and 40% of all testicular cancers.

senile lentigo (se'nǐl len-ti'go) a benign (noncancerous) skin condition, commonly called liver spots, which rarely becomes cancerous.

senograph (se'no-graf) a machine for MAMMOGRAPHY developed in France that uses a special X-ray tube and filters. It can take mammograms using minute amounts of radiation, 0.02 to 0.03 RAD for two views.

sentinel lymph node the first lymph node in a chain or cluster of lymph nodes to receive lymphatic drainage from a tumor.

sentinel lymph-node biopsy a procedure in which the SENTINEL LYMPH NODE is identified, removed, and examined for cancer cells. If no cancer cells are found it can be assumed with a high degree of certainty that cancer cells would not be found in any of the other lymph nodes, since they would travel through the sentinel node first. Thus, a negative (cancer-free) sentinel lymph node would eliminate the need for removal of the entire group of lymph nodes in that region. This has been done most successfully in patients with MELANOMA, and in patients with BREAST CANCER (where removal of all the axillary nodes can have some severe and lasting side effects). Its role in providing information on treatment of the cancer and prognosis is being evaluated and compared with the traditional SURGICAL STAGING PROCEDURES.

serotonin (ser"o-to'nin) a naturally occurring chemical neurotransmitter and vasoconstrictor that plays a major role in inhibiting pain in the gastrointestinal tract. Serotonin-based antidepressants have proven effective in treating a variety of chronic pain conditions. Serotonin has also been implicated in some of the unpleasant side effects of some chemotherapy (anticancer drugs); the release of serotonin triggered by some chemotherapy sets off nerve impulses that may cause nausea and vomiting. Serotonin antagonists may be used to counter this effect. Serotonin is also released by CELLS of CARCINOID TUMORS.

serotonin antagonists (ser"o-to'nin) a type of antiemetic drug given to prevent nausea and vomiting caused by some chemotherapy (anticancer drugs). It acts by blocking SEROTONIN receptors in the intestines and brain, stopping nerve impulses that would otherwise travel to the brain and stimulate an area that causes vomiting.

Sertoli-Leydig tumor See OVARIAN GERM CELL TUMOR AND STROMAL TUMOR.

serum (se'rum) the clear fluid that separates from the blood when it is allowed to clot. Serum retains ANTIBODIES present in the whole blood.

sestamibi breast imaging See MIRALUMA TEST.

sex cord tumor See OVARIAN GERM CELL TUMOR AND STROMAL TUMOR.

sexual activity Sexual functioning for both reproduction and pleasure, for men and women, can be affected by cancer and by its treatment in various ways. However, many problems are temporary or reversible with treatment.

There are still many myths surrounding sex and cancer. One common myth is that sexual intercourse can cause cancer, especially cancer of the sexual organs. A few specific cancers may be caused by a virus that is passed to a partner during sexual contact; however, there has been no link found between the development of most cancers and sexual activity. (AIDS, which is not cancer but can lead to cancer, can be transmitted during sexual activity through the exchange of body fluid.) Another myth is that sexual activity can worsen the cancer or be harmful to the partner.

Sexual activity may be affected by physical side effects that can be irreversible. Both men and women can become infertile as a result of surgery, HORMONAL TREATMENTS, RADIATION THERAPY, and/or CHEMOTHERAPY. Men can become IMPOTENT as a result of treatment and women can experience vaginal dryness which can make sexual intercourse difficult, painful, and potentially harmful. It is

important to note that in many instances there are remedies to alleviate or reduce the problem.

It is not at all unusual for men and women to lose sexual desire during the treatment of cancer. Loss of desire can be a result of anxiety, depression, side effects of therapy such as nausea, pain, tiredness, etc. In addition, many people who have cancer fear that their partner will be turned off by changes in their body. For example, it is not uncommon for a woman who has had a breast removed to feel less attractive and lose self-esteem. Generally, sexual activity presents no problem during or following cancer treatment. If there are concerns they should be discussed with the doctor. For more information, call the American Cancer Society at 1-800-ACR-2345 for two free, excellent publications: *Sexuality and Cancer, For the Woman Who Has Cancer and Her Partner* and *Sexuality and Cancer, For the Man Who Has Cancer and His Partner.*

Sezary syndrome a more advanced form of MYCOSIS FUNGOIDES, a LYMPHOMA affecting the skin in which large numbers of tumor cells are found in the blood.

SGN-30 [chimeric anti-CD30 antibody] a compound being investigated in anaplastic large cell lymphoma (ALCL).

shark cartilage a product made from the pure cartilage that sharks have in their bodies. As very few sharks develop cancer it was theorized that their cartilage could inhibit the development of blood vessels that would supply needed nutrients to tumors. As a result, shark cartilage has been used by some cancer patients as an alternative treatment. To evaluate its safety and effectiveness as a cancer treatment, a clinical trial of shark cartilage was approved by the National Cancer Institute's Office of Alternative Medicine. Its conclusion in 1998 was that shark cartilage was of no benefit to the patients in the study. The Office of Alternative Medicine is now the National Center for Complementary and Alternative Medicine.

shave biopsy (bi'op-se) removal of a small amount of skin to examine microscopically for cancer cells. If the biopsy is positive and all the cancer has been removed, this can also be the treatment.

shingles   a condition in which chicken pox-like blisters occur, usually in a limited area of the skin, confined to an area supplied by a particular nerve. Shingles is caused by the herpes virus *Varicella zoster*. The viral infection travels along the nerve path. A unique characteristic of shingles is that it is the result of the "reawakening" of a virus that has been dormant (inactive) in the body for years. It is an infection that can occur in AIDS patients, in people whose immune systems are lowered as a result of treatment, and in patients who have undergone BONE MARROW TRANSPLANTATION. Chemotherapy and certain cancers, such as NON-HODGKIN'S LYMPHOMA (NHL), may make a person more susceptible to shingles as well as to a more disseminated and serious form of the disease that can be life-threatening.

shunt   to create a link between two blood vessels, from one compartment to another. A shunt may also be devised to drain fluid in the body. For example, a shunt may be used to relieve increased pressure on the brain caused by brain tumors that block the flow of spinal fluid. The shunt device is a catheter (a narrow piece of tubing).

side effect   a secondary and generally undesirable outcome of treatment. Side effects are usually harmful, painful, or just unpleasant. Some typical side effects of CHEMOTHERAPY are nausea, vomiting, and hair loss. Some side effects are so objectionable to a patient that he or she may choose to stop a potentially curative or useful treatment rather than endure the side effects. Methods have been developed to eliminate or decrease different side effects.

See also individual drug listings and side effects in the Subject Index.

sidestream smoke   See PASSIVE SMOKE.

sigmoidoscope   See SIGMOIDOSCOPY.

sigmoidoscopy (sig″moi-dos′ko-pe) [proctosigmoidoscopy]   an examination of the first 10 to 12 inches of the rectum. A sigmoidoscope (a thin, lighted metal or plastic tube about 10 inches long) is inserted through the rectum in order to view the lower interior portion of the colon where POLYPS and cancer are most frequently found. The patient either lies on his or her side, face down, or is in a kneeling position on the examining table. Tissue can be removed for biopsy (microscopic examination for cancer cells). Although a sigmoidoscopy may be uncomfortable, it is usually not painful. A flexible sigmoidoscope, which can be as long as two feet, became available in the early 1980s. It can be bent by the handle and enables a much larger portion of the colon to be viewed. A sigmoidoscopy may be performed as a screening procedure as well as for the diagnosis of COLON/RECTAL CANCER.

See also SCREENING.

silicone gel   or medical-grade silicone rubber gel that has fluid qualities similar to the normal breast.

See SILICONE IMPLANT.

silicone implant (sil′ĭl-kon)   a pouch filled with a gel-like substance used in breast augmentation (plastic surgery to make the breasts larger) and BREAST RECONSTRUCTION (plastic surgery to replace a breast removed because of cancer). About 20% of the implants are done for reconstructive or other corrective purposes.

Silicone implants were first marketed in the early 1960s. Breast reconstruction for cancer patients has been available for women with breast cancer, on a fairly wide basis, since the early 1970s. In 1976, the medical device law was passed, giving the Food and Drug Administration (FDA) the authority to regulate products such as implants. In 1988 it was reported that silicone implants in rats caused cancer. In December 1990, congressional hearings were held on the safety of silicone breast implants. The FDA is now requiring manufacturers of silicone implants to provide scientific data demonstrating their safety.

There are other risks associated with the implants besides the possible risk of cancer. Silicone implants may make it more difficult to see abnormalities in the breast in a MAMMOGRAM. There can be some discomfort or pain resulting from the growth of hard fibrous tissue around the implant. Some of the silicone may leak out of the implant. Another possible hazard is the polyurethane foam that coats some of the implants. In April 1991, there was a report that the coating can dissolve in the body, and that when it does, the chemical 2-toluene diamine (TDA) is produced. TDA has been shown to cause cancer in rats and other research animals.

In February 1992, a panel of experts appointed by the FDA recommended that silicone implants be restricted to women with breast cancer undergoing breast reconstruction and women with serious breast deformities. These women would be in effect part of a large clinical trial to see if the implants do carry a risk. The panel said there is insufficient evidence to conclude that the implants are not safe and effective. In April 1992, the FDA restricted the use of silicone implants to women with breast cancer and women with serious breast deformities. In December 1998, the National Science Panel, medical experts appointed by a U.S. district judge to decide whether silicone breast implants could cause disease, reported that there was no proof that the implants are harmful to health.

The Institute of Medicine (IOM) published a report in 2002 called, *Safety of Silicone Breast Implants,* indicating that breast cancer is no more common in women with breast implants than those without breast implants. While not conclusive, cancer rates have been reported to be slightly higher for some types of cancers. Cancers rates that have been higher in more than one study are LUNG and VULVA. Because these cancers may be related to other factors that were not examined in these studies (such as SMOKING) these studies are not conclusive. More information on cancer and breast implants is available at the NATIONAL CANCER INSTITUTE Web site at: http://www.nci.nih.gov/newscenter/silicone-othercancers, http://www.nci.nih.gov/newscenter/silicone-mortality, and http://www.nci.nih.gov/newscenter/siliconebreast.

Simonton technique   a self-help program of relaxation and IMAGERY intended to be used as an adjuvant therapy (in addition) to conventional treatment. The technique is explained by its developers, Dr. Carl and Stephanie Simonton, in their book *Getting Well Again: A Step-by-Step Help Guide to Overcoming Cancer for Patients and Their Families.* It is based, at least in part, on Dr. Simonton's belief that stress may contribute to the development of cancer. The book was published in 1970 and has been reprinted in more than 20 editions.

Although the program appears to be harmless, with a number of advantages, there are also some disadvantages. Among the advantages are the patient's sense of having some kind of control in a situation that is largely uncontrollable. It can promote a sense of taking an active part in one's recovery—doing something to help, thereby improving the quality of life. It can be done at home, on one's own, with little or no expense.

On the downside, there is no scientific data that the Simonton program has any effect on the outcome of disease. There is no scientific data that supports Dr. Simonton's belief that stress, depression, and hopelessness contribute directly to the development of cancer. That unproven theory can have a negative impact on a patient who starts thinking that he or she caused the cancer or is at fault for having it. There is the danger that some patients, having a sense of "mastery" while doing the exercises, will opt to stop conventional treatment and use only the Simonton program (a choice that is *not* advocated by its authors). And finally, some studies, in which tumors were implanted in animals, suggest that stress may, in fact, have a positive effect by inhibiting the growth of tumors.

See also UNCONVENTIONAL TREATMENT METHODS.

simple mastectomy (mas-tek'to-me) [total mastectomy, complete mastectomy]   a type of MASTECTOMY that requires the removal of only the breast. A few of the underarm LYMPH NODES closest to the breast may also be removed. A simple mastectomy may be followed by radiation therapy. This is one of the surgeries that is performed in the treatment of BREAST CANCER.

simple nephrectomy   See NEPHRECTOMY.

simple vulvectomy (vul-vek'to-me)   surgical removal of the vulva (the fatty folds of flesh surrounding the vaginal opening) and the clitoris (small organ of female genitalia). This may be performed in the treatment of early vulvar cancer.

single blind   a CLINICAL TRIAL in which the doctor knows the treatment each patient is getting, but the patient does not know which treatment he or she is receiving. This is done to prevent personal bias from influencing their reactions and the study results.

See also DOUBLE BLIND.

sinus cancer See PARANASAL SINUS/NASAL CAVITY CANCER.

6-mercaptopurine See 6-MP.

6-MP [Leukerin, 6-mercaptopurine, mercaptopurine, Purinethol] an ANTIMETABOLITE anticancer drug sometimes used in the treatment of acute lymphocytic leukemia (ALL) and chronic myelogenous leukemia (CML). It is taken by mouth. Side effects include occasional nausea and vomiting. Excessive doses may cause BONE MARROW DEPRESSION.

6-TG [6-thioguanine, thioguanine] an ANTIMETABOLIC anticancer drug sometimes used in the treatment of acute nonlymphocytic (ANLL) and chronic myelocytic leukemia (CML). It is taken by mouth. Common side effects may include occasional nausea and vomiting. Occasional and rare side effects may include BONE MARROW DEPRESSION, jaundice, appetite loss, diarrhea, mouth sores, skin rashes, and possible liver damage.

6-thioguanine See 6-TG.

Sjögren's syndrome (sho'grenz) a combination of symptoms such as enlargement of glands in the neck, inflammation of the cornea, and mouth dryness (due to lack of normal secretions). It is a chronic, slowly progressive autoimmune disorder. This syndrome is not cancer, and although a link is not firmly established, there has been the suggestion of an association with the development of some LYMPHOMAS.

skin the largest organ of the body, which covers the body and protects it from heat, light, injury, and infection. It also stores water, fat, and vitamin D. The top layer of skin is composed of BASAL CELLS, SQUAMOUS CELLS, and melanocytes. Cancer can arise in any of them.

skin cancer cancer of the skin. Skin cancer is the most common cancer in the United States, and its incidence has been increasing, most notably MELANOMA. More than 1 million cases of basal cell or squamous cell cancer are diagnosed annually. The American Cancer Society estimated that the most serious form of skin cancer, MALIGNANT MELANOMA, was expected to be diagnosed in 59,580 persons in 2005. Since 1981, the incidence of melanoma has increased a little less than 3% per year. Melanoma is the most common cancer among people 25 to 29 years old. http://www.cdc.gov/chooseyourcover/skin.htm. There are more than 600,000 new cases of nonmelanoma skin cancers diagnosed each year in the United States and 2,000 deaths. Forty to 50% of people who live to age 65 will have at least one skin cancer.

People at the greatest risk of developing skin cancer are those who have fair complexions and skin that tends to burn and freckle rather than tan and who live nearest the equator. Skin cancer incidence among blacks is very low because of the amount of melanin, a pigment, in the skin.

The most common type of skin cancer is BASAL CELL CARCINOMA OF THE SKIN. The second most common kind of skin cancer is SQUAMOUS CELL CARCINOMA. Melanoma is the most serious. There are other, less common skin cancers.

The most frequent cause of skin cancer is ULTRAVIOLET RADIATION from the Sun. Sun-induced skin damage is cumulative and irreversible. Repeated short exposures, even where there is no visible sunburn, can contribute to long-term skin damage.

The rising incidence of skin cancer in the United States has been attributed to a number of different factors. One is the depletion of the ozone layer that protects the earth from solar radiation.

Another major factor in the rising rate of skin cancer in the United States is lifestyle changes including more outdoor activities, more emphasis on tanning, scantier clothing, and a population shift to sunny climates, all of which result in greater exposure to the harmful rays of the Sun. Occupational exposure to coal tar, pitch, creosote, arsenic compounds, or radium are also risk factors for skin cancer.

Following are a number of steps that can be taken to decrease the risk of skin cancer:

- avoid, as much as possible, exposure to the sun when its ultraviolet rays are the strongest—between 10 A.M. and 3 P.M.
- if you are going to be exposed to the sun, use a sunscreen or sunblock; these are rated in strength by sun protection factor (SPF) from 2 to

15 or higher; the higher the number, the greater the protection
- wear protective clothing, such as sun hats, pants, and long sleeves, that can block out the Sun's harmful rays
- avoid the use of tanning devices.

It is particularly important to protect children from overexposure to the sun, as studies indicate that risk of skin cancer is related to the *cumulative* amount of sun exposure as well as the pigmentation of the skin. As much as 50% of a person's lifetime sun exposure occurs by the age of 18.

The American Cancer Society recommends skin self-examination by adults on a monthly basis. This entails checking all parts of the skin for new growth or other changes. The earlier skin cancer is detected the better the chance for a cure. The most common sign of skin cancer is a change on the skin, such as a growth or a sore that won't heal. Sometimes there may be a small lump. This lump can be smooth, shiny, and waxy looking, or it can be red or reddish brown. Skin cancer may also appear as a flat red spot that is rough or scaly.

Treatments used include surgery (electrocautery, cryosurgery, micrographic surgery, laser surgery), chemotherapy, and radiation therapy. These treatments can usually be performed in the doctor's office.

See also ABCD, ACTINIC KERATOSIS, and MELANOMA.

sleep disturbance   disruption of the sleeping pattern. In the United States as much as 25% of the population suffers from some degree of sleep disturbance. In the cancer population the percentage of people with sleep problems is significantly higher.

Insomnia, the inability to sleep, is the most common sleeping disorder among cancer patients. It can be a result of psychological factors relating to the cancer, such as anxiety and depression; side effects of the treatment, such as pain after surgery, nausea, vomiting; or a consequence of the cancer itself. The cancer can cause pain, fever, coughing, shortness of breath, and other symptoms that can make sleeping difficult. Hypnotic drugs can also cause insomnia. Hospitalization can also be a factor because of frequent interruptions of sleep for treatment, by hospital routines, roommates, and so on.

Getting insufficient sleep can be a serious problem for a cancer patient for a variety of reasons. A sleep disturbance can leave a patient irritable and unable to concentrate, which may in turn affect the patient's compliance with treatment requirements, ability to make decisions, and relations with family members, friends, and the medical staff. Depression and anxiety can also result from insufficient sleep. It is therefore very important that there is appropriate intervention to ensure that a patient with a sleep disorder gets help.

The first step in treating a person with a sleep disturbance is determining its cause or causes. Management of a sleep disorder generally involves a combination of different approaches and may include the following:

- alleviating or controlling symptoms of the cancer that are keeping the patient awake
- alleviating or controlling side effects of treatment
- modifying the environment by such methods as dimming or shutting off light, minimizing noise, or in the hospital, performing all the patient care tasks at the same time, whenever possible
- introducing RELAXATION TECHNIQUES and stress-reducing techniques to the patient and helping the patient learn how to cope with the stresses of the illness
- sleep medications.

Patients having difficulty sleeping should tell their doctor. Remedies are available.

slit lamp   a device used to examine the anterior parts of the eye including the cornea and iris. See EYE CANCER.

small cell carcinoma   See SMALL CELL LUNG CANCER.

small cell lung cancer (SCLC)   [oat cell lung cancer, small cell carcinoma, undifferentiated small cell lung cancer]   a disease in which cancer cells are found in the tissue of the lungs. Small cell lung cancer is characterized by cells that are small and round, or oval, or shaped like oat grains when seen microscopically. It is the most aggressive of all the different types of LUNG CANCER.

Small cell lung cancer is usually found in people who smoke or used to smoke. Other risk factors include exposure to certain industrial substances such as arsenic, certain organic chemicals, and ASBESTOS, particularly for smokers, and exposure to radiation from occupational, medical, and environmental sources, such as RADON. Radon in the home may increase the risk, especially for smokers. Passive smoke increases the risk for nonsmokers.

Small cell lung cancer frequently has no symptoms until it is fairly advanced. Symptoms that may be associated with it include a chronic cough, a change in pulmonary (lung) function, blood in the sputum, wheezing unrelated to asthma, repeated episodes of pneumonia, fever, weakness, weight loss, and chest pain. Other symptoms that may accompany more advanced disease include hoarseness, shortness of breath, enlargement of LYMPH NODES in the neck, shoulder and arm pain, difficulty swallowing, and drooping of the upper eyelids. There can also be symptoms in other parts of the body caused by lung cancer that has metastasized (spread). The MYASTHEMIC SYNDROME, a condition characterized by muscle weakness and other symptoms, occurs in about 6% of small cell lung cancer patients.

Procedures used in the diagnosis and evaluation of SCLC may include chest X-RAY, CT SCAN, MRI, BRONCHOSCOPY, MEDIASTINOSCOPY, THORACOTOMY, and a PERCUTANEOUS NEEDLE BIOPSY.

Following is the NATIONAL CANCER INSTITUTE'S (NCI) STAGING for small cell lung cancer:

- Limited—cancer is found in only one lung and nearby lymph nodes
- Extensive—cancer has spread outside the lung to other tissues in the chest or to other parts of the body
- Recurrent—the cancer has returned in the original site or in another part of the body after treatment.

Treatment depends on the stage of the disease, the general state of health of the patient, and other factors. In the 1970s, it was discovered that SCLC could, in some cases of early stage disease, be cured by CHEMOTHERAPY (anticancer drugs). Surgery may be used in an early stage cancer. However, in most cases surgery is of no value and is not recommended. EXTERNAL RADIATION THERAPY may also be used. CLINICAL TRIALS (are available) for all stages of small cell lung cancer. For specific information on the latest state-of-the-art treatment, by stage, call NCI's Cancer Information Service at 1-800-4-CANCER (1-800-422-6237), or for a TTY: 1-800-332-8615.

See also SMOKING.

small intestine cancer   a very rare cancer found in the tissue of the small intestine, a long multifolded tube in the abdomen that connects the stomach to the large intestine (bowel). According to the American Cancer Society, there were about 5,260 new cases of small intestine cancer in the US in 2004, and an estimated 1,130 deaths from the disease in the same year. It affects women and men equally.

A major risk factor is CROHN'S DISEASE, and people with Crohn's disease should be aware of possible signs of small intestine cancer. Although symptoms are not that common, there may be pain or cramps in the abdomen, weight loss, a lump in the abdomen, or blood in the stool. (These can be symptoms of many other disorders, and a doctor should be consulted if they persist.) Procedures used in the diagnosis of small intestine cancer may include an UPPER GI SERIES, CT SCAN, MRI, ULTRASOUND, GASTROSCOPY, and BIOPSY.

Small intestine cancer is classified by cell type. Following are the four types of small intestine cancer:

- adenocarcinoma—starts in the lining of the small intestine and is the most common type of cancer in the small intestine; the tumors occur most often in the part of the small intestine nearest the stomach; they often grow and block the bowel
- carcinoid tumor—a slow-growing tumor that secretes hormones; can cause circulatory and digestive problems (see also GASTROINTESTINAL CARCINOID TUMOR)
- lymphoma—starts from lymph tissue in the small intestine (see also NON-HODGKIN'S LYMPHOMA)
- leiomyosarcoma—starts growing in the smooth muscle lining of the small intestine (see also SOFT-TISSUE SARCOMA).

Treatment depends on the extent of the disease and the cell type. The three treatments that may be used are surgery, radiation, and chemotherapy. For specific information on the latest state-of-the-art treatment, call the National Cancer Institute's Cancer Information Service at 1-800-4-CANCER (1-800-422-6237), or for a TTY: 1-800-332-8615.

smokeless tobacco   tobacco that is chewed or held in the cheeks or lower lip; or snuff, made from powdered or finely cut tobacco leaves and held between the lip or cheek and the gum. Although snuff can be inhaled, it is rarely used that way in the United States. The most dangerous and addictive form is called "dipping snuff," tobacco that has been processed into a coarse, moist powder. It is placed between the cheek and gum, enabling the absorption of nicotine and carcinogens comparable to the level of cigarettes. More than 2,500 chemical compounds have been identified in processed tobacco—among them, three classes of carcinogens: N-nitrosamines, polynuclear aromatic hydrocarbons, and the alpha-emitting polonium.

Smokeless tobacco was used in the American colonies in the early 1600s. Its use was widespread until the end of the 19th century, when it was stymied by antispitting laws and the growing popularity of cigarettes. Smokeless tobacco now appears to be making a comeback. Sales are up, and there are reports that smokeless tobacco—mostly snuff—is being used by young people, predominantly teenage boys.

Smokeless tobacco has been linked to MOUTH CANCER. In its 1986 report, the advisory committee to the U.S. surgeon general concluded that the use of smokeless tobacco poses a significant health hazard, that it can cause cancer and a number of noncancerous oral conditions; and that it can result in nicotine addiction and dependence.

See also SMOKING.

smoking   a major cause of LUNG CANCER, as well as other cancers and diseases. Smoking is considered the single largest unnecessary and preventable cause of disease and early death in the United States.

It is believed that the tobacco plant may date back 7,000 years, originating somewhere between North and South America. Native Americans may have been the first people to smoke, chew, or snuff tobacco and introduced it to European explorers. In the 17th and 18th centuries it increased in popularity. In 1761 John Hill, a physician in London, reported an association between snuff and cancer of the nose. Thirty years later a doctor in Germany reported on a relationship between tobacco use and lip cancer. However, it was not until the 20th century that researchers started seriously investigating the use of tobacco—and its consequences. Studies conducted by scientists in different countries began appearing in different medical journals describing the relationship between cigarette smoking and cancer and other diseases.

The first study in the United States citing conclusive evidence of the association between cigarette smoking and lung cancer was published in 1950. In 1964, the U.S. surgeon general's landmark report *The Health Consequences of Smoking* was released which showed a strong causal relationship between smoking and lung cancer. Since that time researchers have sought and obtained corroborative evidence, from many different sources, that cigarette smoking leads to early death. There are now thousands of studies that detail the many different and severe consequences of smoking. The only organization that maintains that there is no definitive proof of the hazards of smoking is the Tobacco Institute, created and funded by the tobacco industry to lobby and coordinate its public relations.

Research has also been done on the effect of tobacco smoke on nonsmokers. Evidence of its harmful potential is mounting. According to the National Cancer Institute, nonsmokers who live with a smoker are at an increased risk of developing lung cancer. Epidemiological studies indicate that the risk for lung cancer in nonsmokers increases 30% if they are married to a smoker; the risk increases to 70% if the spouse is a heavy smoker. Involuntary smoking may be particularly harmful for specific population groups, such as children. In 1990 the Environmental Protection Agency concluded that secondhand, passive, or involuntary smoking causes over 3,000 lung cancer deaths a year as well as a substantial number of other respiratory illnesses and deaths among the children of smokers. The unborn children of women who smoke, a very special group of passive smokers, weigh less at birth and are at a greater risk for spontaneous abortion, fetal death, and sudden infant death syndrome. Passive smoking also has some non-life-threatening but very annoying side effects, including burning, itching, and tearing eyes, headaches, coughing, irritation of the nose and throat, allergic reactions, and annoyance from the smell.

Smoking is responsible for about 415,000 (nearly one in five) deaths a year in the United States. The American Cancer Society estimates that cigarette smoking is responsible for 85% of the lung cancer deaths among men in the United States, and 75% of the lung cancer deaths among women. The American Cancer Society estimated there would be about 172,570 new cases of lung cancer (93,010 among men and 79,560 among women), with an estimated 163,510 deaths from the disease (90,490 among men and 73,020 among women) in 2005, accounting for around 28% of all cancer deaths. New diagnoses of lung cancer accounts for about 13% of all new cancers. Lung cancer mainly occurs in the elderly. The average age of people diagnosed with lung cancer is 70; fewer than 3% of all cases are found in people under the age of 45. The chance that a man will develop lung cancer is one in 13 and for a woman, it is one in 18. (Note that this figure includes all people and does not take into account whether or not they smoke.)

Lung cancer is the leading cause of cancer death among both men and women. More people die of lung cancer than of colon, breast, and prostate cancers combined. In spite of the large number of people diagnosed with this cancer, as of 2005 there were only about 330,000 long-term survivors.

Smoking is also associated with cancers of the mouth, pharynx, larynx, esophagus, pancreas, cervix, kidney, breast, and bladder. Smoking is a major cause of heart disease and is associated with conditions ranging from colds and gastric ulcers to chronic bronchitis, emphysema, and cerebrovascular disease.

More than 2,500 chemical compounds have been identified in processed tobacco—among them, three classes of carcinogens: N-nitrosamines, polynuclear aromatic hydrocarbons, and the alpha-emitting polonium.

More than 4,000 different chemicals have also been identified in tobacco smoke. Smoke consists of two parts—gas or vapor and particulate or tar. Following are some of the harmful chemicals that have been identified in cigarette smoke, in the surgeon general's reports:

- Gas
  Major toxic agents include:
  — nitrosamines (eight compounds)
  — nitrogen oxides
  — hydrogen cyanide
  — formaldehyde
  — vinyl chloride
  — ammonia
  — carbon monoxide
  — plus eight other agents
- Particulate "Tar"
  Known tumor-causing agents include:
  — benzo(a)pyrene
  — urethane
  — cadmium compounds
  — nickel compounds
  — polonium-210, a radioactive element
  — phenol
  — plus 42 other agents

In 1988, the surgeon general released a report on nicotine addiction. It concluded that cigarettes and other forms of tobacco are addictive, that nicotine is the drug that causes addiction, and that cigarette addiction is similar to the addiction to such drugs as heroin and cocaine.

In 1989, the surgeon general's report found that the prevalence of smoking in the United States decreased from 40% in 1965 to 29% in 1987. From 1976 to 1987 adult male smokers dropped from 42% of the population to 32%, while women dropped from 32% to 27%. It is estimated that as of 1990 there were 38 million ex-smokers and 50 million smokers. Smoking rates are higher among blacks, blue-collar workers, and less-educated people. Children are starting to smoke at earlier ages. In the United States, more than 3,000 teenagers become regular smokers every day.

In 1990, the surgeon general released a report showing that people who quit smoking, regardless of age, live longer than people who continue to smoke. Fifteen to 20 years after quitting, the risk of lung cancer is about the same as a person who never smoked.

smoldering leukemia a form of acute myelocytic leukemia. It begins slowly and, it is believed, involves abnormal changes in more than one type of cell. Smoldering leukemia may eventually become acute nonlymphocytic leukemia.

SNFB See STEREOTACTIC BIOPSY.

snuff See SMOKELESS TOBACCO.

social worker a professional at a hospital or medical center trained to help a patient and his or her family cope with the emotional and practical problems that cancer can present. They can help locate various support resources such as financial aid, transportation for treatment, support groups, and help at home. The social worker can also help a patient sort out, understand, and clarify treatment options.

soft palate (pal'at) the soft part at the back of the roof of the mouth.

soft palate cancer (pal'at) See OROPHARYNGEAL CANCER.

soft-tissue osteosarcoma (os"te-o"sar-ko'mah) a very rare form of OSTEOSARCOMA that occurs most often in the soft tissue.

soft-tissue radiography See XEROGRAPHY.

soft-tissue sarcoma/adult cancer of the tissue that supports, connects, and surrounds other structures and organs in the body, including the muscles, tendons, fat, blood vessels, nerves, fibrous tissues, and synovial tissues (tissues around joints). Soft-tissue sarcomas are relatively rare; according to the American Cancer Society, in 2005 there would be about 9,420 new cases of soft-tissue sarcomas diagnosed in the United States (4,530 cases in males, and 3,890 in females), with some 3,490 (1,910 males and 1,580 females) deaths from the disease in the same year. These statistics include both adults and children. Soft-tissue sarcomas account for less than half of 1% of all new cancer cases.

Soft-tissue sarcomas can develop in virtually any part of the body. About 40% occur in the knee area; 30% arise in the trunk, 15% in the arms and hands, and 15% in the head and neck. Following is a table of the different types of sarcomas in adults—where

ADULT SOFT-TISSUE SARCOMAS

Tissue of Origin	Type of Cancer	Location in the Body
Fibrous tissue	Fibrosarcoma	Arms, legs, trunk
	Malignant fibrous histiocytoma	Legs
Fat	Liposarcoma	Arms, legs, trunk
Muscle		
striated	Rhabdomyosarcoma	Arms, legs
smooth	Leiomyosarcoma	Uterus, digestive tract
Blood vessels	Hemangiosarcoma	Arms, legs, trunk
	Kaposi's sarcoma	Legs, trunk
Lymph vessels	Lymphangiosarcoma	Arms
Synovial tissue (linings of joint cavities, tendon sheaths)	Synovial sarcoma (also called synovioma)	Legs
Peripheral nerves	Neurofibrosarcoma	Arms, legs, trunk
Cartilage and bone-forming tissue	Chondrosarcoma	Legs

Courtesy U.S. Department of Health and Human Services.

they arise, what they are called, and the usual location in the body.

A FIBROSARCOMA occurs most frequently in men in their mid-40s to early 50s. It is often located deep in the thigh and tends to be large when diagnosed. A MALIGNANT FIBROUS HISTIOCYTOMA occurs most frequently in men in their 50s and 60s. A LIPOSARCOMA is usually found in middle-aged men. A RHABDOMYOSARCOMA is equally common in men and women in their 40s and 50s. It tends to be large when discovered. LEIOMYOSARCOMAS, which are very rare, develop in muscles that control organs.

Risk factors include exposure to phenoxyacetic acids in herbicides; chlorphenols in wood preservatives; vinyl chloride, a substance used in the manufacture of plastics; and high levels of radiation for a variety of noncancerous medical problems. Certain viruses have been shown to cause sarcomas in animals, but there is no evidence that they cause cancer in humans. A RETROVIRUS may play a role in the development of KAPOSI'S SARCOMA when it occurs in AIDS patients.

Soft-tissue sarcomas rarely have symptoms in early stages. Tumors can grow fairly large before they can be felt or cause problems. Generally, a biopsy is performed to diagnose soft tissue sarcoma. Other procedures that may be used in the diagnosis and evaluation include XEROGRAPHY, CT SCAN, MRI, ULTRASOUND, and ARTERIOGRAPHY.

Following is the NATIONAL CANCER INSTITUTE'S (NCI) STAGING for adult soft-tissue sarcoma:

- Stage I—cancer cells look very much like normal cells; the cancer can be less than five CENTIMETERS (cm) or more than 5 cm but has not spread to LYMPH NODES or other parts of the body
- Stage II—cancer cells look somewhat different from normal cells; the cancer can be less than 5 cm or more than 5 cm with no spread to the lymph nodes or other parts of the body
- Stage III—cancer cells look different from normal cells; the cancer can be less than 5 cm or larger than 5 cm but has not spread to lymph nodes or other parts of the body
- Stage IV
  IVA—the cancer has spread to the lymph nodes in the area but has not spread to other parts of the body
  IVB—the cancer has spread to other parts of the body such as the lungs
- Recurrent—the cancer has returned to the same site or to another part of the body after treatment.

Treatment depends on the stage of the disease, the general state of health of the patient, and other factors. Surgery is the most common treatment for soft-tissue sarcoma. RADIATION THERAPY and CHEMOTHERAPY may also be used to shrink the cancer so it can be removed without an amputation. For specific information on the latest state-of-the-art treatment, by stage, call NCI's Cancer Information Service at 1-800-4-CANCER (1-800-422-6237), or for a TTY: 1-800-332-8615.

See also SARCOMA and BONE CANCER.

soft-tissue sarcoma/childhood an extremely rare cancer in children, accounting for about 6% of all childhood cancers. It can occur in the same places in the body as adult soft-tissue sarcomas.

The most common form of childhood soft-tissue sarcoma is RHABDOMYOSARCOMA. There are fewer than five new cases for every 1 million children every year in the United States.

Very little is known about the cause of soft-tissue sarcomas in children. Some children seem to be born with them. The cancer occasionally develops after a child has received RADIATION THERAPY for another cancer. The first noticeable sign of this cancer may be a painless lump or mass. Parents or the doctor frequently notice the lump before the child does. A tumor in the genitourinary tract may cause frequent urination, urine retention, or blood in the urine.

Generally, a biopsy is performed to diagnosis soft tissue sarcoma. Other procedures that may be performed in the diagnosis and evaluation include a BONE SCAN, BONE MARROW BIOPSY, SPINAL TAP, XEROGRAPHY, CT SCAN, MRI, ULTRASOUND, and an ANGIOGRAPHY.

Following is the NATIONAL CANCER INSTITUTE'S (NCI) STAGING for soft-tissue sarcoma in children.

- Group I—small tumors completely removed by surgery; tissue removed includes a margin of noncancerous tissue around the tumor; there is no sign of spread to LYMPH NODES or other tissue
- Group II
  IIA—tumors are surgically removed; there is microscopic evidence that sarcoma cells are left in surrounding tissue
  IIB—cancer has spread to regional LYMPH NODES; the tumor and all affected lymph nodes are surgically removed with no evidence that cancer cells remain in the area
  IIC—cancer has spread to regional lymph nodes; there is microscopic evidence that sarcoma cells are left in surrounding tissue
- Group III—tumor not completely removed by surgery; remaining cancerous tissue can be seen without a microscope
- Group IV—the cancer has spread to other parts of the body
- Recurrent—the cancer has returned to the same site or to another part of the body after treatment

CHILDHOOD SOFT-TISSUE SARCOMAS

Tissue of Origin	Type of Cancer	Location in Body	Age
Fibrous tissue	Fibrosarcoma	Arms, legs	Infant–2
Fat	Liposarcoma	Arms, legs	10–15
Muscle striated	Rhabdomyo-sarcoma	Head, neck, genitourinary tract	2–6
		Arms, legs, trunk, genitourinary tract	14–18
smooth	Leiomyo-sarcoma	Trunk	*
Blood vessels	Infant Hemangio-pericytoma	Head, neck, arms, legs, trunk	Infant–1
Synovial tissue (linings of joint cavities, tendon sheaths)	Synovial sarcoma	Legs, arms, trunk	Infant–14
Peripheral nerves	Neurofibro-sarcoma	Arms, legs, trunk	*
Muscular nerve	Alveolar soft part sarcoma	Legs, arms	Infant–10

*no age range established

Courtesy U.S. Department of Health and Human Services.

For information on treatment see SOFT TISSUE SARCOMA/ADULT.

solar keratosis   See ACTINIC KERATOSIS.

solar radiation   See ULTRAVIOLET RADIATION.

solid tumor   long-standing jargon that distinguishes cancer arising from organs other than BONE MARROW. Since LEUKEMIA or "liquid" cancer was initially successfully treated with CHEMOTHERAPY, early pioneering use of these agents against other cancers (lung, breast, colon, etc.) gave rise to a term to distinguish efficacy. Many early cancer hospitals were organized into different services (e.g. "leukemia" v. "solid tumor")

sonogram   See ULTRASOUND.

Serafenib   See BAY43-9006.

speculum   (spek'u-lum)   an instrument used to widen the opening of the vagina so that the cervix can be seen more easily. It is used for the PAP SMEAR and other examinations.

sperm banking   the freezing of sperm, male fertilizing cells, for use at a later date. The first sperm bank in the United States was started in 1950 at the University of Iowa. The first birth of a child conceived from stored sperm was in 1953. Sperm banking may be used by men who face possible infertility as a result of treatment for TESTICULAR CANCER, PROSTATE CANCER, or CHEMOTHERAPY or other disorders.

SPF   See S-PHASE FRACTION.

SPF (sun protection factor)   a number that indicates the effectiveness of a sunscreen that blocks the ULTRAVIOLET RADIATION of the Sun, rays that can cause skin cancer. Sunscreens usually contain para-aminobenzoic acid (PABA) or related compounds. The higher the number, the greater the blockage of the radiation from the Sun. Following are the rating values of SPF:

- SPF 2 to 4—minimal protection, permits tanning; recommended for people who rarely burn and tan easily
- SPF 4 to 6—moderate protection, permits some tanning; recommended for people who tan well with minimal burning
- SPF 6 to 8—extra protection, permits limited tanning; recommended for people who tan gradually and burn moderately
- SPF 8 to 14—maximum protection, permits little or no tanning; recommended for those who always burn easily and tan minimally
- SPF 15 and higher—ultra protection, permits no tanning; recommended for people who always burn easily and never tan

Sunscreen should be applied about 30 minutes before exposure to the Sun. It should be reapplied at least every two hours or after swimming or perspiring heavily. Sunscreen should also be used on overcast days, because 80% of ultraviolet radiation can penetrate a cloudy haze. Sunscreen protection is needed in the winter as well. Snow, ice, sand, and concrete reflect from 10% to 50% of the damaging rays.

Research suggests that regular use of a sunscreen with an SPF of 15, during the first 18 years of life, could reduce the incidence of NONMELANOMA SKIN CANCER (BASAL AND SQUAMOUS CELL) by 78%.

S-phase fraction (SPF)   the percentage of cancer cells that are in a specific stage (the synthesis phase) of division in the CELL CYCLE. A high SPF number means that the cells are dividing rapidly and that the tumor is fast growing. A low SPF indicates that the tumor is indolent or slow growing. The S-phase fraction can be obtained through the relatively new procedure known as FLOW CYTOMETRY.

spinal anesthesia (an"es-the'ze-ah)   injection of an anesthetic into the spinal fluid. It is a type of LOCAL ANESTHESIA. It completely blocks sensation in the part of the body that is served by the nerves at the site of the injection into the spinal cord. It is most commonly used for surgery in the abdominal and pelvic area or procedures involving the lower extremities.

spinal cord   part of the CENTRAL NERVOUS SYSTEM, enclosed within the backbone, that transmits impulses to and from the brain.

spinal cord cancer   See BRAIN CANCER.

spinal puncture   See SPINAL TAP.

spinal tap [lumbar puncture (L.P.), spinal puncture]   removal of a small amount of the fluid that bathes the brain and spinal cord for microscopic examination for cancer cells or other conditions. A spinal tap may also be performed to administer anesthesia or medication.

The procedure can take 10 minutes to half an hour. It can be performed in a doctor's office or in the hospital. The patient lies on his or her side with knees drawn up and head tucked in, or sits on the edge of the bed or examination table, leaning over the bedside table. The patient is usually given a local anesthetic. A needle is then inserted, and fluid is removed.

A spinal tap is a relatively risk-free procedure. Some patients get a headache shortly after its completion, although the headache may occur several days later. A spinal tap may be performed in the diagnosis of BRAIN CANCER, BREAST CANCER, LEUKEMIA, and other cancers and in the diagnosis of METASTATIC CANCER.

spindle cell carcinoma of the lung   See SQUAMOUS CELL LUNG CANCER.

spine cancer   cancer that begins in the spinal columns (backbone) or spinal cord. The spinal column is made up of linked bones called vertebrae. The spinal cord is a column of nerve tissue that runs from the base of the skull down the back. It is surrounded by three protective membranes and is enclosed within the vertebrae. Many different types of cancer may form in the bones, tissue, fluid, or nerves of the spine. While PRIMARY TUMORS of the vertebrae (e.g., MULTIPLE MYELOMA) are uncommon, METASTASES to the spine are frequent. The spine is the most common site for skeletal metastases. At autopsy, 70% of patients who die from cancer demonstrate vertebral metastases, and more than 5% have evidence of metastatic compression of the spinal cord. Injury to the spinal cord and peripheral nerves is a recognized risk of therapeutic RADIATION that may not become manifest for many months, or even years. A transient RADIATION MYELOPATHY primarily involving sensory neurons may occur in 10% to 15% of patients receiving MANTLE RADIATION for HODGKIN'S DISEASE. This condition is usually associated only with sensory symptoms, such as paresthesias and Lhermitte's sign, and resolves in one to nine months. Delayed radiation myelopathy is an irreversible and progressive neurologic condition that may affect motor, sensory, and sphincter functions and has a reported incidence of 1% to 12%.

spiral CT scan   a thin slice, high-resolution version of CT SCAN most useful in evaluating the lung. It is being evaluated as a screening test for LUNG CANCER compared with evaluation by a chest X-RAY. A large, national CLINICAL TRIAL of the spiral

CT scan was completed in 2004 to determine its diagnostic effectiveness in lung cancer, but (at press time) there were no results available.

spirometry (spi-rom'ĕ-tre) a test that measures the breathing efficiency of the lungs. It may be performed on a patient diagnosed with LUNG CANCER to find out how much lung tissue can be safely removed so that the patient can still have relatively normal activities and a good quality of life.

spleen an organ located in the upper part of the abdomen, on the left side. It manufactures, stores, and destroys blood cells. It is an important center for IMMUNE SYSTEM activity.

spleen cancer See HODGKIN'S DISEASE.

splenectomy (sple-nek'to-me) surgical removal of the spleen. This may be performed in the treatment of LYMPHOMA or LEUKEMIA when the spleen enlarges and destroys large numbers of normal blood cells. In the very rare instances that there is cancer in the spleen itself, a splenectomy may be performed. Removal of the spleen does not interfere with normal living. Its normal functions are taken over by other components of the body.

splenomegaly enlargement of the SPLEEN.

spontaneous tumor regression or remission the shrinking or disappearance of a cancerous tumor in an untreated patient for no apparent reason. However, it is not unusual for the tumor to reappear or grow larger.

sporadic a term applied to forms of common cancers not at present known to be associated with a specific familial cause. The term *wild type* is used also. Most of these cancers are thought to be due to acquired genetic instability (mutation).

sporadic intestinal polyps (pol'ips) small, non-cancerous growths that occur in the intestine, most frequently in the rectum and colon, and are not inherited. They may become cancerous if they grow larger than an inch in diameter. The three main kinds are ADENOMATOUS POLYPS (tubular), VILLOUS POLYPS, and INTERMEDIATE POLYPS (tubulovillous). Sporadic intestinal polyps usually do not cause symptoms, but they can cause intermittent bleeding and obstruction of the passage of waste material if they are large enough.

sporadic medullary cancer (med'u-lār"e) an extremely rare cancer of the thyroid. It is likely to occur in only one lobe of the thyroid. It tends to spread to nearby lymph nodes in the neck first. It is the only THYROID CANCER that can be diagnosed by measuring the amount of CALCITONIN in the blood.
See also MEDULLARY CARCINOMA OF THE THYROID.

sputum (spu'tum) material composed of saliva, mucus, cells, and other matter emitted from the lungs, throat, or mouth through spitting.

sputum cytology exam (spu'tum si-tol'o-je) [pulmonary cytology] microscopic examination of the cells in the sputum, material discharged from the mouth, throat, or lungs. It may be performed in the diagnosis of lung cancer. The sputum coughed up by the patient may reveal abnormal cells too small to be seen in an X-RAY. If cancerous cells are found, further tests are performed with an endoscope (a flexible instrument with a lighted tube and viewing system) to locate the cancer. Sputum cytology can provide a definitive diagnosis in as many as 90% of the cases, including patients with microscopic or occult cancer who have normal X-rays. Sputum cytology may also be helpful in the detection of HEAD AND NECK CANCERS.
See also SCREENING.

squamous cell (skwa'mus) a type of cell that is found on the surface of the skin, the lining of hollow organs, and all passages of the respiratory, digestive, and genitourinary system. They have a flattened, scale-like appearance.

squamous cell carcinoma (skwa'mus kar"sin-o'-mah) [epidermoid cell] a cancer containing squamous cells. Squamous cell carcinomas can be found in many parts of the body including the lungs, skin, esophagus, head and neck areas, and cervix.

squamous cell carcinoma of the skin (skwa'mus kar"sin-no'mah) [squamous cell skin cancer] after BASAL CELL CARCINOMA OF THE SKIN, the second most common type of SKIN CANCER. It generally arises in the uppermost layer of the skin. The appearance of squamous cell carcinoma is more varied than basal cell carcinoma. Squamous cell carcinoma also tends to grow more quickly and can, unlike basal cell, spread to other parts of the body, making it more dangerous than basal cell carcinoma.

The people at the greatest risk are those who:

- have fair complexions
- are over 55 years of age
- are male (two to three times more common in men than in women)
- have worked outdoors most of their lives (e.g., farmers, construction workers, sailors, gardeners)
- live in the South.

The main cause of squamous cell carcinoma is exposure to the ULTRAVIOLET RADIATION of the Sun. Other possible contributors to the development of squamous cell skin carcinoma include chronic ulcers, burns, constant friction, and prolonged contact with certain industrial chemicals.

Squamous cell carcinoma can appear on any part of the body exposed to the sun—most frequently the top of the nose, forehead, lower lip, and hands. It can also appear on areas of the skin that have been burned, exposed to chemicals, or had X-RAY therapy.

The major symptom of squamous cell carcinoma is any change in the skin. Squamous cell carcinoma can have many different appearances. It can start out as a small, smooth, shiny, pale, or waxy lump. It may appear as a firm red bump in the skin. The tumor may feel scaly or develop a crust.

Treatment depends on the size of the tumor, its location, and other factors. In general, the treatment is surgical removal of the cancer. Following is a brief description of the ways in which this can be done:

- electrodessication and curettage—the cancer is burned and removed with a sharp instrument
- cryosurgery—the cancer is killed by freezing it
- excision—the cancer is cut from the skin along with some healthy tissue around it
- micrographic surgery (MOHS' MICROGRAPHIC SURGERY)—the cancer is cut from the skin along

with some healthy tissue around it, after which the doctor uses a microscope to examine the area for any remaining cancer cells
- laser surgery—the cancer is removed by a narrow beam of intense light.

Other treatments for squamous cell carcinoma include RADIATION THERAPY and topical CHEMOTHERAPY applied to the site. Biological therapies are being investigated in clinical trials. For the latest state-of-the-art treatment, call the National Cancer Institute's Cancer Information Service at 1-800-4-CANCER (1-800-422-6237), or for a TTY: 1-800-332-8615.

See also SKIN CANCER, CRYOSURGERY, and LASER THERAPY.

squamous cell lung cancer (skwa′mus) [epidermoid, spindle-cell]   a cancer of the lung characterized by cells that are flat and scale-like. Worldwide, squamous cell carcinoma is the most common form of LUNG CANCER. However, in the United States adenocarcinoma of the lung has become more prevalent in some areas. Some reports indicate that squamous cell lung cancer has declined from 50% of all cases in the United States to 30% in the past 20 years. Squamous cell carcinoma often begins in the large bronchi (air passages) and tends to remain localized in the chest for longer periods of time than other types of lung cancer.

SSTN   See OCTREOTIDE.

stage   See STAGING.

staging [clinical staging of cancer]   a way to describe the extent of a cancer, using such characteristics as the size of the tumor, lymph node involvement, and where it has spread. Staging must be done in order to determine the proper treatment. It also is useful in predicting the course the disease will take and its PROGNOSIS. Systems of staging have been "custom designed" for specific cancers. Staging systems for different cancers have evolved over the years, changing as new information on a particular cancer site becomes available. Some staging systems bear the name of the person or persons who developed them, such as Dukes and Astler Coller, which are used to stage colon/rectal cancer.

Many staging systems use initials and are based on the size of the tumor (T), regional lymph node involvement (N), and metastatic involvement (M). (This is known as the TNM classification system.) The T is accompanied by a number from 1 to 4 for the size of the tumor, an X if the tumor cannot be assessed, 0 if there is no evidence of a primary tumor, or IS if the tumor is IN SITU. The larger the number, the larger the tumor. The N is accompanied by the numbers 1 to 4, which indicates whether the tumor has spread to the lymph nodes, the size of the nodes, and the number of nodes. The N may be followe by a 0 (regional lymph nodes are not involved) or X (regional lymph nodes cannot be assessed clinically). The letter M, for metastasis, is followed by 0 (there is no evidence of spread) or 1 (the cancer has metastasized). For example, a breast cancer staged as T3N0M1 would mean it is a large tumor (T3), there are no lymph nodes involved (N0), and the cancer has spread (M1). The numbers are frequently translated, especially for patients, into Stage I, or Stage II, and so on.

For some cancers there are several staging systems using different terms to describe the different stages. While that may seem confusing, they generally correspond to one another. For example, in bladder cancer, stage I, stage A, and T1N0M0 are the same thing—the cancer has spread into the inner lining of the bladder but has not spread to the muscular wall of the bladder. Cancers are staged in different ways to obtain as much precise information on the characteristics of that particular cancer, which is crucial to successful treatment. Usually staging is by number—the larger the number, the more advanced the disease. However, it may be simply called "localized" (confined to the primary site), "metastatic" (spread to other areas of the body), or "recurrent" (cancer that has returned to its original site or to another part of the body after treatment). Bone cancer is generally staged that way. Or, the staging may relate primarily to where the cancer is located, such as in brain cancer.

Depending on the cancer, it may be staged during its diagnosis; but usually additional tests are performed after diagnosis. As many different tests as necessary are used in the staging of cancer, including X-RAY, NUCLEAR SCANS, CT, MRI, ULTRA-SOUND, and BIOPSY. It can take several days to stage a cancer. It generally does not take longer than two weeks.

standard treatment a therapy or intervention used in the treatment of an illness. In the treatment of cancer, CLINICAL TRIALS are conducted to determine the effectiveness of a treatment. A standard treatment is one deemed to be the most effective treatment for a particular type and stage of cancer. There are frequently several standard treatments for a particular type and stage of the disease, which means none appears to be better than the others. When there is more than one standard treatment, the physician will generally decide which one he or she feels would be most effective for that particular person. However, when the physician feels that any of them would be just as effective, it is not unusual for the patient to be told available treatment options and then asked to make a choice of the treatment he or she prefers. Receiving the appropriate standard treatment, which is commonly referred to as state-of-the-art treatment, is crucial because it gives the patient his or her best chance of survival and recovery.

STAR [Study of Tamoxifen and Raloxifene] STAR is a CLINICAL TRIAL (study) sponsored by the NATIONAL CANCER INSTITUTE (NCI) and designed to see how the drug RALOXIFENE (EVISTA) compares with the drug TAMOXIFEN (NOLVADEX) in reducing the incidence of BREAST CANCER in women who are at an increased risk for developing the disease.

It follows the success of the BREAST CANCER PREVENTION TRIAL (BCPT), which showed that high-risk women taking the drug tamoxifen (Nolvadex) reduced their chance of developing breast cancer by 49% The STAR study got under way in 1999 and was scheduled to run for seven years at an estimated 400 sites across the United States and Canada. Women at increased risk for developing breast cancer who had gone through menopause and were at least 35 years old were eligible to participate in STAR. Participants in STAR were randomized (assigned by chance) to receive either tamoxifen or raloxifene.

state-of-the-art treatment when used in cancer, a term that refers to the best treatment currently available for a specific type and stage of cancer. Although the term "state of the art" implies a superior or more advanced treatment, it is virtually the same as STANDARD TREATMENT and is simply another way of saying it.

statin a class of drugs in widespread use as lipid-lowering agents. Statins block the endogenous synthesis of cholesterol and are effective as lipid-lowering agents. Cancer researchers noted that in laboratory studies of colon cancer cells, statins inhibit the growth of these cells. CLINICAL TRIALS suggest they may also reduce the risk of COLON CANCER. Currently, there is no consensus recommending the broad use of statins as chemo-protective agents

See CHEMO-PROTECTIVE.

statistically significant findings in a study believed to be valid because the results could not have occurred purely by chance.

stem cell a common progenitor cell found in bone marrow that at its most primitive state has the capacity to develop into a wide variety of cells. When the stem cells are stimulated by COLONY-STIMULATING FACTORS, they mature into RED BLOOD CELLS, WHITE BLOOD CELLS, and PLATELETS. Stem cells are responsible for generating all the blood cells that arise in the bone marrow and serve the entire body.

A relatively new technology is peripheral stem cell support. It is based on the finding that stem cells can be stimulated to leave the bone marrow and enter the PERIPHERAL blood circulation. Another source of stem cells is cord blood. When the stem cells are in the blood, they can be removed, stored, and then reinfused into the patient at the time of DOSE INTENSIFICATION CHEMOTHERAPY (very high, potentially lethal doses of anticancer drugs). This treatment is seen as an alternative to bone marrow transplantation.

stem cell harvest removal of blood from a patient who will be undergoing stem cell transplantation. Before removal, growth factors may be given to stimulate production of stem cells. After the blood is removed, the stem cells are separated from the blood through a process called apheresis. The stem cells may be purged (treated) to make sure they contain no cancer cells. They are then frozen and stored until they are reinfused into the patient as a rescue from what could be a lethal dose of chemotherapy and/or radiation. See BONE MARROW HARVEST and PERIPHERAL BLOOD STEM CELL TRANSPLANTATION.

stem cell inhibitor a substance that can stop the production of blood cells by stem cells in the BONE MARROW. Anticancer drugs kill cancer cells and normal cells. If too many normal white blood cells are destroyed, the body's immune system is compromised, and the administration of the drugs may be postponed.

stem cell transplantation See PERIPHERAL STEM CELL TRANSPLANTATION.

stereotactic biopsy (ster"e-o-tak'tik bi'op-se) [sometimes referred to as stereotaxy] the use of a scanning device to find a tumor site that is difficult to locate or see in order to obtain a tissue sample for examination for cancer cells. For example, in a brain biopsy (microscopic examination of tissue for cancer cells), the patient undergoes a CT SCAN with his or her head held firmly in a special device to minimize movement. The target, shown on the CT scan, is approached with a needle through a hole made in the skull. Tissue for a biopsy is removed by the needle. This procedure may also be used in breast biopsies.

stereotactic fine needle biopsy See STEREOTACTIC BIOPSY.

stereotactic radiosurgery (ster"e-o-tak'tik) [sometimes referred to as stereotaxy, Roentgen knife] a new procedure using high-energy X-RAYS to destroy deep-seated tumors and other lesions in the brain. While the head is held firmly in place by a specially designed device (a stereotactic headframe), a computer and scanning device (such as a CT or MRI) pinpoint the exact location of the tumor. A single dose of radiation can be directed to that precisely defined spot. At the same time, the exposure of normal

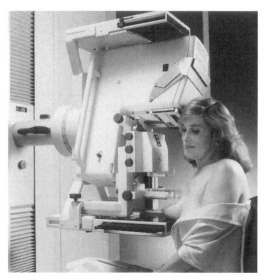

A woman undergoing a stereotactic breast biopsy. The Mammostat 2 pictured here is equipped with a special attachment for performing this type of biopsy. Courtesy Siemens Medical Systems, Inc.

brain cells to the radiation is decreased. The procedure avoids long and potentially dangerous brain surgery and weeks of hospitalization.

Stereotactic radiosurgery has most commonly been performed using a gamma knife, a dedicated and very costly device for stereotactic radiosurgery. In Sweden, gamma knife stereotactic radiosurgery has been performed since 1968. Its use in the United States started in 1987. Cyclotron units which produce charged particles, are also used as stereotactic radiosurgery tools. In 1989 the roentgen knife procedure was developed, combining several advanced medical technologies, including CT SCAN, the ANGIOGRAPHY, and the LINEAR ACCELERATOR. This procedure can be employed by designing a computer program using the existing technology, which makes it more cost effective than the gamma knife.

The role of stereotactic radiosurgery in the treatment of tumors in the brain is still being evaluated. It is currently used predominantly for small, benign (noncancerous) tumors and arteriovenous malformations (a potentially fatal condition). Its usefulness in the treatment of malignant (cancerous) tumors has yet to be determined.

stereotactic surgery (ster″e-o-tak′tik) [sometimes referred to as stereotaxic] a technique used to locate and remove lesions in the brain. The procedure is virtually the same as the STEREOTACTIC BIOPSY but is done as treatment rather than for diagnosis. As much of the tumor as possible is removed.

sternal tap   See BONE MARROW ASPIRATION.

sternotomy (ster-not′o-me) a surgical procedure in which the midline of the sternum (chestbone) is split. This may be performed in the diagnosis of LUNG CANCER. Some doctors feel they can see more easily where the cancer is located on either side of the chest.

steroids   a group of compounds, many of which are normally found in and distributed throughout the body. Many are HORMONES, affecting a variety of body functions. The body produces many different steroids, for example corticosteroids produced by the adrenal gland. Other natural or synthetic hormones used in the treatment of cancer include CORTISONE, hydrocortisone, PREDNISONE, methylprednisolone, and dexamethasone. When hormones are used for cancer treatment, the amount used is generally greater than would be found naturally in the body. Among the cancers that may be effectively treated by steroids are lymphomas, some leukemias, and some breast cancers.

Steroids may also be used in PALLIATIVE TREATMENT. In brain cancer, steroids may be used to reduce the swelling and buildup of fluid surrounding the tumor. The results can be dramatic—restoring speech, thought processes, and body movement. However, the effects of the steroids are often temporary, as the steroids do not slow the growth of the tumor. Steroids may also be given after brain surgery and radiation to suppress swelling. Steroids are sometimes used along with analgesics to relieve or reduce pain.

Side effects of steroids may include an increased appetite, mood changes, fluid retention, acne, increased blood pressure, elevated blood sugar, intestinal ulcers, and lowered resistance to infection.

See ADRENOCORTICOIDS.

stilbestrol diphosphate [diethylstilbestrol diphosphate]   See ESTROGEN.

stilphostrol [diethylstilbestrol diphosphate] See ESTROGEN.

stoma (sto'mah) an artificial opening in the abdominal wall made during surgery for the elimination of body wastes. It is not painful or sensitive to touch. It can be washed gently with mild soap and water. It may bleed slightly, for a short period of time, when it is washed. After the surgery the stoma may be swollen. Over time, usually three to six months, the stoma gets smaller, eventually reaching what is considered to be its "normal" size. Among the procedures that require a stoma are COLOSTOMY, ILEOSTOMY, and OSTOMY. These procedures may be performed in the treatment of COLON/RECTAL CANCER, BLADDER CANCER, and other disorders.

stomach a J-shaped muscular sac located between the ESOPHAGUS and small intestine. The stomach prepares food mechanically and chemically so that it can move into the INTESTINES for further digestion and absorption into the body.

stomach cancer [gastric cancer, gastric carcinoma] cancer of the stomach, the organ in the body located between the end of the esophagus and the beginning of the small intestine, where the digestion of food begins. Stomach cancer used to be fairly prevalent in the United States. The incidence of stomach cancer has been declining. In 1930, there were 33 cases per 1,000, and stomach cancer was the leading cause of death in men. The American Cancer Society estimated that 21,860 Americans (13,510 men and 8,350 women) would be diagnosed with stomach cancer during 2005, with some 11,550 (6,770 men and 4,780 women) deaths from the disease in the same year. This is a disease that mostly affects older people, occurring most often in people between the ages of 50 and 60. Two-thirds of people diagnosed with stomach cancer are older than 65. The risk of developing stomach cancer in a person's lifetime is about one in 100.

Stomach cancer is much more common worldwide, particularly in less developed countries. It is the second-leading cause of cancer deaths in the world, with approximately 700,000 deaths in 2002. Nonwhites develop it twice as often as whites. Men are more likely to develop stomach cancer than women.

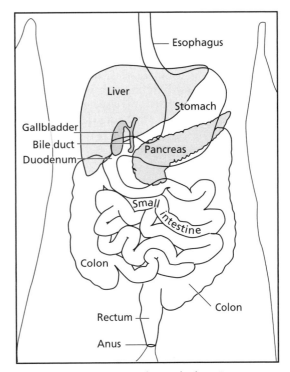

The esophagus, stomach, and digestive system. Courtesy NCI.

Populations at a higher-than-normal risk of developing stomach cancer often use chemicals, such as NITRATE, as food preservatives. There are a number of studies that suggest an association between compounds containing nitrogen and the development of stomach cancer. The availability of refrigeration, which has decreased the need for food preservatives, is thought to be a factor in the decreasing occurrence of stomach cancer in the United States. There have been a few reports of stomach cancer in several first-degree family members, suggesting that genetics may play a role in some stomach cancers.

The role of infection with *H. pylori* (*Helicobacter pylori*, which are bacteria found in the lining of the stomach) has been investigated over the past 10 years.

The major type of stomach cancer is an ADENOCARCINOMA, arising in glandular tissue. Adenocarcinomas account for 97% of the stomach cancers in the United States. They are frequently classified as either intestinal or diffuse. In intestinal stomach cancer, the cells are large and attach to one another to form well-defined, tubular structures. It is similar to cancers that develop in the intestinal organs. In diffuse stomach cancer, clusters of small cells infiltrate the lining of the stomach without a well-defined border. This type is generally found in younger people and in equal numbers of men and women.

Other types of extremely rare tumors that may occur in the stomach include adenoacanthomas, SQUAMOUS CELL CARCINOMAS, LYMPHOMAS, SMALL CELL CARCINOMAS, CARCINOID TUMORS, and KAPOSI'S SARCOMA. Combined, these account for less than 1% of stomach cancers. LEIOMYOSARCOMA develops in the muscle tissue and accounts for 2% of stomach cancer (see SOFT-TISSUE SARCOMA).

The cause of stomach cancer is not fully known. Studies show that there may be a number of factors involved, including environmental factors, socioeconomic status, heredity, certain noncancerous stomach conditions, a history of previous stomach surgery, as well as other factors. Noncancerous conditions that may contribute to the development of stomach cancer include PERNICIOUS ANEMIA, CHRONIC ATROPHIC GASTRITIS, INTESTINAL METAPLASIA, and GASTRIC POLYPS.

Frequently there are no significant symptoms of stomach cancer until the tumor is fairly large, making early detection difficult. The first symptoms are very much like many other stomach problems—persistent indigestion, a feeling of bloated discomfort after eating, slight nausea, loss of appetite, heartburn, and sometimes mild stomach pain. When the disease is more advanced, there may be blood in the stool (either red or black in color), vomiting, weight loss, and pain. Procedures used in the diagnosis of cancer may include tests of the blood, stool, and stomach fluid (anemia and a lack of acid in the stomach can be indications of stomach cancer), an upper GI SERIES, a GASTROSCOPY, and BIOPSY.

Following is the NATIONAL CANCER INSTITUTE'S (NCI) staging for adenocarcinoma stomach cancer:

- Stage 0—cancer has not spread below the limiting membrane of the top layer of tissue
- Stage I—cancer is confined to the stomach wall and LYMPH NODES very close to the tumor

- Stage II—cancer is confined to the entire stomach wall but does not involve adjacent tissue; lymph nodes close to the tumor or in the region around the stomach may be involved
- Stage III—tissue next to the stomach and/or lymph nodes close to the tumor or in the region around the stomach is involved
- Stage IV—cancer has spread to adjacent tissue and to lymph nodes in the region around the stomach or to distant sites (most commonly to the liver or other organs)
- Recurrent—cancer has returned to the original site or to another location after treatment.

Treatment depends on the stage of the disease, the general state of health of the patient, and other factors. Surgery is the only treatment that offers a potential cure when it is performed on a person with very early stage cancer. (Because it is not a vital organ, the entire stomach can be removed.) Other treatment options include RADIATION THERAPY (either before, during, or after surgery), CHEMOTHERAPY, and CLINICAL TRIALS. For specific information on the latest state-of- the-art treatment, by stage, call NCI's Cancer Information Service at 1-800-4-CANCER (1-800-422-6237), or for a TTY: 1-800-332-8615.

stomal therapist (sto'mal) [enterostomal therapist]   a health care specialist (frequently a nurse) trained to help a patient in the use and care of a COLOSTOMY or other STOMA.

stomatitis (sto-mah-ti'tis) [mucostitis, mouth sores] inflammation of the soft tissues in the mouth resulting in mouth sores. Stomatitis can produce a variety of unpleasant symptoms, including dryness of the lips or mouth, a mild burning sensation, soreness, swelling, redness, less saliva, and a change in taste. It is a not uncommon side effect of CHEMOTHERAPY (anticancer drugs), RADIATION THERAPY, and some BIOLOGICAL THERAPIES such as INTERLEUKIN-2. This can be a dangerous condition. A cancer patient who is unable to eat may become malnourished, further weakened, and more susceptible to infections. It is therefore important that this condition be treated. Medication can be taken to reduce the pain while the lining of the mouth heals. Following are some self-help steps patients can take:

- avoid food and juices with a high acid content such as tomato, orange, and grapefruit; apricots, pear nectars, squash, beans, and peas are food that will not sting or burn
- avoid hot or spicy foods
- avoid salty foods such as potato chips, pretzels, and crackers
- avoid carbonated beverages
- eat soft, unseasoned foods such as soft-boiled eggs and oatmeal
- keep mouth and gums clean to prevent infections (rinse or brush teeth within 30 minutes after eating)
- use a soft toothbrush or sponge and a gentle touch
- use a mouth rinse with one teaspoon of baking soda in one cup of warm water; hold rinse in mouth for about a minute
- avoid toothpaste and mouthwash products containing a large amount of salt or alcohol
- for dry lips use lip balm

stool blood test   See OCCULT BLOOD STOOL TEST.

stool guaiac test   See OCCULT BLOOD STOOL TEST.

streptozocin (strep"to-zo'sin) [streptozotocin, Zanosar] an ALKYLATING anticancer drug sometimes used in the treatment of cancers of the pancreas, liver, and colon and HODGKIN'S DISEASE. It is given by IV (injection into a vein). Common side effects include kidney damage, nausea, vomiting, local pain, liver problems, and second malignancies.

streptozotocin   See STREPTOZOCIN.

stress a physical or emotional factor that causes tension in the mind and/or body. Although there have been theories that stress may increase a person's risk of cancer, there has been no convincing evidence that an association exists between stress and cancer. Animal studies have shown that stress can both *stimulate* and *suppress* the IMMUNE SYSTEM. Humans may, in fact, react in the same way. However, it has not been shown that stress-induced changes in the immune system can increase anyone's risk of developing cancer. Researchers continue to investigate the possibility that stress does play a role in cancer. Stress may accompany the diagnosis and treatment of cancer.

See also RELAXATION TECHNIQUES.

stress reduction   See RELAXATION TECHNIQUES.

stromal tumor   See OVARIAN GERM CELL TUMOR.

Sturge-Webber syndrome one of a number of inherited disorders that puts a person at a greater risk of developing KIDNEY CANCER.

subcutaneous (sub"ku-ta'ne-us) a term used to describe medical procedures performed under the skin.

subcutaneous mastectomy (sub"ku-ta'ne-us mas-tek'to-me) removal of the inner breast tissue through an incision under the breast. The breast skin and nipple are left intact. It is primarily performed as a preventive procedure for women who are at a high risk of developing BREAST CANCER. Many physicians are opposed to prophylactic breast removal and instead favor regular and frequent follow-up, as often as every three months, with women who are at a greater risk. Women considering a preventive mastectomy are often advised to seek counseling first. When a subcutaneous mastectomy is done for preventive reasons, the tissue that is removed is examined for cancer. If cancer is found, the remaining skin and nipple are removed. If cancer is not found, a SILICONE IMPLANT may be inserted. Subcutaneous mastectomy is not a satisfactory prophylactic operation because of the danger of residual small amounts of breast tissue in the skin and nipple.

A subcutaneous mastectomy may also be performed in the treatment of breast cancer in its earliest stage, in situ. Most breast surgeons consider a subcutaneous mastectomy an inadequate treatment for any breast cancer because of the risk of leaving cancer cells behind.

See also MASTECTOMY.

subtotal hysterectomy (his-tĕ-rek'to-me) [supracervical hysterectomy] removal of the uterus, with the rest of the female reproductive organs left in place. This may be performed in some cancers of the female organs. Although a woman would not be able to bear children, normal sexual relations are not affected.

subtotal thyroidectomy (thi"roi-dek'to-me) surgical removal of parts of both lobes of the thyroid and of the tissue over the windpipe connecting the two lobes; or removal of a whole lobe and part of the other. A subtotal thyroidectomy may be performed in the treatment of THYROID CANCER.

suction biopsy   See NEEDLE ASPIRATION BIOPSY.

sun protection factor   See SPF.

sunblock   an opaque substance that may be used as a protection from the sun. A sunblock is stronger than a SUNSCREEN because it blocks out all the rays of the Sun, not just the redness-producing rays. Sunblocks usually are thick and white and frequently contain zinc oxide. They are graded according to their SPF, or sun protection factor.

sunlamp   See TANNING BOOTH.

sunscreen   a substance that blocks out redness-producing rays from the Sun. Sunscreens come in different strengths, described as the amount of sun protection factor, or SPF. They do not provide as complete protection as a SUNBLOCK.

superficial spreading melanoma   (mel″ah-no′mah) one of four types of MELANOMA skin cancer. It can start from a preexisting mole or a new growth.

superfractionated radiation therapy   (su″per-frak″shun-a′ted)   administering a dose of RADIATION THERAPY three or more times during the day. The combined doses add up to a greater dose than would be given if only one dose was administered. This decreases the number of days it takes to administer the total dose. This method is being evaluated in clinical trials.

superior sulcus tumor   See PANCOAST TUMOR.

superior vena caval syndrome (SVCS)   obstruction of the blood flow in the superior vena cava, a large vein that empties into the heart. SVCS occurs when there is compression of the blood flow returning to the heart in the superior vena cava. It can be a potentially life-threatening complication of some cancers, mostly SMALL CELL LUNG CANCER and NON-HODGKIN'S LYMPHOMA, as well as other disorders. Its occurrence and diagnosis may result in the diagnosis of cancer in another part of the body.

SVCS can cause a variety of symptoms, including pain when breathing or shortness of breath and a sensation of fullness in the head or facial swelling. Other, less common symptoms include arm swelling, chest pain, cough, and a difficulty or pain in swallowing.

Diagnosis of SVCS may include the use of X-RAYS, CT SCANS, VENOGRAPHY, SPUTUM CYTOLOGY EXAM, THORACENTESIS, BONE MARROW BIOPSY, LYMPH NODE BIOPSY, BRONCHOSCOPY, MEDIASTINOSCOPY, and THORACOTOMY. The goal of treatment in SVCS is usually twofold—relief of the symptoms and an attempt to cure the primary cancer that caused it. The PROGNOSIS of a patient with SVCS correlates strongly with the prognosis of the disease that caused it.

supportive psychotheraphy   a way of treating psychological problems without delving into the unconscious. In cancer patients, its goal is to reassure and encourage the patient in trying to help him or her deal as successfully as possible with the cancer, its side effects, and the emotions it has evoked. Supportive psychotherapy is not confrontational.

supportive treatment   See PALLIATIVE TREATMENT.

supracervical hysterectomy   See SUBTOTAL HYSTERECTOMY.

supraglottic laryngectomy   (su″prah-glot′ik lar″in-jek′to-me)   surgical removal of the tissue in the area above the vocal cords. This is one of the surgical procedures that may be performed in the treatment of LARYNGEAL CANCER.

suprapubic prostatectomy   (su″prah-pu′bik pros″tah-tek′to-me)   surgical removal of all or part of the PROSTATE by cutting through the neck of the bladder. The incision is made above the pubic bone. This results in infertility; however, there is no loss of the ability to sustain an erection.

See also RADICAL PROSTATECTOMY.

suprarenal glands   See ADRENAL GLANDS.

SUR   See SURAMIN.

suramin (su'rah-min) a drug being carefully studied in the treatment of metastatic hormone-refractory prostate cancer as well as several other cancers.

surgery the treatment of disease by removal of tissue, usually by some kind of cutting device. Surgery is the oldest and still most common treatment for cancer. And until fairly recently, surgery was the only treatment that could cure patients with cancer.

Surgery for the removal of tumors was used as early as 1600 B.C., as reported in the Edwin Smith Papyrus from the Egyptian Middle Kingdom. However, surgery today bears virtually no resemblance to that practiced during that period. Tremendous progress has been made. An American, Ephraim MacDowell, can be credited with initiating modern surgery. In 1809, he removed a 22-pound ovarian tumor from a patient who survived for 30 years after the operation. The two major problems in performing surgery—pain and infection—were addressed later in that century. The first operation using general ether ANESTHESIA was performed in 1846 at the Massachusetts General Hospital. Antiseptics to prevent infection were first used in 1867.

Surgery plays multiple roles in cancer management. Following is a brief description of each role:

- *prevention*—In the prevention of cancer, surgery may be performed when known precancerous conditions exist or when a person is known to be at a very high risk of developing a particular cancer. For example, a COLECTOMY is often recommended for people with a genetic trait for familial multiple polyposis of the colon. If a colectomy is not performed in patients with this genetic disorder, about half will develop colon cancer by the age of 40 and virtually all of the rest will develop it by the age of 70. Some women at a very high risk of breast cancer elect to have a BILATERAL MASTECTOMY to prevent the development of breast cancer. While preventive, or prophylactic, surgery is generally successful in preventing disease, it is not 100% successful.
- *diagnosis*—The major role of surgery in the diagnosis of cancer is obtaining tissue for BIOPSY. While avoided whenever possible, exploratory surgery, such as a LAPAROTOMY, may have to be used when a diagnosis can be made in no other way. Surgery such as a laparotomy may also be used, when necessary, in the STAGING of the cancer. Surgery may also be used to determine if cancer cells have spread to other parts of the body.
- *cure*—The removal of cancerous tissue may be the only treatment that is necessary to cure the disease in the case of some IN SITU cancers. However, in general, the best chance of curing the cancer is achieved when surgery is accompanied by another kind of treatment. For example, in breast cancer a LUMPECTOMY is always followed with RADIATION THERAPY to the breast to destroy any cancer cells that may still be in the breast. CHEMOTHERAPY (anticancer drugs) to destroy any microscopic cancer cells that have spread to other parts of the body is frequently recommended for women with breast cancer, even when there is no evidence of spread of the disease. Radiation therapy, chemotherapy, and or BIOLOGICAL THERAPY may be used before surgery to reduce the size of the tumor, or after surgery if it was not possible to remove the entire tumor. Surgery may also be performed when the removal of METASTASES can result in a cure.
- *palliation*—Surgery may be performed just to relieve pain or restore a bodily function in a terminal patient to improve his or her quality of life, even when no cure is possible.
- *reconstruction/rehabilitation*—Surgery may be performed to correct functional and cosmetic defects resulting from the original cancer surgery. This is a rapidly progressing field enhanced by the development of microsurgical techniques.

The most common way of performing surgery remains the use of a knife. A number of other techniques are now available, for both radical and minor surgery, including LASER THERAPY, CRYOSURGERY, and ELECTROSURGERY.

See Subject Index for specific surgical procedures included in this volume.

surgical biopsy (bi'op-se) removal of body tissue for microscopic examination of cancer cells. An EXCISIONAL BIOPSY is sometimes called a surgical biopsy; however, a surgical biopsy can be performed in other ways, such as in a NEEDLE ASPIRATION BIOPSY or a CORE NEEDLE BIOPSY. See BIOPSY.

surgical conization   See CONIZATION.

surgical oncologist   (ong-kol'o-jist)   a physician who specializes in performing operations for the treatment of cancer. Surgical oncologists have experience in dealing with unusual or difficult problems in cancer treatment and can perform surgical procedures not commonly performed by general surgeons.

survival rate   percentage of people alive for a given period of time after the diagnosis of a disease (e.g., cancer). This can be given as the observable survival rate, which considers deaths from all causes, cancer or otherwise. In cancer, this rate is commonly expressed in terms of five-year survival. Relative survival rate is calculated by adjusting the observed survival rate to remove the effects of all causes of death *except* cancer. This rate is also commonly expressed in terms of five-year survival.

suspected   carcinogens   (kar-sin'-o-jenz)   substances that have not been proven to cause cancer, but are believed to do so. There are several hundred chemicals that have resulted in malignant (cancerous) tumors in animals exposed to them in studies. Because substances that cause cancer in animals frequently cause cancer in humans, those substances are suspected of being carcinogens. For example, the chemicals diethylstilbestrol (DES) and vinyl chloride were shown to cause cancer in mice and rats before it was known that humans exposed to them also had increased cancer rates.
See also CARCINOGENS.

SVCS   See SUPERIOR VENA CAVAL SYNDROME.

sweat gland cancer   an extremely rare cancer that may spread to LYMPH NODES or distant sites. It usually occurs near the anus, eyelids, ears, armpits, or scrotum, but can arise from any gland.

synchronous disease   in cancer, two or more tumors appearing *at the same time* in the primary site location. This is different from metastatic disease, cancer that has spread.

syngeneic bone marrow transplant   (sin"jĕ-ne'ik) using perfectly matched, genetically identical tissue in a transplant. Perfectly matched tissue is generally only available in an identical twin. It is extremely rare for anyone other than an identical twin to be able to provide a syngeneic graft. Because identical twins represent only 0.3% of all births, this type of transplant, which has the highest success rate, is relatively rare.
See also BONE MARROW TRANSPLANTATION.

synovial cell carcinoma   See SYNOVIAL SARCOMA.

synovial sarcoma   (sĭ-no've-al sar-ko'mah) [synovioma, synovial cell carcinoma] a cancer tumor arising near joints and tendons (tissues that connect muscles to bones), most often in the leg, between the thigh and knee. It also occurs in the hands and feet. Adults in their 20s and 30s are most commonly affected. See SOFT TISSUE SARCOMA.

synovioma   See SYNOVIAL SARCOMA.

syringoma   (sir"in-go'mah)   a benign (noncancerous) tumor on the skin caused by an enlarged sweat gland.

systemic treatment   treatment that reaches and affects cells all over the body. This type of treatment is commonly used for cancers that are known to be systemic, cancers that can spread and affect any part of the body. Treatment is accomplished by CHEMOTHERAPY, anticancer drugs that travel through the bloodstream throughout the body. Depending on the drug and the type of cancer, the chemotherapy may be injected into a vein, or into a muscle or taken by mouth.

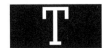

T cell [T lymphocytes] one of the two major types of lymphocytes, which are white blood cells. (The other major type is the B CELL.) T cells are processed in the thymus and are part of the body's IMMUNE SYSTEM. Regulatory T cells play a major role in orchestrating the very complex immune system. The most important T cells are the "helper/ inducer" cells (identified by the T4 marker), which activate B cells, other T cells, NATURAL KILLER CELLS, and MACROPHAGES. Another regulatory T cell (identified by the T8 marker) turns off or suppresses those same cells. The killer cytotoxic T cells (also identified by the T8 marker) rid the body of cells that are perceived as harmful—cells infected by a virus or transformed by cancer—and reject foreign substances such as tissue and organ grafts as well.

See WHITE BLOOD CELLS.

TAC TAXOL (Docitaxel), ADRIAMYCIN (doxorubicin), and cyclophosphamide combination being investigated as active adjuvant chemotherapy for the treatment of BREAST CANCER.

Tace See ESTROGEN.

tachycardia (tak″ĕ-kar′de-ah) an excessively rapid heartbeat. There are many causes of tachycardia. It can be a side effect of INTERLEUKIN-2 treatment.

TAH See TOTAL ABDOMINAL HYSTERECTOMY.

TAHBSO See TOTAL ABDOMINAL HYSTERECTOMY and BILATERAL SALPINGO-OOPHORECTOMY.

TAM a slang term for TAMOXIFEN.

tamoxifen (tah-moks′ĭ-fen) [Nolvadex, TAM] a nonsteroidal ANTIESTROGEN drug used extensively in the treatment of BREAST CANCER as ADJUVANT THERAPY following surgery. It is also front-line hormonal treatment for both premenopausal and postmenopausal women with advanced breast cancer. In 1998, a worldwide meta-analysis of tamoxifen studies concluded that the drug significantly reduces the rates of breast cancer recurrence and death. It found that tamoxifen was of benefit to women of any age with breast cancer; that it was effective whether the cancer was confined to the breast or was found in the axillary lymph nodes. According to the study, tamoxifen could save 2,500 lives a year in the United States and prevent recurrence in 5,000 women a year. Tamoxifen is believed to work by preventing the estrogen in the body from stimulating the growth of breast cancer tumors that are estrogen receptor positive. It helps to shrink the tumor in about half the cases.

Results of some studies show additional advantages to tamoxifen treatment. A study completed in 1990 indicated that tamoxifen may reduce the overall risk of heart disease by as much as 40%. Data from other studies indicate that tamoxifen may prevent bone loss, thereby reducing the risk of osteoporosis (a decrease in the amount and strength of bone tissue).

The use of tamoxifen in the treatment of other cancers, including PROSTATE, SKIN (MELANOMA), and KIDNEY CANCER, is also being explored. Its use as a possible fertility drug is also being examined.

Tamoxifen is far less toxic than most anticancer drugs. It is generally well tolerated. For most patients there are no side effects. Some of the side effects that may occur, if uncommon, include mild nausea, hot flashes, subtle weight gain, and visual changes. Very uncommon side effects may include mild BONE MARROW DEPRESSION, vaginal bleeding and discharge, menstrual irregularity, bone and tumor pain, skin rashes, depression, light-headedness, and headaches. Tamoxifen increases slightly the risk of uterine cancer and potentially fatal blood clots. But the benefits of tamoxifen are considered to outweigh those risks. Tamoxifen is in a pill taken by mouth.

See also BREAST CANCER PREVENTION TRIAL.

Tamoxifen and Raloxifene Study   See STAR.

tamoxifen prevention trial   See BREAST CANCER PREVENTION TRIAL.

tanning booth   a place where ultraviolet lights are used to induce an artificial tan. Although many tanning salons now have sunlamps that emit predominantly UVA radiation, they are still considered a skin cancer risk. UVA radiation is no longer considered generally harmless. And the small amount of the more dangerous, faster-burning UVB radiation that is emitted can cause a significant increase in cancer risk. As of 1990 the Federal Trade Commission had taken action against three major importers and manufacturers of tanning devices for misrepresenting the safety of their products.

Tarceva   [erlotinib]   an   oral   tyrosine   kinase inhibitor (antiangiogenesis agent) approved for treatment of patients with locally advanced or metastatic NSCLC (NON-SMALL CELL LUNG CANCER) after failure of at least one prior chemotherapy regimen.

targeted therapy   use of one of the newer drugs (as of 2005) directed against a specific molecular target or receptor, eg anti-VEGF, EGFR, etc.

TAX   See TAXOL.

taxane   family name of a group of active anticancer drugs. See TAXOL and TAXOTERE.

Taxol (tax'ol) [paclitaxel] a major anticancer drug produced initially in small quantities from the bark of the Pacific yew tree. It can now be produced in much greater amounts through a semisynthetic process. It is indicated for the treatment of advanced ovarian cancer, metastatic breast cancer, and AIDS-related KAPOSI'S SARCOMA. It is also being used to treat other cancers, including lung cancer. Ongoing clinical trials are being conducted to find other cancers that could be treated effectively with Taxol.

Taxol shares many of the common side effects of chemotherapy, such as bone marrow suppression and hair loss. It also is associated with an unusual hypersensitivity reaction, which can be prevented using a variety of premedications, including corticosteroids and antihistamines. This is due to the agent cremophor used to solubilize the product. It is given by IV (into a vein).

Taxotere   [docetaxel]   an   anticancer   drug   FDA-approved in the treatment of metastatic or locally advanced BREAST CANCER. It is active also in LUNG CANCER, HEAD AND NECK CANCER, as well as in others. In 2005, it is being widely used in PROSTATE CANCER, as the CHEMOTHERAPY of choice in HORMONE insensitive METASTATIC DISEASE. Its usefulness in the treatment of other cancers is being investigated. Side effects may include BONE MARROW SUPPRESSION and an unusual hypersensitivity reaction, which can be prevented using a variety of premedications, including corticosteroids and antihistamines. In 2005, Taxotere was FDA-approved in combination with doxorubicin and cyclophosphamide (the "TAC" regimen) in the adjuvant treatment of women with operable, NODE-POSITIVE CANCER.

TBI (total-body irradiation)   See WHOLE-BODY RADIATION.

TC   a combination of the anticancer drugs 6-TG and ARA-C sometimes used in the maintenance therapy of ALL. See individual drug listings for side effects.

See also COMBINATION CHEMOTHERAPY.

TCC See TRANSITIONAL CELL CANCER OF THE RENAL PELVIS AND URETER.

T-cell leukemia a type of acute lymphocytic leukemia (ALL) affecting immature STEM CELLS. It accounts for about 12% of ALL cases. It occurs primarily in older adolescents and young adults.

T-cell lymphoma See MYCOSIS FUNGOIDES.

T-cell prolymphocytic leukemia a form of LEUKEMIA in which the cell of origin is a T CELL as shown by FLOW CYTOMETRY. A small percentage of prolymphocytic leukemias are derived from T cells and are thus managed differently from diseases not derived from T cells.
See also PROLYMPHOCYTIC LEUKEMIA.

Teceleukin See INTERLEUKIN-2.

technesium (tek-ne′ze-um) a radioactive substance that may be used in some NUCLEAR SCANS.

tegafur [Florafur, 5-fluoro-1-tetrahydro-2-furyluracil] an anticancer drug being investigated for its use in the treatment of gastrointestinal cancers. It is administered by IV (injected into a vein) or taken by mouth. Common side effects may include nausea, vomiting, flushing, dizziness, and apprehension with rapid administration. Occasional or rare side effects may include mouth sores, loss of muscle coordination, diarrhea, lethargy, and confusion.

teletherapy See EXTERNAL RADIATION THERAPY.

Temodar [temozolomide] capsules an oral chemotherapeutic agent indicated in combination with radiotherapy in newly diagnosed patients with GLIOBLASTOMA MULTIFORME and as maintenance after combined therapy.

10-EDAM See EDATREXATE.

teniposide [VM-26 Vunom] an anticancer drug used in the induction treatment of REFRACTORY childhood acute lymphoblastic leukemia (ALL). It is being investigated for the treatment of lymphoma, melanoma, and cancers of the brain, bladder, lung, ovary, breast, and kidney. BONE MARROW DEPRESSION may be a side effect. Other, less common side effects may include nausea, vomiting, hair loss, fever, liver problems, and loss of reflexes. It is administered by IV (injected into a vein).

TENS See TRANSCUTANEOUS ELECTRICAL NERVE STIMULATION.

tension relaxation See RELAXATION TECHNIQUES.

teratoma a neoplasm (abnormal growth of tissue) composed of a number of different types of tissue. One type of TESTICULAR CANCER is called teratoma, as is one type of congenital BRAIN CANCER.

terminal in cancer, a term used to characterize a patient with progressive advanced disease with vital organ involvement who has a very limited life expectancy in the absence of any useful further therapy. Duration of life has been defined in various ways, but most understand "terminal" to be six months or less left to live.

Teslac [testolactone] See ANDROGEN.

Teslascan the first liver-cell specific contrast agent approved for the detection, localization, characterization, and evaluation of liver lesions.

testes (tes′tēz) [testicles] the male sperm-producing glands encased in the scrotum (a sac of loose skin) located directly under the penis. They are round and a little smaller than golf balls.
See also TESTICULAR CANCER.

testicular cancer (tes-tik′u-lar) cancer of the TESTES, the male reproductive glands, and is one of the most curable forms of cancer. It is a rare cancer, accounting for about 1% of all the cancers occurring in men. It usually arises in just one testicle. The American Cancer Society estimated that in the year 2005, about 8,010 new cases of testicular cancer would be diagnosed in the United States, with 390 deaths from the disease in the same year. The rate of testicular cancer has been increasing in many countries including the United States. The increase is mostly of SEMINOMAS. Experts have not been able to find reasons for this increase.

Testicular cancer is the most common cancer occurring in men aged 20 to 34, and it accounts for 19% of all the cancers diagnosed in men in that age group. Four times as many white men as black men develop testicular cancer.

There are two major kinds of testicular cancer, seminoma and NONSEMINOMA, which arise from the cells that produce sperm. They account for about 95% of testicular tumors. Other, very rare types of nonseminomas are EMBRYONAL CELL carcinomas, TERATOMAS, yolk sac tumors, and CHORIOCARCINOMAS.

The cause of testicular cancer is not clear. One known risk factor is the congenital condition CRYPTORCHIDISM, in which one or both testes fail to descend. Studies indicate that men with cryptorchidism have as much as 17 times more risk than normal of developing this cancer. There is also an indication that the risk becomes normal if men with that condition have it surgically repaired before the age of six. Other conditions that have been associated with testicular cancer include KLINEFELTER'S SYNDROME (characterized by men with small testes, enlarged breasts, and lack of secondary sex characteristics, such as low voice and beard growth); gonadal aplasia (failure of the testes to develop); and various forms of HERMAPHRODITISM (development of both male and female sex characteristics). Low birth weight, under five pounds, may also be a risk factor, as well as a mother's history of unusual bleeding or spotting during pregnancy, use of alcohol or sedatives, or exposure to X-RAYS while pregnant.

It is recommended that men do a monthly TESTICULAR SELF-EXAMINATION for the following warning signs of testicular cancer:

- a lump in either testicle
- any enlargement of a testicle
- a feeling of heaviness in the scrotum
- pain or discomfort in a testicle or in the scrotum
- enlargement or tenderness of the breasts

These signs can be symptoms of other disorders as well. A doctor should be consulted if any of the warning signs lasts longer than two weeks.

Diagnostic procedures include BLOOD TESTS and URINALYSIS. In most other cancers a diagnosis is made by removing a small tissue sample for biopsy. However, a testicular biopsy is not done because cutting through the outer capsule of the testis may contribute to the spread of the cancer cells. Since most lumps are malignant (cancerous), and because of the risk of the cancer spreading during a biopsy, the standard procedure to evaluate a lump is removal of the entire affected testis. Other procedures that may be used to evaluate the extent of the disease include X-RAYS, CT SCANS, IVP, LYMPHANGIOGRAPHY, ULTRASOUND, and MRI. levels of ALPHA-FETOPROTEIN and LACTATE DEHYDROGENASE in the blood are TUMOR MARKERS for nonseminomas and can be useful in monitoring a patient after treatment.

Following is the NATIONAL CANCER INSTITUTE'S (NCI) STAGING for testicular cancer:

- Stage I—cancer is found only in the testicle
- Stage II—cancer has spread to the LYMPH NODES in the abdomen
- Stage III—cancer has spread beyond the lymph nodes in the abdomen and may have metastasized (spread) to other parts of the body, such as the lungs and liver
- Recurrent—cancer has returned in the same place or in another part of the body after treatment

Treatment depends on the stage of the disease, the type (seminoma or nonseminoma), the general state of health of the patient, and other factors. Surgery is a common treatment for most stages of cancer. A RADICAL INGUINAL ORCHIECTOMY is the most frequently performed surgery. RADIATION THERAPY and CHEMOTHERAPY may also be used. For specific information on the latest state-of-the-art treatment, by stage and type, call NCI's Cancer Information Service at 1-800-4-CANCER (1-800-422-6237), or for a TTY: 1-800-332-8615.

testicular self-examination (TSE) (tes-tik'u-lar) an examination, by a man, of his testicles. It should be done after a warm bath or shower. The heat relaxes the scrotum, making it easier to feel anything unusual. Testicular self-examination should be done once a month. It is simple to do and takes just a few minutes. Following are the guidelines for doing TSE:

- While standing in front of a mirror, look for any swelling in the skin of the scrotum.
- Examine each testicle with both hands. The index and middle fingers should be placed under

Position of Testicles

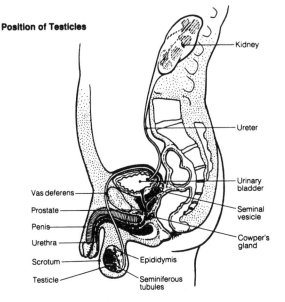

Testicular cancer is the most common cancer occurring in men aged 20 to 34. Courtesy NCI.

the testicles, the thumbs on top. Gently roll one testicle at a time between the thumb and fingers checking for lumps, swelling, or other changes. A normal testicle feels smooth, egg shaped, and rather firm.

• Find the epididymis, the soft, tubelike structure at the back of the testicle that collects and carries sperm; this should not be mistaken for an abnormal lump.

If a lump is found, a physician should be consulted as soon as possible.

See also SCREENING.

testolactone   See ANDROGEN.

testosterone (tes-tos'tĕ-rōn)   the most powerful of the male sex hormones. It is produced by the testes, the male reproductive glands. Small amounts are produced by the adrenal glands. Its major role is inducing the secondary sex characteristics, such as a deep voice or facial hair. On rare occasion it may be used in the treatment of BREAST CANCER. Women produce a very small amount of testosterone.

testosterone propionate   See ANDROGEN.

tetrahydrocannabinol   See MARIJUANA.

TGF   See TUMOR GROWTH FACTORS.

thalidomide [Thalidomid]   an agent originally developed to combat morning sickness that was withdrawn when it was found to cause developmental abnormalities in newborns. In 1998, it was in clinical trials to investigate its effectiveness as an antiangiogenesis agent (inhibiting the formation of blood vessels). This property could allow thalidomide to block the growth of cancer. Most activity has been seen in AIDS-KAPOSI'S SARCOMA, PROSTATE CANCER, and GBM (GLIOBLASTOMA MULTIFORME). It is being investigated for use in the treatment of relapsed multiple myeloma as an ANTIANGIOGENESIS agent.

THC   See MARIJUANA.

therapeutic radiologist   See RADIATION THERAPIST.

thermography (ther-mah'graf-e) [contact thermograph, graphic stress telethermometry]   examination of body tissue using an infrared camera to measure and display heat patterns. Abnormalities may show up as "hot" spots in the film, since the temperature of diseased or abnormal tissue is frequently higher than that of normal tissue.

Thermography in the detection of BREAST CANCER can be performed in several ways. The woman can put her hands in ice water, or can disrobe and sit in a cool room for about ten minutes. Heat emitted from the breast is measured by an infrared sensor and then recorded by a camera. In contact thermography the breasts are held against or wrapped with a material that changes color with changes in temperature. The heat emissions are recorded by a camera.

Thermography is not a very accurate test, missing as many as 30% of cancers, and compares unfavorably with MAMMOGRAPHY. It does not use radiation. A mammogram, with low exposure to radiation, is the preferred method of mass screening for breast cancer.

thioguanine   See 6-TG.

thiotEPA (thi"o-te'pah) [TSPA, triethylene thiophosphoramide]   an ALKYLATING anticancer drug that may be used in the treatment of HODGKIN'S DISEASE and cancers of the BREAST, OVARY, and BLADDER. It can be administered by IV (injected into a vein), intramuscularly (injected into a muscle), subcutaneously (under the skin), or intrathecally (injected into the cerebro spinal fluid). Common side effects may include nausea, vomiting, and BONE MARROW DEPRESSION. Occasional or rare side effects may include headaches, fever, allergic reaction, dizziness, and local pain.

13-CRA   See ACCUTANE.

thoracentesis (tho"rah-sen-te'sis) [pleural   tap] a procedure that may be used in the diagnosis of cancer and other conditions. A small amount of fluid is removed from the chest cavity, the space between the lungs and chest wall. The fluid is then biopsied (microscopically examined for cancer cells). Thoracentesis is performed by inserting a needle into the chest cavity between the ribs and removing some fluid by suction. This procedure may also be performed to relieve symptoms, such as shortness of breath or pain, that can be caused by the accumulation of fluid. This is usually performed in the hospital and can take between 15 minutes and half an hour.

thoracic surgeon (tho-ras'ik)   a medical doctor who specializes in performing operations in the chest area, including the lungs and esophagus. Certification by the American Board of Thoracic Surgery requires certification by the American Board of Surgery, two additional years of training in thoracic surgery, and successful completion of the board's written and oral exams.

thoracoscopy (tho"rah-kos'ko-pe)   a procedure used to examine the chest wall and surface of the lung. After the patient has been anesthetized, an incision is made between two ribs. An endoscope (a long, thin tubular instrument) is inserted and used to examine the lung and retrieve some tissue to be biopsied. This procedure may be performed in the diagnosis of LUNG CANCER.

See also ENDOSCOPY.

thoracotomy (tho"rah-kot'o-me)   surgical opening of the chest. A thoracotomy may be performed in the diagnosis of LUNG CANCER when all other diagnostic procedures have failed to produce a diagnosis. It is considered major surgery and is performed under anesthesia. When the chest is opened, a small part of lung containing a nodule or other mass is removed and examined for cancer cells. This procedure is usually not done if the surgeon thinks that surgical removal of the tumor would not be possible. However, that cannot always be determined before the surgery. A thoracotomy and resection (surgical removal) of the cancer in the lung is the most likely treatment to result in a cure.

thorax   the part of the body between the neck and ABDOMEN.

thorazine   See ANTIEMETIC.

thorium dioxide   See CARCINOGENS.

throat cancer   See OROPHARYNGEAL CANCER.

thrombocytapheresis   See PLATELETPHERESIS.

thrombocythemia   See   ESSENTIAL   THROMBOCYTHEMIA.

thrombocytopenia (throm"bo-si"to-pe'ne-ah)   a drop in the level of PLATELETS, the blood cells that are responsible for clotting. Platelets are produced by megakaryocytes in the BONE MARROW. The reduction in the production of platelets in the bone marrow can be a side effect of RADIATION THERAPY, CHEMOTHERAPY, or other factors. Thrombocytopenia may also be the result of the destruction of platelets that are circulating in the bloodstream by certain types of cancer as well as other factors. Depending on its severity, thrombocytopenia can be a very dangerous condition. A simple paper cut or nosebleed can have major repercussions.

People with thrombocytopenia should take precautions to avoid any situations that could result in internal or external bleeding. Following are some simple precautionary guidelines:

- Do not take aspirin, which can exacerbate bleeding. Instead, take acetaminophen, e.g., Tylenol or Datril.
- Avoid alcohol, which decreases platelet function.
- Drink a lot of liquids, at least eight to ten glasses a day.
- Eat high-protein foods and beverages; protein is essential for the production of megakaryocytes.
- Avoid spicy and hot foods and foods such as popcorn and pretzels that can irritate the mouth; bland and mild foods should be eaten instead.
- Use a toothbrush with soft bristles (or a sponge-tipped applicator or a piece of gauze moistened with salt water wrapped around a finger) and a mouthwash with a low-alcoholic content.
- Keep lips lubricated.
- Consult a doctor before having any dental work.
- Use stool softeners whenever necessary.
- Avoid enemas, suppositories, harsh laxatives, and the use of rectal thermometers.
- Take steroids with an antacid or milk to help prevent irritation.
- Avoid forcefully blowing the nose; if necessary, blow gently through both nostrils.
- Use an electric shaver instead of a razor.
- Take extra care when using knives or tools.
- Avoid contact sports and other activities that could result in injury.
- Wear heavy gloves when working in the garden or with thorny plants.

Treatment of thrombocytopenia depends on the cause and the extent of the condition. In severe cases, platelet transfusions, intravenous gamma-globulin, and other drugs, as well as removal of the spleen, may be used to boost the platelet count. If the thrombocytopenia is a result of chemotherapy or radiation therapy, it may be reversible, on its own, in a relatively short period of time.

thrombopoietin See INTERLEUKIN-6.

thymoma (thi-mo′mah) [malignant thymoma] a rare cancer in the tissues of the thymus (a small organ that lies under the breastbone). Symptoms of this cancer may include a cough that will not go away, weakness in the muscles, or chest pains. Diagnostic procedures may include an X-RAY of the chest and CT SCAN.

Following is the NATIONAL CANCER INSTITUTE's STAGING for thymoma:

- Stage I—cancer found only within the thymus gland and its sac
- Stage II—cancer invasion into surrounding fat or lining of lung cavity
- Stage III—cancer invasion into organs near the thymus
- Stage IVa—greater spread of cancer into sac around heart or lungs
- Stage IVb—greater spread of cancer through vessels carrying blood or lymph
  (Stage I malignant thymoma may be referred to as noninvasive malignant thymoma. Stages II through IVb malignant thymoma may be referred to as invasive malignant thymoma.)
- Recurrent—the cancer has returned to the same site or to another part of the body after treatment

Treatment depends on the stage of the disease, the general state of health of the patient, and other factors. Surgical removal of the tumor is the most common treatment. The lymph nodes or tissue around the tumor may also be removed. RADIATION THERAPY, CHEMOTHERAPY, and HORMONE THERAPY may also be used.

thymosin (thi′mo-sin) [thymic humoral factor (THF)] a hormone produced by the thymus gland that promotes the maturation of T CELLS.
See also BIOLOGICAL RESPONSE MODIFIERS.

thymus (thi′mus) a gland located high in the chest that produces the hormone thymosin (thymic humoral factor [THF]) and controls the production and function of T CELLS, small white blood cells that are important in the IMMUNE SYSTEM. T cells, which are produced in the BONE MARROW, migrate to the thymus, where they multiply.

thyroglobulin (thi-ro-glob′u-lin) the protein in which the thyroid hormone is stored. A high level of thyroglobulin in the blood could be an indication of a recurrence or metastasis (spread) of THYROID CANCER.

thyroid (thi′roid) a gland at the base of the neck with two lobes, one on either side. The thyroid produces important hormones used in regulating the body's metabolism as well as other body functions. It is also plays a role in the IMMUNE SYSTEM.

thyroid cancer (thi'roid)   a disease in which cancer cells are found in the tissue of the thyroid gland. According to the American Cancer Society, there were 23,600 new cases of thyroid cancer diagnosed in the United States in 2004 (5,960 in males, and 17,640 in females), with approximately 1,460 deaths from the disease. It accounts for about 1% of all the cancers diagnosed in the United States. It occurs in women two to three times more often than in men, particularly women of childbearing age, and generally affects people between the ages of 25 and 65. People at the highest risk of developing thyroid cancer are those who, as children, had radiation treatments to the head and neck. Before the availability of antibiotics, in the 1920s, doctors routinely used X-RAYS to treat such infectious diseases as tonsillitis and adenoiditis as well as conditions such as ear inflammations and ringworm of the scalp. Radiation was also used on newborn infants with breathing difficulties. The effect that radiation could have on the thyroid gland was not known until some 25 years later. The National Cancer Institute recommends that anyone who received radiation to the head or neck in childhood be examined by a doctor every one to two years.

There are four major types of thyroid cancer. Papillary adenocarcinoma is the most common type of thyroid cancer, accounting for about 60%. It is slow growing and rarely metastasizes (spreads to other parts of the body). The other types are follicular carcinoma, which occurs less frequently than papillary; medullary; and anaplastic, which grows faster than the other three.

The major symptom of thyroid cancer is an enlarged thyroid, a swelling or lump in the neck in the vicinity of the Adam's apple. Other symptoms, such as discomfort in swallowing, may be caused by the size of the tumor; there may also be symptoms associated with a disturbance in the functioning of the thyroid. Procedures used in the diagnosis of thyroid cancer may include blood tests, a THYROID SCAN, ULTRASOUND, and BIOPSY. Most thyroid tumors are benign (noncancerous), as many as 90%. Unless a benign tumor is causing a problem, it does not have to be removed other than for cosmetic purposes.

Following is the NATIONAL CANCER INSTITUTE'S (NCI) STAGING for papillary and follicular thyroid cancer:

- Stage I—cancer is only in one or both lobes of the thyroid
- Stage II—cancer has spread to the LYMPH NODES around the thyroid
- Stage III—cancer has spread outside the thyroid but not outside the neck
- Stage IV—cancer has spread to other parts of the body such as the lungs and bones
- Recurrent—cancer has returned to the same site or to another part of the body after treatment

Following is NCI's staging for medullary thyroid cancer:

- Stage I—cancer is less than one centimeter (about $1/2$ inch) in size
- Stage II—cancer is between one and four centimeters (about $1/2$ to $1 1/2$ inches) in size
- Stage III—cancer has spread to the lymph nodes
- Stage IV—cancer has spread to other parts of the body
- Recurrent—the cancer has come back (recurred) after it has been treated. It may come back in the thyroid or in another part of the body

There is no staging system for anaplastic cancer of the thyroid. This type grows faster than the other types.

Treatment depends on the stage of disease and other factors. Surgery is the most common treatment. Near-total thyroidectomy removes all of the thyroid except for a small part. Total thyroidectomy removes the entire thyroid. A lobectomy, removal of one side of the thyroid, may be performed if the cancer is found on only one side. RADIATION THERAPY, CHEMOTHERAPY, and HORMONE THERAPY may also be used. CLINICAL TRIALS are also being conducted in the treatment of thyroid cancer. For specific information on the latest state-of-the-art treatment, by stage, call NCI's Cancer Information Service at 1-800-4-CANCER (1-800-422-6237), or for a TTY: 1-800-332-8615.

thyroid scan (thi'roid)   an examination of the THYROID after a RADIOACTIVE IODINE or another radioactive substance has been administered by IV (injected into a vein) to the patient. The images that are obtained, showing distribution of the radioactive material, can indicate possible problems in the thyroid. If every part of the thyroid uses the iodine uniformly, the picture will be normal. An abnormal picture will result if the distribution is not uniform. Malignant (cancerous) tissue usually does not absorb iodine in a normal way. However, other conditions could cause that result as well. A thyroid scan can be a good indicator of cancer in the thyroid, but it cannot be used for a definitive diagnosis.

See also NUCLEAR SCAN.

thyroidectomy (thi″roi-dek′to-me) surgical removal of all or part of the THYROID gland. The procedure is called lobectomy when only the side of the thyroid where cancer has been found is removed. In a near-total thyroidectomy, nearly all of the thyroid is removed. In a total thyroidectomy, the entire thyroid is removed.

thyroid-stimulating hormone (TSH) a substance produced by the pituitary gland, which controls the activity of the thyroid gland.

TICE BCG See BCG.

TIF See TUMOR INHIBITORY FACTORS.

Tigan See ANTIEMETIC.

TIL See TUMOR-INFILTRATING LYMPHOCYTES.

tissue typing See HISTOCOMPATIBILITY TESTING.

TLI See THYMIDINE LABELING INDEX.

TNF See TUMOR NECROSIS FACTOR.

TNM classification system a method of STAGING cancer developed by the American Joint Committee on Cancer. The *T* stands for tumor; the *N* stands for lymph node involvement; the *M* stands for metastases. A number following the letter indicates the size of the tumor; the extent of lymph node involvement; and the extent of metastatic disease. A 0 following an N would mean there is no lymph node involvement; a 0 following an M would mean the cancer has not metastasized to other parts of

the body. For example the staging for a breast cancer might be T3N0M1—which would translate to a large tumor with no lymph node involvement but evidence present of cancer in another part of the body.

TNS See TRANSCUTANEOUS ELECTRICAL NERVE STIMULATION.

tobacco See SMOKING.

tomogram See TOMOGRAPHY.

tomography (to-mog′rah-fe) a general term referring to a diagnostic procedure in which multiple cross-sectional X-RAYS are taken of a specific section of the body. Originally tomography was used primarily for X-rays of the chest. With the advent of computerization and nuclear scanning, the use of tomography has been greatly broadened and is commonly used in the diagnosis and evaluation of many different cancers as well as many other disorders. The CT SCAN, MRI, and the PET SCAN are examples of tomography.

tongue cancer See MOUTH CANCER.

tonsil a small, rounded mass of (mostly) lymphoid tissue, located at the back of the throat. It is one of the LYMPHOID ORGANS, the organs of the immune system, which are involved in the growth, development, and distribution of LYMPHOCYTES (a type of white blood cell).

tonsil cancer See MOUTH CANCER.

topical anesthesia (an″es-the′ze-ah) deadening of sensation by administration of an anesthetic (numbing agent) directly to the area involved. It is sprayed or "painted" on. Topical anesthesia may be used for procedures involving the eye, nose, or throat. It is also commonly used when tubes are inserted in the trachea (windpipe) or esophagus (tube connecting the stomach to the throat).

topical chemotherapy application of an anticancer drug (a cream or solution) to a surface of the body. For example, topical CHEMOTHERAPY may be used in the treatment of early stage skin cancer.

The drug is applied to the growth daily for several weeks.

topical photochemotherapy   See PUVA THERAPY.

TOPO   See HYCAMTIN.

Toposar   See ETOPOSIDE.

topotecan   See HYCAMTIN.

Torecan   See ANTIEMETIC.

toremifene (Fareston)   a hormonal treatment for metastatic BREAST CANCER in postmenopausal women with estrogen receptor positive or receptor unknown tumors. Possible side effects may include nausea and vomiting, stomach pain, loss of or increased appetite, diarrhea, constipation, dry eyes, cataracts, dizziness, sleeplessness, hot flashes, sweating, vaginal discharge or bleeding. Toremifene is taken orally.

Tositumomab   See Bexxar.

total abdominal hysterectomy (TAH) (ab-dom′ĭ-nal his″ter-ek′to-me) surgical removal of the uterus through an incision made in the abdomen. This surgery may be performed in the treatment of CERVICAL CANCER.
    See also HYSTERECTOMY.

total abdominal hysterectomy and bilateral salpingo-oophorectomy (TAHBSO) (ab-dom′ĭ-nal his″ter-ek′to-me sal-ping′o o″of-o-rek′to-me) surgical removal of the uterus, both ovaries, and the fallopian tubes through an incision in the abdomen. This surgery may be performed in the treatment of ENDOMETRIAL CANCER and UTERINE SARCOMA. LYMPH NODES in the pelvis may also be removed.
    See also HYSTERECTOMY.

total biopsy (bi′op-se)   See EXCISIONAL BIOPSY.

total gastrectomy (gas-trek′to-me) surgical removal of the entire stomach, portions of the esophagus or small intestine, any obvious sites of metastases, and part of the peritoneum. The spleen may also be removed. A substitute stomach may be made, either during the surgery or after the patient has spent some time recovering from the initial surgery. A total gastrectomy may be performed in the treatment of STOMACH CANCER.
    See also GASTRECTOMY.

total hysterectomy (his″ter-ek′to-me) surgical removal of the cervix and uterus. This surgery may be performed in the treatment of CERVICAL CANCER.
    See also HYSTERECTOMY.

total laryngectomy (lar″in-jek′to-me) surgical removal of the entire larynx (voice box). After this extensive surgery, breathing is done through a TRACHEOSTOMY, an opening made in the windpipe. This surgery may be performed in the treatment of LARYNGEAL CANCER.

total mastectomy   See SIMPLE MASTECTOMY.

total mastectomy with axillary dissection   See MODIFIED RADICAL MASTECTOMY.

total pancreatectomy (pan″kre-ah-tek′to-me) surgical removal of the entire pancreas, part of the small intestine, part of the stomach, the bile duct, the gallbladder, spleen, and most of the lymph nodes in the area. The total pancreatectomy was created to improve the survival rate of the WHIPPLE PROCEDURE and to ensure that as many cancer cells as possible were removed. This extensive surgery may be performed in the treatment of PANCREATIC CANCER. Patients who have undergone this surgery are given replacement enzymes.

total parenteral nutrition (TPN)   See PARENTERAL NUTRITION.

total pelvic exenteration   surgical removal of the bladder, prostate, seminal vesicles, and rectum. A total pelvic exenteration may be performed in the treatment of colon cancer when the tumor is large. It is very radical surgery.

total prostatectomy (pros″tah-tek′to-me) surgical removal of the prostate gland. This surgery may be performed in the treatment of PROSTATE CANCER.
    See also RADICAL PROSTATECTOMY.

total skin electronic beam radiation therapy (TSEB) the use of special rays of tiny particles called electrons to treat the entire surface of the skin. The radiation penetrates only the outer layers of the skin. TSEB may be performed in the treatment of MYCOSIS FUNGOIDES.

total thyroidectomy (thi″roi-dek′to-me) surgical removal of the entire thyroid gland. This surgery may be performed in the treatment of THYROID CANCER.

total-body irradiation (TBI) See WHOLE-BODY RADIATION.

toxicity refers to the undesirable and harmful side effects of a drug. Based on the toxicity, the amount of the drug a person can safely take can be determined. For example, too much of the anticancer drug Adriamycin can cause damage to the heart. The maximum total dose for any patient is based on its toxicity. One function of CLINICAL TRIALS is to determine the toxicity of drugs being investigated for their use in the treatment of cancer.

TPN (total parenteral nutrition) See PARENTERAL NUTRITION.

TPT See HYCAMTIN.

trachea (tra′ke-ah) the windpipe; the tube that extends from the voice box to the bronchi, the tubes through which air is inhaled in the nose and mouth.

tracheostomy (tra″ke-os′to-me) a stoma (hole) that is made in the trachea for breathing, which may be temporary or permanent, depending on the extent of the surgery. In a partial laryngectomy, the metal tube that is inserted in the stoma is removed usually within a few days, and the stoma then closes. When a total laryngectomy (removal of the entire voice box) is performed, the tube is permanent.

transcutaneous electrical nerve stimulation (TENS) (trans″ku-ta′ne-us) [TNS] the use of electrical stimulation to relieve or control pain. A small power pack is used to apply mild electric currents to specific sites on the skin. The electric impulses appear to block the transmission of pain. The degree of current can be adjusted. The pain relief can last for a period of time after the current is stopped.

See also PAIN MANAGEMENT.

transdermal nicotine patch See NICOTINE PATCH.

transillumination (trans″ĭlu″mĭ-na′shun) [diaphanography, light scanning] a procedure that may be used in the diagnosis of BREAST CANCER. A strong, cold beam of light is focused on the breast in a darkened room. An infrared camera is used, which will show, on a screen, differences that distinguish a solid tumor from a cyst that is filled with fluid. It cannot detect very small tumors and has not proved to be useful in breast cancer screening. When used, it is usually with other diagnostic procedures, such as MAMMOGRAPHY, to get additional information. Transillumination was first used in 1929.

transitional cell cancer of the renal pelvis and ureter (TCC) (re′nal pel′vis u-re′ter) cancer arising in the cells in the kidney that collect urine (the renal pelvis) and/or in the tube that connects the kidney to the bladder (ureter). Most of the cells lining the urinary system are transitional cells. There may be no symptoms in the early stages of the disease. When there are symptoms, they are similar to those of KIDNEY CANCER and other kidney disorders—blood in the urine, back pain, a mass in the flank or abdomen, high blood pressure, and fever.

Diagnostic procedures may include a URETEROSCOPY, CT SCAN, MRI, and BIOPSY.

Following is the NATIONAL CANCER INSTITUTE'S (NCI) STAGING:

- Localized—the cancer is only in the primary site and has not spread outside the kidney or ureter
- Regional—the cancer has spread to the tissue around the kidney or to LYMPH NODES in the pelvis
- Metastatic—the cancer has spread to other parts of the body
- Recurrent—the cancer has returned to the original site or to another part of the body after treatment.

Treatment depends on the stage of the disease, the general state of health of the patient, and other factors. Surgery is the treatment most often performed. The types of surgery used include NEPHROURETERECTOMY (removal of the kidney, ureter, and top part of the bladder), segmental resection (removal of part of the kidney or ureter), ELECTROSURGERY, and LASER SURGERY. RADIATION THERAPY, CHEMOTHERAPY, and BIOLOGICAL THERAPY may also be used. Clinical trials are also being performed. For specific information on the latest state-of-the-art treatment, by stage, call NCI's Cancer Information Service at 1-800-4-CANCER (1-800-422-6237), or for a TTY: 1-800-332-8615.

transperineal biopsy (trans-per"ĭ-ne'al bi'op-se) insertion of a needle between the scrotum and rectum to obtain a tissue sample for biopsy (microscopic examination of cancer cells). This may be performed in the diagnosis of PROSTATE CANCER.

transphenoidal hypophysectomy (trans"fĕ-noi'dal hi"po-fi-sek'to-me) surgical removal of a PITUITARY TUMOR by making an incision in the nasal passage to get to the pituitary gland below the brain. Besides being a treatment for pituitary tumors, this was once performed in the treatment of BREAST CANCER and PROSTATE CANCER to eliminate HORMONES produced by the pituitary gland that may stimulate breast and prostate tumors.

transplant a term, when used in a cancer context, that implies infusion of stem cells (no matter how acquired) into a patient to reconstitute bone marrow function after marrow ablative chemotherapy or radiation. See TRANSPLANTATION.

transplantation the removal of a body organ or tissue and its replacement in another part of the body or in another person's body.

transrectal biopsy (trans-rek'tal bi'op-se) insertion of a special needle through the rectum to obtain a tissue sample for microscopic examination for cancer cells. This may be performed in the diagnosis of PROSTATE CANCER.

transrectal ultrasound (trans-rek'tal) an examination of the prostate. This procedure is commonly performed in the diagnosis of PROSTATE CANCER, primarily in the detection of early-stage disease. In the procedure a probe is inserted in the rectum and an ultrasound is taken. This procedure takes a short time and can be done in a doctor's office. See ULTRASOUND.

transurethral resection (TUR) (trans"u-re'thral) a procedure that may be used in the treatment of bladder and prostate cancer. A cystoscope (a lighted, tubular instrument) is put through the urethra into either the bladder or prostate gland. The cancer is either cut away with a small wire loop that is on the end of the cystoscope, or it is burned away with high-energy electricity (fulguration). This treatment can be repeated as often as necessary.

transvaginal sonography See TRANSVAGINAL ULTRASONOGRAPHY.

transvaginal ultrasonography (trans-vaj'ĭ-nal ul"trah-son-og'rah-fe) [transvaginal sonography] the use of an internal vaginal probe in combination with ULTRASOUND for the detection of OVARIAN CANCER. The vaginal probe, available since the late 1980s, can visualize the ovaries on an ultrasound screen better than the traditional external abdominal probe.

transverse abdominal island flap See BREAST RECONSTRUCTION.

transverse loop colostomy (ko-los'to-me) a two-step surgical procedure involving removal of a malignant (cancerous) tumor in the colon—creating an artificial opening through which body wastes are collected outside the body—then rejoining the colon so that the device outside the body is no longer needed and normal functioning is resumed.

See also COLOSTOMY.

trastuzumab See HERCEPTIN.

Treatment IND a program of the Food and Drug Administration that makes certain experimental drugs available to seriously ill people, generally people for whom there is no other available treatment. Drug companies may charge for the drug.

See COMPASSIONATE DRUG.

treatment port the exact place on the body where radiation treatment will be administered. It is determined by X-RAY.

See EXTERNAL RADIATION THERAPY.

treatment-related leukemia a form of LEUKEMIA, usually myeloid (See myelodysplastic syndromes), thought to be a direct consequence of previous exposure to anticancer treatment, either radiotherapy or chemotherapy.

tretinoin See ALL-TRANS RETINOIC ACID.

triamcinolone See ADRENOCORTICOIDS.

triethylene thiophosphora See THIOTEPA.

true cords See VOCAL CORDS.

TSE See TESTICULAR SELF-EXAMINATION.

TSEB See TOTAL SKIN ELECTRON BEAM RADIATION THERAPY.

TSH See THYROID-STIMULATING HORMONE.

TSPA See THIOTEPA.

tuberous sclerosis a genetic disorder in which BENIGN (noncancerous) TUMORS form in the kidneys, brain, eyes, heart, lungs, and skin. This disease can cause seizures, mental disabilities, and different types of skin LESIONS.

tubular ductal breast cancer a relatively rare form of BREAST CANCER occurring about 1% of the time. The tumor has tube-shaped structures ringed with a single layer of cells. It is a well-differentiated carcinoma. It generally has a favorable PROGNOSIS.

tubulovillous polyps See INTERMEDIATE POLYPS.

tumor an abnormal tissue growth or mass on or in the body that serves no useful purpose. A tumor can be benign (noncancerous) or malignant (cancerous). It can be a MIXED TUMOR, meaning it has two or more cell types. Most tumors do not become cancerous. Following are the characteristics that distinguish a benign tumor from a malignant tumor:

- a *benign* tumor grows slowly, has limited growth, and does not destroy normal cells; a *malignant* tumor grows rapidly, destroys normal cells, and has unlimited growth potential
- a *benign* tumor continues to grow in the place where it originated; a *malignant* tumor can spread to other parts of the body
- a *benign* tumor usually does not have serious side effects (the major exception being brain tumors, which grow in a confined space); *malignant* tumors are life threatening
- *benign* tumors grow in an orderly way; *malignant* tumors grow in a disorderly way, unpredictably.

Some tumors are characterized as precancerous. Precancerous tumors do not always become cancerous, but they should be removed, if possible, to avert the possibility of cancer developing.

tumor barrier barriers developed by tumors that prevent chemotherapy (anticancer drugs) from reaching many of the cancer cells in the tumor. An example of a barrier would be an area of collapsed blood vessels. The anticancer drugs that travel through the bloodstream would not be able to reach an area with few or no normal blood vessels. Therefore, the chemotherapy may be able to destroy the outer parts of the tumor but would not be able to eradicate the entire tumor.

tumor debulking surgical removal of as much of a tumor as possible. This is particularly important in the treatment of OVARIAN CANCER.

tumor embolization (em"bo-li-za'shun) obstruction of blood vessels by a tumor. This condition can prevent CHEMOTHERAPY (anticancer drugs) from reaching parts of the tumor.

tumor growth factors (TGF) hormone-like proteins secreted by a cancerous tumor that stimulate the growth of identical cancer cells. MONOCLONAL ANTIBODIES can bind to the substances and inactivate them. Researchers have identified TGF associated with different cancers. For example, TGF-alpha, epidermal growth factor, and fibroblast growth factors are produced by human breast cancer cells that have been stimulated by estrogen.

tumor inhibitory factors (TIF) substances secreted by a cancerous tumor that inhibit the growth of identical cancer cells.

tumor lysis syndrome (li'sis) a side effect that can occur as a result of the administration of chemotherapy (anticancer drugs) to certain very bulky tumors. The tumors grow rapidly and are very sensitive to chemotherapy. A large amount of the tumor may shrink in days, and the products of the breakdown of the tumor can cause potentially dangerous, life-threatening side effects. These side effects can be anticipated, and generally measures are taken to control them.

tumor marker a chemical substance found in increased amounts in the body fluids of some cancer patients. The presence, or elevated level, of a tumor marker in the blood for a specific cancer can be an indication that cancer is present in the body. Tumor markers can be used as part of the diagnostic process but generally cannot provide a definitive diagnosis. Tumor markers are also used to monitor the progress of treatment as well as possible recurrence of cancer after treatment. They may also be used to screen people who have no symptoms of disease. Some tumor markers now in use are:

- alpha-fetoprotein (ALF)—for LIVER, TESTICULAR, STOMACH, PANCREAS, LUNG, and OVARIAN CANCER
- CEA—for COLON/RECTAL CANCER—levels may also be elevated by MELANOMA, LYMPHOMA, and cancers of the breast, lung, pancreas, stomach, cervix, bladder, kidney, thyroid, liver, and ovary
- calcitonin—for medullary cancer of the thyroid, multiple endocrine neoplasia, and myeloma
- prostate-specific antigen (PSA) and prostatic acid phosphatase (PAP)—for prostate cancer
- CA 19-9—for pancreatic cancer
- CA-125—for ovarian cancer—levels may also be elevated by cancers of the uterus, cervix, pancreas, liver, colon, breast, lung, and digestive tract
- lactate dehydrogenase (LDH)—for monitoring treatment of testicular cancer, NON-HODGKIN'S LYMPHOMA, Ewing's sarcoma, and some types of leukemia
- CA 15-3—for recurrent breast cancer—elevated levels may be found in cancers of the ovary, lung, and prostate

- Human chorionic gonadotropin (HCG)—for choriocarcinoma—elevated HCG levels may also indicate the presence of cancers of the testis, ovary, liver, stomach, pancreas, and lung cancer
- CA 27-29—found in the blood of most breast cancer patients—levels may also be elevated by cancers of the colon, stomach, kidney, lung, ovary, pancreas, uterus, and liver
- neuron-specific enolase (NSE)—for neuroblastoma; small cell lung cancer
- pancreatic oncofetal antigen (POA)—an elevated level has been found in about 75% of patients with pancreatic cancer
- thyroglobulin—a high level could be an indication of a recurrence of metastasis of thyroid cancer

tumor necrosis factors (TNF) (ně-kro'sis) TNF is a protein produced in the body that has an important role in immune and inflammatory functions. Its place in the treatment of cancer is being investigated.

tumor nuclear grade a measure of the DIFFERENTIATION of a cancer and its probable aggressiveness. This is assessed by examining nuclei under a microscope to determine the number that are actively undergoing cell division. The PATHOLOGIST also assesses the degree to which structural features of the nuclei differ from normal cells. The grade is on a scale of one to three. The higher the grade number, the more aggressive the cancer and the poorer the PROGNOSIS.

tumor registry [cancer registry] a database created for the collection of information on cancer cases. Most registries are based in hospitals or other medical institutions. Estimates of cancer incidence and survival rates are derived from tumor registry data.

tumor suppressor genes genes in the body that can suppress or block the development of cancer. Suppressor genes have been identified for breast, prostate, lung, and bone cancer. Attempts to exploit this very new discovery in cancer treatment are still in very early stages of investigation.

tumor-infiltrating lymphocytes (TIL) lymphocytes, a type of WHITE BLOOD CELL, that can invade or infiltrate growing tumors and kill cancer cells while sparing normal cells. TIL can be produced in a laboratory by treating the malignant (cancerous) tumor, which has been removed from the patient, with INTERLEUKIN-2 (IL-2). The IL-2 stimulates TIL production and results in an expanded number of lymphoid cells, or TIL. As the TIL increases, the number of cancer cells decreases. Eventually there is a sufficient number of TIL produced to return or transfer to the patient, along with additional IL-2. This is a type of BIOLOGICAL THERAPY under investigation that has shown promise.

TUR   See TRANSURETHRAL RESECTION.

Turcot's syndrome   an inherited condition in which there are multiple POLYPS in the colon. It is a very rare condition and may be associated with BRAIN CANCER (glioma) in some people.

2CdA   See LEUSTATIN.

2-naphthylamine   See CARCINOGENS.

two-step procedure   a term commonly used in BREAST CANCER treatment, referring to the practice of performing a biopsy and, if it is positive (cancerous), surgical treatment on a different day. Until the mid-to late 1970s, a "one step" procedure was routinely performed. A woman would undergo general anesthesia. If the biopsy was positive, the surgeon would then perform a MASTECTOMY. The woman would go into the procedure not knowing if she would awake with a breast removed.

One reason, at the time, for the one-step procedure was that doctors believed the cancer would spread unless the breast was removed immediately. Research has shown that a reasonable delay of several weeks between the biopsy and treatment will do no harm. In addition, the one-step procedure meant the woman would not have to undergo general anesthesia, which involves some risk, two times. At that time a NEEDLE ASPIRATION BIOPSY, which does not require general anesthesia, was rarely performed.

In June 1979, the National Institutes of Health held an International Concensus Development Conference. It was unanimously recommended that diagnostic biopsies and additional treatment be done at different times. Today many women

choose the two-step procedure. It has a number of advantages:

- The biopsy can frequently be done with local anesthesia in a doctor's office or on an outpatient basis at a hospital; since most lumps are benign (noncancerous), the woman avoids unnecessary general anesthesia, which has a risk factor and is also more costly.
- The slides used for the biopsy can be given to another pathologist for a second opinion before follow-up treatment is performed.
- The woman can get a second opinion on treatment options and has the time to make a decision on what treatment she wants.
- Other tests can be performed that may influence the treatment options.
- Plans can be made to have BREAST RECONSTRUCTION performed at the same time that the surgery to remove the breast is performed.
- Last, but not least, the woman has time to emotionally prepare for the loss of a breast.

Proponents of the one-step procedure—performing surgical treatment at the time of the biopsy—say it has its own advantages:

- It spares the woman the anxiety and stress of waiting to have the surgery.
- The risk of any infection in the biopsy wound is eliminated.
- Those women who have to have the biopsy performed under general anesthesia will not have to undergo it twice.

Although Congress has failed to do so, more than a dozen states have passed "informed consent" laws requiring doctors to inform women of all the treatment options in BREAST CANCER including the two-step procedure.

TWSST   stands for *Time Without Symptoms of Disease and Systemic Treatment*. A method of evaluating the efficacy of ADJUVANT TREATMENT of BREAST CANCER based on a measure of quality of life and the recognition that both CHEMOTHERAPY and relapse alter quality of life.

tylectomy   See LUMPECTOMY.

Tylenol   See ANALGESIC and ACETAMINOPHEN.

tyrosine kinase receptors receptors belonging to the tyrosine kinase family (for example, EGFR, PDGFR). They are activated through the auto- or transphosphorylation of tyrosine residues in the cytoplasmic region of the receptors. Protein and peptide hormones, catecholamines like epinephrine, and eicosanoids such as prostaglandins, find their receptors decorating the plasma membrane of target cells. Binding of HORMONE to receptor initiates a series of events, which leads to generation of so-called second messengers within the cell (the hormone is the first messenger). The second messengers then trigger a series of molecular interactions that alter the physiologic state of the cell. Another term used to describe this entire process is *signal transduction*. The receptors for several protein hormones are themselves protein kinases that are switched on by binding of hormone. The kinase activity associated with such receptors results in phosphorylation of tyrosine residues on other proteins. Insulin is an example of a hormone whose receptor is a tyrosine kinase. The hormone binds to domains exposed on the cell's surface, resulting in a conformational change that activates kinase domains located in the cytoplasmic regions of the receptor. In many cases, the receptor phosphorylates itself as part of the kinase activation process. The activated receptor phosphorylates a variety of intracellular targets, many of which are enzymes that become activated or are inactivated upon phosphorylation.

U

UA (urine analysis)   See URINALYSIS.

ultrasonography   See ULTRASOUND.

ultrasound (US) [sonogram, ultrasonography] a relatively new way to locate and measure solid tumors in the body using very high frequency sound waves, which the human ear cannot hear. A small, handheld device called a transducer is used to transmit the sound waves to a site in the body. The transducer is rubbed firmly back and forth over the site after the skin has been lubricated with a special gel. The gel provides the fluid needed to make contact for transmitting the echoes to a computer. When the echoes are produced, they are transformed into pictures (sonograms) by the computer. Tumors, which give off different echoes than normal tissue, can be detected in the pictures.

Ultrasound is noninvasive, painless, without risk, of short duration (generally five minutes to half an hour), and can be done in a doctor's office. While ultrasound can show the presence of a tumor, it cannot tell whether it is benign (noncancerous) or malignant (cancerous).

Ultrasound may be used in the diagnosis of many different cancers, including breast, eye, liver, gallbladder, bile duct, pancreatic, testicular, prostate, kidney, ovarian, uterus, pelvis, thyroid, spleen and in HODGKIN'S DISEASE. It is useful in breast cancer because it can distinguish between a solid lump and a cyst.

ultraviolet radiation (UV)   high-frequency radiation from the Sun that covers the wavelengths between 0 and 400 nanometers. The group of wavelengths between 290 and 330, which are called UV-B, reach the Earth. Because of the depletion of the Earth's ozone layer, more and more of this potentially harmful radiation is reaching the Earth's surface. Exposure to too much UV can cause BASAL and SQUAMOUS CELL SKIN CANCER. It is a major cause of MELANOMA on the skin.

See also SUNSCREEN.

unconventional treatment method [unproven treatment method, unsound treatment method, unorthodox treatment method, alternative treatment] treatment that falls outside the bounds of "mainstream" medicine. In general, unconventional treatments have not undergone scientific testing to establish their benefits and effectiveness. Critics of unconventional treatments may refer to them as unproven, questionable, dubious, unsound, and quackery. Proponents refer to them as alternative, complementary, nontoxic, holistic, natural, and noninvasive. *Unorthodox* is a term that may be used by both critics and opponents. Unconventional methods of treatment continue to be a major area of controversy in the treatment of cancer.

Although most patients in the United States use conventional treatment, there are thousands of patients who follow unconventional treatment. Many patients use an unconventional treatment along with conventional treatment. And there are patients who use unconventional treatment instead of conventional treatment. Among their reasons for using unconventional treatments are:

- for many cancers, especially in advanced stages of the disease, there is no effective treatment
- conventional treatment is frequently very toxic, with side effects ranging from unpleasant to life threatening
- long-term survival may be questionable even after "successful" treatment.

In addition, many patients feel that some unconventional medical treatments offer them more humane care—compassion and psychological support. For some patients, choosing a course of treatment on their own can give them a sense of control at a time when they have very little control over what is happening to their body.

A 1991 study comparing two groups of patients with ADVANCED CANCER, half of whom received unconventional treatment, found no difference in length of survival. However, the report found that the patients receiving conventional treatment had a better quality of life than those getting the unconventional treatment. (It had been hypothesized that the patients getting the less toxic, unconventional treatment would have a better quality of life.)

The questioning and controversy surrounding unconventional treatments came into prominence in the 20th century as a result of several factors. During this century, physicians and their organizations, such as the American Medical Association (AMA), became the "experts" in health care and medical research and set up standards and methods of evaluation for both. In addition, medical advances that led to longer lives also resulted in an increase in chronic diseases with longer and more unpredictable courses. That created a need for new treatments as well as methods to evaluate their effectiveness.

The AMA has been a leader on this front—not only supporting a structured approach to research and enhancing the authority of physicians, but also fighting alleged health fraud, frequently in cancer treatment. In 1962 it formed the Committee on Quackery and the Department of Investigation. The American Cancer Society has also played a major role in discouraging the use of unconven-

tional treatment methods. Its Unproven Methods List is used by doctors as well as insurance companies to determine whether patients should be reimbursed for medical costs.

The Federal Food, Drug and Cosmetic Act (FDCA) and other laws regulate the manufacture, sale, and advertising of medical products. Approval by the Food and Drug Administration (FDA) is required before a drug can be offered to the public. Although in the United States there are generally no legal restrictions on a patient's right to choose a particular treatment, some treatments are simply not available because they involve the use of substances that are not approved and therefore not legally available. In the late 1970s, the U.S. Supreme Court ruled that even terminally ill patients should be protected from potentially unsafe and ineffective medicines.

Unconventional treatments usually fall into four general categories:

- psychological/behavioral
- dietary
- herbal/pharmacological
- biological

The increasing interest in these methods and their possibilities has prompted an increased amount of research into their potential effectiveness. The research has generally focused on whether these methods can have an impact on the immune system and on cancer.

Among the psychological and behavioral methods are IMAGERY and visualization, behavior modification, and psychotherapy. It is commonly accepted that many of these activities can improve the quality of life of the cancer patient. And many physicians accept, support, or even encourage their patients in this direction as long as it is practiced along with conventional therapy. Many advocates of these methods also state that these psychological approaches are *not* a substitute for conventional treatment. However, claims have been made by some that by practicing some of these techniques alone one can boost the immune system and be cured. There is no data that establishes a link between psychological and behavioral methods and the onset or progression of cancer

Among the unconventional dietary treatment methods are the GERSON TREATMENT and the MAC-

ROBIOTIC DIET. As with psychological and behavioral methods, many physicians accept, support, or advocate a nutritional approach *along with* conventional treatment. The American Cancer Society has issued dietary guidelines for cancer prevention that include more fruits, vegetables, and whole grains and less fat, salt-cured, and smoked foods. Unconventional dietary methods can be a problem whey they are used *instead* of conventional treatment. They frequently recommend just a few foods and totally eliminate others; they may recommend the same regimen for all cancer patients regardless of the condition of the patient, type of disease, or stage; or they may claim the diet reverses the course of the disease and improves the quality of life. There is no dietary method that has proven to be a more effective cancer treatment than conventional cancer treatment.

Among the unconventional herbal treatments is Hoxey's herbal tonic treatment, which was declared ineffective by a federal court in the 1950s. Examples of pharmacological and biological treatments include LAETRILE, Revici's "BIOLOGICALLY GUIDED CHEMOTHERAPY," Burton's IMMUNOAUGMENTATIVE THERAPY (IAT), and Burzyncki's treatment with antineoplastons. There have been no controlled studies that have proven these treatments to be effective methods of treatment for cancer.

An unconventional treatment, when used in place of a conventional treatment, can pose a potential risk for patients on several fronts. Valuable time in the treatment of a life-threatening disease may be lost when using an unconventional treatment instead of a conventional treatment that has been proven to be of benefit in CLINICAL TRIALS. Many cancers have a good chance of being cured when detected and *treated* early. Besides not curing or controlling cancer, an unconventional treatment may in itself be harmful and can result in greater suffering. For example, one clinic that was offering "immune system augmentation" was shut down when it was discovered that some of the serum being used in the treatment contained the deadly AIDS virus.

The NATIONAL CANCER INSTITUTE recommends that cancer patients remain in the care of physicians who use "accepted and proven methods"; it warns that the use of unconventional cancer treatments may result in a loss of time and reduce the chance for a cure or control of the cancer; and it points out the availability of experimental or investigational forms of treatment for patients where there is no STANDARD TREATMENT available, or when the standard treatment has not been effective, and advises those patients to ask their doctors about clinical trials.

The American Society of Clinical Oncology developed the following questions for consideration in regard to any unproven cancer treatments:

- Is the treatment based on an unproven theory?
- Is there a purported need for *special nutritional support?*
- Is there a claim for *painless, nontoxic* treatment?
- Are claims published only in the mass media and not in reputable peer-review scientific journals?
- Are claims for benefit merely compatible with a PLACEBO EFFECT?
- Are the major proponents *recognized experts* in cancer treatment?
- Do proponents claim benefit for use with proven methods of cancer treatment? for prolongation of life? for use as a cancer preventative?
- Is there a claim that only specially trained physician can produce results with the drug?
- Is the method of drug preparation a secret?
- Is there an attack on the medical and scientific establishment?
- Is there a demand by promoters for "freedom of choice" regarding drugs?

Unproven methods can be dangerous and deadly when a person forgoes conventional treatment for a treatment that has not been proven to be effective. It can also be very costly, as insurance companies do not reimburse for unproven treatments.

See NATIONAL CENTER FOR COMPLEMENTARY AND ALTERNATIVE MEDICINE.

undifferentiated cells cells that lack specialization in structure and function. As cells "mature" they take on distinct characteristics and their adult function. As cancer cells reproduce, the new cells are undifferentiated, unable to carry on normal activity. The more undifferentiated, or abnormal, the cells appear under a microscope, the more malignant (cancerous) the cells are, and the more active and uncontrollable the cancer is likely to be.

undifferentiated large cell lung cancer See NON-SMALL CELL LUNG CANCER.

undifferentiated small cell lung cancer See SMALL CELL LUNG CANCER.

unilateral salpingectomy (sal"pin-jek'to-me) surgical removal of one fallopian tube. This may be performed in the treatment of cancer of the female reproductive organs as well as other disorders.

unilateral salpingo-oophorectomy surgical removal of an ovary that is malignant (cancerous) and the fallopian tube on the same side. This may be performed in the treatment of OVARIAN CANCER.

unknown primary [occult primary, carcinoma of unknown primary (CUP)] a condition in which cancer has been diagnosed, but it is not known where it originated. This is more common in cancers that may not have symptoms in the early stage of disease. Most large studies have shown that an unknown primary cancer often starts in the lungs or pancreas. Less often, it may start in the colon, rectum, breast, or prostate. For example, prostate cancer may not be found until it has metastasized (spread) to the bone. When pain is experienced in the bone, metastatic cancer may be found in the bone, and additional diagnostic testing reveals that the cancer started in the prostate. In as many as 9% of the cancers that are diagnosed with an unknown primary site, the site of origin is never discovered. Cancer with an unknown primary does not have a good PROGNOSIS. Treatment usually depends on where the metastatic cancer was found and the cell type. Many different treatments are used either alone or in combination. Some of the treatments that are used are surgery, radiation therapy, chemotherapy, and hormonal therapy.

unorthodox treatment method See UNCONVENTIONAL TREATMENT METHOD.

unproven treatment method See UNCONVENTIONAL TREATMENT METHOD.

unsound treatment method a treatment that is unsafe or ineffective in treating disease.
See also UNCONVENTIONAL TREATMENT METHOD.

upper GI series (UGIS) [barium swallow, barium milkshake] an examination of the esophagus, stomach and/or small intestine by X-RAY using the CONTRAST MEDIUM BARIUM. Before the procedure is started the stomach must be completely empty. X-rays are taken as the patient swallows small amounts of barium. When only the esophagus is being examined this procedure may be referred to as an ESOPHAGOGRAPHY, in which case the stomach does not have to be empty. An upper GI series can be done at the doctor's office or at the hospital on an outpatient or inpatient basis and can take anywhere from 30 to 90 minutes. It may be performed in the diagnosis of cancer of the stomach, small intestine or esophagus as well as other illnesses such as ulcers and esophagitis (an inflammation of the esophagus).

ureteral cancer (u-re'ter-al) cancer of the tubes going from the kidneys to the bladder. This is a fairly rare cancer occurring most frequently in people over the age of 60. The American Cancer Society estimates there were 2,450 new cases for ureter/other urinary organ cancer in the United States in 2004 (1,570 new male cases and 880 new female cases), with about 690 deaths from the disease in that year. It is about four times more likely to appear in men as in women. SMOKING appears to be a risk factor since most people who develop ureteral cancer are smokers.

Symptoms may include blood in the urine and pain or cramps in the back. Frequent and painful urination occurs in about half the people diagnosed with ureteral cancer. Procedures used in the diagnosis of ureteral cancer may include URINALYSIS, CYSTOSCOPY, URETEROPYLOSCOPY, and IVP.

Treatment depends on the stage of the disease, the general state of the patient's health, and other factors. Surgery is generally performed. RADIATION THERAPY may be used as a palliative treatment. CHEMOTHERAPY has been used very rarely. For the latest state-of-the-art treatment, call the National Cancer Institute's Cancer Information Service at 1-800-4-CANCER (1-800-422-6237), or for a TTY: 1-800-332-8615.

ureteropyloscope See URETEROPYLOSCOPY.

ureteropyloscopy (u-re"ter-o-pi"ĕ-los'sko-pe) an examination of the urinary tract, bladder, ureters, and kidney with a lighted instrument (ureteropyloscope) that allows access to that part of the body. A ureteropyloscope can remove tissue for microscopic examination for cancer cells. It may also be used to remove small tumors. A ureteropyloscopy may be used in the diagnosis of KIDNEY CANCER and URETERAL CANCER as well as other disorders.

ureterosigmoidostomy (u-rē″ter-o-sig″moi-dos′to-mē) a surgical technique used in the treatment of BLADDER CANCER that creates a urinary diversion using a lower portion of the large bowel. This averts the need for an outside STOMA (surgical opening) for removal of urine from the body. The procedure carries the risk of some side effects. There is an increased possibility of infection in the kidney and biochemical blood changes.

ureters (u-rē′ters) tubes that carry urine from the kidneys to the bladder.

urethra (u-rē′thra) the tube in the body that carries urine from the bladder to the openings through which it passes out of the body. In women, the urethra is about one and a half inches long and opens above the vaginal opening. In men, it is about eight inches long and goes through the prostate and the penis to the outside of the body.

urethral cancer a very rare cancer arising in the tube that empties urine from the bladder. Women develop urethral cancer about twice as often as men, which makes it the only cancer of the urinary tract to occur more often in women.

Women are at the greatest risk in their 60s. Infection and chronic irritation may be predisposing factors. There may be no early signs of urethral cancer. When symptoms do occur, they may include urethral or vaginal bleeding, urinary frequency, burning, pain, vaginal discharge, and painful intercourse. These can be symptoms of other disorders as well.

Urethral cancer can occur in men starting in their teenage years through their 80s, although it occurs most commonly in men aged 55 to 60. Predisposing factors may include a history of chronic infection, irritation, and obstruction of the urethra. Venereal disease or frequent urethral dilations may also be significant. Symptoms may include urethral bleeding, a bloody or foul-smelling discharge, difficulty in urination, and pain in the groin. These can be symptoms of other disorders.

A physical exam for a lump in the urethra will be done if there are symptoms. In men, a CYSTOSCOPY may be performed. The NATIONAL CANCER INSTITUTE (NCI) stages urethral cancer by location and whether it has spread:

- Anterior—cancer in the part of the urethra that is closest to the outside of the body; these tumors are likely to be noninvasive
- Posterior—cancer in the part of the urethra that connects to the bladder; this tumor is more likely to invade nearby tissue
- Urethral cancer associated with invasive bladder cancer—the patient also has bladder cancer
- Recurrent—cancer has returned to the same site or to another part of the body after treatment

Treatment depends on the stage of the disease and other factors. Surgical treatments that may be used include FULGURATION, LASER THERAPY, CYSTOURETHRECTOMY, PENECTOMY (in men), CYSTOPROSTATECTOMY (in men), or ANTERIOR EXENTERATION (in women). For specific information on the latest state-of-the-art treatment, by stage, call NCI's Cancer Information Service at 1-800-4-CANCER (1-800-422-6237), or for a TTY: 1-800-332-8615.

urethrogram (u-rē′thro-gram) See URETHROGRAPHY.

urethrography (u-rē″throg′rah-fe) examination of the urethra by X-RAY for the presence of a TUMOR or suspicious area. This procedure may be used in the diagnosis of cancer in the URETHRA of men.

urinalysis (u″rĭ-nal′ĭ-sis) [urine analysis (UA)] examination of urine. It may be performed in the diagnosis of KIDNEY CANCER as well as in many benign disorders. The degree of concentration of the urine compared with plain water is called specific gravity (SG) and can be an indication of a urinary obstruction. The amount of acidity, protein, sugar, and ketones (organic compounds) in the urine can indicate acidosis or alkalosis, kidney damage, diabetes, and other disorders. A urine sediment exam checks for red cells, white cells, kidney cells, crystals, and microorganisms. It may be used in the diagnosis of urinary tract cancers, especially bladder cancer, as well as kidney damage, urinary tract infection, or gout.

urinary diversion   creation of a new way to eliminate urine when the bladder and/or URETHRA has been removed. The standard procedure used to be formation of a STOMA, or surgical opening through which urine passed. The urine would be emptied into a flat bag located outside the body. Newer forms of urinary diversion have made an external urinary device unnecessary in many cases. Surgeons try to use the newer techniques whenever possible. See CONTINENT ILEAL RESERVOIR, BRICKER'S POUCH, CAMEY PROCEDURE, ILEAL BLADDER, and URETEROSIGMOIDOSTOMY.

urinary tract cancer   cancer occurring in any of the organs in the urinary tract (kidneys, bladder, urethra). See KIDNEY CANCER, BLADDER CANCER, URETERAL CANCER, URETHRAL CANCER, and PROSTATE CANCER.

urine sediment test   See URINALYSIS.

urogram   See UROGRAPHY.

urography (u-rog'rah-fe)   an X-RAY examination of the kidneys, bladder, ureters, and urethra. This may be performed in patients who cannot tolerate an IVP. It may be used in the diagnosis of urinary tract cancers as well as other disorders.

urologist (u-rol'o-jist)   a medical doctor who specializes in diseases that affect the kidneys, ureters, urethra, bladder, prostate gland, and male sex organs. A urologist is an expert in diagnosis and in surgical treatment in the urologic area. A board-certified urologist has two years of postmedical training, three years of training in urologic surgery, and 18 months of independent practice. In addition, he or she has passed the written and oral exams given by the board.

uroprotective   a drug given to protect the urinary bladder from the irritative effects of some CHEMOTHERAPEUTIC agents. See MESNA.

urostomy   See OSTOMY.

urticaria (ur"tĭ-ka're-ah) [hives]   an allergic reaction marked by itching welts. This may be a side effect of CHEMOTHERAPY. They may appear at the site of a chemotherapy (anticancer drug) injection or on other parts of the body. The hives may develop along the vein through which the chemotherapy was administered as well as other locations. The hives usually disappear within several hours.

US   See ULTRASOUND.

uterine cancer   See ENDOMETRIAL CANCER.

uterine sarcoma (u'ter-ine sar-ko'mah)   an extremely rare type of ENDOMETRIAL CANCER. It accounts for between 1 and 5% of all endometrial (uterine) cancers. Symptoms include bleeding after menopause (the time when women no longer have menstrual periods) or bleeding that is not part of menstruation. Following are the NATIONAL CANCER INSTITUTES (NCI) STAGINGS for uterine sarcoma:

- Stage I—cancer is found only in the main part of the uterus (it is not found in the cervix)
- Stage II—cancer cells have spread to the cervix
- Stage III—cancer cells have spread outside the uterus but have not spread outside the pelvis
- Stage IV—cancer cells have spread beyond the pelvis, to other body parts, or into the lining of the bladder (the sac that holds urine) or rectum
- Recurrent—the cancer has come back (recurred) after it has been treated

Treatment for uterine sarcoma is based on the guidelines used in the treatment of SARCOMA in any part of the body.

uterography   See HYSTEROGRAPHY.

uterus [womb]   a hollow organ in the body of a woman in which the fetus develops.

uterus cancer   See ENDOMETRIAL CANCER.

UV   See ULTRAVIOLET RADIATION.

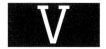

VAB a combination of the anticancer drugs VIN-BLASTINE, COSMEGEN, BLEOMYCIN, CISPLATIN, and CYTOXAN sometimes used in the treatment of KIDNEY, BLADDER, and PROSTATE CANCER. See individual drug listings for side effects.

See also COMBINATION CHEMOTHERAPY.

VAC a combination of the anticancer drugs VIN-CRISTINE, ADRIAMYCIN, and CYTOXAN sometimes used in the treatment of SMALL CELL LUNG CANCER. See individual drug listings for side effects.

See also COMBINATION CHEMOTHERAPY.

vaccine tumor vaccines are another form of biological therapy currently under study. Vaccines for various diseases are effective because the immune system can develop acquired immunity to disease after initial exposure to it. This occurs because when T cells and B cells are activated, some of them become memory cells. The next time the same antigen enters the body, the immune system remembers how to destroy it. Researchers are developing tumor vaccines that may encourage the immune system to recognize cancer cells in this way. Tumor vaccines may help the body reject tumors and also help prevent cancer from recurring. Researchers are also investigating ways that tumor vaccines can be used in combination with biological response modifiers (BRMs). Tumor vaccines are being studied in treating melanoma, renal cell cancer, colorectal cancer, breast cancer, prostate cancer, and lymphomas.

vacuum aspiration See ENDOMETRIAL ASPIRATION.

vacuum curettage (ku″rĕ-tahzh′) See ENDOMETRIAL ASPIRATION.

VAD See VENOUS ACCESS DEVICE.

VAD a combination of the anticancer drugs VIN-CRISTINE, ADRIAMYCIN, and DECADRON sometimes used in the treatment of MYELOMA. See individual drug listings for side effects.

See also COMBINATION CHEMOTHERAPY.

vagina the passageway in a woman's body between the cervix and the vulva. Menstrual fluid passes out of the body through the vagina and a baby travels through the vagina during childbirth. The vagina is sometimes called the birth canal.

vaginal cancer (vaj′in-al) a rare cancer accounting for less than 2% of gynecological cancers. It occurs most often in women over the age of 50. In 2004, there were about 2,160 new cases of vaginal cancer and 790 deaths resulting from the disease, according to the American Cancer Society. However, an even more rare form of vaginal cancer called CLEAR CELL ADENOCARCINOMA may be found in young women and adolescents. This type of cancer is strongly associated with DES (diethylstilbestrol). It is believed that daughters of women who took DES (to prevent miscarriage) between 1945 and 1971 are at a risk of developing clear cell adenocarcinoma. DES daughters should have regular gynecological checkups for any signs of precancerous changes.

Symptoms of vaginal cancer may include bleeding or discharge not related to menstruation, difficult or painful urination, pain during sexual intercourse, and pain in the pelvic area. These can be symptoms of other disorders as well. Procedures that may be used in the diagnosis of vaginal cancer include a PELVIC EXAM, PAP SMEAR, and BIOPSY. Whitish, raised patches on the surface of the vagina may be a precancerous condition.

Following is the NATIONAL CANCER INSTITUTE'S (NCI) STAGING for vaginal cancer:

- Stage 0 (carcinoma in situ)—cancer is only in the vagina in a few layers of cells
- Stage I—cancer is in the vagina but has not spread outside it
- Stage II—cancer has spread to the tissues just outside the vagina but has not gone into the bones of the pelvis
- Stage III—cancer has spread into the bones of the pelvis; it may also have spread to other organs and the LYMPH NODES in the pelvis
- Stage IV
  IVA—cancer has spread into the bladder or rectum
  IVB—cancer has spread to other parts of the body, such as the lungs
- Recurrent—cancer has returned to the same site or to another part of the body after treatment.

Treatment depends on the stage of the disease, the general state of health of the patient, and other factors. Surgery is the most common treatment for all stages of vaginal cancer. The various surgical options include LASER THERAPY, wide local excision (removal of the cancer and tissue around it), VAGINECTOMY, RADICAL HYSTERECTOMY, and EXENTERATION. RADIATION THERAPY and CHEMOTHERAPY may also be used. For specific information on the latest state-of-the-art treatment, by stage, call NCI's Cancer Information Service at 1-800-4-CANCER (1-800-422-6237), or for a TTY: 1-800-332-8615.

vaginal estrogen cream   See ESTROGEN CREAM.

vaginal fibrosis (vaj'in-al fi-bro'sis) the growth of adhesions from fibrous tissue in the vagina. This can be a result of RADIATION THERAPY or the cancer itself. Vaginal fibrosis can make sexual intercourse difficult and painful for a woman.

vaginal hysterectomy (vaj'in-al his"ter-ek'to-me) surgical removal of the uterus and cervix through the vagina. It has the advantage of not leaving a scar. Its major disadvantage is that the surgeon is unable to see the full extent of the cancer. For that reason, a vaginal hysterectomy is generally not recommended for women with cancer.

vaginal pool aspiration   See ENDOMETRIAL ASPIRATION.

vaginal reconstruction (vaj'in-al) the use of plastic surgery to make an artificial vagina using segments of the intestine. A woman's ability to have sexual intercourse is usually restored with this surgery. Surgical removal of the vagina in the treatment of cervical, vaginal, and urethral cancers necessitates the reconstruction.

vaginectomy (vaj"ĭ-nek'to-me) surgical removal of the vagina. This procedure may be performed when it is the only way to remove all the cancer in the vagina VAGINAL RECONSTRUCTION may be needed.

vaginoscopy   See COLPOSCOPY.

valium   See ANTIEMETIC.

VAP a combination of the anticancer drugs VINCRISTINE, L-ASPARAGINASE, and PREDNISONE sometimes used in the treatment of childhood ALL. See individual drug listings for side effects.

See also COMBINATION CHEMOTHERAPY.

vascular leak syndrome an adverse drug reaction characterized by leaking of PLASMA from within the blood vessels into the surrounding tissue, and by two or more of three clinical findings: hypotension (low blood pressure), edema (tissue swelling), and decreased serum albumin. This is caused by many of the drugs classified as MONOCLONAL ANTIBODIES, among others. It is a serious shocklike condition requiring urgent treatment.

vasectomy (vah-sek'to-me) a minor surgical procedure in which a man is sterilized. The passageway through which the sperm must pass in ejaculation is cut. A study in Scotland found TESTICULAR CANCER in eight of 3,079 men who had a vasectomy. Only about two cases would be expected to be found in a group of that size. Other studies have found no association between vasectomy and testicular cancer. It is not known why vasectomy would promote tumor growth.

VATH a combination of the anticancer drugs VINBLASTINE, ADRIAMYCIN, and THIOTEPA sometimes used in the treatment of BREAST CANCER. See individual drug listings for side effects.

See also COMBINATION CHEMOTHERAPY.

VB a combination of the anticancer drugs VINBLASTINE and BLEOMYCIN sometimes used in the treatment of KIDNEY, BLADDER, and PROSTATE CANCER. See individual drug listings for side effects.

See also COMBINATION CHEMOTHERAPY.

VBAP a combination of the anticancer drugs VINCRISTINE, BCNU, ADRIAMYCIN, and PREDNISONE sometimes used in the treatment of MYELOMA. See individual drug listings for side effects.

See also COMBINATION CHEMOTHERAPY.

VBC a combination of the anticancer drugs VINBLASTINE, BLEOMYCIN, and CISPLATIN sometimes used in the treatment of MELANOMA. See individual drug listings for side effects.

See also COMBINATION CHEMOTHERAPY.

VBP a combination of the anticancer drugs VINBLASTINE, BLEOMYCIN, and PREDNISONE sometimes used in the treatment of KIDNEY, BLADDER, and PROSTATE CANCER. See individual drug listings for side effects.

See also COMBINATION CHEMOTHERAPY.

VC a combination of the anticancer drugs ETOPOSIDE and CARBOPLATIN sometimes used in the treatment of SMALL CELL LUNG CANCER. See individual drug listings for side effects.

See also COMBINATION CHEMOTHERAPY.

VCAP a combination of the anticancer drugs VINCRISTINE, CYTOXAN, ANDRIAMYCIN, and PREDNISONE

sometimes used in the treatment of MYELOMA. See individual drug listings for side effects.

See also COMBINATION CHEMOTHERAPY.

VDP a combination of the anticancer drugs VINBLASTINE, DTIC, and CISPLATIN sometimes used in the treatment of MELANOMA. See individual drug listings for side effects.

See also COMBINATION CHEMOTHERAPY.

VEGF (vascular endothelial growth factor) on a molecular level, the VEGF Pathway is considered one of the key regulators of ANGIOGENESIS, the formation of new BLOOD vessels. The pharmaceutical industry has actively been working to develop agents that block VEGF and its receptor, as drugs that would have ANTIANGIOGENESIS properties. Among the agents in this category are AVASTIN and BAY43-9006.

Velban See VINBLASTINE.

vena caval syndrome (ve'nah ka'val) See SUPERIOR VENA CAVAL SYNDROME.

venacavography (ve"nah-ka-vog'rah-fe) an X-RAY of the renal (kidney) vein. This may be done in the diagnosis of KIDNEY CANCER.

venography (ve-nog'rah-fe) an X-RAY of any of the blood veins after administration by injection of a dye into a vein. The dye is injected into the site to be examined. It generally takes less than an hour and usually can be done by a radiologist. This procedure may be used in the diagnosis of different types of cancer, including kidney cancer, as well as to outline points of blood flow obstruction caused by clots or various tumors (e.g., ovarian, rectal).

venous of or relating to veins.

venous access device (VAD) (ve'nus) a general term to describe the use of a soft, plastic catheter in the treatment of a cancer patient. The catheter is placed in a vein for a variable duration of time to allow the administration of treatment with chemotherapy (anticancer drugs), antibiotics, nutritional support, or other medical products as well as the drawing of blood from the body. In a sense, any intravenous (IV) procedure is a VAD in that it provides access into the bloodstream. However, the term is generally applied to those newer materials that may be able to remain in place for longer periods of time—weeks, months, or indefinite periods. These IVs for long-term use are placed in one of the larger veins in the body (e.g., the subclavian under the collarbone) and are usually inserted by a surgeon.

There are two basic kinds of VADs. One type, such as the HICKMAN CATHETER, extends slightly out of the body; the other type, such as a MEDIPORT, is completely under the skin and a special (Huber) needle is used for access. A VAD may be removed at any time.

VADs do present some risk, in performing the procedure and possible infection and blood clotting after insertion. However, they have several advantages. Frequent blood drawing, for example, which is necessary in the care of a person with leukemia, may be done without pain. Certain anticancer drugs must be given through one of these "deep" veins (a large vein so opposed to a hand or arm vein) because of the irritation they can cause to the skin when given in a more superficial vein.

ventriculography (ven-trik"u-log'rah-fe) an X-RAY examination of the heart chambers or brain. When the heart is being examined, a special CONTRAST MEDIUM is injected into an artery before the X-ray is taken. If the brain is being examined, X-rays are taken after the cerebral spinal fluid has been displaced by the injection of air into the ventricles of the brain. Asymmetrical air patterns may indicate brain cancer.

VePesid   See ETOPOSIDE.

verapamil (ver-ap'ah-mil) [VPAM]   a drug traditionally used to treat high blood pressure that is being investigated for its use in treating cancer in combination with CHEMOTHERAPY (anticancer drugs). It appears that verapamil may help alleviate the resistance of some cancer cells to chemotherapy in the following way. Some normal cells and cancer cells contain what is described as a pump called P-glycoprotein. When an anticancer drug enters the cell, the pump pushes it out again. The pumps push out other drugs as well, such as verapamil. In an early trial verapamil was used on some patients who

had not been helped by chemotherapy. When large doses of verapamil were administered, along with the chemotherapy, many of the patients went into remission. Researchers believe that while the pumps are busy pushing out the verapamil, the chemotherapy can enter the cell (through the back door, so to speak) and do its job—kill the cancer cell. The use of verapamil to overcome drug resistance is still investigational and promising. It is not, as yet, part of any standard therapy.

See MULTIDRUG RESISTANCE.

Vesanoid   See ALL-TRANS RETINOIC ACID.

vesicant   an intravenous drug that causes tissue blistering and/or tissue death if it leaks into the surrounding tissue (muscle, skin). A VENOUS ACCESS DEVICE (VAD) is recommended for the administration of these agents.

VH gene   in CHRONIC LYMPHOCITIC LEUKEMIA (CLL), the variable region of the immunoglobulin heavy chain gene, when mutated, imparts a favorable prognosis. The CLL patients with an unmutated VH gene have progressive disease and a shorter survival time than those with the mutated gene. Thus the VH gene status may be used as a prognostic test. The test is, however, not universally available for routine clinical use (as of 2005).

Vidaza [Azacytadine or AZC]   the first chemotherapy drug FDA-approved (2004) for treatment of MYELODYSPLASTIC SYNDROME (MDS). It is given intravenously (IV).

video surgery   a fairly new technique that enables a surgeon to operate by viewing the site in the body via a very tiny TV camera and monitor. This surgery greatly reduces the amount of cutting that is traditionally required for surgery. Surgical tools are inserted into the body through very small incisions. The surgeon guides the instrument by watching the monitor screen, which is enlarged up to 18 times. The recovery time after this procedure is much faster. The patient may be able to leave the day the surgery is performed instead of spending a week or more in the hospital. Video surgery has been used in the diagnosis and treatment of a number of different cancers including cancers of the prostate, lung, colon, gallbladder, pancreas, and ovaries.

villous polyps (vil'us pol'ips) small, benign (noncancerous) growths found in the colon that may become cancerous. About 3 to 4% of the people in the United States have villous polyps. An estimated 40% become malignant (cancerous). Villous polyps bleed easily and may cause the passage of mucus with bowel movements. When present, the polyps should be removed, and patients should be monitored for their reappearance. The polyps return in about 50% of the cases.

vinblastine (vin-blas'tēn) [Velban] an anticancer drug sometimes used in the treatment of cancers in the head and neck, breast, kidney, and testes and LYMPHOMA and KAPOSI'S SARCOMA. It is given by IV (injection into a vein). A common side effect is BONE MARROW DEPRESSION, along with the burning pain where the needle was inserted if any of the drug leaks out during its administration. Occasional or rare side effects may include nausea, vomiting, hair loss, mouth sores, loss of reflexes, severe constipation, skin rashes, mental depression, headaches, and diarrhea. Vinblastine is an important anticancer drug in the treatment of a variety of cancers.

vinblastine amide sulfate   See VINDESINE.

vincristine (vin-kris'tēn) [Oncovin] an anticancer drug derived from the periwinkle plant that is sometimes used in the treatment of cancers of the breast, brain, testes, and cervix as well as LYMPHOMA, acute leukemias (ALL), WILMS' TUMOR, NEUROBLASTOMA, and RHABDOMYOSARCOMA. It is given by IV (injection into a vein). Hair loss is a common side effect, along with a burning pain where the needle was inserted if any of the drug leaks out during its administration. Occasional or rare side effects may include arm, leg, jaw, or stomach pain, numbness or tingling in hands or feet, BONE MARROW DEPRESSION, severe constipation, metallic taste, hoarseness, and mental depression. Vincristine is a widely used anticancer drug and important in the treatment of cancer.

vindesine (vin'dĕ-sēn) [Eldisine, vinblastine amide sulfate] a drug under investigation for its use in the treatment of LYMPHOMA, MELANOMA, LEUKEMIA, and cancers of the lung, colon, breast, and testes. It is given by IV (injection into a vein). Common side effects may include BONE MARROW DEPRESSION, burning pain where the needle was inserted if the drug leaks out during IV, loss of reflexes, and loss of hair. Occasional or rare side effects may include nausea, vomiting, jaw pain, constipation, loss of taste, fatigue, tiredness, skin rash, mouth sores, loss of appetite, and diarrhea.

vinorelbine   See NAVELBINE.

vinyl chloride   See CARCINOGENS.

viral oncology (ong-kol'o-je) the study of the role of viruses in the development of cancer.

Virchow's node   a LYMPH NODE in the left side of the neck. An enlarged and firm node is a possible sign and site of spread of STOMACH CANCER.

virtual colonoscopy [computed tomography] an alternative method for evaluation of the colon (searching for COLON CANCER or potentially PRE-CANCEROUS conditions, such as bleeding or polyps) using X-RAY technology instead of the traditional colonoscope.

virus   a submicroscopic microbe that causes infectious disease. Viruses can reproduce only in living cells. Scientists estimate that as many as 5% of the cases of cancer in the United States are related to a virus.

The role of viruses in the development of cancer is not completely understood. The first evidence of a virus causing cancer was observed in 1908 in Denmark in the transmission of avian leukemia in chickens. However, it was not until the 1950s that there was a real interest in the role of viruses in cancer, which prompted a surge in research.

It does not appear that viruses in and of themselves cause cancer; rather, it is likely that the presence of other factors, such as an infection with a second virus, a compromised immune system, or exposure to environmental factors, makes the person more susceptible to the virus-linked cancers.

Viruses that have been associated with cancer include the HERPES SIMPLEX, EPSTEIN-BARR VIRUS, the HUMAN PAPILLOMA VIRUS, and the RETROVIRUSES, including HTLV and HIV. Cancers thought to be linked, in some way, to a virus are hepatocellular carcinoma (see LIVER CANCER), BURKITT'S LYM-PHOMA, immunoblastic lymphoma, NASOPHARYN-GEAL CANCER, cervical neoplasia, skin cancer, adult T-cell leukemia-lymphoma (ATLL), and HAIRY CELL LEUKEMIA.

visualization   See IMAGERY.

vitamins   chemicals found in foods that play a role in body function. These chemicals are essential in minute quantity for normal health. For example, the absence of vitamin C can cause scurvy. There is evidence that some vitamins may contribute to cancer prevention as well as to cure. Investigations into the use of naturally occurring and synthetic vitamins are being conducted worldwide. There are still many unanswered questions, including dosage and side effects. Following are some of the vitamins being investigated:

- vitamin A—found in liver, eggs, and milk. Vitamin A has been found to play a role in the treatment of skin cancers and is being investigated for its use in the treatment of MYELOID LEUKEMIA. Beta carotene (a dietary source of vitamin A) is found in carrots, winter squash, broccoli, spinach, and cantaloupe. Beta-carotene appears to have a part in cancer prevention (see ACCUTANE).
- vitamin B—LEUCOVORIN is a synthetic form of vitamin B.
- vitamin C—found in many fruits and vegetables. Vitamin C has been investigated for its role in both preventing and treating cancer. Preliminary evidence from animal experiments and human population studies suggests that vitamin C may inhibit the development of some forms of cancer, in particular, cancer of the ESOPHAGUS, COLON, LUNG, and STOMACH. However, two large studies supported by the National Cancer Institute found that patients with advanced cancer derived no benefits from vitamin C therapy.
- vitamin D—preliminary findings indicate that vitamin D may play a role in the prevention of colon CANCER. It is being investigated, along with vitamin A, for its use in the treatment of MYELOID LEUKEMIA.
- vitamin E—laboratory studies suggest that vitamin E may inhibit the formation of some natural cancer-causing agents. There is no strong evidence for a protective effect of vitamin E.

The American Cancer Society recommends including foods rich in vitamins A, C, and E in the daily diet.

VM-26   See TENIPOSIDE.

vocal cords [true cords]   the two small shelves of muscular tissue adjacent to the LARYNX that vibrate against each other to generate sound.

voice box cancer   See LARYNGEAL CANCER.

voice-button fistula procedure   a technique for speech for people who have had a laryngectomy (voice box removed). A small rubber device (voice button) is surgically inserted in the back of the throat. Sounds can then be made by expelling air through the esophagus.

vomiting   See EMESIS.

VP-16   See ETOPOSIDE.

VP-16213   See ETOPOSIDE.

VPAM   See VERAPAMIL.

VP/L asparaginase   a combination of the anticancer drugs VINCRISTINE, PREDNISONE, and L-ASPARAGINASE. See individual drug listings for side effects.
     See also COMBINATION CHEMOTHERAPY.

VP/Vidaribine   See PENTOSTATIN.

vulva   the external parts of the female genitalia; the fatty folds of flesh surrounding the opening of the vagina.

vulvar cancer   a rare cancer accounting for 3 to 4% of gynecological cancers. The women most commonly affected are over the age of 50 or 60. However, it is now being seen more frequently in women under the age of 40. The American Cancer Society estimated that 3,870 women would be diagnosed with vulvar cancer in 2005, with 870 deaths from the disease in that year. Many patients who develop vulvar cancer have had a history of chronic vulvar dystrophy, a thickened, whitish area associated with chronic irritation. LEUKOPLAKIA in the vulva may also develop into cancer. Many doctors consider leukoplakia a PRECANCEROUS CONDITION and advocate treatment. Other doctors think regular follow-up exams are sufficient.

Symptoms of vulvar cancer may include itching, burning, pain, and bleeding. These symptoms may also be caused by an INFECTION. Procedures used in the diagnosis of vulvar cancer may include a PAP SMEAR, COLPOSCOPY, and BIOPSY. Following is the NATIONAL CANCER INSTITUTE's STAGING for vulvar cancer:

- Stage 0 or in situ—cancer is located entirely in the vulva
- Stage I—cancer is confined to the vulva, is less than two CENTIMETERS (cm) in diameter; there is no evidence of spread to the LYMPH NODES
- State II—cancer is confined to the vulva, is larger than 2 cm; there is no evidence of spread to the lymph nodes

- Stage III—cancer has spread to adjacent tissues such as the urethra, vagina, and anus or to the lymph nodes
- Stage IV—cancer has invaded the mucosa of the bladder or rectum; it has spread to other areas of the body such as the lungs
- Recurrent—cancer has returned to the same site or to another part of the body after treatment.

Treatment depends on the stage of the disease and other factors. The most common form of treatment is surgery, which may include a wide local excision (removal of the cancer and some tissue surrounding it), LASER THERAPY, VULVECTOMY, or PELVIC EXENTERATION. RADIATION THERAPY may also be used.

vulvectomy (vul-vek'to-me)   removal of the vulva.
See SIMPLE VULVECTOMY and RADICAL VULVECTOMY.

Vunom   See TENIPOSIDE.

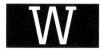

Waldenstrom's macroglobulinemia (vahl'den-stremz mak"ro-glob"u-lǐ-ne'me-ah) an extremely rare, chronic form of lymphoproliferative (a rapid, abnormal growth of lymphoid tissue) disorder affecting B LYMPHOCYTES (a type of WHITE BLOOD CELL). The abnormal cell resembles a lymphocyte and a PLASMA CELL and produces an abnormal protein that is responsible for many of its symptoms. In many aspects, the illness behaves like MYELOMA in that it arises in a BONE MARROW cavity and causes bone defects and the protein products also impair health. It occurs primarily in men over the age of 60. It progresses very slowly.

Symptoms may include weakness, fatigue, drowsiness, paleness, a tendency to bleed easily, fever, weight loss, dizziness, headaches, and LYMPH NODE enlargement. Some patients may develop a condition known as hyperviscosity (thickening of the blood). This can result in a sluggish blood flow leading to a stroke and other problems. Treatment for Waldenstrom's macroglobulinemia is very similar to that for MYELOMA. RITUXAN is also used, as is INTERFERON.

warning signs (of cancer) general symptoms in the body that may be an indication of cancer. Following are the most common warning signs of cancer:

- a change in bowel or bladder habits
- a sore that does not heal
- unusual bleeding or discharge
- a thickening or lump in the breast or elsewhere
- indigestion or difficulty in swallowing
- an obvious change in a wart or mole
- a nagging cough or hoarseness.

These are *very general* and can be an indication of many other disorders. A doctor should be consulted for any problem that lasts two weeks. See individual cancers for specific warning signs or symptoms.

wart a BENIGN (NONCANCEROUS) growth on the skin caused by a VIRUS.

wasting syndrome See CACHEXIA.

WBC See WHITE BLOOD COUNT.

wedge resection surgical removal of a cancerous lump and the tissue surrounding it. It is used in the early stages of some cancers. When appropriate, it is the treatment of choice because the entire ORGAN is not removed. The term "wedge resection" is frequently associated with a LUMPECTOMY for the treatment of breast cancer, but it is performed in the treatment of many other cancers as well.

Wellcovorin See LEUCOVORIN CALCIUM.

Wellferon See ALPHA INTERFERON and INTERFERON.

Wertheim's operation   See RADICAL HYSTERECTOMY.

Whipple procedure   surgical removal of the head of the PANCREAS, part of the SMALL INTESTINE, and some of the surrounding tissue. Enough of the pancreas is left to continue making digestive juices and insulin. However, there is concern that cancer cells may be left behind when this surgery is performed. The Whipple procedure is the oldest and least-extensive operation for PANCREATIC CANCER.

white blood cells [leukocytes]   a general term for a variety of cells in the blood that play a major role in the body's immune system, which defends the body against disease. White blood cells are produced primarily in the bone marrow, but other organs, such as the lymph nodes, the spleen, and the thymus, can produce some as well. Many white blood cells are known as phagocytes—which is simply a term used for any large white blood cell that can engulf and destroy microorganisms and foreign particles. MONOCYTES and MACROPHAGES are two important PHAGOCYTES.

There are three major types of white blood cells: monocytes, granulocytes, and lymphocytes. Following is a brief description of each group and their subgroups.

Monocytes make up 5 to 10% of the circulating white blood cells. They help defend the body against bacterial infection. Monocytes circulate through the blood before entering tissue, where they develop into macrophages. Macrophages engulf and destroy foreign substances, such as bacteria, in the body. They secrete chemical substances including enzymes, proteins, and regulatory factors such as interleukin-1. Macrophages, which are often called "scavengers," rid the body of worn-out cells and debris.

Granulocytes (also called myelocytes and polymorphonuclear cells) fight bacteria by engulfing and destroying them. They contain potent chemicals that enable them to digest microorganisms. There are three major types of granulocytes:

- neutrophils—account for 60% of all the circulating white blood cells and are the most prevalent of the granulocytes. They can pass through capillary walls to engulf and destroy invading bacteria. They play a major role in the body's defense against bacteria, viruses, and fungi.

- basophils—account for less than 1% of the white blood cells in the body. They contribute to inflammatory reactions and allergic reactions.
- eosinophils—make up a very small part of the white blood cells. They contain chemicals that are damaging to parasites and enzymes that damp down inflammatory reactions.

Lymphocytes make up between 20 and 40% of the circulating white cells and are the most important cells in the immune system. They are responsible for regulating and carrying out most of its activities. The major types of lymphocytes are:

- T CELLS (also called T lymphocytes)—attack and destroy virus-infected cells, foreign tissues, and cancer cells. They work mainly by secreting substances known as cytokines or, more specifically, lymphokines—powerful chemicals that play a major role in the immune system. Gamma interferon is one lymphokine. There are a number of different types of T cells
   — regulatory T cells—play a major role in regulating the immune system. They activate B cells, other T cells, natural killer cells, and macrophages
   — cytotoxid T cells (also called killer cells)—directly attack infected or malignant (cancerous) cells. However, they also reject tissue and organ grafts
- B CELLS (also called B lymphocytes)—produce antibodies that help destroy foreign substances. The antibodies fight foreign substances in the body that could cause infections, disease, or poisoning. Each B cell produces one specific antibody. For example, one B cell may produce antibodies to fight a particular bacteria, while another B cell may produce antibodies to fight a flu virus
- natural killer cells (NK cells)—a type of lymphocyte that contains potent chemicals capable of killing tumor cells. NK cells bind to the "target" cell and then release a lethal burst of the chemicals. They are thought to play a major role in cancer prevention by destroying abnormal cells before they have a chance to pose a real threat

white blood count (WBC)   the number of white blood cells in a sample of blood. This is important because a low level of white blood cells can make a person susceptible to infections. When a white blood count is too low, the administration of anticancer drugs may be postponed.

See also COMPLETE BLOOD COUNT.

whole-body irradiation [total-body irradiation (TBI)] external RADIATION THERAPY administered to the entire body. This has been used in the past as a treatment for some forms of LEUKEMIA. Its role in the current treatment of cancer is not certain. Whole body radiation may also be a treatment performed during a BONE MARROW TRANSPLANTATION. Side effects may include sterility, early menopause, or cataracts.

wide core needle biopsy See CORE NEEDLE BIOPSY.

Wilms' tumor [nephroblastoma]   the most common KIDNEY CANCER occurring in children. It was first described by Dr. Max Wilms in 1899. About 500 new cases of Wilms' tumor are diagnosed in the United States every year. It accounts for between 6 and 8% of childhood cancer, affecting one child in about 10,000. It generally occurs in young children, under the age of seven, with most cases in children aged one to four. Boys and girls are equally affected.

The cause is not known. Wilms' tumor seems to be unrelated to race, climate, or environment and does not appear to be linked to birth order or weight or other factors associated with birth, such as the mother's age or a history of previous stillbirths. About 10% of children with the disease have some kind of CONGENITAL abnormality. Researchers believe that there are both hereditary (caused by a defective gene) and nonhereditary forms of the disease. The hereditary type is more likely to arise in younger children and in both kidneys. It is not known if the children of people who have had Wilms' tumor are at a greater risk of developing the cancer.

The major symptom of Wilms' tumor is a swelling on one side of the upper abdomen. Other symptoms may include blood in the urine, low-grade fever, loss of appetite, paleness, weight loss, and lethargy. These symptoms can be signs of other disorders. Procedures used in the diagnosis and evaluation of Wilms' tumor may include blood test

and URINALYSIS, IVP, CT SCAN, SELECTIVE RENAL ARTERIOGRAPHY, URETEROPYLOSCOPY, ULTRASOUND, BONE MARROW TEST, and MRI.

Following is the NATIONAL CANCER INSTITUTE's (NCI) STAGING for Wilms' tumor:

- Stage I—cancer is confined to the kidney and is completely removed by surgery
- Stage II—cancer extends beyond the kidney and is not completely removed with surgery
- Stage III—cancer extends beyond the kidney and is not completely removed during surgery; residual cancer cells are known to have been left in the abdomen after surgery
- Stage IV—cancer has spread from the kidney to other structures in the body such as the bones, lungs, liver, or brain
- Stage V—cancer involves both kidneys
- Recurrent—cancer has returned to the original site or to another part of the body after treatment

Treatment depends on the stage of the disease, the general state of health of the child, and other factors. Treatment frequently requires the use of surgery, RADIATION THERAPY, and CHEMOTHERAPY. For specific information on the latest state-of-the-art treatment, by stage, call NCI's Cancer Information Service at 1-800-4-CANCER (1-800-422-6237), or for a TTY: 1-800-332-8615.

womb See UTERUS.

womb cancer See ENDOMETRIAL CANCER.

workup jargon, generally applied to a diagnostic evaluation which may require blood tests, scans, and other diagnostic tests.

Womens Health Study (WHS) An ongoing NUTRITIONAL INTERVENTION STUDY launched in the United States in 1993. The study enrolled 38,876 women 45 years of age or older, and examined the effects of ASPIRIN, Vitamin E, and/or beta-carotene on cardiovascular disease and cancer. The part of the study examining the effects of beta-carotene was discontinued in 1996, because of concerns over a negative impact of beta-carotene, but the other components of the study continue (as of 2006).

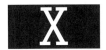

Xeloda [capecitabine]   Xeloda is an anticancer medicine (CHEMOTHERAPY) used for treating cancer of the colon after surgery (adjuvant). Xeloda is also used to treat COLORECTAL or BREAST CANCER that has spread to other parts of the body (METASTATIC CANCER).

xeroderma pigmentosum (ze"ro-der'mah pig-men-to'sum)   a rare hereditary disease in which the skin and eyes are extremely sensitive to light. People with xeroderma pigmentosum are 1,000 times more likely to develop MELANOMA than the general population.

xerogram   See XEROGRAPHY.

xerography (ze-rog'rah-fe) [soft tissue radiography, xeroradiography]   an X-RAY that produces detailed images of fat, muscle, blood vessels, and other soft tissues. The pictures are printed on a special photographic paper instead of on film. This type of X-RAY can be used in the diagnosis of SOFT TISSUE SARCOMA and BREAST CANCER as well as other disorders.

xeromammography (ze"ro-mam-mog'rah-fe)   an examination of the breast similar to MAMMOGRA-PHY, but the pictures are produced on a special paper instead of film. It uses less radiation than the conventional mammography.

See also XEROGRAPHY.

xerostomia (ze"ro-sto'me-ah)   a condition characterized by a dry mouth that occurs when saliva production is inadequate or absent. It can be a side effect of radiation therapy or chemotherapy. RADIATION THERAPY to the salivary glands is a major cause. Xerostomia usually begins seven to ten days after the start of treatment and in some cases is permanent. Other causes of xerostomia may include a tumor in the salivary region, dehydration, antihistamines, narcotics, drugs containing atropine, infections inside the mouth, and the use of tobacco and alcohol.

Insufficient saliva can result in an inadequate amount of starches. It can also irritate or damage the mucous membranes in the mouth, cause mouth sores and infections, make chewing solid food difficult, cause an alteration in the taste of foods, and cause difficulty in speaking.

Following are some things people with xerostomia can do to eliminate or reduce the problem:

- drink water and other nonirritating beverages several times an hour
- lubricate the lips with a water-based lubricant, cocoa butter, or a lip balm
- suck on smooth, flat sugarless candy, lozenges, or ice chips
- eat moist foods like ice cream and fruit, moisten dry foods with butter, gravy, sauces, and/or broth
- dunk dry foods in liquids such as coffee, tea, milk

- humidify the air with a pan of water near a heater, a cold water vaporizer, or a humidifier

If saliva impairment is permanent, artificial saliva, available by prescription, may be necessary. One artificial saliva is Salivart.

X-ray [Roentgen ray] high-energy electromagnetic waves of very short length that can penetrate the body and produce pictures. X-rays can be used in the diagnosis of disease as well as treatment (see RADIATION THERAPY). Since the first X-rays were discovered by William Roentgen, in 1895, there have been tremendous technological advances in diagnostic X-rays, and today they play a major role in the diagnosis of virtually every type of cancer as well as many other diseases. Between 1970 and 1980 the use of X-rays increased substantially. In 1980, an estimated 180 million were performed in the United States. The number increased to more than 265 million in 1985.

The risks involved in diagnostic X-rays have decreased with the improvement of X-ray machines and techniques. Possible risks associated with diagnostic X-rays include the development of leukemia, genetic mutations that will affect future generations, and effects on an embryo and fetus due to exposure during pregnancy. Based on data collected by the United Nations Scientific Committee on the Effects of Atomic Radiations (UNSCEAR), it is estimated that a few thousand deaths per year may be a result of diagnostic X-rays. That is less than 1% of the 1 million cancers diagnosed in the United States each year. It is widely felt in the medical field that the benefits greatly outweigh any risk when a diagnostic X-ray is performed for an important medical reason.

Diagnostic X-rays can be done with or without the injection or ingestion of a contrast medium, frequently radioactive. A hot spot (an area of the body seen on the X-ray film where the radioactive substance has accumulated) may be an indication of a cancerous area.

Following are X-rays used in the diagnosis of cancer (as well as other disorders):

- ANGIOGRAPHY—examination of blood vessels with a contrast medium
- BRONCHOGRAPHY—examination of the lungs and windpipe branches with a contrast medium
- CHOLANGIOGRAPHY—examination of the liver's bile ducts with a contrast medium
- CHOLECYSTOGRAPHY—examination of the gallbladder and bile ducts with a contrast medium
- CT SCAN—a combination of X-ray and computer to obtain a cross-sectional picture of an organ
- CYSTOGRAPHY—examination of the bladder with a contrast medium
- DUODENOGRAPHY—examination of the part of the small intestine that connects with the stomach and pancreas with a contrast medium
- ENDOSCOPIC RETROGRADE CHOLANGIOPANCREATOGRAPHY (ERCP)—examination of the pancreas with a contrast medium
- FLUOROSCOPY—an X-ray that can show tissues and organs "in action" on a screen similar to a television screen
- HYSTEROGRAPHY—examination of the uterus and fallopian tubes with a contrast medium
- INSUFFLATION—an X-ray taken after powder, vapor, gas, or air is blown into a hollow space in the body
- IVP—examination of the urinary tract with a contrast medium
- LOWER GI SERIES—examination of the colon with barium, a contrast substance
- LYMPHANGIOGRAPHY—examination of the lymph system and lymph nodes with a contrast dye
- MAMMOGRAPHY—examination of the breasts
- MYELOGRAPHY—examination of the spinal cord with a contrast medium
- NEPHROTOMOGRAPHY—examination of the kidneys with a contrast medium
- PERITONEOGRAPHY—examination of the membrane lining the abdomen
- PNEUMOALVEOLOGRAPHY—examination of the air sacs of the lungs
- PNEUMOANGIOGRAPHY—examination of lung blood vessels with a contrast substance
- PNEUMOGRAPHY—examination of a specific part of the body such as the bladder, stomach, brain, spinal column, and mediastinum after injection of a gas such as oxygen
- PORTOGRAPHY—examination of the veins that carry blood to the liver from the stomach, intestine, spleen, and pancreas with a contrast medium
- RETROGRADE PANCREATICODUODENOGRAPHY—examination of part of the small intestine and pancreas with a contrast medium

- RETROGRADE PYELOGRAPHY—examination of the urinary system with a contrast medium
- UROGRAPHY—examination of the kidneys, bladder, urethra, and ureters
- VENOGRAPHY—examination of the blood veins with a contrast medium
- VENTRICULOGRAPHY—examination of the brain after injection of oxygen into the ventricles

- XEROGRAPHY—examination of fat, muscles, blood vessels, and other soft tissue.

See individual listings for details about each procedure.

X-ray therapy or treatment   See RADIATION THERAPY.

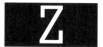

Zanosar See STREPTOZOCIN.

ZAP-70 an intracellular protein rarely present in normal B lymphocytes, but has been found in B CELLS from some patients with CLL (chronic lymphocitic leukemia). The measurement of this protein in patients with CLL can serve as a clinical test (2004) and predict for a more aggressive course of this disease. Some practitioners use the measurement of this protein as a guide for when to recommend RX in CLL.

ZDV See AZT.

ZDX See ZOLADEX.

Zevalin (Ibritumomab Tiuxetan) A RADIOPHARMACEUTICAL used in treatment of relapsed or refractory low grade, follicular or transformed B-cell NON-HODGKINS LYMPHOMA (NHL). The material links the MONOCLONAL ANTIBODY IBRITUMOMAB (directed against the CD-20 ANTIGEN found on the surface of normal and malignant B lymphocytes) with radioactive Indium-III and Yttrium-90. The material is given by INTRAVENOUS (IV) INFUSION in several steps over several days usually by nuclear medicine personnel as the injectable Zevalin therapeutic regimen. The regimen consists of several steps, two low doses of RITUXIMAB, an imaging dose, two or three whole body scans, and a therapeutic dose (Yttrium-90). Thus radiation is brought directly to the tumor cells.

The major toxicities are infusion-related allergic symptoms and MYELOSUPPRESSION. One to 2% of patients develop a HUMAN ANTI-MOUSE ANTIBODY (HAMA).

zidovudine See AZT.

Zinecard [dexrazoxane] An iron-chelating agent used to prevent or reduce the incidence and severity of doxorubicin cardiomyopathy (a condition affecting the heart muscle). It may be given to women whose doctors feel they would benefit from continuing therapy with ADRIAMYCIN. Common side effects may include mild nausea, vomiting, and hair loss. Occasional or rare side effects may include bone marrow depression, diarrhea, skin rash, flu-like symptoms, mouth sores, and headache. It is given by IV (injected into a vein).

zinostatin [neocarzinostatin] a drug being investigated for its use in the treatment of acute leukemia (ALL), MELANOMA, and cancers of the pancreas, bladder, and stomach. It is administered by IV (injected into a vein), IM (injected into a muscle), or subcutaneously (under the skin). Possible side effects may include BONE MARROW DEPRESSION and burning pain where the needle was inserted if the drug leaks out during IV. Occasional or rare side effects may include nausea, vomiting, diarrhea, loss of appetite, fever, liver problems, skin rash, chills, headache, mouth sores, fatigue, and lung problems.

Zofran [ondansetron] an ANTIEMETIC drug that has proven to be of benefit to some patients taking the toxic anticancer drug CISPLATIN. It is one of a new class of drugs that blocks SEROTONIN. Zofran appears to dramatically reduce episodes of nausea and vomiting that generally follow the administration of cisplatin. Zofran may also have side effects including headache, constipation, fatigue, and diarrhea, although they are not common. It is given by IV (injected into a vein).

Zoladex [ZDX, goserelin, acetate] a drug that blocks the production of male hormones by the testes. Zoladex is administered by depot (a pellet of the drug is injected beneath the skin of the abdomen, where it slowly releases the drug over a month's time). Side effects may include impotence and hot flashes. Zoladex may be used in the treatment of PROSTATE CANCER. It is also indicated as a PALLIATIVE TREATMENT of advanced BREAST CANCER in pre- and postmenopausal women.

Zometa Zoledronic Acid Injection a bisphosphonate given via IV injection, indicated to treat malignant HYPERCALCEMIA. It is also indicated as an adjunct in patients with MULTIPLE MYELOMA and other cancers with proven BONE METASTASIS to delay further bone destruction.

zoster an encircling structure or pattern. Zoster is used to describe an infection with the herpes zoster virus, which is a cause of SHINGLES.

Zyloprim See ALLOPURINOL SODIUM.

APPENDIXES

NOTEWORTHY WEB SITES OF NATIONAL ORGANIZATIONS FOR CANCER AND AIDS

AIDS Info
http://www.actis.org
Toll free: 1-800-HIV-0440 (1-800-448-0440)
Fax: 1-301-519-6616
Outside U.S.: 1-301-519-0459
TTY: 1-888-480-3739
Spanish-speaking health information specialists are
available.

A service of the U.S. Department of Health and
Human Services (HHS), Information on AIDS
Treatment, Prevention, and Research, including
clinical trials, guidelines, and vaccines. AIDS Info's
comprehensive Web site offers a "Search" option,
along with live help, as well as help for Spanish-
speaking people.

AMC Cancer Research Center
http://www.amc.org
1600 Pierce Street
Denver, CO 80214
Toll free: 1-800-321-1557
Tel: 1-303-233-6501

AMC Cancer Research Center is a 501(c)(3) not-
for-profit research institute dedicated to the prevention and control of cancer and other chronic
diseases. AMC was founded in 1904 as the Jewish
Consumptives Relief Society (JCRS), a tuberculosis sanitarium in Denver, Colorado. JCRS treated
all tuberculosis patients, including the indigent. It
was a self-sustaining hospital community, with its
own farm, dairy, printing press, etc., and the JCRS
received financial aid from a nationwide network
of volunteers collecting donations on its behalf. In
the 1950s, AMC helped to finally bring tuberculosis under control. JCRS leaders decided to devote
their resources to conquering cancer, and became
AMC Cancer Research Center. Information is provided on the causes, prevention, detection, diagnosis, and treatment of cancer, as well as treatment
facilities, rehabilitation, and counseling services.

American Brain Tumor Association
http://hope.abta.org/site
2720 River Road
Des Plaines, IL 60018
Tel: 1-847-827-9910
Toll free/Patient line: 1-800-886-2282
Fax: 1-847-827-9918
E-mail: info@abta.org

ABTA offers a searchable Web site on the association and its services, including patient education,
advocacy, meetings and events, donation options,
as well as information on support groups and
investigational treatment, and research.

American Cancer Society (ACS)
http://www.cancer.org

Toll free: 1-800-ACS-2345
TTY: 1-866-228-4327

The ACS Web site is a comprehensive, searchable site (including information in Spanish as well as Asian language materials) that offers a tremendous amount of information for patients, families, survivors, friends, and supporters. The site even offers searchable information and key statistics for each type of cancer. It also offers free registration for the site. Visitors who register get access to personalized features, including the special "tools," that enable you to join online communities of people who share similar interests. You can also track appointments, save important articles, and keep tabs on local ACS events you're interested in for the ACS network of volunteers, supporters, and survivors. ACS is a nationwide voluntary health organization with 13 chartered divisions throughout the United States and a presence in most communities. The ACS has more than 3,400 local offices nationwide that are organized to deliver cancer prevention, early detection, and patient services programs at the community level. It supports and funds research; provides education on cancer prevention, early detection, and treatment; and provides services for cancer patients and their families. Among the programs sponsored by the ACS are Reach to Recovery, Road to Recovery, I Can Cope, Look Good . . . Feel Better, Can Surmount, Man to Man, Hope Lodge, and the "tlc" catalog at (800) 850-9445. ACS has numerous free publications.

American Urological Association
http://www.afud.org
1000 Corporate Boulevard
Linthicum Heights, MD 21090-2260
Toll free: 1-800-242-2383
Tel: 1-410-689-3700
E-mail: admin@afud.org

The American Urological Association Foundation is a partnership of physicians, researchers, healthcare professionals, patients, caregivers, families and the public established to support and promote research, patient/public education and advocacy that improve the prevention, detection, treatment and cure of urologic disease. Patients can browse the UrologyHealth.org site for the doctor-created source for reliable urological information. Referrals to a urologist in your area are also available on UrologyHealth.org. Free pamphlets on prostate and bladder cancer; sponsors US TOO support groups for prostate cancer patients.

American Institute for Cancer Research (AICR)
http://www.aicr.org
1759 R Street NW
Washington, DC 20009
Toll free: 1-800-843-8114 (weekdays 9:00 A.M. to 5:30 P.M. EST)
Local: 1-202-3288-77
Fax: 1-202-328-7226
E-mail: aicrweb@aicr.crg.

The American Institute for Cancer Research provides information on nutrition and cancer; registered dieticians are available to talk with callers.

American Liver Foundation
http://www.liverfoundation.org
75 Maiden Lane, Suite 603
New York, NY 10038
Toll free: 1-800-GO-LIVER (1-800-465-4837)
Toll free: 1-888-4HEPUSA (1-800-443-7872)
Tel: 1-212-668-1000
Fax: 1-212-483-8179

The American Liver Foundation (ALF) is the nation's leading nonprofit organization promoting liver health and disease prevention. ALF provides research, education and advocacy for those affected by hepatitis and other liver-related disease. Although liver disease is among the 10 major causes of death in the United States, there was no national voluntary health agency devoted exclusively to combating liver diseases until 1976, when the American Liver Foundation was formed. The Web site is comprehensive, offering information on liver health, the different chapters around the country, news and events, and clinical trials; visitors to the Web site may also order materials from the foundation.

American Heart Association
http://www.americanheart.org

National Center Mailing Addresses:
American Heart Association
National Center

7272 Greenville Avenue
Dallas, TX 75231
AHA: 1-800-AHA-USA-1 (1-800-242-8721)

American Stroke Association (ASA)

National Center
7272 Greenville Avenue
Dallas, TX 75231
Toll free: 1-888-4-STROKE (1-888-478-7653)

This comprehensive Web site offers a wealth of information, ranging from diet and nutrition help to summaries of key research and a means to access free scientific journal content; the American Heart Association (AHA) also focuses on issues relating to strokes. Visitors to the Web site who take the AHA's "Learn and Live" quiz can receive a free cookbook with heart-healthy recipes; you can also access a free online "Heart and Stroke Encyclopedia" and search for local events via your zip code, among many other resources. The Web site has an interactive feature, is searchable, and is accessible in Spanish. You can also contact the AHA with any questions via the Web site.

American Lung Association

http://www.lungusa.org
61 Broadway, 6th Floor
New York, NY 10006
Tel: 1-212-315-8700
Toll free: 1-800-LUNG-USA (1-800-586-4872)
To speak to a lung health professional, contact the American Lung Association Call Center at 1-800-548-8252.

The American Lung Association (ALA) offers this comprehensive, full-service Web site that enables visitors to access a tremendous amount of information on lung cancer, asthma, hay fever, and chronic obstructive pulmonary disease (COPD), among other issues. You can search for your local ALA chapter, get information on news and events (including local smoking cessation programs, lectures, and fundraising events), sign up for an e-newsletter, and make your voice heard via the ALA's "take action" activities. The Web site has an interactive feature, is searchable, and is accessible in Spanish.

American Medical Association

http://www.ama-assn.org

515 North State Street
Chicago, IL 60610
Toll free: 1-800-621-8335

Primarily a Web site for its physician members, the AMA has expanded the patient section to include patient education materials, advocacy information, a searchable database to help patients find doctors ("Doctor Finder"), and online access to a bookstore, among many other functions. The AMA has also created "doctor appreciation cards," that patients can download and personalize for their own physicians.

American Society for Dermatologic Surgery (ASDS)

http://www.asds-net.org
5550 Meadowbrook Drive Suite 120
Rolling Meadows, IL 60008
Tel: 1-847-956-0900
Fax: 1-847-956-0999
E-mail: info@asds.net

Toll free (800) 441-2737 for requesting information only; you can leave your name and address and specify which procedures you are interested in, and information will be mailed to you.

The Web site offers information on dermatologic surgery in a special section for patients. The Web site also offers information on the various stages of skin aging, facts sheets, "before and after" photos, and links to other related Web sites.

American Society of Plastic and Reconstructive Surgeons

http://www.plasticsurgery.org
Plastic Surgery Educational Foundation
444 East Algonquin Road
Arlington Heights, IL 60005
Plastic Surgeon Referral Service: 1-888-4-PLASTIC (1-888-475-2784)

This Web site provides names of board-certified plastic surgeons in a specific area as well as free publications. It has many excellent features, including a special section honoring people who have shown tremendous courage when facing reconstructive surgery under the most difficult circumstances, including breast cancer.

Bone and Marrow Transplant Newsletter (BMTN)

http://www.bmtinfonet.org/newsletters

BMT InfoNet
2310 Skokie Valley Road, Suite 104
Highland Park, IL 60035
Tel: 1-847-433-3313
Fax: 1-847- 433-4599
E-mail: help@bmtinfonet.org
Toll free: 1-888-597-7674 to subscribe to blood and marrow transplant newsletter, order other publications, or reach a member of the staff.

BMT InfoNet publishes a quarterly newsletter for bone marrow, peripheral stem cell, and cord blood transplant patients, and has all of the newsletters online, going back to 1992; access is free; on the site you will also find many other resources, including information on transplant centers, how to receive e-newsletters, and a listing of "helpful services."

Bone Marrow Foundation
http://www.bonemarrow.org
337 East 88th Street, Suite 1B
New York, NY 10128
Tel: 1-212-838-3029
Toll free: 1-800-365-1336

There is also a Bone Marrow Transplant Family Support Network—1-800-826-9376—where you can leave a message; matches up by telephone newly diagnosed cancer patients with patients with a similar diagnosis who have undergone the treatment.

Brain Tumor Society
http://www.tbts.org
84 Seattle Street
Boston, MA 02134-1245
Tel: 1-617-783-0340
E-mail: info@tbts.org
Toll free: 1-800-770-8287

The Brain Tumor Society provides educational materials and professional support; it also runs a network of peer-support volunteers.

CancerCare
http://www.cancercare.org
275 Seventh Avenue
New York, NY 10001
Tel: 1-212-712-8400

Toll free: 1-800-813-HOPE (4673)
E-mail: info@cancercare.org

CancerCare is a national nonprofit social service agency that provides services (usually free of charge) to help patients and family members cope with the emotional and financial consequences of cancer. The CancerCare Web site is comprehensive and offers a gateway to all of the services offered by the organization, including counseling, education, an online newsletter, financial assistance and practical help, as well as information on workshops and events. The Web site divides the services into different categories: CancerCare Connect, CancerCare Counseling, CancerCare Inform, and CancerCare Assist. All are free of charge and provided by trained oncology social workers CancerCare.

CancerCare offers toll-free teleconferences on various cancer issues, and and provides free publications including its *Connect Booklet, Coping With Cancer: Tools to Help You Live,* for help in understanding the challenges that are a part of living with cancer. This booklet offers concrete tips to help you deal with some of the most common cancer questions. You may also request a free printed version by e-mailing publications@cancercare.org with your name, address, and the title of the booklet. Healthcare professionals may order the booklet in packets of 10.

Cancer Information Service
http://cis.nci.nih.gov

In the United States: contact the National Cancer Institute's Cancer Information Service (CIS) at 1-800-4-CANCER (1-800-422-6237) Monday through Friday from 9:00 A.M. to 4:30 P.M. local time to speak with a Cancer Information specialist.
Toll free: 1-800-332-8615

From outside the United States, contact the International Union Against Cancer (UICC). A list of international resources is also available.
E-mail: cancernet@icicb.nci.nih.gov

The National Cancer Institute's (NCI's) Cancer Information Service (CIS) is a national information and education network. The CIS is a free public service of the NCI, the U.S. agency for cancer research. The CIS site is fully searchable and contains fact sheets, as well as news about cancer research and findings. The site also offers free booklets, either online or via mail, and offers assistance to smokers who want to quit smoking.

Candlelighters Childhood Cancer Foundation
http://www.candlelighters.org
P.O. Box 498
Kensington, MD 20895-0498
Tel: 1-301-962-3520
Toll free: 1-800-366-CCCF (1-800-366-2223)
Fax: 1-301-962-3521
E-mail: staff@candlelighters.org

This organization was founded by the parents of children with cancer to help families cope with the emotional stresses of their experience. It has various publications available and provides bereavement counseling, pain management information, and a program on insurance concerns. There are about 50,000 members of the national offices and some 100,000 members across the country.

CanSurmount
http://www.cancer.ca/ccs
Peer Support Assistant: 1-204-786-0616
Toll free: 1-800-263-6750.
E-mail: infor@cis.cancer.ca

CanSurmount is the Web site for the Manitoba division of the Canadian Cancer Society.

Centers for Disease Control and Prevention (CDC)
http://www.cdc.gov
1600 Clifton Road NE
Atlanta, GA 30333
Tel: 1-404-639-3311
Public inquiries: 1-800-311-3435
E-mail: netinfo@cdc1.cdc.gov

The CDC is a federal agency and one of the 13 major operating components of the Department of Health and Human Services (HHS), the principal agency in the U.S. government charged with protecting the health and safety of Americans. The CDC has a comprehensive, fully searchable Web site, with links to other Web sites of interest, a searchable job database, news, and even a link to information on the latest health-related hoaxes or rumors that may be circulating around the Internet. The CDC also provides information on different forms of cancer, cancer research, and community resources.

Chemotherapy.com
http://www.chemotherapy.com

Chemotherapy.com is a Web site created by Amgen, a biotechnology company that manufactures chemotherapy drugs, along with many other therapeutic drugs. The tagline for the Web site is "easing the chemotherapy journey." The site is thus organized for people with cancer and their caregivers and families as a central resource for people undergoing chemotherapeutic treatment. There are also links to other resources, including resources for people choosing not to undergo chemotherapy. The site offers a ChemoCoach feature that patients/caregivers/family members can register for and receive updates for preparing for or managing the process of chemotherapy.

Children's Hospice International (CHI)
http://www.chionline.org
901 North Pitt Street, Suite 230
Alexandria, VA 2231
Tel: 1-703-684-0330
Toll free: 1-800-2-4-CHILD (1-800-242-4453)
E-mail: chiorg@aol.com

CHI provides a network of support for terminally ill children and their families. It serves as a clearinghouse on research programs and support groups. Pain management publications are available on a variety of topics, including home care for children with cancer.

Children's Oncology Camping Association International
http://www.coca-intl.org

Children's Oncology Camping Association International (C.O.C.A.) is an international assembly of people providing camping programs for children with cancer. The association is made up of member camps that serve a broad range of special needs populations but that share the common thread of working with children with cancer. The site offers information for members, volunteers, and those interested in the services, as well as conferences, events, and links to various resources.

Conversations: The International Newsletter for Those Fighting Ovarian Cancer
http://www.ovarian-news.org

P.O. Box 7948
Amarillo, TX 79114-7948
Tel: 1-806-355-2565
Fax: 1-806-467-9757

This Web site offers information and a connection for those fighting ovarian cancer. Pen-pal and phone-pal networks are available.

Corporate Angel Network (CAN)

http://www.corpangelnetwork.org
Westchester County Airport
One Loop Road
White Plains, NY 10604-1215
Tel: 1-914-328-1313
Fax: 1-914-328-3938
Toll free patient line: 1-866-328-1313
E-mail: info@corpangelnetwork.org

CAN finds free air travel on corporate jets for cancer patients and one attendant or family member in need of transportation for treatment, consultations, or checkups. CAN is supported entirely by contributions from individuals, foundations, and corporations. Its tagline is, "An empty seat is a lost opportunity. Give a cancer patient a lift." The Web site offers information for patients, potential donors, and all interested in the CAN services.

DES Cancer Network (DCN)

http://www.descancer.org
Tel: 1-800-DES-NET (1-800-337-6384)

The DES Cancer Network is an organization that addresses the special needs of women who have had clear cell adenocarcinoma of the vagina and/or cervix—a cancer linked to exposure to DES before birth. Current statistics indicate that 746 women in the United States are registered as having had this cancer, 62% of whom were DES exposed in utero. Membership is available to any individual interested in participating in the work of the DES Cancer Network. The mission of the DES Cancer Network is providing recovered patients with ways to contact one another and to support new patients who have been diagnosed or are undergoing treatment. The DCN is also a support group to the family and friends of DES daughters who are clear cell cancer survivors as well as those who have lost loved ones to the disease. DCN also serves as a resource to health care professionals and attorneys whose patients/clients have had

clear cell cancer. To get in touch with someone working for the DES Cancer Network, e-mail the organization at DESnetwrk@aol.com.

ENCORE

http://www.encore.net.au
YWCA of Australia
P.O. Box 1022
Dickson, ACT 2602
Toll free: 1800 305 150
E-mail: encore@ywca.org.au

Encore (of the YWCA, Australia) is an exercise program designed specifically for women who have experienced mastectomy, lumpectomy, or breast reconstruction surgery at any time in their lives. It is based around floor and pool exercises and relaxation techniques. The program includes water-resistance exercises that are gentle but effective, and the warm water relaxes and relieves affected muscles. Encore can help strengthen and tone arms, shoulders, and chest, regain mobility, and improve general fitness. Encore is funded throughout Australia by AVON.

Gilda Radner Familial Ovarian Cancer Registry

http://www.ovariancancer.com
Roswell Park Cancer Institute
Department of Gynecologic Oncology
Elm and Carlton Streets
Buffalo, NY 14263
1-716-845-3110.
Toll free: 1-800-OVARIAN (1-800-682-7426)

This Web site keeps track of/monitors families in which two or more members have had ovarian cancer; provides general counseling, support groups, and help with genetic screening. In addition to ovarian cancer research, the registry offers a help line and education, information, and peer support for women with a high risk of ovarian cancer. It is named after Gilda Radner, the comedienne who died in 1989 at age 43 of ovarian cancer. The Web site offers many links to resources as well.

Hereditary Cancer Institute (HCI)

http://medicine.creighton.edu/hci
Creighton University School of Medicine
California at 24th
Omaha, NE 68178
Tel: 1-402-280-2942

HCI studies family linked cancer and provides free cancer-risk information, genetic counseling, and cancer and nutrition information.

Hole in the Wall Gang Camp
www.holeinthewallgang.org
565 Ashford Center Road
Ashford, CT 06278
Tel: 1-860-429-3444
Fax: 1-860-429-7295
E-mail: ashford@holeinthewallgang.org

The Hole in the Wall Gang Camp, founded by Paul Newman in 1988, is a nonprofit residential summer camp in northeastern Connecticut, where some 1,000 children with cancer and other life-threatening illnesses, between the ages of seven and 15 from across the country and abroad get to "be kids" and participate in a full range of camping activities and form loving, supportive friendships with both campers and staff, all free of charge. The camp provides year-round activities for campers and other seriously ill children and their siblings at camp and in their own communities. Camp-sponsored programs provide health care professionals and social workers with support and training. Retreats are organized for the children's parents at resorts around the country, offering respite, counseling, mutual support, and positive activities, free of charge. More than 3,500 family members take part in the fall to spring programs.

HospiceLink
http://www.rideforlife.com
1-800-331-1620

HospiceLink helps people seeking information and education about hospice care and makes referrals to hospices in all 50 states and the District of Columbia. HospiceLink is a service of the Hospice Education Institute, an independent nonprofit organization founded in 1985. There is no charge for any HospiceLink service. Since taking its first call in 1986, HospiceLink has helped hundreds of thousands of people in facing the challenges of coping with end-of-life issues.

International Myeloma Foundation (IMF)
http://www.myeloma.org

Hotline: 1-800-452-CURE (1-800-452-2873)
E-mail: TheIMF@myeloma.org

The IMF cites its mission as being "dedicated to improving the quality of life of myeloma patients while working toward prevention and a cure." The Web site offers up-to-date information and services in many languages for treatment and management, of all forms of myeloma, along with quarterly newsletter *Myeloma Today.*

I Can Cope
(accessible through http://www.cancer.org)

This patient education program of the American Cancer Society (ACS) is designed to help patients, families, and friends cope with the day-to-day issues of living with cancer. An eight-session course taught by health professionals from the hospital and community is usually offered through the local hospital. For information on this program, contact the ACS: 1-800-ACS-2345 (1-800-227-2345).

International Association of Laryngectomees (IAL)
http://www.larynxlink.com
Tel: 1-317-570-4568

IAL helps people who have lost their voice as a result of cancer; provides information on the skills needed by laryngectomees; and works toward total rehabilitation of patients. Offers free publications; more than 257 local organizations are in the United States; clubs go by the names "Lost Chord," "New Voice," or "Anamilo."

Leukemia Society of America
http://www.leukemia.org
Tel: 1-800-955-4572

This organization has free publications on leukemia and related diseases, all lymphomas, and multiple myeloma; provides information on referrals to other means of local support for patients with leukemia and other diseases; offers some supplemental financial assistance for outpatient care for chemotherapy and radiation treatment not covered by insurance and for transportation.

Look Good . . . Feel Better
http://www.cancer.org (part of the Support for
    Survivors and Patients section)
Toll free: 1-800-395-LOOK (1-800-395-5665)

This program was developed by the Cosmetic, Toiletry and Fragrance Association Foundation in cooperation with the American Cancer Society (ACS); it teaches cancer patients skills to improve their appearance while undergoing treatment.

Make-A-Wish Foundation

http://www.wish.org
3550 North Central Avenue, Suite 300
Phoenix, AZ 85012-2127
Tel: 1-602-279-WISH (9474)
Toll free: 1-800-722-WISH
Fax: 1-602-279-0855

The foundation grants wishes for young people up to the age of 18 who are suffering from a life-threatening illness; the "wish fulfillment" is free of charge for the young person and includes the immediate family and all expenses.

Mautner Project, The National Lesbian Health Organization

http://www.mautnerproject.org
1707 L Street NW, Suite 230
Washington, DC 20036
Tel: 1-202-332-5536
Toll free: 1-866-MAUTNER (1-866-628-8637)
Fax: 1-202-332-0662
E-mail: mautner@mautnerproject.org

The Mautner Project improves the health of lesbians and their families through advocacy, education, research, and direct service.

National AIDS Hotline

http://www.thebody.com/hotlines/national.html
Hotline: 1-800-514-0301
TTY: 1-800-514-0383
International: 1-202-541-0301

This Web site's tagline is "the complete HIV/AIDS resource," and it includes extensive listings of organizations such as the Americans With Disabilities Act.

National Alliance of Breast Cancer Associations (NABCO)

http://www.nabco.org
9 East 37th Street
10th Floor
New York, NY 10016
Toll free: 1-888-806-2226
Fax: 1-212-689-1213
E-mail: nabcoinfo@aol.com

NABCO provides information and educational materials on breast cancer, promotes affordable and accessible detection and treatment, advocates legislation for the rights and concerns of breast cancer patients. NABCO provides the latest information about breast health and breast cancer to medical professionals and organizations, patients and their families, and media. NABCO is also an experienced champion of women's and men's breast cancer needs and concerns.

National Association of Hospital Hospitality Houses, Inc. (NAHHH)

http://www.nahhh.org
P.O. Box 18087
Asheville, NC 28814-0087
Tel: 1-828-253-1188
Toll free: 1-800-542-9730
Fax: 1-828-253-8082
E-mail: helpinghomes@nahhh.org

The National Association of Hospital Hospitality Houses, Inc. is a nonprofit corporation serving facilities that provide lodging and other supportive services to patients and their families when confronted with medical emergencies. NAHHH facilities strive to provide a homelike environment for people traveling to be with a patient or to receive necessary outpatient care.

National Bone Marrow Transplant Link (BMT Link)

http://www.nbmtlink.org
20411 West 12 Mile Road, Suite 108
Southfield, MI 48076
Toll free: 1-800-LINK-BMT (1-800-546-5268)
Tel: 1-248-358-1886
E-mail: library@nbmtlink.org

This organization provides referrals, publications, and patient advocacy for people undergoing bone marrow and/or stem cell transplants; publishes a resource guide, available from the organization (for a fee), or available free online in downloadable format: *Resource Guide for Bone Marrow/Stem Cell Transplant; Including Bone Marrow, Peripheral Blood and Cord Blood: Friends Helping Friends.*

National Brain Tumor Foundation (NBTF)

http://www.braintumor.org
22 Battery Street, Suite 612

San Francisco, CA 94111-5520

E-mail: nbtf@braintumor.org

Toll free: 1-800-934-CURE (1-800-934-2873)

The NBTF Web site is designed to help patients, friends, and families cope with brain tumors by providing information about brain tumors and treatment, malignant and benign brain tumors, brain tumor medical centers, the latest brain tumor clinical trials, along with a network of brain tumor survivors. Information on the Web site is available in multiple languages. Information is also available about supporting brain tumor research by participating in Angel Adventures across the country.

National Breast Cancer Coalition (NBCC)

http://www.natlbcc.org

1101 17th Street NW

Suite 1300

Washington, DC 20036

Toll free: 1-800-622-2838

Tel: 1-202-296-7477

Fax: 1-202-265-6854

This an advocacy group is made up of breast cancer grassroots groups throughout the United States that seek to promote research into breast cancer, improve quality of care for all women, provide education, and motivate greater participation in the fight against breast cancer.

Cancer Genetics Network (CGN)

http://epi.grants.cancer.gov/CGN

The Cancer Genetics Network (CGN) is a national network of centers specializing in the study of inherited predisposition to cancer. It is part of the Epidemiology and Genetics Research Program (EGRP) under the umbrella of the National Cancer Institute (NCI). The EGRP manages a comprehensive program of grant-supported, population-based research that brings to bear the expertise of scientists to increase understanding of cancer etiology and prevention. Scientists from throughout the United States and internationally are supported. The resource is available to the research community at large to support studies on the genetic basis of human cancer susceptibility, integration of this information into medical practice, and behavioral, ethical, and public health issues associated with human genetics. The growing database has information on some 24,000 individuals (16,000 families) with cancer and/or a family history of cancer. CGN makes the data available to researchers, including demographic information, relevant medical history, and a four-generation cancer family history on each enrollee. The population enrolled makes possible research on both common and uncommon tumors. The CGN infrastructure enables studies on genes of moderate and low penetrance, as well as the more easily identified high penetrance genes.

The Cancer Genetics Network seeks to enroll individuals from minority populations; individuals at high risk for breast, ovarian, and colon cancer; and families with multiple tumors.

Contact one of the eight centers to discuss participating (see listing below). Volunteers do not need to live near a CGN center in order to join. Some centers have hospital affiliates through which one can enroll, and much of the contact can be by telephone, mail, or e-mail.

For additional information on the program:

Division of Cancer Control and Population Sciences

National Cancer Institute

6130 Executive Boulevard

Room 6134

Executive Plaza North

Rockville, MD 20852

Tel: 1-301-594-6776

Fax: 1-301-594-6787

Following are the individual centers of the CGN:

Carolina-Georgia Center of the Cancer Genetics Network

Duke University Medical Center, Durham, NC, in collaboration with the University of North Carolina at Chapel Hill and Emory University, Atlanta, GA. CGN Web site: http://cancer.med. unc. edu/cancergenetics

Duke University Medical Center

Tel: 1-866-681-4762

University of North Carolina at Chapel Hill

Tel: 1-877-692-6960

Emory University
Tel: 1-888-946-7447

Lombardi Cancer Center Cancer Genetics Network
Georgetown University Lombardi Cancer Center, Washington, DC
CGN Web site: http://lombardi.georgetown.edu/research/areas/cancercontrol/CGN.htm
Lombardi Clinic: 1-202-444-2223
General information: 1-202-444-4000

Mid-Atlantic Cancer Genetics Network
Johns Hopkins University, Baltimore, in collaboration with the Greater Baltimore CGN
Web site: http://www.macgn.org
Tel: 1-877-880-6188

Northwest Cancer Genetics Network
Fred Hutchinson Cancer Research Center, Seattle, in collaboration with the University of Washington School of Medicine, Seattle, WA
CGN Web site: http://www.fhcrc.org/science/phs/cgn
Tel: 1-800-616-8347

Rocky Mountain Cancer Genetics Coalition
University of Utah, Salt Lake City, in collaboration with the University of Colorado, Aurora, and University of New Mexico, Albuquerque
CGN Web site: http://www.rmcgc.org

University of Utah
Tel: 1-877-585-0473

University of New Mexico
Tel: 1-800-303-4503

University of Colorado
Tel: 1-877-700-0697

Texas Cancer Genetics Consortium
University of Texas MD Anderson Cancer Center, Houston, in collaboration with the University of Texas Health Science Center at San Antonio Southwestern Medical Center at Dallas, and Baylor College of Medicine, Houston, TX
CGN Web site: http://texas.cgnweb.org
Tel: 1-877-900-8894

UCI-UCSD Cancer Genetics Network Center
University of California at Irvine and University of California at San Diego
https://www.cgn.epi.uci.edu
Tel: 1-888-666-6002
University of California–Irvine
Department of Medicine/Epidemiology
224 Irvine Hall
Irvine, CA 92697

University of Pennsylvania Cancer Genetics Network
University of Pennsylvania Cancer Center, Philadelphia
Tel: 1-888-666-6002

Informatics Infrastructure

The CGN also has an Informatics and Information Technology Group to meet its information exchange and data management and statistical needs. The participating institutions and principal investigators are the University of California at Irvine, with Hoda Anton-Culver, Ph.D.; Massachusetts General Hospital, Boston, with Dianne M. Finkelstein, Ph.D.; and Yale University, New Haven, CT, with Prakash M. Nadkarni, Ph.D.

National Cancer Institute Information Resources

You may want more information for yourself, your family, and your doctor. The following National Cancer Institute (NCI) services are available to help you.

Telephone
Toll free: 1-800-4-CANCER (1-800-422-6237)
TTY: 1-800-332-8615

Cancer Information Service (CIS) Provides accurate, up-to-date information on cancer to patients and their families, health professionals, and the general public. Information specialists translate the latest scientific information into understandable language and respond in English, Spanish, or on TTY equipment.

Internet

http://cancer.gov—Cancer.gov is the NCI's primary Web site and provides immediate access to critical cancer information and resources. It contains material for health professionals, patients, and the public, including informationc from PDQ about cancer treatment, screening, prevention, genetics, supportive care, and clinical trials, and CANCERLIT, a bibliographic database. Cancer.gov also includes information on understanding trials, deciding whether to participate in trials, finding specific trials, plus research news and other resources.

CancerMail

Includes NCI information about cancer treatment, screening, prevention, genetics, and supportive care. To obtain a contents list, send e-mail to cancermail@cips.nci.nih.gov with the word *help* in the body of the message.

CancerFax

Includes NCI information about cancer treatment, screening, prevention, genetics, and supportive care. To obtain a contents list, dial 1-301-402-5874 or 1-800-624-2511 from a touch-tone telephone or fax machine handset and follow the recorded instructions.

National Cancer Institute (NCI)

http://cancernet.nci.nih.gov
Office of Cancer Communication
Building 31, Room 10A24
9000 Rockville Pike
Bethesda, MD 20892
Tel: (301) 496-5583.
E-mail: cancernet@icib.nic.nih.gov

This U.S. government agency conducts and supports research on cancer; it sponsors the Physicians Data Query (PDQ), an up-to-date computerized listing of cancer information and resources; the cancer information service (1-800-4-CANCER), providing state-of-the-art cancer information and free publications; Cancerfax 1-301-402-5874; Internet access (Cancernet).

National Center for Complementary and Alternative Medicine (NCCAM)

http://nccam.nih.gov
P.O. Box 8218
Silver Spring, MD 20907-8218.
Toll free: 1-888-NIH-OCAM (1-888-644-6226)
Fax: 1-301-495-4947

This federal agency has information packages, fact sheets, and a newsletter on complementary and alternative medical practices; gives grants for research; does *not* advise about specific therapies or provide referrals.

National Childhood Cancer Foundation (NCCF)

http://www.curesearch.org
Children's Oncology Group
Research Operations Center
440 East Huntington Drive
P.O. Box 60012
Arcadia, CA 91066-6012
Toll free: 1-800-458-6223
E-mail: info@curesearch.org

The NCCF is now part of "CureSearch," which unites the world's largest childhood cancer research organization, the Children's Oncology Group, and the National Childhood Cancer Foundation through their shared missions to cure childhood cancer. Their slogan is "Research is the key to cure." The groups provide referrals to Children's Cancer Group (CCG) treatment centers and information on clinical trials.

National Coalition for Cancer Survivorship— (NCCS)

http://www.canceradvocacy.org
1010 Wayne Avenue, Suite 770
Silver Spring, MD 20910
Tel: 1-301-650-9127
Fax: 1-301-565-9670
E-mail: info@canceradvocacy.org

NCCS is network of independent groups and individuals offering support to cancer survivors, family members, and friends; provides information and resources on support and life after a cancer diagnosis. The NCCS is the oldest survivor-led cancer advocacy organization in the country.

National Foundation for Facial Reconstruction (NFFR)

http://www.nffr.org
317 East 34th Street
Room 901
New York, NY 10016
Tel: 1-212-263-6656
Fax: 1-212-263-7534

People who cannot afford facial reconstruction may be eligible to get treatment through NFFR.

National Hospice and Palliative Care Organization (NHPCO)
http://www.nhpco.org
1700 Diagonal Road, Suite 625
Alexandria, VA 22314
Tel: 1-703-837-1500
Fax: 1-703-837-1233
E-mail: nhpco_info@nhpco.org
Helpline: 1-800-658-8898—provides free consumer information on hospice care and puts you in direct contact with hospice programs.

The National Hospice and Palliative Care Organization (NHPCO) is the largest nonprofit membership organization representing hospice and palliative care programs and professionals in the United States. The organization is committed to improving end-of-life care and expanding access to hospice care with the goal of profoundly enhancing quality of life for people dying in America and their loved ones.

National Kidney Cancer Association (NKCA)
http://www.curekidneycancer.org
1234 Sherman Avenue
Evanston, IL 60202
Toll free: 1-800-850-9132
Fax: 1-847-332-2978
E-mail: office@curekidneycancer.org

NKCA funds, promotes, and collaborates on research on kidney cancer; the association also provides information and referral, in addition to educating physicians about the disease and advocating for patients on the state and federal levels.

National Lymphedema Network (NLN)
http://www.lymphnet.org
Latham Square
1611 Telegraph Avenue, Suite 1111
Oakland, CA 94612-2138
Hotline: 1-800-541-3259
Tel: 1-510-208-3200
Fax: 1-510-208-3110
E-mail: nln@lymphnet.org

NLN provides information on lymphedema.

National Marrow Donor Program (NMDP)
http://www.marrow.org
3001 Broadway Street NE, Suite 500
Minneapolis, MN 55413-1753
General Information: 1-800-MARROW2
   (1-800-627-7692)
The Office of Patient Advocacy: 1-888-999-6743

NMDP is the hub of a worldwide network of more than 500 medical facilities in marrow and blood cell transplantation. Through this network, NMDP facilitates an average of 200 marrow or blood cell transplants each month and has helped give more than 20,000 patients a second chance at life. NMDP maintains a searchable registry of bone marrow donors, provides support for the doctors, patient and family during the transplant process, and works to match patients with the optimal donor or cord blood.

NMDP also offers information on how to become a donor, and produces relevant publications.

National Organization for Rare Disorders (NORD)
http://www.rarediseases.org
55 Kenosia Avenue
P.O. Box 1968
Danbury, CT 06813-1968
Toll free: 1-800-999-6673 (voicemail only)
TDD: 1-203-797-9590
Fax : 1-203-798-2291
E-mail: orphan@rarediseases.org
For questions related to providing care or accessing services for someone with a rare disease.
E-mail: RN@rarediseases.org.
For questions related to genetic testing or the inheritance patterns of diseases
E-mail: genetic_counselor@rarediseases.org.

NORD, a clearinghouse for information on rare diseases, offers networking and a medication assistance program.

National Ovarian Cancer Coalition (NOCC)
http://www.ovarian.org/
500 NE Spanish River Boulevard, Suite 8
Boca Raton, FL 33431
Tel: 1-561-393-0005
Fax: 1-561-393-7275

Toll free:1-888-OVARIAN
E-mail: NOCC@ovarian.org

NOCC is the leading ovarian cancer public information and education organization in the United States. NOCC initiated the first toll-free ovarian cancer information line (1-888-OVARIAN), maintains a comprehensive Web site for ovarian cancer support around the world, and has built a network of many state divisions across the United States. NOCC has a board of directors made up of diverse professionals from around the country, as well as a medical advisory board comprising physicians and researchers active in the discovery of new treatments and early detection for ovarian cancer. The Web site is comprehensive and offers many different resources and publications.

National Patient Air Transport Helpline (NPATH)

http://www.npath.org and http://mercymedical.org
Mercy Medical Airlift
4620 Haygood Road, Suite 1
Virginia Beach, VA 23455
Tel: 1-757-318-9174
Fax: 1-757-318-9107
E-mail: mercymedical@erols.com
Toll-free helpline: 1-800-296-1217

Immediate, live online response runs from 9 A.M. to 5 P.M Eastern Time Monday through Friday. Contact with the helpline outside normal business hours allows the caller to either leave a routine message that will be answered next normal business hours or to leave an urgent message that will receive a response within 10 minutes at any time. Calls may be made by patient friends, social or medical workers, or by patient's themselves. NPATH will discuss a need with anybody or give further detailed information about how charitable medical air transportation is provided nationally—to anybody. The Web Site and Helpline service are provided by Mercy Medical Airlift, a national charity.

NPATH provides information about all forms of charitable, long-distance medical air transportation and provides referrals to all appropriate sources of help available in the national charitable medical air transportation network.

National Rehabilitation Information Center

http://www.naric.com/naric

4200 Forbes Boulevard, Suite 202
Lanham, MD 20706-4829
E-mail: naricinfo@heitechservices.com
Fax: 1-301-459-4263 (for information or document requests; please include your contact information)
Toll free: 1-800-346-2742
Local and international callers: 1-301-459-5900
TTY: 1-301-459-5984

An information specialist will answer your call. If no information specialists are available, you may leave a message, including your telephone number with area code, and an information specialist will return your call.

NARIC has resource guides and information on prosthetics and rehab equipment. NARIC is a federally funded library with no medical professionals on staff and cannot offer diagnoses or treatment.

Patient Advocate Foundation (PAF)

http://www.patientadvocate.org
700 Thimble Shoals Boulevard, Suite 200
Newport News, VA 23606
E-mail: help@patientadvocate.org
Fax: 1-757-873-8999
Toll free: 1-800-532-5274

PAF provides help, advocacy, and many resources for patients.

RESOLVE

http://www.resolve.org
7910 Woodmont Avenue, Suite 1350
Bethesda, MD 20814
Toll free: (888) 623-0744 (help in Spanish available during select hours)
Tel: 1-301-652-8585
Fax: 1-301-652-9375
E-mail: info@resolve.org

This organization helps people who are infertile; offers sexual therapy, support groups, physician referral, a member-to-member contact system, a newsletter, and support services through local chapters.

Ronald McDonald House Charities (RMH)

http://www.rmhc.org
One Kroc Drive
Oak Brook, IL 60523

Tel: 1-630-623-7048
Fax: 1-630-623-7488

RMH provides temporary lodging in Ronald McDonald Houses in many states and cities for families of children who are undergoing treatment for cancer or other serious illnesses.

Skin Cancer Foundation (SCF)

http://www.skincancer.org
245 5th Avenue, Suite 1403
New York, NY 10016
Toll free: 1-800-SKIN-490 (1-800-754-6490)
E-Mail: info@skincancer.org
Fax: 1-212-725-5751

The mission of the foundation is to decrease the incidence of disease by means of public and professional education, medical training, and research. The SCF Web site is extensive, searchable, and interactive with a host of information and resources.

Starlight Starbright Children's Foundation

http://www.starlight.org
1850 Sawtelle Boulevard, Suite 450
Los Angeles, CA 90025
Toll free: 1-800-315-2580
Local: 1-310-479-1212
Fax: 1-310-479-1235
E-mail: info@starlight.org

This foundation grants special wishes of critically, chronically, and/or terminally ill children around the world; the Web site is a comprehensive, searchable, interactive resource with a tremendous amount of information on this international organization and the many services it offers.

Tuberous Sclerosis Alliance

http://tsalliance.easycgi.com
801 Roeder Road, Suite 750
Silver Spring, MD 20910
Toll free: 1-800-225-6872
Tel: 1-301-562-9890
Fax: 1-301-562-9870
E-mail: info@tsalliance.org

The Tuberous Sclerosis Alliance is dedicated to finding a cure for tuberous sclerosis while improving the lives of those affected.

United Ostomy Associations of America (UOAA)

http://www.uoaa.org
Toll free: 1-800-826-0826
E-mail: info@uoaa.org

UOAA is a national network for bowel and urinary diversion support groups in the United States. Its goal is to provide nonprofit association that will serve to unify and strengthen its member support groups, which are organized for the benefit of people who have, or will have, intestinal or urinary diversions and their caregivers.

US TOO

http://www.ustoo.com
Support Hotline: 1-800-80-US TOO
   (1-800-808-7866)
5003 Fairview Avenue
Downers Grove, IL 60515
Tel: 1-630-795-1002
Fax: 1-630-795-1602
M–F 9A.M.–5P.M. Central Time
E-mail: ustoo@ustoo.org

This organization provides support groups and services through local chapters for men who have prostate cancer.

Visiting Nurse Association of America (VNAA)

http://www.vnaa.org
99 Summer Street, Suite 1700
Boston, MA 02110
Tel: 1-617-737-3200
Fax: 1-617-737-1144
E-mail: vnaa@vnaa.org

The Visiting Nurse Association of America (VNAA) is the official national association for not-for-profit, community based home health organizations known as Visiting Nurse Associations (VNAs). VNAA gives referrals to local offices that can supply information on all forms of home health care, including physical, occupational, and speech therapy; medical social services; home health aide and homemaker services; nutritional counseling and hospice care; and meals on wheels.

Y-Me Breast Cancer Support Program

http://www.y-me.org

212 West Van Buren Street
Chicago, IL 60607-3908
Tel: 1-312-986-8338
Fax: 1-312-294-8597
E-mail: info@yme.org
24-hour Y-ME National Breast Cancer Hotline:
1-800-221-2141

(Staffed by trained peer counselors who are breast cancer survivors; interpreters available in 150 languages)

This program provides breast cancer patients with pretreatment counseling, treatment information, peer support, self-help counseling, and free literature; has a wig and prosthesis bank.

APPENDIX II

COMPREHENSIVE CANCER CENTERS BY STATE—AS OF JANUARY 2006

The Cancer Centers Program of the National Cancer Institute (NCI) supports major academic and research institutions throughout the United States. The NCI's mission is the advancement of cancer research to reduce the incidence of cancer, and to reduce the rates of morbidity and mortality from the disease.

NCI reviews requests from eligible institutions via a peer review process. Successful institutions are awarded a Cancer Center Support Grant (CCSG) to fund the scientific infrastructure of the cancer center.

Each institution receiving a CCSG award is recognized as an NCI-designated Cancer Center. There are two types of designations: **Cancer centers** have a scientific agenda that is primarily focused on basic, population sciences, or clinical research, or any two of the three components. **Comprehensive cancer centers** integrate research activities across three major areas: laboratory, clinical, and population-based research. Although the CCSG is mainly limited to support of research infrastructure, a majority of centers also provide clinical care and service for cancer patients. In addition, comprehensive cancer centers have extensive ancillary cancer-related activities such as outreach, education, and information dissemination.

Following is a list of the 39 comprehensive cancer centers (as of January 2006) by state. You can also find an integrated list of these cancer centers (both comprehensive cancer centers and clinical cancer centers) on the World Wide Web at: http://www3.cancer.gov/cancercenters/centerslist.html

ALABAMA
University of Alabama Comprehensive Cancer Center
1824 Sixth Avenue South
Room 237
Birmingham, AL 35293-3300
Tel: 1-205-934-5077
Fax: 1-205-975-7428
http://www.ccc.uab.edu

ARIZONA
University of Arizona Cancer Center
1501 North Campbell Avenue
Tucson, AZ 85724
Tel: 1-520-626-7925
Fax: 1-520-626-2284
http://www.azcc.arizona.edu

CALIFORNIA
The Kenneth Norris Jr. Comprehensive Cancer Center
University of Southern California

1441 Eastlake Avenue
Los Angeles, CA 90033-0804
Tel: 1-323-865-0816
Fax: 1-323-865-0102
http://www.ccnt.hsc.usc.edu

Jonsson Comprehensive Cancer Center
University of California at Los Angeles
Factor Building, Room 8-684
10833 Le Conte Avenue
Los Angeles, CA 90095-1781
Tel: 1-310-825-5268
Fax: 1-310-206-5553
http://www.cancer.mednet.ucla.edu

UCI Cancer Center/Chao Family Comprehensive Center
University of California at Irvine
101 The City Drive
Building 23, Route 81, Room 406
Orange, CA 92868
Tel: 1-714-456-6310
Fax: 1-714-454-2240
http://www.ucihs.uci.edu/~cancer

UCSF Comprehensive Cancer Center & Cancer Research Institute
University of California San Francisco
2340 Sutter Street
P.O. Box 0128
San Francisco, CA 94115-0128
Tel: 1-415-502-1710
Fax: 1-415-502-1712

Rebecca and John Moores UCSD Cancer Center
University of California at San Diego
3855 Health Sciences Drive
Room 2247
La Jolla, CA 92093-0658
Tel: 1-858-822-1222
Fax: 1-858-822-1207

City of Hope National Medical Center & Beckman Research Institute
1500 East Duarte Road
Duarte, CA 91010
Tel: 1-626-256-HOPE (4673)
Fax: 1-626-930-5394
http://www.cityofhope.org

COLORADO
University of Colorado Cancer Center
RC1-South Tower
Mail Stop 8111, P.O. Box 6511
Aurora, CO 80045-0511
Tel: 1-303-724-3155
Fax: 1-303-315-3304
http://www.uccc.info

CONNECTICUT
Yale Cancer Center
Yale University School of Medicine
333 Cedar Street
New Haven, CT 06520-8028
Tel: 1-203-785-4371
Fax: 1-203-785-4116
http://info.med.yale.edu/ycc/welcome.html

DISTRICT OF COLUMBIA
Lombardi Cancer Research Center
Georgetown University Medical Center
3800 Reservoir Road, NW
Washington, DC 20057
Tel: 1-202-687-2110
Fax: 1-202-687-6402
http://lombardi.georgetown.edu

FLORIDA
H. Lee Moffitt Cancer Center & Research Institute at the University of South Florida
12902 Magnolia Drive, MCC-CEO
Tampa, FL 33612-9497
Tel: 1-813- 615-4261
Fax: 1-813-615-4258
http://www.moffitt.usf.edu

ILLINOIS
Robert H. Lurie Cancer Center
Northwestern University
676 North Saint Clair Street
Suite 1200
Chicago, IL 60611
Tel: 1-312-908-5250
Fax: 1-312-908-1372
http://www.nums.nwu.edu/lurie

IOWA
Holden Comprehensive Cancer Center at the University of Iowa
5970 "Z" JPP

200 Hawkins Drive
Iowa City, IA 52242
Tel: 1-319-353-8620
Fax: 1-319-353-8988
http://www.uihealthcare.com/depts/cancercenter

MARYLAND
**The Sidney Kimmel Comprehensive Cancer
    Center at Johns Hopkins**
401 North Broadway
The Weinberg Building
Suite 1100
Baltimore, MD 21231
Tel: 1-410-955-8822
Fax: 1-410-955-6787
http://ww2.med.jhu.edu/cancerctr

MASSACHUSETTS
Dana-Farber/Harvard Cancer Center
Dana-Farber Cancer Institute
44 Binney Street
Room 1628
Boston, MA 02115
Tel: 1-617-632-4266
Fax: 1-617-632-2161
http://www.dfci.harvard.edu

MICHIGAN
**Comprehensive Cancer Center, University of
    Michigan**
6302 CGC/0942
1500 East Medical Center Drive
Ann Arbor, MI 48109-0942
Tel: 1-734-936-1831
Fax: 1-734-615-3947
http://www.cancer.med.umich.edu

The Barbara Ann Karmanos Cancer Institute
Wayne State University School of Medicine
4100 John R. Street
Detroit, MI 48201
Tel: 1-313-576-8660
Fax: 1-313-576-8661
http://www.karmanos.org

MINNESOTA
University of Minnesota Cancer Center
MMC 806
420 Delaware Street, SE

Minneapolis, MN 55455
Tel: 1-612-624-8484
Fax: 1-612-626-3069
http://www.cancer.umn.edu

Mayo Clinic Cancer Center
Mayo Clinic Rochester
200 First Street, SW
Rochester, MN 55905
Tel: 1-507-284-3753
Fax: 1-507-284-9349
http://mayoresearch.mayo.edu/mayo/research/
    cancercenter

MISSOURI
Siteman Cancer Center
Washington University School of Medicine
660 South Euclid Avenue
Campus Box 8109
St. Louis, MO 63110
Tel: 1-314-362-8020
Fax: 1-314-454-1898
http://www.siteman.wustl.edu

NEW HAMPSHIRE
**Norris Cotton Cancer Center, Dartmouth-
    Hitchcock Medical Center**
One Medical Center Drive
Hinman Box 7920
Lebanon, NH 03756-0001
Tel: 1-603-653-9000
Fax: 1-603-653-9003
http://www.cancer.dartmouth.edu

NEW JERSEY
The Cancer Institute of New Jersey
Robert Wood Johnson University Hospital
Robert Wood Johnson Medical School
195 Little Albany Street
Room 2002B
New Brunswick, NJ 08903
Tel: 1-732-235-8064
Fax: 1-732-235-8094
http://www.cinj.org

NEW YORK
Roswell Park Cancer Institute
Elm & Carlton Streets
Buffalo, NY 14263-0001

Tel: 1-716-845-5772
Fax: 1-716-845-8261
http://rcpi.med.buffalo.edu

Memorial Sloan-Kettering Cancer Center
1275 York Avenue
New York, NY 10021
Tel: 1-212-639-2000 or (800) 525-2225
Fax: 1-212-717-3299
http://www.mskcc.org

Herbert Irving Comprehensive Cancer Center
College of Physicians & Surgeons
Columbia University
161 Fort Washington Avenue
11th Floor, Room 1153
New York, NY 10032
Tel: 1-212-305-5201
Fax: 1-212-305-6813
http://www.ccc.columbia.edu

NORTH CAROLINA
UNC Lineberger Comprehensive Cancer Center
University of North Carolina Chapel Hill
School of Medicine, CB-7295
102 West Drive
Chapel Hill, NC 27599-7295
Tel: 1-919-966-3036
Fax: 1-919-966-3015
http://cancer.med.unc.edu

Duke Comprehensive Cancer Center
Duke University Medical Center
P.O. Box 3843
Durham, NC 27710
Tel: 1-919-684-5613
Fax: 1-919-684-5653
http://cancer.duke.edu

Comprehensive Cancer Center
Wake Forest University
Medical Center Boulevard
Winston-Salem, NC 27157-1082
Tel: 1-336-716-7971
Fax: 1-336-716-0293
http://www1.wfubmc.edu/cancer

OHIO
Case Comprehensive Cancer Center
Case Western Reserve University

11100 Euclid Avenue, Wearn 151
Cleveland, OH 44106-5065
Tel: 1-216-844-8562
Fax: 1-216-844-4975
http://cancer.case.edu

Comprehensive Cancer Center Arthur G. James Cancer Hospital & Richard J. Solove Research Institute
Ohio State University
A458 Starling Loving Hall
320 West 10th Avenue
Columbus, OH 43210
Tel: 1-614-293-7521
Fax: 1-614-293-7522
http://www.jamesline.com

PENNSYLVANIA
Fox Chase Cancer Center
333 Cottman Avenue
Philadelphia, PA 19111
Tel: 1-888-FOX-CHASE
http://www.fccc.edu.

Abramson Cancer Center of the University of Pennsylvania
16th Floor Penn Tower
3400 Spruce Street
Philadelphia, PA 19104-4283
Tel: 1-215-662-6065
Fax: 1-215-349-5325
http://www.penncancer.org

University of Pittsburgh Cancer Institute
UPMC Cancer Pavilion
5150 Centre Avenue, Suite 500
Pittsburgh, PA 15232
Tel: 1-412-623-3205
Fax: 1-412-623-3210
http://www.upci.upmc.edu

TENNESSEE
Vanderbilt-Ingram Cancer Center
Vanderbilt University
691 Preston Research Building
Nashville, TN 37232-6838
Tel: 1-615-936-1782
Fax: 1-615-936-1790
http://www.vicc.org

TEXAS

The University of Texas M.D. Anderson Cancer
    Center
1515 Holcombe Boulevard
Houston, TX 77030
Tel: 1-713-792-2121
Fax: 1-713-799-2210
http://www.mdanderson.org

VERMONT

Vermont Cancer Center
University of Vermont
149 Beaumont Avenue
HRSF326
Burlington, VT 05405
Tel: 1-802-656-4414
Fax: 1-802-656-8788
http://www.vermontcancer.org

WASHINGTON

Fred Hutchinson Cancer Research Center
P.O. Box 19024, D1-060
Seattle, WA 98109-1024
Tel: 1-206-667-4305
Fax: 1-206-667-5268
http://www.fhcrc.org

WISCONSIN

Comprehensive Cancer Center
University of Wisconsin
600 Highland Avenue
Room K4/610
Madison, WI 53792-0001
Tel: 1-608-263-8610
Fax: 1-608-263-8613
http://www.cancer.wisc.edu

APPENDIX III

CLINICAL CANCER CENTERS BY STATE—AS OF JANUARY 2006

Clinical cancer centers, funded by the National Cancer Institute (NCI), have a scientific agenda that is primarily focused on basic, population sciences, or clinical research, or any two of the three components (see more information in Appendix II). As of January 2006, there were 22 NCI-designated Clinical Cancer Centers, as follows:

CALIFORNIA

Salk Institute Cancer Center
10010 North Torrey Pines Road
La Jolla, CA 92037
Tel: 1-858-453-4100 X1386
Fax: 1-858-457-4765
http://www.salk.edu

The Burnham Institute for Medical Research
10901 North Torrey Pines Road
La Jolla, CA 92037
Tel: 1-858-646-3100
Fax: 1-858-646-3199
http://www.burnhaminstitute.org

UC Davis Cancer Center
4501 X Street, Suite 3003
Sacramento, CA 95817
Tel: 1-916-734-5800
Fax: 1-916-451-4464
http://www.ucdmc.ucdavis.edu/cancer

HAWAII

Cancer Research Center of Hawaii
University of Hawaii at Manoa
1236 Lauhala Street
Honolulu, HI 96813
Tel: 1-808-586-3013
Fax: 1-808-586-3052
http://www.crch.org

ILLINOIS

University of Chicago Cancer Research Center
5841 South Maryland Avenue, MC 2115
Chicago, IL 60637-1470
Tel: 1-773-702-6180
Fax: 1-773-702-9311
http://uccrc.org

INDIANA

Indiana University Cancer Center
Indiana Cancer Pavilion
535 Barnhill Drive
Room 455
Indianapolis, IN 46202-5289
Tel: 1-317-278-0070
Fax: 1-317-278-0074
http://iucc.iu.edu

Purdue University Cancer Center
Hansen Life Sciences Research Building
South University Street
West Lafayette, IN 47907-1524
Tel: 1-765-494-9129

Fax: 1-765-494-9193
http://www.cancer.purdue.edu

MAINE
The Jackson Laboratory
600 Main Street
Bar Harbor, ME 04609-0800
Tel: 1-207-288-6041
Fax: 1-207-288-6044
http://www.jax.org

MASSACHUSETTS
**Massachusetts Institute of Technology Center
for Cancer Research**
77 Massachusetts Avenue
Room E17-110
Cambridge, MA 02139-4307
Tel: 1-617-253-8511
Fax: 1-617-253-0262
http://web.mit.edu/ccr

MINNESOTA
Mayo Cancer Center
200 First Street SW
Rochester, MN 55905
Tel: 1-507-284-3753
Fax: 1-507-284-9349
http://www.mayo.edu/cancercenter

NEBRASKA
**University of Nebraska Medical Center/Eppley
Cancer Center**
600 South 42nd Street
Omaha, NE 68198-6805
Tel: 1-402-559-4238
Fax: 1-402-559-4652
http://www.unmc.edu/cancercenter

NEW MEXICO
UNM Cancer Research & Treatment Center
MSC 08 4630
1 University of New Mexico
2325 Camino de Salud NE
Albuquerque, NM 87131
Tel: 1-505-272-5622
Fax: 1-505-272-4039
http://cancer.unm.edu

NEW YORK
Albert Einstein Cancer Center
Chanin Building, Room 209
1300 Morris Park Avenue
Bronx, NY 10461
Tel: 1-718-430-2302
Fax: 1-718-430-8550
http://www.aecom.yu.edu/cancer

Cold Spring Harbor Laboratory
P.O. Box 100
Cold Spring Harbor, NY 11724
Tel: 1-516-367-8383
Fax: 1-516-367-8879
http://www.cshl.org

NYU Cancer Institute
New York University Medical Center
550 First Avenue
New York, NY 10016
Tel: 1-212-263-8950
Fax: 1-212-263-8210
http://www.nyucancerinstitute.org

OREGON
OHSU Cancer Institute
Oregon Health & Science University
3181 S.W. Sam Jackson Park Road, CR145
Portland, OR 97201-3098
Tel: 1-503-494-1617
Fax: 1-503-494-7086
http://www.ohsu.edu

PENNSYLVANIA
The Wistar Institute
3601 Spruce Street
Philadelphia, PA 19104-4268
Tel: 1-215-898-3926
Fax: 1-215-573-2097
http://www.wistar.org

Kimmel Cancer Center
Thomas Jefferson University
233 South 10th Street
BLSB, Room 1050
Philadelphia, PA 19107-5799
Tel: 1-215-503-4645
http://www.kcc.tju.edu

TENNESSEE
St. Jude Children's Research Hospital
332 North Lauderdale
Memphis, TN 38105-2794
Tel: 1-901-495-3982
Fax: 1-901-495-3966
http://www.stjude.org

TEXAS
San Antonio Cancer Institute
University of Texas Health Science Center at San
    Antonio
7703 Floyd Curl Drive, MSC 7772
San Antonio, TX 78229-3900
Tel: 1-210-567-2710
Fax: 1-210-567-2709
http://saci.uthscsa.edu

UTAH
Huntsman Cancer Institute
University of Utah
2000 Circle of Hope
Salt Lake City, UT 84112-5550
Tel: 1-801-585-3281
Fax: 1-801-581-3389
http://www.hci.utah.edu

VIRGINIA
University of Virginia Cancer Center
Jefferson Park Avenue
Room 617E
Charlottesville, VA 22908
Tel: 1-434-924-9333
Fax: 1-434-982-0918
http://www.healthsystem.virginia.edu/internet/
    cancer

Massey Cancer Center
Virginia Commonwealth University
P.O. Box 980037
Richmond, VA 23298-0037
Tel: 1-804-828-0450
Fax: 1-804-828-8453
http://www.vcu.edu/mcc

SUBJECT INDEX

Antiemetics

allopurinol
Anzemet
Ativan (see ANTIEMETIC)
Compazine (see ANTIEMETIC)
Decadron
dexamethasone (see DECACRON)
dolasetron (see ANZEMET)
dronabinol (see MARIJUANA)
granisetron hydrochloride (see KYTRIL)
Kytril (granisetron hydrochloride)
marijuana
Marinol (see MARIJUANA)
metoclopramide
odansetron (see ZOFRAN)
Reglan (see METOCLOPRAMIDE)
tetrahydrocannabinol (see MARIJUANA)
THC (see MARIJUANA)
thorazine (see ANTIEMETIC)
Tigan (see ANTIEMETIC)
Torecan (see ANTIEMETIC)
Valium (see ANTIEMETIC)
Zofran

Biological Therapy

Actimmune (see INTERFERON GAMMA 1-B)
aldesleukin (see INTERLEUKIN-2)
allovectin-7
B-cell stimulatory factor-1 (see INTERLEUKIN-4)
B-cell stimulatory factor-2 (see INTERLEUKIN-6)
biological response modifiers
Biological Response Modifiers Program
biological therapy
chimeric antibody
eosinphil colony-stimulating factor (see INTERLEUKIN-5)
eosinphil CSF (see INTERLEUKIN-5)
EPO (see EPOGEN)
Epogen
epoetin (see EPOGEN)
epoetin alpha (see EPOGEN)
Eprex (see EPOGEN)
erythropoietin (see EPOGEN)
filgrastim (see G-CSF)
gamma interferon
G-CSF
gene therapy
GM-CSF
granulocyte colony-stimulating factor (see G-CSF)
granulocyte macrophage–colony-stimulating factor (see GM-CSF)
growth factor (see COLONY-STIMULATING FACTORS)
hematopoietic growth factors (see COLONY-STIMULATING FACTORS)
hematopoietin-1 (see INTERLEUKIN-1)
Herceptin
IL-1 (see INTERLEUKIN-1)
IL-2 (see INTERLEUKIN-2)
IL-2/LAK
IL-2/TIL

IL-3 (see INTERLEUKIN-3)
IL-4 (see INTERLEUKIN-4)
IL-5 (see INTERLEUKIN-5)
IL-6 (see INTERLEUKIN-6)
IL-11 (see INTERLEUKIN-11)
immune system
immunomodulation
immunotherapy
interferon
interferon alpha-2A
interferon alpha-2b
interferon alpha-2c
interferon alpha-2d
interferon beta
interferon gamma 1-b
interleukin
interleukin-1
interleukin-2
interleukin-3
interleukin-4
interleukin-5
interleukin-6
interleukin-11
Opreluekin (see INTERLEUKIN-11)
leukine (see GM-CSF)
MoAb (see MONOCLONAL ANTIBODY)
molecular cell biology
monoclonal antibody
multicolony-stimulating factor (see INTERLEUKIN-3)
multi-CSF (see INTERLEUKIN-3)
Neupogen (see G-CSF)
Numega (see INTERLEUKIN-11)
Procrit (see EPOGEN)
Prokine (see GM-CSF)
Proleukin (see INTERLEUKIN-2)
recombinant (see INTERLEUKIN-2)
r-IFN-beta (see INTERFERON BETA)
rIL-2 (see INTERLEUKIN-2)
Rituxan
Rituximab (see RITUXAN)
Roferon-A (see INTERFERON ALPHA-2A)
Teceleukin (see INTERLEUKIN-2)
trastuzumab (see HERCEPTIN)

Cancer Sites/Types

abdominal cancer
acinar cell carcinoma

acoustic neuroma (noncancerous)
acquired immune deficiency syndrome (see AIDS)
    [NONCANCEROUS]
acral-lentiginous melanoma
acute erythroleukemia
acute granulocytic leukemia (see AML)
acute lymphatic leukemia (see ALL)
acute lymphoblastic leukemia (see ALL)
acute lymphocytic leukemia (see ALL)
acute monocytic leukemia (see AML)
acute myelocytic leukemia (see AML)
acute myelogenous leukemia (see AML)
acute myelomonocytic leukemia (see AML)
acute nonlymphocytic leukemia (AML)
acute promyelocytic leukemia (AML)
adamantinoma
adenocarcinoma
adenocarcinoma of the lung
adenoid cystic carcinoma
adrenal cancer
adrenocortical cancer
adult Hodgkin's disease (see HODGKIN'S
    DISEASE/ADULT)
adult non-Hodgkin's lymphoma (see NON-
    HODGKIN'S DISEASE/ADULT)
adult soft-tissue sarcoma (see SOFT-TISSUE SAR-
    COMA/ADULT)
adult T-cell leukemia (see CCL)
adult T-cell leukemia-lymphoma (see ATLL)
aggressive non-Hodgkin's lymphoma
AIDS (noncancerous)
ALL
alveolar cell lung cancer (see BRONCHIOLOAVEOLAR)
alveolar soft part sarcoma
AML
anal cancer
anaplastic astrocytoma
anaplastic oligodendroglioma (see BRAIN CANCER)
anaplastic thyroid carcinoma
angiosarcoma
ANLL (see AML)
astrocytoma
ATLL
B-cell acute lymphocytic leukemia
basal cell carcinoma of the eye (see EYE CANCER)
basal cell carcinoma of the skin
basaloid carcinoma (see CLOACOGENIC CANCER)
bile duct cancer
bladder cancer

bone cancer

bowel cancer (see COLON/RECTAL CANCER)

Bowen's disease

brain cancer

brain stem glioma (see BRAIN CANCER)

breast cancer

bronchioloalveolar lung cancer

bronchogenic carcinoma

Burkitt cell acute lymphocytic leukemia (see B-CELL ACUTE LYMPHOCYTIC LEUKEMIA)

Burkitt's lymphoma

carcinoma

carcinoma in situ

carcinoma in situ of the breast

carcinoma of unknown primary (see UNKNOWN PRIMARY)

cervical cancer

CGL (see CML)

cheek cancer (see MOUTH CANCER)

childhood leukemia (see ALL)

childhood non-Hodgkin's lymphoma (see NON-HODGKIN'S LYMPHOMA/CHILDHOOD)

childhood rhabdomyosarcoma (see RHABDOMYOSARCOMA)

cholangiocarcinoma

cholesteatoma (see CONGENITAL BRAIN TUMORS)

chondrosarcoma

choriocarcinoma

chronic granulocytic leukemia (see CML)

chronic lymphatic leukemia (see CLL)

chronic lymphocytic leukemia (see CLL)

chronic lymphogenous leukemia (see CLL)

chronic lymphoid leukemia (see CLL)

chronic myelocytic leukemia (see CML)

chronic myelogenous leukemia (see CML)

chronic myeloid leukemia (see CML)

chronic myelosis leukemia (see CML)

clear cell adenocarcinoma

CLL

cloacogenic cancer

CML

colon/rectal cancer

colon cancer

comedocarcinoma

congenital brain tumors

connective tissue cancer (see SOFT-TISSUE SARCOMA)

cutaneous melanoma (see MELANOMA)

DCIS (see DUCTAL BREAST CANCER IN SITU)

DHL (see DIFFUSE HISTIOCYTIC LYMPHOMA)

diffuse histiocytic lymphoma

diffuse large cell lymphoma (see DIFFUSE HISTIOCYTIC LYMPHOMA)

DiGugliemo's syndrome (see ERYTHROLEUKEMIA)

ductal breast cancer in situ

endocrine cancers

endometrial cancer

endometrial carcinoma (see ENDOMETRIAL CANCER)

endothelioma

eosinophilic leukemia

ependemoblastoma (see BRAIN CANCER)

ependymoma

epidermoid cancer of mucus membranes

epidermoid carcinoma of the lung (see SQUAMOUS CELL CARCINOMA OF THE LUNG)

epithelioma

erythroleukemia

esophageal cancer

Ewing's sarcoma

eye cancer

fibrosarcoma of soft tissue

follicular cell thyroid cancer

gallbladder cancers

gastric cancer (see STOMACH CANCER)

gastric carcinoma (see STOMACH CANCER)

gastrointestinal cancer

germ cell tumors

gestational trophoblastic tumor

giant cell tumor of the bone

glioblastoma multiforme

glioma

glomus tumor

glucagonoma

Grawitz's tumor (see KIDNEY CANCER)

hairy cell leukemia

HCL (see HAIRY CELL LEUKEMIA)

head and neck cancer

hemangioblastoma

hemangiopericytoma

hemangiosarcoma

hepatoblastoma (see LIVER CANCER/CHILDHOOD)

hepatocellular carcinoma (see HEPATOMA)

hepatoma

histiocytic non-Hodgkin's lymphoma

Hodgkin's disease/adult

Hodgkin's disease/childhood

hypopharyngeal cancer

indolent non-Hodgkin's lymphoma

osteosarcoma
ovarian cancer
ovarian germ cell tumor and stromal tumor
Paget's disease
pancoast tumor
pancreatic cancer
paranasal sinus/nasal cavity cancer
parathyroid gland cancer
parosteal osteosarcoma
parosteal sarcoma (see PAROSTEAL OTEOSARCOMA)
parotoid gland cancer
penile cancer
peripheral neuroepithelioma
pharyngeal cancer (see OROPHARYNGEAL CANCER)
pharynx cancer (see OROPHARYNGEAL CANCER)
pheochromocytoma
pineal gland tumors (noncancerous)
pituitary adenoma (see PITUITARY TUMOR)
pituitary tumor
plasma cell dyscrasias (see MULTIPLE MYELOMA)
plasma cell leukemia (see LEUKEMIA)
plasma cell neoplasm (see MULTIPLE MYELOMA)
plasma cell tumor (see PLASMACYTOMA)
plasmacytoma
primary cancer
prostate cancer
rectal cancer
renal cell cancer (see KIDNEY CANCER)
renal cell carcinoma (see KIDNEY CANCER)
renal pelvis tumors (see TRANSITIONAL CELL CAN-
    CER OF THE RENAL PELVIS AND URETER)
reticulum cell sarcoma (see BONE CANCER)
retinoblastoma
rhabdomyosarcoma
salivary glands cancer
sarcoma
SCLC (see SMALL CELL LUNG CANCER)
secondary liver cancer (see METASTATIC LIVER
    CANCER)
secondary tumor (see METASTATIC CANCER)
seminoma
Sezary syndrome
sinus cancer (see PARANASAL SINUS/NASAL CAVITY
    CANCER)
skin cancer
small cell carcinoma (see SMALL CELL LUNG
    CANCER)
small cell lung cancer small intestine cancer
soft palate cancer (see OROPHARYNGEAL CANCER)

soft-tissue sarcoma/adult
soft-tissue sarcoma/childhood
spinal cord cancer (see BRAIN CANCER)
spindal cell carcinoma of the lung (see SQUAMOUS
    CELL LUNG CANCER)
spleen cancer
squamous cell carcinoma
squamous cell carcinoma of the skin
squamous cell lung cancer
stomach cancer
superficial spreading melanoma
superior sulcus tumor (see PANCOAST TUMOR)
sweat gland cancer
synovial cell carcinoma (see SYNOVIAL SARCOMA)
synovial sarcoma
T-cell leukemia
T-cell lymphoma (see MYCOSIS FUNGOIDES)
TCC (see TRANSITIONAL CELL CANCER OF THE
    RENAL PELVIS AND URETER)
testicular cancer
thymoma
thyroid cancer
tongue cancer (see MOUTH CANCER)
tonsil cancer (see MOUTH CANCER)
transitional cell cancer of the renal pelvis and
    ureter
tubular ductal breast cancer
undifferentiated large cell lung cancer (see NON-
    SMALL CELL LUNG CANCER)
undifferentiated small cell lung cancer (see SMALL
    CELL LUNG CANCER)
unknown primary
ureteral cancer
urethral cancer
uterine sarcoma
uterus cancer (see ENDOMETRIAL CANCER)
vaginal cancer
voice box cancer (see LARYNX CANCER)
vulvar cancer
Waldenstrom's macroglobulinemia
Wilms' tumor
womb cancer (see ENDOMETRIAL CANCER)

Carcinogens/Suspected Carcinogens

Agent Orange
aflatoxins (see CARCINOGENS)
4-aminobiphenyl (aminodiphenyl) (see
    CARCINOGENS)

arsenic

asbestos

aspartame (see ARTIFICIAL SWEETENERS)

azathioprine (see CARCINOGENS)

benzene (see CARCINOGENS)

benzidine (see CARCINOGENS)

bis(chloromethyl) ether (see CARCINOGENS)

butanediol dimethylsulfonate (Myleran, Busulfan) (see CARCINOGENS)

carcinogens

chewing tobacco (see SMOKELESS TOBACCO)

chlorambucil (see CARCINOGENS)

chromium hexabalent (see CARCINOGENS)

cigar smoking

coal tar, creosote (coal and wood) (see CARCINOGENS)

coke oven emissions (see CARCINOGENS)

conjugated estrogens (see CARCINOGENS)

cyclamate (see ARTIFICIAL SWEETENERS)

cyclophosphamide—(Cytoxan, CTX, Endoxan, Neosar) (see CARCINOGENS)

cyclosporin A (cyclosporine A; ciclosporin) (see CARCINOGENS)

diethylstilbestrol (DES) (see CARCINOGENS)

electromagnetic fields

environmental tobacco smoke (see PASSIVE SMOKE)

erionite (see CARCINOGENS)

fat

food additives

formaldehyde

4-aminobiphenyl

hair dye

herbicide

indoor air quality (IAQ)

involuntary smoking (see SECONDHAND SMOKING)

melphalan (see CARCINOGENS)

methoxsalen with ultraviolet A therapy (see CARCINOGENS)

microwave oven

mineral oils (see CARCINOGENS)

mouthwash

mustard gas

nitrates

nitrites (see NITRATES)

nitrosamines (see NITRATES)

nuclear power plants

mustard gas

—1-(2-chloroethyl)-3-4-methylcyclohexyl)-1-nitrosourea (MeCCNU) (see CARCINOGENS)

passive smoke

passive smoking (see SECONDHAND SMOKING)

phenacetin

radon

secondhand smoke (see PASSIVE SMOKE)

secondhand smoking

smoking

smokeless tobacco

suspected carcinogens

thiotepa (see CARCINOGENS)

thorium dioxide (see CARCINOGENS)

2-naphtylamine (see CARCINOGENS)

ultraviolet radiation

UV (see UTRAVIOLET RADIATION)

vinyl chloride (see CARCINOGENS)

Chemotherapy Agents

(NOTE: Drugs with initial capital letters are trademark or brand names; drugs spelled with all lowercase letters are the chemical or generic agent names)

Accutane (isotretinoin)

actinomycin D (see COSMEGEN)

adrenocorticoids

Adriamycin

Adrucil (see 5-FU)

AGT (see CYTADREN)

alkaloids

Alkeran

alkylating agents

allopurinol sodium (Zyloprim)

all-trans retinoic acid

altretamine (see HEXAMETHYLMELAMINE)

amethopterin (see METHOTRAXATE)

amifostine (see ETHYOL)

aminoglutethimide (see CYTADREN)

AMSA (see M-AMSA)

amsacrine (see M-AMSA)

anagrelide (see ARGYLIN)

anastrozole (see ARIMIDEX)

antiandrogen drug

antibiotic

antimetabolite

arabinosylcytosine (see ARA-C)

ara-C

Arimidex

ASP (see L-ASPARAGINASE)

asparaginase (see L-ASPARAGINASE)

azidothymidine (see AZT)

AZT
bacillus Calmette-Guérin (see BCG)
BCG (bacillus Calmette-Guérin)
BCNU
betamethasone (see ADRENOCORTICOID)
bicalutamide (see CASODEX)
BiCNU (see BCNU)
Blenoxane (see BLEOMYCIN)
BLEO (see BLEOMYCIN)
bleomycin
bromfenac sodium capsules (see DURACT)
BU (see BUSULFAN)
busulfan
calcium leucovorin (see LEUCOVORIN CALCIUM)
Camptosar
capecitabine (see XELODA)
carboplatin
carboxmide (see DTIC)
carmustine (see BCNU)
Casodex
CBDCA (see CARBOPLATIN)
CCNU
CDDP (see CISPLATIN)
CeeNU (see CCNU)
Cerubidine (see DAUNOMYCIN)
CF (see LEUCOVORIN CALCIUM)
CLB (see LEUKERAN)
chemo
chemoembolization
chemoprevention
chemoprophylaxis (see CHEMOPREVENTION)
chemosensitivity assay
chemosurgery
chlorambucil (see LEUKERAN)
chlorodeoxyadenosine (see LEUSTATIN)
cis-diammine-dichloroplatinum (see CISPLATIN)
cis-platinum (see CISPLATIN)
cisplatin
cladribine (see LEUSTATIN)
CLB (see LEUKERAN)
clomiphene
combination chemotherapy
corticosteroid (see ADRENOCORTICOIDS)
cortisone (see ADRENOCORTICOIDS)
Cosmegen
CPT-11
crossover chemotherapy
cross resistance (see DRUG RESISTANCE)
CTX (see CYTOXAN)

cyclobutane dicarboxylate platinum (see CARBOPLATIN)
cyclophosphamide (see CYTOXAN)
Cytadren
cytarabine (see ARA-C)
Cytosar-U (see ARA-C)
cytosine arabinoside (see ARA-C)
Cytovene (see GALLIUM NITRATE)
cytotoxic drug
Cytoxan
dacarbazine (see DTIC)
DACT (see COSMEGEN)
dactinomycin (see COSMEGEN)
DAN (see DANOCRINE)
danazol (see DANOCRINE)
Danocrine
daunomycin
daunorubicin (see DAUNOMYCIN)
DaunoXome (see LIPOSOMAL DAUNORUBICIN)
DAVA (see VINDESINE)
DBD (see DIBROMODULCITOL)
DCF (see PENTOSTATIN)
DDD Lysodren (see MITOTANE)
DDP (see CISPLATIN)
Deca-Durabolin (see ANDROGEN)
Decadron (see DEXAMETHASONE)
Delalutin (see PROGESTERONE)
Deltasone (see PREDNISONE)
dexamethasone (see DECADRON)
deoxycoformycin (see PENTOSTATIN)
Depo-Provera (see PROGESTERONE)
Depo-Testosterone
DES
DESP (see DIETHYLSTILBESTROL DIPHOSPHATE)
dexamethasone (see DECADRON)
dexrazoxane (see ZINECARD)
DHAD (see MITOXANTRONE)
dibromodulcitol
Didronel (see ETIDRONATE)
diethylstilbestrol (see DES and ESTROGEN)
diethylstilbestrol diphosphate (see ESTROGEN)
DM (see DECADRON)
DNR (see DAUNOMYCIN)
DOX (see ADRIAMYCIN)
doxorubicin (see ADRIAMYCIN)
Drolban (see ANDROGEN)
dromostanolone propionate (see ANDROGEN)
DTIC
DTIC-Dome (see DTIC)

Leucovorin Calcium
leucovorin rescue
Leukeran
Leukerin (see 6-MP)
LEUP (see LUPRON)
leuprolide (see LUPRON)
Leustatin
LEV (see LEVAMISOLE)
levamisole
LHRH (see LUTEINIZING HORMONE-RELEASING HOR-
   MONE)
lomustine (see CCNU)
liposomal daunorubicin
L-PAM (see ALKERAN)
L-phenylalanine mustard (see ALKERAN)
L-Sarcolysin (see ALKERAN)
Lupron
luteinizing hormone-releasing hormone
Lysodren (see MITOTANE)
M-AMSA
Macleron (see ANDROGEN)
Masteril (see ANDROGEN)
Matulane (see PROCARBAZINE)
mechlorethamine (see MUSTARGEN)
meddroxyprogesterone (see PROGESTERONE)
MEG (see MEGACE)
Megace
megestrol (see MEGACE)
melphalan (see ALKERAN)
mercaptopurine (see 6-MP)
mesna
Mesnex (see MESNA)
Methosarb (see ANDROGEN)
methotrexate
methotrexate with leucovorin rescue (see LEUCO-
   VORIN RESCUE)
methoxsalen
methoxsalen with ultraviolet A therapy (see PUVA)
methyl-G (see METHYL-GAG)
methyl-GAG
methylglyoxal-bis-guanylhydrazone (see METHYL-
   GAG)
methylprednisolone (see ADRENOCORTICOIDS)
methylprednisone (see ADRENOCORTICOIDS)
meticorten (see PREDNISONE)
Mexate (see METHOTREXATE)
MGBG (see METHYL-GAG)
mifepristone (see RU486)

MITH (see MITHRACIN)
Mithracin
Mithramycin (see MITHRACIN)
MITO (see MUTAMYCIN)
mitoguazone (see METHYL-GAG)
mitolactol (see DIBROMODULCITOL)
mitomycin (see MUTAMYCIN)
mitomycin C (see MUTAMYCIN)
mitotane
mitoxantrone
MP (see 6-MP)
MTP-PE
MS Contin
multidrug chemotherapy (see COMBINATION
   CHEMOTHERAPY)
muramyl tripeptide phosphatidylethanolamine
   (see MTP-PE)
Mustargen
Mutamycin
M-VAC
MVAC (see M-VAC)
Myleran (see BUSULFAN)
MYX (see METHOTREXATE)
nandrolone phenpropionate (see ANDROGEN)
nandrolone decanoate (see ANDROGEN)
Navelbine
neocarzinostatin (see ZINOSTATIN)
neo-hombreol (see ANDROGEN)
Neosar (see CYTOXAN)
Nilandrone (see NILUTAMIDE)
nilutamide
Nipent (see PENTOSTATIN)
nitrogen mustard
Nizoral (see KETOCONAZOLE)
Nolvadex (see TAMOXIFEN)
Novantrone (see MITOXANTRONE)
O,p'-DDD lysodren (see MITOTANE)
octreotide (see SANDOSTATIN)
Oncaspar (see PEGASPARGASE)
Oncovin (see VINCRISTINE)
Orasone (see PREDNISONE)
Oreton (see ANDROGEN)
paclitaxel (see TAXOL)
Pallace (see MEGACE)
paramethasone (see ADRENOCORTICOIDS)
Paraplatin (see CARBOPLATIN)
PCB (see PROCARBAZINE)
pegaspargase

pentostatin
Permastril (see ANDROGEN)
Photofrin
phymoyoxin
plant alkaloid (see ALKALOIDS)
Platinol (see CISPLATIN)
platinum (see CISPLATIN)
plicamycin (see MITHRACIN)
polychemotherapy
porfimer sodium (see PHOTOFRIN)
predinsolone (see ADRENOCORTICOIDS)
prednisone
Premarin (see ESTROGEN)
procarbazine
Proscar
Provera (see PROGESTERONE)
Psoralen (see METHOXSALEN)
Purinethol (see 6-MP)
raloxifene
Retrovir (see AZT)
rubidomycin (see DAUNOMYCIN)
RU486
Sandostatin
6-mercaptopurine (see 6-MP)
6-TG
6-thioguanine (see 6-TG)
SSTN (see SANDOSTATIN)
Stilbestrol diphosphate (see ESTROGEN)
Stilphostrol (see ESTROGEN)
streptozocin
streptozotocin (see STREPTOZOCIN)
SUR (see SURAMIN)
suramin
Tace (see ESTROGEN)
TAM (see TAMOXIFEN)
tamoxifen
TAX (see TAXOL)
Taxol
tegafur
10-EdAM (see EDATREXATE)
teniposide
Teslac (see ANDROGEN)
testolactone (see ANDROGEN)
testosterone
testosterone propionate (see ANDROGEN)
thioguanine (see 6-TG)
thiotepa
13-CRA (see ACCUTANE)
TOPO (see HYCAMTIN)

Toposar (see ETOPOSIDE)
topotecan
toremifene
TPT (see HYCAMTIN)
trastuzumab (see HERCEPTIN)
tretinoin (see ALL-TRANS RETINOIC ACID)
triamcinolone (see ADRENOCORTICOIDS)
triethylene thiophosphoranide (see THIOTEPA)
TSPA (see THIOTEPA)
VBL (see VINBLASTINE)
Velban (see VINBLASTINE)
VePesid (see ETOPOSIDE)
verapamil
Vesanoid (see ALL-TRANS RETINOIC ACID)
Videx (see DDL)
vinblastine amide sulfate (see VINDESINE)
vinblastine
vincristine
vindesine
vinorelbine (see NAVELBINE)
VM-26 (see TENIPOSIDE)
VP-16 (see ETOPOSIDE)
VP-16213 (see ETOPOSIDE)
VPAM (see VERAPAMIL)
VP/Vidaribine (see PENTOSTATIN)
Xeloda
Zanosar (see STREPTOZOCIN)
ZDV (see AZT)
ZDX (see ZOLADEX)
zidovudine (see AZT)
Zinecard
zinostatin
Zoladex

Combination Chemotherapy (and cancers with which they may be used)

ABVD—Hodgkin's disease
AC—myeloma and bone cancer
ACOPP—childhood Hodgkin's
AP—ovarian cancer
ASHAP—non-Hodgkin's lymphoma
AVDP—ALL
BACON
BACOP—non-Hodgkin's lymphoma
B-CAVe—Hodgkin's disease
B-DOPA—Hodgkin's disease
BCP—myeloma

BHD—melanoma
CAF—breast cancer
CAMP—non-small cell lung cancer
CAP—non-small cell lung, kidney, bladder, and
   prostate cancers
CD—ANLL
CDC—ovarian cancer
CF—gestational trophoblastic tumor
CFL—gestational trophoblastic tumor
CFM—breast cancer
CFPT—breast cancer
CHAD—ovarian cancer
CHEX-UP—ovarian cancer
CHOP—non-Hodgkin's lymphoma
CHOP-BLEO—non-Hodgkin's lymphoma
CISCA—kidney, bladder, and prostate cancers
CMF—breast cancer
CMFP—breast cancer
CMFVP—breast cancer
COAP—AML
COB—head and neck cancers
COMLA—non-Hodgkin's lymphoma
COP—non-Hodgkin's disease
COP-BLAM—non-Hodgkin's lymphoma
COPE—leukemia
COPP—non-Hodgkin's lymphoma
CP—ovarian cancer
CT—childhood ANNL
CV—small cell lung cancer
CVEB—kidney, bladder, and prostrate cancers
CVI—non-small cell lung cancer
CVP—non-Hodgkin's lymphoma
CVPP—Hodgkin's disease
CYADIC—soft-tissue sarcoma
CYVADIC—sarcomas
DC—childhood ANLL
DCPM—childhood AML
DCT—AML
DMC—gestational trophoblastic tumor
DTIC-ACTD—melanoma
DVP—ALL
E-SHAP—non-Hodgkin's lymphoma
FAC—breast cancer
FAM—stomach and non-small cell lung cancer
FCE—stomach cancer
F-CL—colon cancer
FL—kidney, bladder, and prostate cancers
Fle—colon cancer
FMS—pancreatic cancer

FOMi/CAO—non-small cell lung cancer
ID—soft-tissue sarcoma
IMAC—bone cancer
IMF—breast cancer
IMVP—non-Hodgkin's lymphoma
L-VAM—kidney, bladder, and prostate cancers
MACC—non-small cell lung cancer
m-BACOD—non-Hodgkin's lymphoma
m-BACOS—non-Hodgkin's lymphoma
MBC—head and neck cancers
MC—ANLL
M-2—myeloma
M-VAC—kidney, pancreas and bladder cancers
MAP—head and neck cancers
MBC—head and neck cancers
MF—head and neck cancers
MINE—non-Hodgkin's lymphoma
MM—ALL
MOPP—Hodgkin's disease
MP—myeloma
MV—ANLL
MVPP—Hodgkin's disease
NOVP—Hodgkin's disease
OPEN—non-Hodgkin's lymphoma
PAC—ovarian cancer
ProMACE—non-Hodgkin's lymphoma
TC—ALL
VAB—kidney, bladder, and prostate cancers
VAC—small cell lung cancer
VAD—myeloma
VAP—childhood ALL
VATH—breast cancer
VBAP—myeloma
VB—kidney, bladder, and prostate cancers
VBC—melanoma
VBP—kidney, bladder, and prostate cancers
VC—small cell lung cancer
VCAP—myeloma
VDP—melanoma

Diagnosis/Evaluation

acid phosphatase test
AFP (see ALPHA-FETOPROTEIN TEST)
air-contrast X-rays
alkaline phosphatase test
alpha-fetoprotein test
angiography

gastrointestinal series (see GI SERIES)

GI series

gonioscopy

graphic stress telethermometry (see THERMOGRA-PHY)

guaiac test (see OCCULT BLOOD STOOL TEST)

HCG (see HUMAN CHORIONIC GONADOTROPIN)

hormone assay

human chorionic gonadotropin hysterography

immunoassay

intravenous pyelography (see IVP)

isotope scan (see NUCLEAR SCAN)

kidney scan

lactate dehydrogenase

laparoscopy

laryngeal tomography (see LARYNGOGRAPHY)

laryngography

laryngoscopy

lienography

light scanning (see TRANSILLUMINATION)

lower GI series

L.P. (see SPINAL TAP)

lumbar puncture (see SPINAL TAP)

lung function test (see PULMONARY FUNCTION TEST)

lung scan

lymphadenectomy

lymphangiography

lymphography (see LYMPHANGIOGRAPHY)

magnetic resonance imaging (see MRI)

mammography

mediastinoscopy

mediastinotomy

metastatic workup

metrography (see HYSTEROGRAPHY)

miraluma test

MRI

myelography

nasopharyngoscopy

needle aspiration biopsy

needle biopsy (see CORE NEEDLE BIOPSY)

needle localization

nephroureterectomy

neurological workup or exam

nuclear scan

occult blood stool test

oncor test

oncofetal antigen (see CEA)

opthalamoscopy

oral gallbladder test (see CHOLECYSTOGRAPHY)

palpate

pancreas scan

PAP smear

PAP test (see PROSTATIC ACID PHOSPHATASE TEST)

paracentesis

PCR (see POLYMERASE CHAIN REACTION)

pelvic exam

pelvic lymph node dissetion

percutaneous needle biopsy

percutaneous transhepatic cholangiography

peritoneocentesis (see PARACENTESIS)

peritoneoscopy

permanent section biopsy

PET scan

PFT (see PULMONARY FUNCTION TEST)

pleural tap (see THORACENTESIS)

pleuroscopy

polymerase chain reaction (PCR)

portography

positron emission tomography (see PET SCAN)

procto exam

progesterone receptor test

prostate-specific antigen test

PSA test (see PROSTATE-SPECIFIC ANTIGEN TEST)

pulmonary cytology

punch biopsy (see EXCISIONAL BIOPSY)

pyelography (see IVP)

quadrantectomy (see LUMPECTOMY)

radioactive iodine

radioactive isotope

radioactive scan (see NUCLEAR SCAN)

radioisotope scan (see NUCLEAR SCAN)

rectal exam (see DIGITAL RECTAL EXAM)

Reed-Sternberg cell

renal arteriography (see SELECTIVE RENAL ARTERI-OGRAPHY)

renal scan (see KIDNEY SCAN)

retrograde pyelography

retrograde urography (see RETROGRADE PYELOGRA-PHY)

scintimammography (see MIRALUMA TEST)

sestamibi breast imaging (see MIRALUMA TEST)

scan

Schiller test

scintigraphy

scintiscan (see SCINTIGRAPHY)

screening

second-look laparotomy
second-look surgery
selective renal arteriography
self-examination of the breast (see BREAST SELF-
    EXAMINATION)
self-examination of the testicles (see TESTICULAR
    SELF-EXAMINATION)
sentinel lymph node biopsy
shave biopsy
sigmoidoscopy
soft-tissue radiography (see XEROGRAPHY)
spinal tap
spirometry
stereotactic biopsy
stool blood test (see OCCULT BLOOD STOOL TEST)
stool guaiac test (see OCCULT BLOOD STOOL TEST)
suction biopsy (see NEEDLE ASPIRATION BIOPSY)
surgical biopsy (see EXCISIONAL BIOPSY)
surgical conization (see CONIZATION)
teslascan
testicular self-examination
thoracentesis
thoracoscopy
total biopsy (see EXCISIONAL BIOPSY)
transillumination
transperineal biopsy
transrectal biopsy
TSE (see TESTICULAR SELF-EXAMINATION)
UA (see URINE ANALYSIS)
ultrasonography (see ULTRASOUND)
ultrasound
upper GI series
ureteropyloscopy
urethrography
urinalysis
urine sediment test (see URINALYSIS)
urography
US (see ULTRASOUND)
uterogography (see HYSTEROGRAPHY)
vacuum aspiration (see ENDOMETRIAL ASPIRATION)
vaginal pool aspiration (see ENDOMETRIAL
    ASPIRATION)
vaginoscopy (see COLPOSCOPY)
venacavography
venography
wide core needle biopsy (see CORE NEEDLE
    BIOPSY)
X-ray
xerography
xeromammography

Medical Support

American Board of Surgeons
care giver
board certification
dietician
dosimetrist
endoscopist
enterostomal therapist (see STOMAL THERAPIST)
gynecologic oncologist
hematologist
hematopathologist
maxillofacial prosthodontist
medical oncologist
neurologist
neuroradiologist
neurosurgeon
oncologist
oncology nurse
ophthalmogist
opthalmogist
orthopedic surgeon
otolaryngologist
pathologist
pediatric oncologist
physiatrist
physical therapist
proctologist
radiation oncologist
radiation physicist
radiation therapist
radiologist radiotherapist (see RADIATION THERAPIST)
reconstructive surgeon
social worker
stomal therapist
surgical oncologist
therapeutic radiologist (see RADIATION THERAPIST)
thoracic surgeon
urologist

Pain Management

acetaminophen
acupressure
Actiq
acupuncture
Advil (see NONSTEROIDAL ANTI-INFLAMMATORY
    DRUGS)

analgesic drug
analgesic pump
aspirin
brompton cocktail
codeine
cordotomy
Datril (see NONSTEROIDAL ANTI-INFLAMMATORY DRUGS)
Demerol
Dilaudid
Dolophine (see METHADONE)
Dronabinol (see MARIJUANA)
endorphins
enkaphalines
epidural catheter
epidural dorsal column stimulator
Fentanyl
heroin
hospice mix (see BROMPTON COCKTAIL)
hydromorphone (see DILAUDID)
hypnosis
ibuprofen (see NONSTEROIDAL ANTI-INFLAMMATORY DRUGS)
imagery
infusion pump
Levo-Dromoran
levorphanol (see LEVO-DROMORAN)
marijuana
meperidine (see DEMEROL)
methadone
morphine
Nuprin (see NONSTEROIDAL ANTI-INFLAMMATORY DRUGS)
narcotic
nerve block
nerve root clipping
nonsteroidal anti-inflammatory drugs
NSAIDS (see NONSTEROIDAL ANTI-INFLAMMATORY DRUGS)
Numorphan
oxycodone (see PERCODAN)
oxymorphone (see NUMORPHAN)
pain
pain management
Percodan
percutaneous cordotomy
phantom pain
Quadramet (samarium Sm-153 lexidronam injection)
rhizotomy

Rufen (see NONSTEROIDAL ANTI-INFLAMMATORY DRUGS)
SCA (see PAIN MANAGEMENT)
self-controlled analgesic (see PAIN MANAGEMENT)
serotonin
serotonin antagonists
TENS (see TRANSCUTANEOUS ELECTRICAL NERVE STIMULATION)
TNS (see TRANSCUTANEOUS ELECTRICAL NERVE STIMULATION)
transcutaneous electrical nerve stimulation
Tylenol (see ACETAMINOPHEN)

Precancerous Conditions

achlorhydria
actinic keratosis
adenomatous hyperplasia
adenomatous polyps
adrenal medullary tumors
AIDS
ataxia telangiectasia
benign prostatic hyperplasia
Bowen's diseases
chronic atrophic gastritis
chronic ulcerative colitis (see CROHN'S DISEASE)
chronic vulvar dystrophy
Crohn's disease
dysplasia
dysplastic nevi
dysplastic nevus syndrome (see DYSPLASTIC NEVI)
EBV (see EPSTEIN-BARR VIRUS)
endometrial hyperplasia
Epstein-Barr virus
erythroplakia
erythroplasia (see ERYTHROPLAKIA)
genital herpes virus
giant cell tumor of the bone
gonadal aplasia
HPV (see HUMAN PAPILLOMAVIRUS)
human papillomavirus
hyperkeratosis
intermediate polyps
intestinal metaplasia
leukoplakia
MDS (see MYELODYSPLASTIC SYNDROMES)
moles
myelodysplastic syndromes

Prevention

Reconstruction/Rehabilitation

Risk Factors

familial atypical multiple mole melanoma syndrome
familial polyposis (see FAMILIAL MULTIPLE POLYPO-
SIS OF THE COLON)
familial multiple polyposis of the colon
FAPC (see FAMILIAL MULTIPLE POLYPOSIS OF THE
COLON)
Gardner's syndrome (see FAMILIAL MULTIPLE POLY-
POSIS OF THE COLON)
gastric polyps
genital herpes virus
HER-2/neu gene
hereditary pancreatitis
hereditary polyposis of the colon (see FAMILIAL
MULTIPLE POLYPOSIS OF THE COLON)
hermaphroditism
high risk
hormonal replacement therapy (see ESTROGEN
REPLACEMENT THERAPY)
HPV (see HUMAN PAPILLOMAVIRUS)
human papillomavirus
hyperkeratosis
intermediate polyps
intestinal metaplasia
involuntary smoking (see SECONDHAND SMOKING)
Klinefelter's syndrome
leukoplakia
LFS (see LI-FRAUMENI SYNDROME)
Li-Fraumeni syndrome
MDS (see MYELODYSPLASTIC SYNDROMES)
microcalcifications
moles
mouthwash
multiple basal cell carcinoma syndrome
myasthemia
myelodysplastic syndromes
Oldfield's syndrome
oncogene
papillomavirus (see HUMAN PAPILLOMAVIRUS)
passive smoke
passive smoking (see SECONDHAND SMOKING)
pernicious anemia
photosensitivity
pigmented nevi (see MOLES)
Plummer-Vinson syndrome
polyps
radiation therapy
radiology (see RADIATION THERAPY)
von Recklinghausen's neurofibromatosis
regional enteritis (see CROHN'S DISEASE)

regional ileitis (see CROHN'S DISEASE)
sebaceous hyperplasia
secondhand smoke (see PASSIVE SMOKE)
secondhand smoking
senile lentigo
smoking
smokeless tobacco
sporadic intestinal polyps
stress
tubulovillous polyps (see INTERMEDIATE POLYPS)
Turcot's syndrome
ultraviolet radiation
UV (see ULTRAVIOLET RADIATION)
vasectomy
villous polyps
X-ray therapy or treatment (see RADIATION
THERAPY)

Side Effects

agranulocytosis (see NEUTROPENIA)
aleukemia
allopurinol
alopecia
amyloidosis
anemia
anorexia
anticipatory nausea and vomiting
aplastic anemia
atrophy
bone marrow depression
cachexia
chloromas
diarrhea
drug tolerance
dry heaves (see RETCHING)
dumping syndrome dyspnea
edema
effusion
erythema
fatigue
graft versus host disease
hair loss (see ALOPECIA)
hemolysis
hypercalcemia
hyperviscosity syndrome
infections
jaundice
leukostasis

Symptoms

Treatment

cobalt treatment
cold knife conization (see CONIZATION)
combination therapy
combined modality therapy (see COMBINATION
    THERAPY)
complete mastectomy (see SIMPLE MASTECTOMY)
conization consolidation therapy
contact thermography (see THERMOGRAPHY)
continent illeal reservoir
continuation therapy (see MAINTENANCE THERAPY)
continuous infusion chemotherapy
craniotomy
cryosurgery
cryotherapy (see CRYOSURGERY)
curettage
differentiation therapy
distal pancreatectomy
double-barrel colostomy
electric needle (see ELECTROCAUTERY)
electrocautery
electrofulguration (see FULGURATION)
electron beam therapy
electrosurgery
embolization
endocrine therapy (see HORMONE THERAPY)
endoscopic resection and fulguration (see
    TRANSURETHAL RESECTION OR SURGERY)
esophagectomy
enteral feeding
excisional biopsy
exenteration
experimental treatments (see CLINICAL TRIALS)
external beam radiation therapy
extrapleural pneumonectomy (see PLEUROPNEU-
    MONECTOMY)
freezing surgery (see CRYOSURGERY)
gastrectomy
gene therapy
Gerson treatment
Halsted mastectomy (see RADICAL MASTECTOMY)
heat treatment (see HYPERTHERMIA THERAPY)
hemilaryngectomy (see PARTIAL LARYNGECTOMY)
hemimastectomy (see LUMPECTOMY)
herbal treatment
holistic medicine
hormone therapy
hospice
hyperalimentation
hyperfractionated radiation therapy

hyperthermia therapy
hysterectomy
hystero-oophorectomy
hysterography
IAT (see IMMUNOAUGMENTATIVE THERAPY)
illeal bladder
ileostomy
immunoaugmentative therapy
immunomodulation
immunotherapy (see BIOLOGICAL THERAPY)
induction therapy
indwelling catheter
infuse-a-port infusion pump
infusion therapy
internal radiation
interstitial implant (see INTERSTITIAL RADIATION)
interstitial radiation
intra-arterial infusion (see INFUSION THERAPY)
intracavitary radiation
intraoperative radiation therapy
intraperitoneal chemotherapy
intraperitoneal radiotherapy
intrathecal chemotherapy
intravesical chemotherapy
investigational treatment (see CLINICAL TRIALS)
intravesical immunotherapy
IORT (see INTRAOPERATIVE RADIATION TREATMENT)
iridectomy
iridocyclectomy
iridotrabulectomy
irradiation (see RADIATION THERAPY)
isolation perfusion
Laetrile
laminectomy
laparotomy
laryngectomy
laser therapy
leukapheresis
limb sparing surgery
liver transplant
lobectomy
localized radiation
lumpectomy
lymphadenectomy
macrobiotic diet
maintenance therapy
mastectomy
Mediport (see INFUSE-A-PORT)
micrographic surgery

total abdominal hysterectomy
total abdominal hysterectomy and bilateral
    salpingo-oophorectomy
total hysterectomy
total laryngectomy
total mastectomy (see SIMPLE MASTECTOMY)
total mastectomy with axillary dissection (see
    MODIFIED RADICAL MASTECTOMY)
total pancreatectomy
total parenteral nutrition (see HYPERALIMENTATION)
total prostatectomy
total thyroidectomy
TPN (see HYPERALIMENTATION)
tracheostomy
transphenoidal hypophysectomy
transurethral resection or surgery (TUR)
transverse loop colostomy
tumor debulking
two step procedure
unilateral salpingectomy
unconventional treatment method
unproven treatment method (see UNCONVENTIONAL
    TREATMENT METHOD)
unsound treatment method
uterosigmoidostomy
urinary diversion
vaginal hysterectomy

vaginectomy
vulvectomy
wedge resection
whipple procedure
X-ray therapy (see RADIATION THERAPY)

Tumor Markers

AFP (see ALPHA-FETOPROTEIN)
alpha-fetoprotein
CA 15-3
CA 19-9
CA 27-29
CA 125
calcitonin
CEA
carcinoembryonic antigen (see CEA)
human chorionic gonadotropin (HCG)
HCG (see HUMAN CHORIONIC GONADOTROPIN)
neuron-specific enolase (NSE)
NSE (see NEURON-SPECIFIC ENOLASE)
PAP (see PROSTATIC ACID PHOSPHATASE)
pancreatic oncofetal antigen (POA) (see PANCRE-
    ATIC ONCOFETAL ANTIGEN)
prostate-specific antigen
prostatic acid phosphatase
PSA (see PROSTATE-SPECIFIC ANTIGEN)
thyroglobulin

BIBLIOGRAPHY

This is a list of books, broken down loosely by topic, that offer additional information on different aspects of cancer. Many of the books are in paperback, and many can be found in the public library. In addition, there are many free publications available. As you have seen in the text and in the Appendices, the National Cancer Institute offers many free publications either on the NCI Web site (http://www.cancer.gov) or by calling (1-800-4-CANCER). In addition, Appendix I offers a comprehensive listing of noteworthy Web sites of National Organizations for Cancer and AIDS.

General Cancer/Medical Information

Advice for the Patient: Drug Information in Lay Language. Vol. 2. Rockville, Md.: The United States Pharmacopeial Convention, Inc., 1991. (to order call US Pharmacopeia, 1-800-227-8772, press 5 for a product catalog); also see http://www.usp.org.

Ammer, Christine. *The New A-Z of Women's Health.* New York: Facts On File, 1995.

Bloch, Richard, and Annette Bloch. *Fighting Cancer: A Step-by-Step Guide to Helping Yourself Fight Cancer.* R. A. Bloch Cancer Foundation; Revised edition (January 1, 1992) Kansas City, Mo.: Cancer Connection, Inc., 1985.

Bognar, David, *Cancer: Increasing Your Odds for Survival—A Resource Guide for Integrating Mainstream, Alternative and Complementary Therapies.* Alameda, Calif.: 1996. (Paperback edition, Hunter House Publishers.)

Boston Women's Health Collective. *Our Bodies, Ourselves: A New Edition for a New Era.* New York: Touchstone, 2005.

DeVita, Vincent, Jr., Samuel Hellman, and Steven Rosenberg. *Cancer: Principles and Practice of Oncology.* Philadelphia: Lippincott, 1999. Lippincott Williams & Wilkins, 7th Bk&cdr edition, 2004. A textbook written for doctors that covers all aspects of cancer. It can be difficult for the layperson but does offer a great deal of information.

Diamond, John, M.D., and Lee Cowden, M.D., with Burton Goldberg. *An Alternative Medicine Definitive Guide to Cancer.* Tiburon, Calif.: Future Medicine Publishing, 1997. Second edition, available in paperback. Ten Speed Press, June, 2002.

Directory of Pain Treatment Centers in the United States and Canada. Phoenix, Ariz.: Oryx Press, 1989.

Holub, Arthur, ed. *The American Cancer Society Book: Prevention, Detection, Diagnosis, Treatment, Rehabilitation, Cure.* New York: Doubleday, 1986.

Morra, Marion, and Eve Potts, *Choices: Realistic Alternatives in Cancer Treatment.* New York: Avon, 1994. Written in easy-to-understand question and answer format for the layperson.

Murphy, Gerald, M.D., Lois Morris, and Diane Lange. *American Cancer Society's Informed Decisions; The*

Complete Book of Cancer Diagnosis, Treatment and Recovery. New York: Viking, 1997. (For additional information on American Cancer Society publications, see: http://www.cancer.org or call: 1-800-ACS-2345 (1-800-227-2345) [TTY 1-866-228-4327 for hearing-impaired].)

Schlessel Harpham, Wendy, M.D. *Diagnosis Cancer: Your Guide to the First Months of Healthy Survivorship.* New York: Norton, 1998; expanded and revised edition (paperback), Norton, 2003.

Shtasel, D. O. *Medical Tests and Diagnostic Procedures: A Patient's Guide to Just What the Doctor Ordered.* New York: Harper Perennial, 1990.

Sontag, Susan. *Illness as Metaphor.* New York: Random House, 1977; paperback edition, *Illness as Metaphor & AIDS and Its Metaphors*, New York: Picador, 2001.

Weinbert, Robert. *One Renegade Cell: How Cancer Begins.* New York: Basic Books, 1998, paperback, 1999.

Zakarian, Beverly. *The Activist Cancer Patient: How to Take Charge of Your Treatment.* New York: John Wiley & Sons, 1996.

Body/Mind/Psychological/Emotional/Self-Help

Babcock, Elise NeeDell. *When Life Becomes Precious: A Guide for Loved Ones and Friends of Cancer Patients.* New York: Bantam, 1997.

Benjamin, Harold. *From Victim to Victor: The Wellness Community Guide to Fighting for Recovery for Cancer Patients and Their Families.* Los Angeles: Jeremy Tarcher, 1987, revised edition, 1995.

Benson, Herbert, and Miriam Klipper. *The Relaxation Response.* New York: Avon, 1990.

Cousins, Norman. *Anatomy of an Illness as Perceived by the Patient.*, New York: Bantam, 1991; W. W. Norton, reprint edition, 2005.

———. *The Healing Heart: Antidotes to Panic and Helplessness.* New York: W. W. Norton, 1983; Random House, hardcover, 1986.

Garrison, Judith, and Scott Shepherd. *Cancer and Hope: Charting a Survival Course.* Minneapolis: CompCare Publishers, 1989.

Johnson, Judi, and Linda Klein. *I Can Cope: Staying Healthy with Cancer.* New York: John Wiley & Sons, 1994.

Kalter, Suzy. *Looking Up: The Complete Guide to Looking and Feeling Good for the Recovering Cancer Patient.* New York: McGraw Hill, 1987. Advice on hair care, wigs, makeup, and exercise.

Kushner, Harold. *When Bad Things Happen to Good People.* New York: Avon, 1994; 20th anniversary edition, Schocken, 2001.

LeShan, Lawrence. *Cancer as a Turning Point: A Handbook for People with Cancer, Their Families and Health Professionals.* New York: Plume, 1994.

———. LeShan, Lawrence. *You Can Fight for Your Life.* New York: M. Evans, 1977; paperback, 1980.

Noyes, Diane. *Beauty and Cancer: Looking and Feeling Your Best.* Dallas: Taylor Publishers, 1992.

Rossman, Martin. *Healing Yourself: A Step-by-Step Program for Better Health through Imagery.* New York: Pocket Books, 1987.

Guided Imagery for Self-Healing: An Essential Resource for Anyone Seeking Wellness (paperback), H. J. Kramer, 2nd edition, 2000.

Schlessel Harpham, Wendy, M.D. *Diagnosis: Cancer: Your Guide to the First Months of Healthy Survivorship.* New York: W. W. Norton, 1994; expanded and revised edition (paperback), W. W. Norton, 2003.

Siegel, Bernie. *Love Medicine and Miracles.* New York: HarperCollins, 1990.

———. *Peace, Love and Healing.* New York: Harper and Row, 1989.

Simonton, O. C., S. Mathews-Simonton, and J. Creighton. *Getting Well Again. The Bestselling Classic About the Simontons' Revolutionary Life-saving Self-Awareness Techniques.* New York: Bantam, 1992.

Breast Cancer

Altman, Roberta. *Waking Up, Fighting Back: The Politics of Breast Cancer.* New York: Little, Brown and Company, 1996.

Baron-Faust, Rita. *Breast Cancer: What Every Woman Should Know.* New York: Hearst, 1995.

Greenberg, Mimi. *Invisible Scars: A Guide to Coping with the Emotional Aspects of Breast Cancer.* New York: Walker, 1988; St. Martin's mass market paperback, 1989.

Kushner, Rose. *Alternatives: New Developments in the War on Breast Cancer.* New York: Warner Books, 1986.

————. *Rose Kushner's If You've Thought about Breast Cancer . . . (And Have Found Something You're Worried About),* revised and updated, 2002. Published by Rose Kushner, Breast Cancer Advisory Center, c. 2002 Harvey D. Kushner. For a free copy of the book, see the Web site for the Rose Kushner Breast Cancer Advisory Center (formerly the Women's Breast Cancer Advisory Center) at http://www.rkbcac.org or write to the RKBCAC at Rose Kushner Breast Cancer Advisory Center, P.O. Box 757, Malaga Cove, CA 90274.

Love, Susan, and Karen Lindsey. *Dr. Susan Love's Breast Book.* Reading, Mass.: Perseus, 1995; *Dr. Susan Love's Breast Book: New Edition, 2005* (paperback) Da Capo Lifelong Books; 4th rev. ed. 2005.

McGinn, Kerry. *Keeping Abreast: Breast Changes That Are Not Cancer.* Palo Alto, Calif.: Bull Publishing Co., 1987.

McLean, Marsha. *If You Find a Lump in Your Breast.* Palo Alto, Calif.: Bull Publishing Co., 1986.

Seltzer, V. L. *Every Woman's Guide to Breast Cancer.* New York: Viking, 1987.

Snyder, Marilyn. *Informed Decision: Understanding Breast Reconstruction.* New York: W. W. Norton, 1989; M. Evans, reprint, 1990.

Walter, Carol, with Leonore Miller. *Moving Free: A Total Program of Post-Mastectomy Exercises.* New York: Bobbs-Merrill, 1981; MacMillan paperback edition, 1981.

Colon Cancer

Miskovitz, Raul, M.D., and Marian Betancourt. *What to Do If You Get Colon Cancer. A Specialist Helps You Take Charge and Make Informed Choices.* New York: John Wiley & Sons, 1997.

Chemotherapy

Blumberg, Rena. *Headstrong: A Story of Conquests and Celebrations . . . Living through Chemotherapy.* New York: Crown, 1982; HB Press, 2nd edition, 1991.

Skeel, Roland, M.D., and Neil Lachant, M.D. *Handbook of Cancer Chemotherapy.* New York: Little, Brown, 1995; Lippincott Williams & Wilkins, 6th edition, 2003.

Slayton-Mitchell, Joyce. *Winning the Chemo Battle.* New York: W. W. Norton, 1991.

Children

Adams, David, and Eleanor Deveau. *Coping with Childhood Cancer: Where Do We Go from Here?* Reston, Va.: Reston Publishing, 1984; Kinbridge; new revised edition, 1993.

Baker, Lynn, Charles Roland, and Gerald Gilchrist. *You and Leukemia: A Day at a Time.* Philadelphia: Saunders, 1978; 2nd edition, 2001.

Fine, Judylaine. *Afraid to Ask: A Book for Families to Share about Cancer.* New York: Lothrop, Lee and Shepard, 1984. Information for children on the physical and emotional impact of cancer.

Gaes, Jason. *My Book for Kids with Cancer: A Child's Autobiography of Hope.* Aberdeen, Md.: Melius & Peterson, 1987. Written by a child for other children with cancer.

Keene, Nancy. *Childhood Leukemia: A Guide for Families, Friends and Care Givers.* Sebastopol, Calif.: O'Reilly & Associates, 1997; Patient Centered Guides, 3rd edition, 2002.

Kellerman, Jonathan, ed. *Psychological Aspects of Childhood Cancer.* Springfield, Ill.: Charles C. Thomas, 1980.

Koocher, Gerald, and John O'Malley. *The Damocles Syndrome: Psychosocial Consequences of Surviving Childhood Cancer.* New York: McGraw Hill, 1981.

Miles, Margaret. *The Grief of Parents: When a Child Dies.* Oak Brook, Ill.: Compassionate Friends, 1980. Suggestions on how to respond and cope with the death of a child.

Nutrition

Bradley, Jane, and Susan Nass. *Nutrition of the Cancer Patient.* Dallas: NRC Publishing, 1988.

Fishman, Joan, and Barbara Anrod. *Something's Got to Taste Good: The Cancer Patient's Cookbook.* New York: Signet Paperback, 1982.

Margie, Joyce, and Abby Block. *Nutrition and the Cancer Patient.* Radnor, Pa.: Chilton, 1984. A guide to nutrition and recipes.

Ovarian Cancer

Piver, M. Steven, M.D., with Gene Wilder. *Gilda's Disease.* New York: Prometheus Books, 1996; Broadway Books, reprint edition, 1998.

Personal Stories

Bloch, Richard, and Annette Bloch. *Cancer, There's Hope.* Kansas City, Mo.: Cancer Connection, Inc., 1981; hardcover, Putnam, 1983. Lung cancer experience of the founder of H & R Block.

Ford, Betty, and Chris Chase. *The Times of My Life.* New York: Harper and Row, 1978; Ballantine Paperbacks, 1979. Former first lady's experience with breast cancer.

Gunther, John. *Death Be Not Proud.* New York: Harper and Row, 1949; Harper Perennial Modern Classics; 1st Perennial Classics edition, 1998. A father's account of his son's battle with a brain tumor.

Ipswitch, Elaine. *Scott Was Here.* New York: Dell, 1979. A mother's account of her son's battle with Hodgkin's disease.

Ireland, Jill. *Life Wish.* Boston: Little, Brown, 1987; Jove Books, reissue edition, 1988. Actress's experience with breast cancer.

Lohmann, J. *Gathering a Life: A Journey of Recovery.* Santa Barbara, Calif.: John Daniel & Co.: 1989. Experience of the wife of a brain-tumor patient.

Mullan, Fitzhugh. *Vital Signs: A Young Doctor's Struggle with Cancer.* New York: Farrar, Straus & Giroux, 1975; Dell reprint, 1984.

Pepper, Curtis. *We the Victors: The Inspiring Stories of People Who Conquered Cancer and How They Did It.* New York: Doubleday, 1984.

Pringle, Terry. *This Is the Child: A Father's Story of His Young Son's Battle with Leukemia.* New York: Alfred A. Knopf, 1983; Southern Methodist University Press, 1992.

Radner, Gilda. *It's Always Something.* New York: Simon & Schuster, 1989; Harper Paperbacks, First Harper Entertainment edition, 2000. Actress/comedienne's experience with ovarian cancer.

Rollin, Betty. *First, You Cry.* New York: Harper and Row, 1976; mass market paperback, Signet, 1978. TV reporter's experience with breast cancer.

Shook, Robert. *Survivors: Living with Cancer.* New York: HarperCollins, 1983. Experience of 12 people who survived cancer.

Spingarn, Natalie Davis. *Hanging in There: Living Well on Borrowed Time.* Lanham, Md.: Madison Books, 1982. Experience of an award-winning journalist's bout with breast cancer.

———. *The New Cancer Survivors: Living with Grace, Fighting with Spirit.* Baltimore: Johns Hopkins University Press, 1999.

Trull, Patti. *On with My Life.* New York: Putnam, 1983. Experience of long-term survivor of osteogenic sarcoma.

Tsongas, Paul. *Heading Home.* New York: Alfred A. Knopf, 1984; Vintage reissue edition, 1992. Experience of the former senator's bout with lymphoma.

Radiation Therapy

Cukier, Daniel, M.D., and Virginia McCullough. *Coping with Radiation Therapy.* Los Angeles, Calif.: Lowell House, 1996; McGraw Hill, 4th edition, 2004.

Sexual Issues

Johnson, Jacquelyn. *Intimacy: Living as a Woman after Cancer.* Toronto: NC Press Ltd., 1987.

Schover, Leslie. *Sexuality and Cancer: For the Man Who Has Cancer, and His Partner.* Atlanta, Ga.: American Cancer Society, 1988. (See the American Cancer Society Web site at http://www.cancer.org.)

———. *Sexuality and Cancer: For the Woman Who Has Cancer, and Her Partner.* Atlanta, Ga.: American Cancer Society, 1988.

INDEX

Page numbers in **boldface** indicate main articles.

aflatoxins, 62
AFP test, **8**
after loading, **8**
AG 013736, 8
age-adjusted rate, **8**
Agent Orange, 8, 95
aggressive non-Hodgkins lymphoma, **8**
agnogenic myeloid metaplasia, 209
agranulocytosis, 8, 216–217
AGT, **8**
AIDS, 8–9, 27, 138, 162, 350
AIDS encephalopathy, 104
AIDS Info Web site, **343**
AIPC, **9**
air quality, 152
air-contrast X-rays, 9–10, 155
albinism, 10
ALCL, 10
alcohol, 10
aldesleukin, 10, 155
alemtuzumab, 10
aleukemia, 10
Alferon, 10, 155
alkaline phosphatase, 10
alkaline phosphatase test, 10
alkaloids, **10–11**
Alkeran, 11, 63
alkylating, 11, 37
ALL, **11–12**
allogenic bone marrow transplants, 12, 41, 131–132
allogenic stem cell transplant, 12
allopurinol sodium, 12
allovectin-7, 12
all-trans retinoic acid, 12
alopecia, 12–13
alpha interferon, 13, 33
alpha-fetoprotein (ALF), 13, 316
alteramine, 137
alternative treatment, 13, 212, 319–321
altretamine, 13
alveolar cell lung cancer, 4, 13
alveolar ridge cancer, 13
alveolar soft part sarcoma, 13
alveoli, 13
AMC Cancer Research Center, 343
American Board of Certified Specialties, 37
American Board of Surgeons, 13
American Brain Tumor Association, 343
American Cancer Society, 343–344
American Heart Association, 344–345
American Liver Foundation, 344
American Lung Association, 345

American Medical Association, **345**
American Society for Dermatologic Surgery (ASDS), **345**
American Society of Plastic and Reconstructive Surgeons, **345**
American Urological Association (AUA), **344**
amethopterin, 13, 197
amifostine, 13, 113
4-aminobiphenyl, **123**
aminoglutethimide, 6, **13**, 88
AML, 13
AMSA, 13
amsacrine, 13, 189
amyloidosis, 13–14
anagrelide, 14, 22
anal cancer, 14, 76
analgesic pump, 15
analgesics, 14–15, 55, 234. *See also* Patient controlled analgesia
anaplasia, 15
anaplastic, 15
anaplastic adenocarcinoma, 310
anaplastic astrocytoma, 15
anaplastic large cell lymphoma, 10
anaplastic oligodendroglioma, 15
anaplastic thyroid carcinoma, 15
anastomosis, 15
anastrozole, 15, 22
androgen, 6, **15–16**, 59, 91, 305
androgen-independent prostate cancer, 9
anecdotal evidence, 16
anemia, 16, 119, 125, 246
anesthesia, 16
  caudal, 64–65
  epidural, 108
  general, 128
  intravenous, 158
  local, 177
  regional, 267
  saddle block, 274
  spinal, 291
  topical, 311
anesthetic, 16
aneuploid, 16, 251
angiogenesis, 16
angiogenesis inhibitors, 16, 19
angiogram, 16
angiography, 16, 336
angiosarcomas, 16, 36, 175
angiostatin, 17
ANLL (acute nonlymphocytic leukemia), **17–18**
anorexia, 18
anoscopy, 18
anterior exteneration, 18

anthracycline, 19
antiandrogens, 19, 122, 217
antiangiogenesis agents, 17, **19**, 26, 107, 258, 304
antibiotic, **19**
antibodies, **19–20**. *See also* monoclonal antibodies (MAB)
  auto-, 26
  B-cells and, 28
  chimeric, 72, 272
  cytotoxicity and, 20
  human anti-mouse, 133–134, 201, 338
  immune system and, 19
antibody-dependent cell-mediated cytotoxicity, 20
anticipatory nausea and vomiting, 20
anticoagulants, 135
anticonvulsants, 95
antidepressant drug, 20
antiemetics, 20, 22, 81, 104, 198, 339
antiestrogen, 20, 76, 113, 303–304
antigen, 20
antimetabolites, 20–21, 121, 197, 283
antineoplastic, 21, 36
antineoplastons, 21, 56
antioxidants, 21, 212, 279
antipyretic, 21
antiretroviral therapy, 21
antisense therapy, 21, 26, 224
antiserotonin, 21
antithymocyte globulin, 21
antiviral, 21
anus, 21
ANV, 21
Anzemet, 21
AP, 21
APC 8015, 21
apheresis, 21
APL, 21, 23
aplasia, 21, 131
aplastic, 21
aplastic anemia, 21–22
apoptosis, 22, 30
appendix, 22
appetite loss, 22
APR, 22
Aprepitant, 22, 104
arabinosyl cytosine, 22
ara-C, 22
Aredia, 22
areola, 22
argon lasers, 169
Argylin, 22
Arimidex, 22
aromatase inhibitors, 22–23, 119
arsenic, 23, 62

mastectomy (continued)
   subcutaneous, 299
   total, 312
Masteril, 16, 97, **192**
Matulane, **192**, 253
Mautner Project, The National
  Lesbian Health Organization, **350**
maxillofacial prosthetics, **192**
maxillofacial prosthodontists, **192**
m-BACOD, **192**
m-BACOS, **192**
MBC, **192**
MC, **192**
MDR, **192**
MDS, **192**
MeCCnu, 62
mechlorethamine, **192**, 206
mediastinoscopes, **192**
mediastinoscopy, **192–193**
mediastinotomy, **193**
mediastinum, **193**
medical oncologists, **193**
medical physicists, **193**, 261
MediPort, 154, **193**, 328
Medrol, 7, **193**
medroxyprogesterone, 19, **193**, 253
medullary cancer, 48, 118, **193**, 292,
  310
medullary carcinoma of the breast,
  193
medullary carcinoma of the thyroid,
  65, **193**
medulloblastoma, 44, 45, 131, 154,
  193–194
MEG, **194**
Megace, 18, **194**, 253
megavoltage linear accelerators, 174,
  194
megestrol, 19, 194, **194**
melanin, 10, **194**
melanomas, 3, 118, 157–158,
  194–195, 300
melphalan, 63, **195**
MEN, **195**
meningeal carcinomatosis, **195**
meningioma, 44, **195**
meperidine, **195**
mercaptopurine, **195**, 283
Merkel cell carcinoma, **195**
mesenchymoma, **195**
mesna, 147–148, **195–196**
mesna rescue, 147–148, **196**
mesna uroprotection, **196**
Mesnex, **196**
mesothelioma, 10, **196**
mesothelium, **196**

meta-analysis, **196**
metastases, 87, **196**
metastasis, 42, **197**
metastasize, **197**
metastatic brain tumors, **197**
metastatic cancers, **197**
metastatic liver cancer, **197**
metastatic workups, **197**
metastic melanoma, 12
methadone, **197**
Methosarb, 16, 59, **197**
methotrexate, 21, 69, 73, 138,
  197–198
methotrexate with leucovorin rescue,
  171, **198**
methoxsalen, 63, **198**, 248
methoxsalen with ultraviolet light,
  198
8-methoxypsoralen, 102, **198**
methyl-G, **198**
methyl-GAG, **198**
methylglyoxal-bis-guanylhydrazone,
  198
methylprednisolone, 193, **198**
methylprednisone, **198**
meticorten, 198, 252
metoclopramide, **198**
metrography, 145, **198**
metronomic chemotherapy, **198**
mets, **198**
MeV linear accelerators, 174
Mexate, 197, **198**
MF, **198**
MFG, **194**
MFH, **198**
MGBG, **198**
MGUS, **198**, 208
microcalcifications, 47, **198–199**
micrographic surgery, 29, **199**, 200
micrometastases, **199**
microsatellite instability, 203–204
microstaging, 55, 195, **199**
microwave ovens, **199**
Mifepristone, **199**, 273
MINE, **199**
minipill, 227–228
Miraluma tests, **199**, 276
MITH, **199**
Mithracin, **199**
mithramycin, **199**
MITO, **199**, 206
mitoguazone, **199**
mitolactol, 92, **199**
mitomycin, **199**, 206
mitomycin-C, **199**, 206
mitosis, **199**

mitotane, **200**
mitotic inhibitors, **200**
mitoxantrone, **200**
mixed cellularity, **200**
mixed gliomas, 44
mixed tumors, **200**
MM, **200**
MoAb, **200**
modified radical mastectomy, 192,
  200
modulation, 121
Mohs' micrographic surgery, 29, **200**
molar pregnancy, 129, **200**
molecular (cell) biology, **200–201**
molecular targets, 304
moles, 99–100, 118, 194, **200**
monoclonal antibodies (MAB), 31, 33,
  130, 136, **201**
monocytes, **201**, 333
monocytic leukemia, **201**
monokines, **201**
mononucleosis, 109
8-MOP, 102, 198
MOPP, 2, **201**
morbidity, **201**
morbidity rate, **201**
morphine, 202, 204
mortality rate, **202**
Motrin, **202**
mouth cancer, 69, 110, 174, **202–203**,
  251, 286
mouth sores, 203, 298–299
mouthwash, **203**
MP, **203**
6-MP, **283**
M-Protein, **203**
MRI (magnetic resonance imaging),
  203–204
MS Contin, **204**
MSI (microsatellite instability),
  204–205
MTP-PE, **205**
MTX, 197, **205**
mucinous carcinoma, 48, **205**, 231
mucositis, **205**, 298–299
mucous membranes, **205**
mullerian tumors, **205**
multicentric disease, **205**
multicolony-stimulating factor, 156,
  205
multi-CSF, **205**
multidrug resistance (MDR), **205**, 258
multifocal osteosarcoma, **205**, 230
multi-modality treatment, **205**
multiple basal cell carcinoma
  syndrome, **205**